PRINCIPLES OF

CLINICAL ELECTROMYOGRAPHY

CASE STUDIES

PRINCIPLES OF CLINICAL ELECTROMYOGRAPHY *CASE STUDIES*

Shin J. Oh, MD
Professor of Neurology and Pathology
Medical Director, Department of Clinical Neurophysiology
Director, EMG and Evoked Potentials Laboratory
Director, Muscle and Nerve Histopathology Laboratory
The University of Alabama at Birmingham
Department of Veterans Affairs Medical Center
Birmingham, Alabama

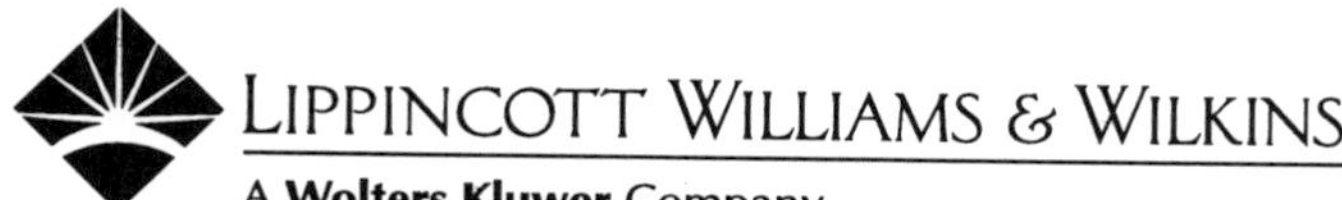

A **Wolters Kluwer** Company
Philadelphia • Baltimore • New York • London
Buenos Aires • Hong Kong • Sydney • Tokyo

Editor: Charles W. Mitchell
Managing Editor: Keith Rhett Murphy
Marketing Manager: Lori Smith
Production Coordinator: Raymond E. Reter
Project Editor: Karen Ruppert
Designer: Graphic World
Cover Designer: Graphic World
Typesetter: Maryland Composition
Printer: McNaughton and Gunn
Digitalized Illustrations: Graphic World

351 West Camden Street
Baltimore, Maryland 21201-2436 USA

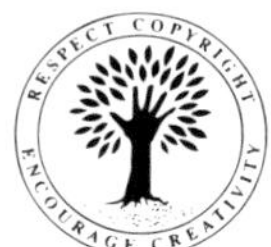

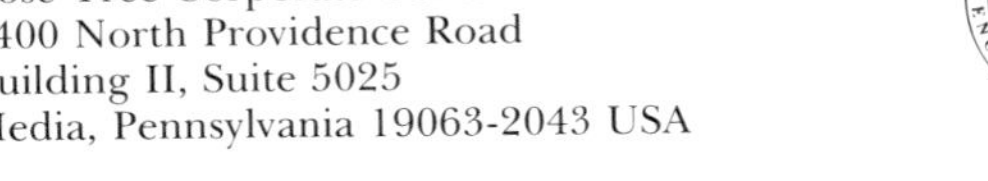

Rose Tree Corporate Center
1400 North Providence Road
Building II, Suite 5025
Media, Pennsylvania 19063-2043 USA

Accurate indications, adverse reactions and dosage schedules for drugs are provided in this book, but it is possible that they may change. The reader is urged to review the package information data of the manufacturers of the medications mentioned.

Printed in the United States of America

Library of Congress Cataloging-in-Publication Data

Oh, Shin J.
Principles of clinical electromyography : case studies / Shin J. Oh.
p. cm.
Includes bibliographical references and index.
ISBN 0-683-18106-8
1. Electromyography—Case studies. 2. Neuromuscular diseases--Diagnosis—Case studies. I. Title.
[DNLM: 1. Neuromuscular Diseases—diagnosis case studies. 2. Peripheral Nervous System Diseases—diagnosis case studies. 3. Electromyography—methods. WE 550 036p 1998]
RC77.5.036 1998
616.7′407547—dc21
DNLM/DLC
for Library of Congress 98-10426
CIP

The publishers have made every effort to trace the copyright holders for borrowed material. It they have inadvertently overlooked any, they will be pleased to make the necessary arrangements at the first opportunity.

To purchase additional copies of this book, call our customer service department at **(800) 638-0672** or fax orders to **(800) 447-8438.** For other book services, including chapter reprints and large quantity sales, ask for the Special Sales department.

Canadian customers should call **(800) 665-1148,** or fax **(800) 665-0103.** For all other calls originating outside of the United States, please call **(410) 528-4223** or fax us at **(410) 528-8550.**

***Visit Williams & Wilkins on the Internet*: http://www.wwilkins.com** or contact our customer service department at **custserv@wwilkins.com.** Williams & Wilkins customer service representatives are available from 8:30 am to 6:00 pm, EST, Monday through Friday, for telephone access.

99 00 01 02
3 4 5 6 7 8 9 10

Cover Graphic: John Bavosi/SciencePhoto Library.

This book is dedicated to my wife, Dr. M. Kim Oh, Associate Professor of Pediatrics at the University of Alabama at Birmingham, and to my sons, David and Michael, and my daughter-in-law, Bryn, all MIT graduates.

PREFACE

Principles of Clinical Electromyography is written for the clinician-electromyographer who wants to learn the basic principles and techniques of electromyography (EMG) and know how these principles and techniques are applied to actual cases in practice.

The first six chapters explain the basic principles, techniques, and clinical applications of the various EMG techniques. Thus, these chapters provide basic step-by-step methods for the more common electrophysiological techniques, tables of normal values, and guides for the interpretation of the data.

The second nine chapters present 111 actual cases spanning the entire gamut of neuromuscular diseases. Because these were actual case studies, none were straightforward, but every case provided the clinician-electromyographer with a challenge regarding the correct diagnosis and treatment. Thus, these cases provide the basis for the clinical EMG correlations and up-to-date information on various diseases. The clinical EMG correlations are facilitated by illustrations of actual tracings of electrophysiological responses. Maxims are provided to highlight the most important clinical and EMG caveats. Only those references that provide the most informative knowledge of specific subjects are cited.

It is my hope that this book contains sufficient basic and practical information on the EMG tests and their clinical correlations to enable every clinician-electromyographer to solve everyday problems in the EMG laboratory with efficiency and accuracy.

ACKNOWLEDGMENTS

First, I want to thank Dr. M. Kim Oh, my wife, friend, and companion for 31 years, who provided me with emotional and intellectual support at home so that I could fully devote myself to the authorship of this book.

Second, I want to thank Dr. Mary Ward, my administrative assistant for 20 years, who made the present manuscripts readable.

Third, I have to give credit to Adobe Photoshop 3.0, with which I was able to do all the illustrations in this book myself.

Fourth, I owe the production of this book to the editorial staff of Williams & Wilkins —Charley Mitchell, editor; Keith Murphy, managing editor; Ray Reter, production coordinator; and Karen Ruppert, project editor—who provided valuable technical support from the conception to the printing of this book.

And finally, I want to thank all my patients whoses stories have made this book instructive.

CONTENTS

CHAPTER 1

Anatomical and Physiological Basis for Electromyography Studies

MOTOR UNIT

The lower motor neuron system consists of the anterior horn cells, the peripheral nerves, neuromuscular synapses, and muscles. A motor neuron together with its axon and all muscle fibers that it innervates is called a motor unit (Fig. 1.1).

Stimulation of a single motor neuron causes contraction of all its subservient muscle fibers. The average size of a motor unit, as measured by determination of the innervation ratio (number of muscle fibers:number of motor axons), varies in different muscles. The ratio is 2:1 to 3:1 for the laryngeal muscle and 1934:1 for the gastrocnemius. In general, muscles that control finer or smaller movements have a smaller motor unit than those that control gross movements.

There are two types of muscle fibers: type I (red) and type II (white) (Table 1.1). These types can be easily distinguished by adenosine triphosphatase (ATPase) staining: type I is ATPase-poor and type II is ATPase-rich. Type I ("red" and "slow") muscle fibers contain more myoglobin, have less evident striations, respond more slowly, and have a longer latency than type II fibers (Fig. 1.2). They are adapted for long, slow, posture-maintaining contractions. The soleus of the cat is a typical example. Type II ("white" and "fast") muscle fibers have fewer fibers per motor unit and short, "twitch" durations. They are specialized for fine and skilled movements. The gastrocnemius of the cat belongs in this category. In human muscles, type I and II fibers are well intermixed at a ratio of 4:6. Anatomical, histochemical, and physiological differences in the properties of type I and type II fibers are listed in detail in Table 1.1 and Figure 1.3.

It now seems that the character of the muscle is determined in part by its innervation. All the constituent muscle fibers of a motor unit are of the same type, indicating a strong trophic control of nerves and muscles. In a crossed innervation experiment, the nerves to fast and slow muscles were crossed and allowed to regenerate. When regrowth was complete and the nerve that had previously supplied the slow muscle innervated the fast muscle, the fast muscle became slow. The reverse change occurred in the previously slow muscle. It seems, therefore, that even the biochemical characteristics of muscles depend in part on the type of innervation they receive.

Recent studies have shown that muscle fibers under the control of a single motor unit are scattered among other muscle fibers, not grouped as previously thought. This finding agrees with the mosaic intermixing of type I and II fibers in human muscles.

With a very weak voluntary contraction, the needle electromyography (EMG) electrode records activity from single motor units. These action potentials are called motor unit potentials (MUPs). Usually several MUPs fire together. However, a single MUP can be isolated and recorded with good cooperation from the patient and careful manipulation of the needle electrode.

The motor unit is the basic anatomical substrate for the MUP. Recent studies have suggested that the spike component of MUP recorded with a concentric needle having a 150×580-μm recording surface is generated from 5 to 12 muscle fibers within a radius of 1 mm.

The amplitude, duration, and phase of the MUP are important in the differential diagnosis of various neuromuscular diseases (Fig. 1.4). When recorded with a concentric needle elec-

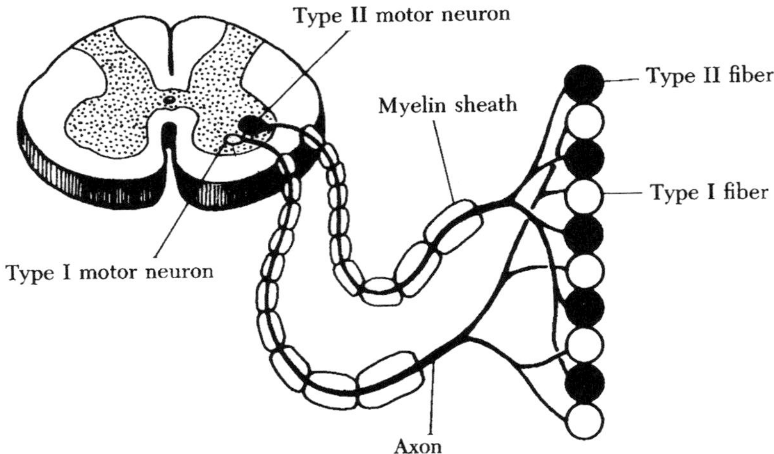

FIGURE 1.1. A single motor unit: motor neuron (anterior horn cell), peripheral nerve fiber (axon and myelin sheath), and all muscle fibers innervated by the nerve fibers.

TABLE 1.1. Properties of Type I and II Fibers

	Type I Fibers	**Type II Fibers**
Color	Red	White
Myoglobin content	High	Low
Muscle fiber diameter	Smaller	Larger
Enzymes		
Myofibrillar ATPase	Low	High
Mitochondrial oxidative enzymes	High	Low
Glycolytic enzymes	Low	High
Energy source	Fatty acids, glucose	Glycogen
Metabolic characteristics	Aerobic oxidative phosphorylation	Anaerobic glycolysis
Twitch contraction time	Slow	Fast
Tetanus tension output	Low	High
Resistance to fatigue	High	Low
Motor units		
Size	Small	Large
Intensity required for activation	Low	High
Axon conduction velocity	Slower	Faster
Anatomical location	Deep muscle; axial portion of surface muscle	Superficial portion of surface muscle

trode, normal MUPs usually have a duration of from 3 to 15 ms, a peak-to-peak amplitude of 300 μV and 3 mV, and a bi- or triphasic configuration. The small-amplitude short-duration MUPs are characteristic in patients with myopathy, whereas in patients with denervated disorders, the high-amplitude long-duration MUPs are typical (Fig. 1.5). High-amplitude (giant) MUPs (with greater than 5 mV amplitude) are classically noted in the denervated disorders. It is likely that high-amplitude MUPs result from reinnervation of denervated muscle fibers by sprouts from intact motor axons.

Fasciculation is the normal-duration spontaneous muscle twitching commonly seen in anterior horn cell diseases (e.g., amyotrophic lateral sclerosis). Fasciculation is thought to be a spontaneous discharge (depolarization) of the motor unit irritated by the disease process. Thus, the various parameters of fasciculation are not different from those of the MUP (Fig. 1.6).

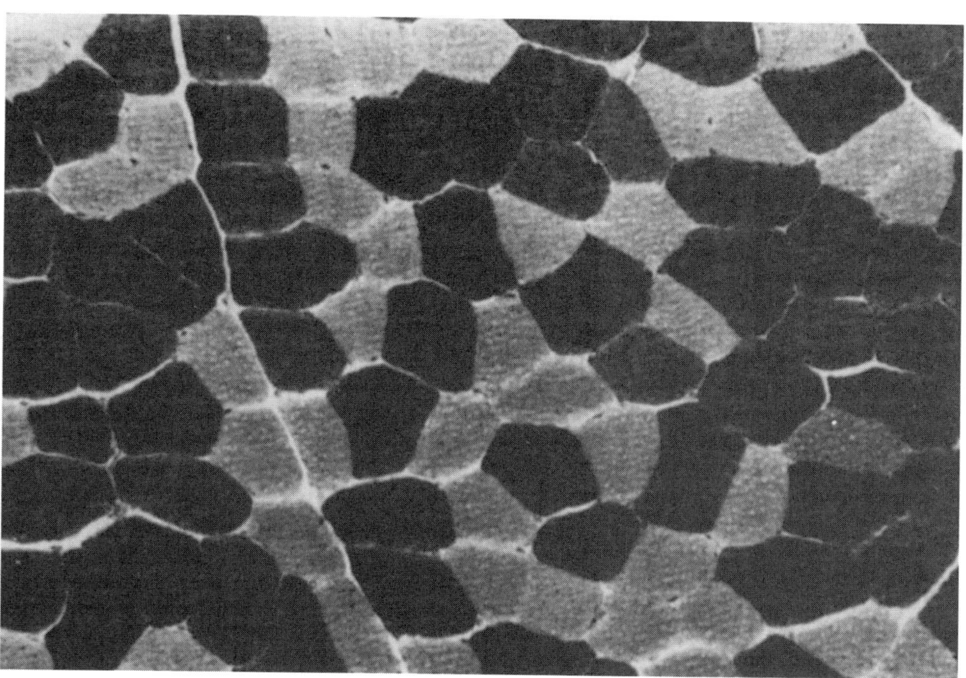

FIGURE 1.2. Normal muscle stained with myosin ATPase at pH 9.4. Dark fibers are type II fibers; light fibers are type I fibers.

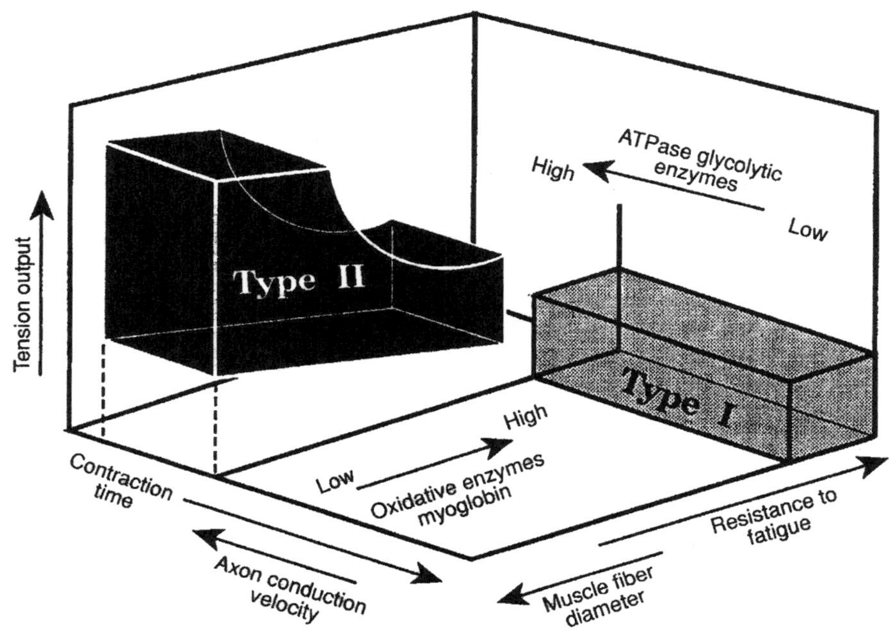

FIGURE 1.3. Relationship between physiological and histochemical properties of type I and II fibers. (Modified from Burke R. Motor units in mammalian muscle. In: Summer A, ed. The physiology of peripheral nerve disease. Philadelphia: WB Saunders, 1980:133–194.)

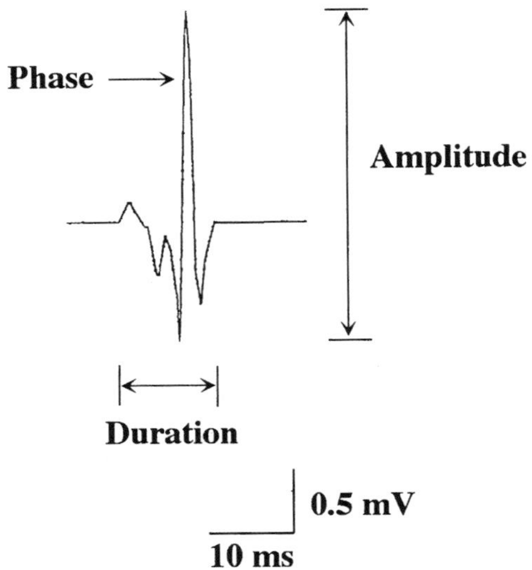

FIGURE 1.4. Various components of the motor unit potential.

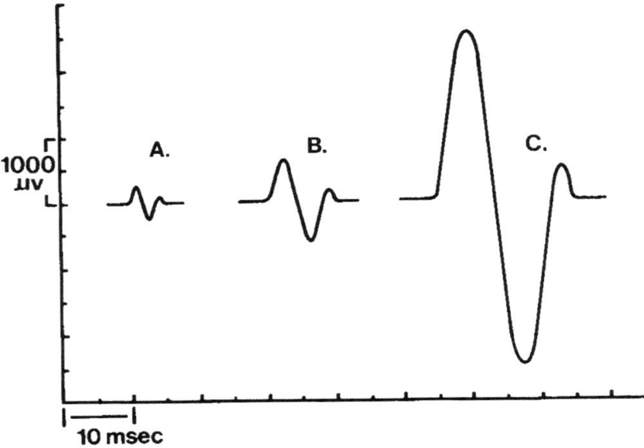

FIGURE 1.5. MUP in the various neuromuscular diseases: trace *A*, small-amplitude short-duration MUP in myopathy; trace *B*, normal MUP; trace *C*, high-amplitude long-duration MUP in denervation process.

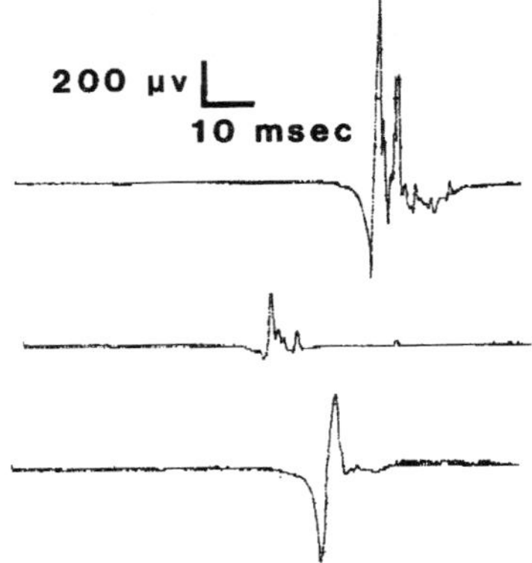

FIGURE 1.6. Fasciculation.

Recently, an attempt was made to record the action potential within the whole motor unit using the entire cannula as an active electrode in a modified single-fiber EMG needle (the macro EMG needle). The single-fiber action potential was used to trigger a digital averager to which the signal from the larger recording surface, the cannula, was fed and averaged, usually 128 to 512 impulses. The shape of the macro EMG action potential was determined by the temporal and spatial summation of the individual single-fiber potentials within the motor unit. The amplitude of the macro EMG action potential ranged from 10 to 290 μV in normal individuals, was usually increased in those with neurogenic disorders, and was normal or decreased in those with myopathies.

EXCITABILITY OF THE NERVE AND MUSCLE

In most cells, there is a difference in potential between the interior and the exterior of the cell. When the cell is in a resting state, the membrane potential is called the resting potential. The resting potential is always negative in nerve and muscle (i.e., negative on the inside as compared with the outside of the membrane). The resting potential is −70 mV in the nerve and −80 mV in the muscle. When the nerve and muscle work, brief positive changes in the membrane potential occur that are called the action potential.

The terms for the various phases of the action potential are given in Figure 1.7. The action potential in a particular cell always follows a constant sequence of depolarization and repolarization of the membrane, which occurs whenever the membrane is depolarized at or beyond the threshold level. The action potential is therefore "all or none" in character and is said to obey the "all-or-none law" of excitation.

Cells in which action potentials can be triggered are called excitable. Excitability is a typical property of nerve and muscle cells. Thus, excitation occurs as a result of depolarization of the membrane to the threshold level. This depolarization is also called stimulation. When a depolarizing electrical current crosses the threshold, an excitation is triggered. The electrical current pulse that generates such a change in potential is called a stimulating current, or stimulus. Both the intensity (strength) and the duration of the stimulating current are important in the generation of excitation. The relationship between the strength and the duration of the stimulating current is called the strength-duration curve (Fig. 1.8).

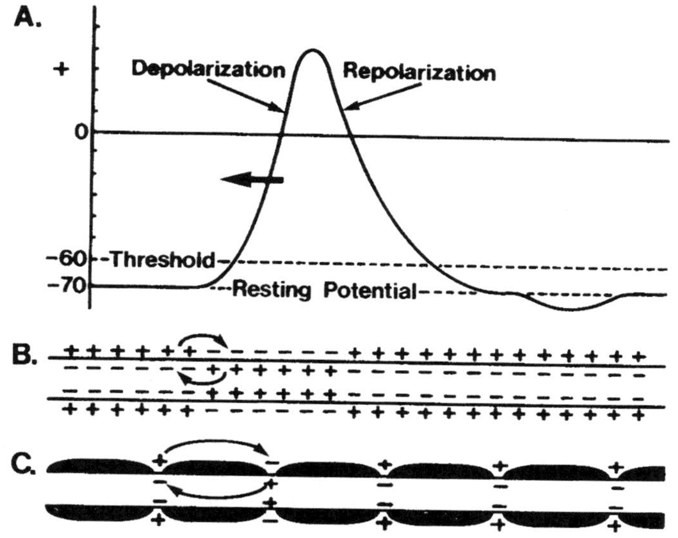

FIGURE 1.7. Phases of the action potential and its propagation. **A.** Terms for the various phases of the action potential. It also shows the action potential propagating from right to left. **B.** Mechanism of conduction in unmyelinated fiber: local circuit conduction. **C.** Mechanism of conduction in a myelinated fiber: saltatory conduction.

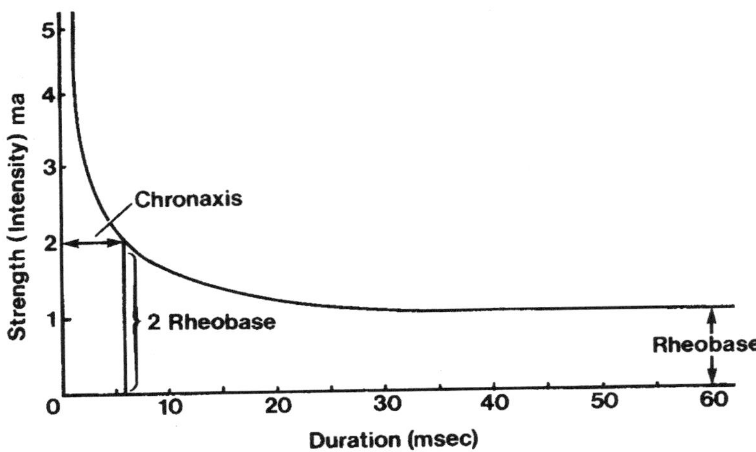

FIGURE 1.8. Relationship between the strength (intensity) and duration of the stimulating current and the terms for the excitability.

The rheobase is defined as the strength of a stimulating current of very long duration that is just large enough to trigger an excitation. However, chronaxie is more commonly used as a measure of the excitability of muscle or nerve. Chronaxie is defined as the necessary duration of a stimulating current of twice the rheobase strength.

The strength-duration curve on the nerve is called nerve excitability. Nerve excitability becomes abnormal 72 hours after severe nerve injury and is the earliest electrophysiological abnormality observed after a nerve injury. The nerve excitability test is still used in the evaluation of Bell's palsy (idiopathic facial palsy) to predict the prognosis in the early stages.

On the fifth day after severe nerve injury, the strength-duration curve of the muscle becomes abnormal. The strength-duration curve on muscle has been used extensively in the past as an electrodiagnostic test in muscle. However, because of its limited value, it has not been used in many laboratories in recent years.

PROPAGATION OF ACTION POTENTIAL

The actual task of the nerve and muscle is the propagation of excitation (action potential). The action potential, once initiated, is self-propagating and spreads like a wave over the membrane until it has moved along the entire cell.

The mechanism of propagation of the action potential differs in unmyelinated and myelinated nerve fibers. There is "local circuit" conduction in unmyelinated fibers and "saltatory" conduction in myelinated fibers.

For an unmyelinated axon, the mechanism of propagation occurs as diagramed in Figure 1.7. During the peak of the action potential in a segment of nerve, the membrane potential reverses polarity, the inside becoming positive in regard to the outside. The reversal of polarity leads to a local current flow from positive to negative, as indicated by the arrows in Figure 1.7. The outward current flow through the resting membrane in front of the action potential (which is depicted as moving from right to left) depolarizes the membrane. The newly activated membrane, in turn, explodes into an action potential, generates local currents, depolarizes the next segment, and so on until the action potential has moved along the full length of the axon.

The conduction speed is determined by the diameter of the unmyelinated fibers (Table 1.2). Larger fibers conduct more rapidly than small fibers because they have a lower resistance. Because of the continuous local circuit conduction, the nerve conduction velocity (NCV) of

TABLE 1.2. Conduction Velocity in Various Nerve Fiber Types in Mammalian Nerve

Fiber Type: Erland and Gasser's System	Fiber Type: Lloyd's System for Sensory Fibers	Function	Fiber Diameter (μm)	Conduction Velocity (m/s)	Most Susceptibility to Conduction Block by Agents
Myelinated fibers					
A	Ia	Proprioception; primary muscle spindle afferents; motor to skeletal muscles	12–20	70–120	Pressure
	Ib	Afferents from Golgi tendon organ			
	II	Cutaneous touch and pressure	5–12	30–70	
		Motor to muscle spindle	3–6	15–30	
	III	Cutaneous temperature and pain	2–5	12–30	
B		Sympathetic preganglionic	3	3–15	Hypoxia
Unmyelinated fibers					
C	IV	Cutaneous pain	0.4–1.2	0.5–2	Local anesthetic
		Sympathetic postganglionic	0.3–1.3	0.7–2.3	

unmyelinated fibers is relatively slow. In human unmyelinated pain fibers, the NCV is 1 m/s. The giant axon of squid, which is 0.7 mm in diameter, has a speed of conduction of 25 m/s. In general, the NCV of unmyelinated fibers can be calculated by the following formula:

$$\textit{NCV of unmyelinated fibers (m/s)} = \sqrt{\textit{diameter of unmyelinated fiber (axon) } (\mu m)}$$

In myelinated fibers, the myelin sheath acts as an insulator and prevents transmembrane current flow in the internodes. The movement of the current occurs only at the nodes of Ranvier, spaced at intervals of about 2 mm in larger fibers (Fig. 1.7). The impulse hops from one node to the next. This is called saltatory conduction in myelinated fibers. In vertebrates, all fibers that conduct at velocities of propagation in excess of 3 m/s are myelinated. For myelinated fibers, the following formula is applied in the calculation of the NCV:

$$\textit{NCV of myelinated fibers (m/s)} = \textit{conversion factor} \times \textit{outer diameter of myelinated fiber } (\mu m)$$

The NCV that we measure in the human subject is predominantly contributed by the large-diameter fibers of the nerves. Thus the NCV reflects the fastest conduction velocity of the nerve. The conversion factor varies according to the nerve and to the animal (e.g., 4.4 for the human sural nerve, 5.2 for the baboon median and ulnar nerves, and 6.0 for the cat saphenous nerve).

Slowing in NCV is caused either by loss of large fibers or by segmental demyelination. When it is the axons that are predominantly affected by the disease process, the NCVs are minimally affected. On the other hand, when it is the myelin that is predominantly involved, marked slowing in NCV is seen because of the loss of saltatory conduction. In fact, in axonal neuropathy, the NCVs are either normal or slowed by less than 40% of normal. In contrast, in demyelinating neuropathy, the NCVs are slowed by more than 40% of normal.

NEUROMUSCULAR TRANSMISSION

By nerve impulse, the action potential of the muscle is generated at the motor end plate (neuromuscular junction) where the nerve makes contact with the muscle fibers. The structure of the motor end plate is illustrated in Figure 1.9. The axon ends in the presynaptic terminal that is separated from the postsynaptic membrane of muscle fibers by the synaptic cleft (200 to 500 Å). The presynaptic terminal contains mitochondria and many synaptic vesicles. Many experiments indicate that these vesicles contain acetylcholine (ACh). The postsynaptic membrane has repeated synaptic folding where the ACh receptors are located.

The action potential of the nerve terminal triggers the release of ACh from the vesicles into the synaptic cleft (Fig. 1.10). The released ACh diffuses across the gap and attaches to the ACh receptors on the postsynaptic membrane. This induces the depolarization that leads to the generation of action potential of the muscle membrane.

This depolarization at the end plate is called an end-plate potential (EPP). The EPP is nonpropagated and graded, rather than following the all-or-none law. The EPP induces a sink for current flow through the adjacent muscle cell membrane, depolarizing it to the threshold value required to initiate an action potential, which then propagates along the fiber by local circuit current flow. In healthy muscles, the EPPs are always far above the threshold. Each presynaptic action potential triggers a contraction in the muscle fibers. Thus, neuromuscular transmission is normally obligatory.

The end-plate membrane is special in containing acetylcholinesterase, which breaks down ACh into inactive choline and acetic acid. Choline and acetic acid are, for the most part, reabsorbed by the presynaptic terminal and, with the aid of ACh transferase, recombined

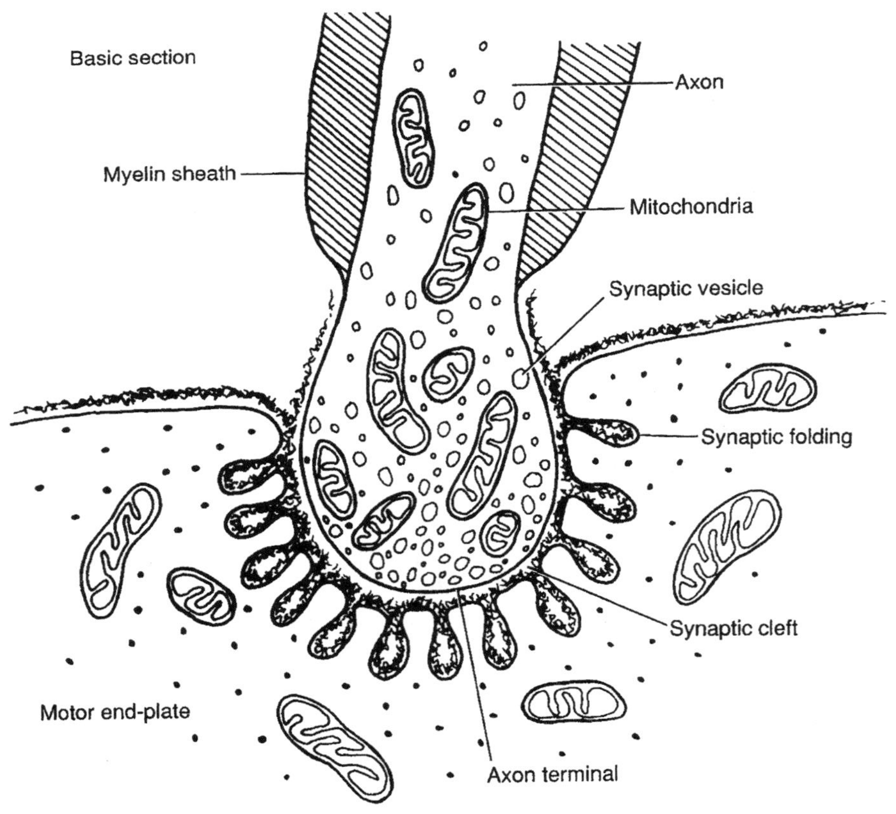

FIGURE 1.9. Neuromuscular junction.

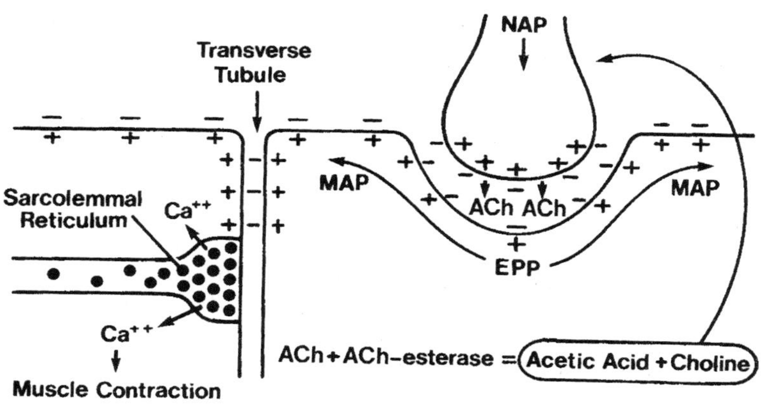

FIGURE 1.10. Physiological sequences at the neuromuscular junction and muscle for muscle contraction. *MAP,* Muscle action potential.

into ACh. This ACh is then stored in the synaptic vesicles of the presynaptic terminal until it is released once more.

At rest, the presynaptic terminal releases single quanta (the nearly equal-sized packets) of ACh at irregular intervals, producing the spontaneous potentials called miniature end-plate potentials (MEPPs). The MEPPs are similar in their time course to normal EPPs, but their amplitude is very much smaller than that of the EPP. The pharmacological properties of the EPP and MEPP are also identical. Studies show that the EPP is the summation of multiple MEPPs; that is, the normal EPP is generated by the simultaneous release of a large number of ACh quanta. It has been estimated that about 100 to 200 quanta or synaptic vesicles in amphibians and about 60 in human subjects are released per presynaptic nerve action potential.

When the needle electrode is inserted near the end plate of a muscle, end-plate noise is often recorded. These potentials are the EMG equivalent of the MEPP.

The presence of Ca^{++} ions is absolutely essential for the normal course of quantal release of ACh triggered by a presynaptic action potential. The Mg^{++} ion has the opposite effect of Ca^{++} at the presynaptic membrane. Presumably, Mg^{++} ions compete with Ca^{++} ions for their site of action.

Botulinus toxin inhibits the release of ACh, producing the neuromuscular blocking that is seen with botulism. A similar mechanism is postulated in antibiotic-induced myasthenia, in which intravenous calcium gluconate is the recommended treatment because Ca^{++} ions facilitate the release of ACh.

There are two classic diseases that are caused by a defect in neuromuscular transmission. In myasthenia gravis, the basic defect lies in the postsynaptic membrane: ACh receptor antibody-induced decrease of the functioning ACh receptors. Anticholinesterase (e.g., Mestinon) relieves myasthenic symptoms because of slowed breakdown of ACh at the postsynaptic membrane and permits a more prolonged depolarization of the end plate. In the Lambert-Eaton myasthenic syndrome (Eaton-Lambert syndrome), which is commonly associated with small cell lung carcinoma, the main defect is the insufficient release of ACh at the presynaptic membrane induced by the antibody against voltage-gated calcium channels. Guanidine and aminopyridine, which facilitate a release of ACh, are effective in relieving myasthenic symptoms in this disorder.

The MEPPs recorded in the muscle of patients with myasthenia gravis show a greatly reduced amplitude but a normal frequency. A reduced amplitude of the MEPP was originally thought to be due to a reduced amount of ACh in each ACh packet. However, a recent study has shown that this was caused by the reduced number of postsynaptic ACh receptors. On the other hand, in the Lambert-Eaton myasthenic syndrome, the amplitude of the MEPP was normal but the frequency of the MEPP did not increase as it normally does when the motor nerve terminals were depolarized by increasing the external potassium ion concentration. This observation led to the conclusion that a very low number of ACh packets are released by a nerve action potential in this disorder.

When a muscle fiber is denervated, its sensitivity to ACh increases by as much as 100-fold over a period of 1 to 2 weeks. This is called denervation hypersensitivity: a muscle fiber contracts in response to a smaller amount of ACh than is normally effective. This phenomenon is due to the development of multiple, highly sensitive sites in the nonjunctional membrane. Fibrillation, which is usually detectable by a needle EMG study in the muscle 2 weeks after denervation, is thought to represent denervation hypersensitivity. Thus, fibrillation is the spontaneous twitching of the hypersensitive muscle fiber in response to a small quantity of ACh in the bloodstream that is normally ineffective. Fibrillations are usually indicative of axonal degeneration and are absent or few in number in patients with demyelination.

MUSCLE CONTRACTION

A skeletal muscle consists of many thousands of muscle fibers (Fig. 1.11). Muscle fibers contain bundles of myofibrils. Each fibril is comprised of many filaments and is divided into many "sarcomeres," or units, between two Z-lines. Thin filaments (actin-troponin-tropomyosin) are anchored securely to Z-lines and extend less than half the length of the sarcomere. On the

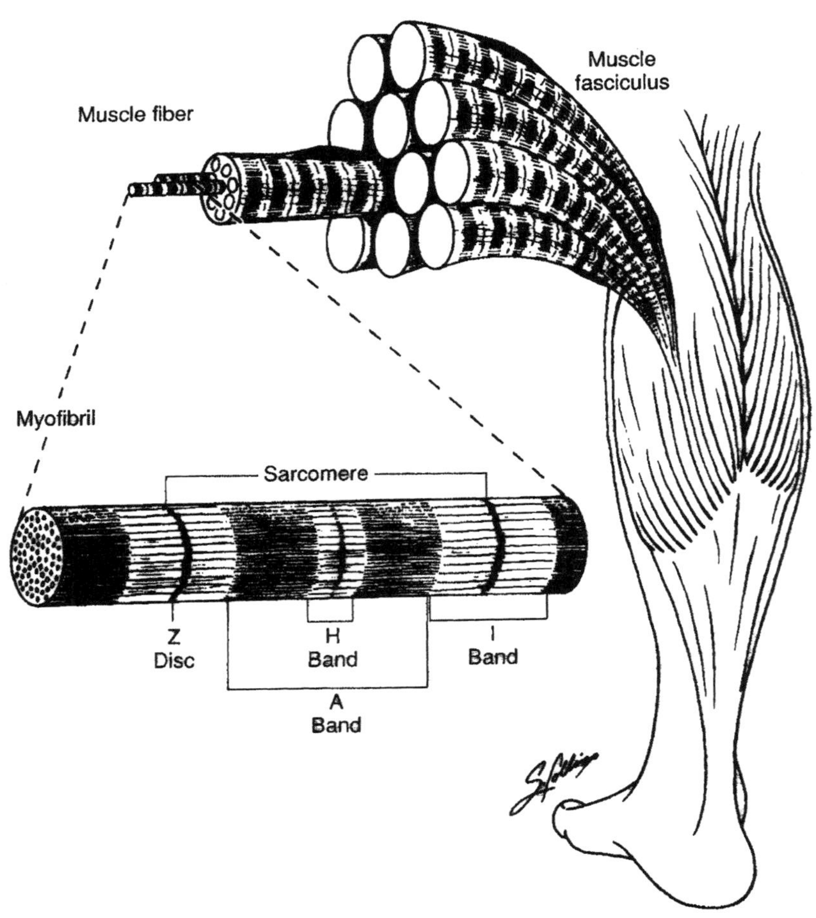

FIGURE 1.11. Histological and molecular structure of skeletal muscle.

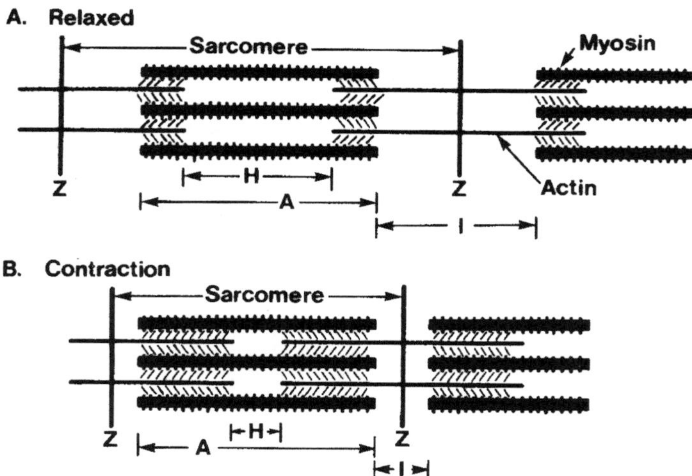

FIGURE 1.12. Mechanism of contraction. Note the arrangement of the myosin and actin filaments in a sarcomere and of the bridges between these filaments. It is thought that changes in the configuration of the bridges produce a shear force that moves the actin filaments between the myosin filaments. **A.** Arrangement of filaments at the relaxed state. **B.** Arrangement of filaments at the time of maximal contraction. The sarcomere becomes shorter because of shortening of the H and I bands.

other hand, the thick filaments (myosin) in the middle part of the sarcomeres are interdigitated between the free ends of the thin filaments (actin). The various bands of the sarcomere are indicated in Figure 1.12.

During muscle contraction (shortening), the I and H bands decrease in thickness. This thinning is due to a sliding of the thin filaments (actin) between the thick filaments (myosin), thus shortening the sarcomere at the expense of the I and H bands (Fig. 1.12).

The initial event in muscle contraction is a depolarization of the muscle fiber membrane, which starts at the end plate. The action potential is propagated by local circuit current flow along the membrane. The conduction speed is only about 5 m/s, which is much slower than that in the axons. The depolarization is conducted into the depths of the muscle fibers through the transverse tubular system (Fig. 1.10). This results in a release of calcium from the sarcoplasmic reticulum, the ends of which abut the transverse tubules. The free calcium ions in the sarcoplasm of the muscle cell then initiate the formation of bridges between the thin and thick filaments, leading to contraction. As the action potential wanes, the sarcoplasmic reticulum rapidly resequesters the Ca^{++}, ATP breaks the bridge-coupling filaments, and the fibers relax. The energy for this movement is provided by the hydrolysis of ATP by myosin ATPase.

Myotonia is a typical example of a disorder of the muscle fiber membrane. Myotonia is characterized clinically by a difficulty of contracted muscle to relax. Myotonic response is detected very easily by a needle EMG because of the typical waxing and waning of high-frequency discharges associated with a "dive-bomber" sound. The disturbance appears to be due to an abnormally low threshold of the muscle fiber membrane, so that it fires repetitively in response to the depolarization produced by ACh release.

McArdle's disease affects the contractile mechanism because of a lack of phosphorylase, which is involved in the breakdown of muscle glycogen to glucose-6-phosphate. The most prominent symptom is painful exertional cramp. The needle EMG study in the shortened muscle in cramp shows electrical silence. Thus, this cramp fits the physiological definition of contracture. In this disorder, contracture is attributed to a critical shortage of ATP during strenuous exercise, when most of the energy for normal muscle contraction derives from glycogen. A shortage of ATP could impair muscle relaxation by inhibiting the energy-dependent calcium uptake of the sarcoplasmic reticulum. Although one study disputed this mechanism, it is possible that the technique used in the study was not sophisticated enough to detect a local defect in the ATP of sarcoplasmic reticulum.

The single-fiber EMG (SFEMG) electrode, with a 25-μm recording surface, records the action potential generated from one or two muscle fibers within a radius of about 300 μm. The single-fiber action potentials have an amplitude of 0.2 to 20 mV and a duration of less than 300 μs. They give information about the individual muscle fiber (propagation velocity), its motor end-plate function (jitter), and the focal characteristics in the topography of the motor unit (fiber density). The SFEMG is used predominantly in the detection of abnormal jitter in patients with myasthenia gravis and related disorders.

CHAPTER 2

Basic Components of the EMG Machine and Its Setups for Testing

The modern basic electromyography (EMG) machine consists of an amplifier, displaying and storage oscilloscopes, an audio-amplifier and speaker, a stimulator, a signal averager, and recording apparatus (Fig. 2.1). In many advanced EMG machines, there is also the capability of storing the EMG signal and data, automatically measuring and analyzing the various potentials, and generating reports.

AMPLIFIER

The potentials picked up by the recording electrodes are usually very small in amplitude and consequently must be augmented by an amplifier before they can be displayed or recorded. Another role of the amplifier is to reject any unnecessary interference signals. The amplifier has control modes for sensitivity and frequency filter selection.

Sensitivity

The sensitivity control determines the amplitude of potentials, which are usually measured in microvolts per centimeter. The usual range of sensitivity in most EMG machines is from 1 μV to 10 mV. For the near-nerve needle sensory nerve conduction study, a sensitivity higher than 1 μV is sometimes required.

Frequency Filter Selection

An amplifier usually has low- and high-filter selection modes. This component is introduced to ensure distortion-free recording of actual potentials and to maintain the noise level as low as possible. Consequently, a high- or low-filter setting is carefully chosen on the basis of the frequency characteristics of the EMG potentials for each test (Table 2.1). Thus, it is important to follow the low- and high-frequency selections recommended for a particular test; otherwise, the shape of potentials, amplitude, and latency will be distorted. In some basic EMG machines, the frequency setting is preselected for given tests for the convenience of the electromyographer.

OSCILLOSCOPE

The cathode ray oscilloscope displays the potentials instantaneously on a linear time scale. New potentials are displayed and old potentials are erased with each sweep. On the needle EMG, many electromyographers recognize the moving potentials on the oscilloscope and interpret their clinical significance.

The storage oscilloscope permits the potentials to be stored on the screen until the erase button is pushed or the potentials are recorded. This feature is essential to basic EMG workups for detailed analysis of motor unit potentials (MUPs), measurement of latency and amplitude of potentials in the nerve conduction test, and analysis of decrement or increment in the repetitive nerve stimulation test.

There is usually a selection mode for needle EMG and the nerve conduction studies. For needle EMG study, the time base (triggering mode) is allowed to run freely, sweeping repetitively from left to right. In this setup, the sweep seems to be frozen because of the fast repetition of the sweep. In the nerve conduction study, the stimulus is made to trigger a single sweep on the time base. Thus, measurement of latency can be made from the onset

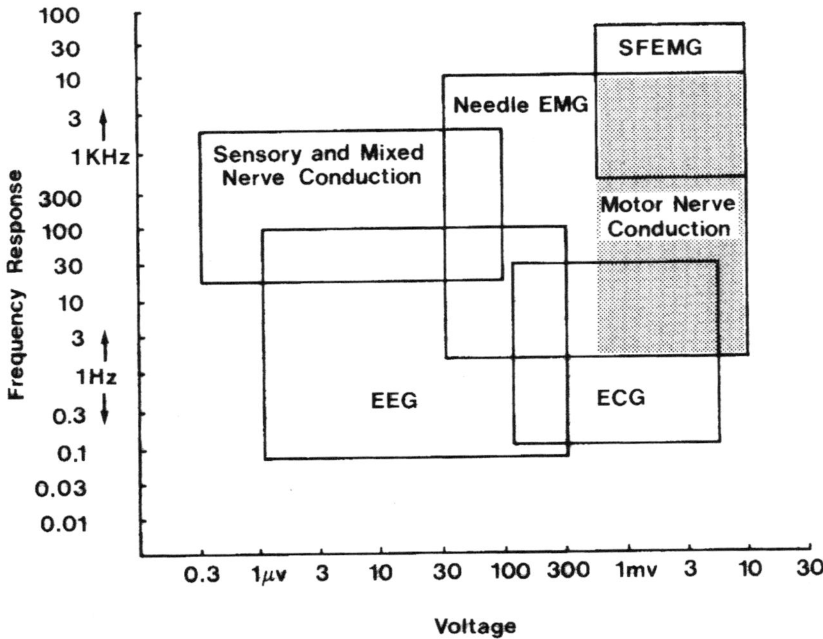

FIGURE 2.1. Basic components of the EMG machine. *EEG*, electroencephalogram; *ECG*, electrocardiogram; *SFEMG*, single-fiber EMG.

of the sweep. There is also a selection mode for the sweep speed. The sweep speed (time base) usually ranges from 0.1 to 500 ms/cm and should be selected according to the kind of test being performed (Table 2.1).

There is also an electronic latency indicator that automatically reads the latency of potentials when the marker is set at any particular point of the potentials or is adjusted manually to read the latency of potentials, for example, the onset of deflection of the compound muscle action potentials (CMAPs) in the motor nerve conduction test. Latency is usually read in milliseconds. The delay line is useful in capturing the potentials on the oscilloscope. Any selected point of the potential can trigger the single sweep (trigger level or point). Accordingly, the same potentials can be displayed on the oscilloscope repeatedly. This feature is used in the single-fiber EMG (SFEMG) study and in the quantitative analysis of MUPs in the needle EMG. In most EMG machines, the calibration signal, consisting of a square pulse, can be easily displayed. The amplitude and duration of potentials can thus be calibrated. It is important to check the accuracy of the amplifier and oscilloscope with the calibration signal as often as possible to ensure the accuracy of the EMG studies.

AUDIO-AMPLIFIER AND SPEAKER

The audio-amplifier and speaker comprise a unique system present only in the EMG machine. In addition to the display of potentials on the oscilloscope for visual analysis, the potentials are also fed from the amplifier to an audio-amplifier and then to a loudspeaker, producing characteristic sounds. This system is essential for the recognition of many EMG potentials (e.g., the "dive-bomber" sound of myotonic potentials). In the nerve conduction study, a single stimulus sound is heard with each stimulation.

STIMULATOR

For the nerve conduction study, it is necessary to stimulate the nerves electrically. As a result, the stimulator generates, for a brief period of time, a square-wave electrical current (stimulus)

TABLE 2.1. Typical EMG Machine Settings for Various Procedures

	Needle EMG									
Setting	**At Rest**	**Minimal Contraction**	**Maximal Contraction**	**Motor Nerve Conduction**	**Sensory or Mixed Nerve Conduction**	**H-reflex**	**F-wave**	**Repetitive Nerve Stimulation Test**	**SFEMG**	**Other Reflexes**
Sweep velocity (ms/division)	10	10	100	2	1	10	5–10	2 or 200	0.5–1.0	5–10
Sensitivity (μV)	100	500–1000	1000	2000	10	500	200	2000	500–1000	100–200
Filter										
High (KHz)	10	10	10	10	2	10	10	10	30	10
Low (Hz)	2–20	2–20	2–20	2–20	20	20	20	2–20	500	20
Audio	On	On	On	On or off	On	On or off	On or off	On or off	On	On or off
Stimulus duration (ms)	N/A	N/A	N/A	Start with 0.05–0.1; increase to obtain SMS	Start with 0.05–0.1; do not increase beyond 0.2	0.5 or 1.0	Start with 0.05–0.1; increase to SMS	Start with 0.05–0.1; increase to SMS	N/A	Start with 0.05–1.0; increase to SMS
Stimulus rate	N/A	N/A	N/A	1 Hz	1 Hz	Every 2 or 5 s	Every 2 s	2 Hz, 3 Hz, 5 Hz, 50 Hz	N/A	Every 2 s

SMS, supramaximal stimulation; N/A, not applicable.

that stimulates the nerve at the cathode electrode. The stimulator has three control modes: the duration of the stimulus, the intensity of the stimulus, and the rate of stimulation. The stimulus duration usually ranges from 0.05 to 1 ms. The longer the duration of the stimulus, the more pain the patient feels. It is best to start with the shortest stimulus duration in the nerve conduction study. The intensity of stimulation can be gradually increased from 0 to 500 V or from 0 to 100 mA. In most modern EMG machines, the exact intensity of the stimulus is displayed on the stimulator as milliamperes or volts. Display of the stimulus intensity is helpful for the examiner to achieve the supramaximal stimulation. Again, the higher the intensity of the stimulus, the more painful it is. Therefore, a gradual increase of intensity from zero to above the maximal intensity to achieve the maximum amplitude of potentials (called supramaximal stimulation) is recommended in the nerve conduction study and in the repetitive nerve stimulation test for myasthenia gravis. The rate of stimulation can be varied from 1 to 50 Hz. In the nerve conduction study, one stimulation per second is often recommended because it is usually well tolerated by patients. The higher the rate of stimulation, the more painful it is. A low rate of stimulation (2 to 5 Hz) is needed to test the functions of neuromuscular transmission, especially in myasthenia gravis. A high rate of stimulation (above 20 Hz) is needed to document the facilitation phenomenon in myasthenic syndrome (Lambert-Eaton myasthenic syndrome). There is also a selection mode for the number of repetitive nerve stimulations. This feature is especially useful in the repetitive nerve stimulation test because it reduces the unnecessary pain associated with prolonged stimulation. Five or six potentials are needed in most repetitive nerve stimulation tests. Even at a high rate of stimulation (e.g., 50 Hz), 1-second stimulation is sufficient to yield the necessary information.

The signal averager is a standard item on EMG machines. The basic aim of the signal averager is to improve the signal-to-noise ratio. It is impossible to record very small sensory compound nerve action potentials (CNAPs) without an averager because they are of the order of a few microvolts, which is about the same as or even lower than the noise level of the EMG amplifier or the electrode. With the use of the signal averager, the random noises cancel each other out, and only the time-locked sensory or mixed CNAPs are clearly recorded. As a general rule, the signal-to-noise ratio improves proportionally as the square root of the number of signal averagings. Therefore, the more averaging is done, the better the record will be. There are usually two control modes on the signal averager: the number of the averaging sweeps and the analysis time. Averaging up to 256 signals and an analysis time of 20 ms are sufficient for most nerve conduction studies.

RECORDING APPARATUS

EMG machines are equipped with paper recording systems. Some EMG machines have the capability of storing EMG potentials on a hard disk or a tape, using an analog magnetic tape recorder or a digital audiocassette. Four modes of recording are usually available on the major EMG machines: single shot; superimposed shots; continuous recording; and raster recording (Fig. 2.2). The single shot records an actual display of potentials on the oscilloscope screen. The superimposed shots record four or five tracings superimposed on a common baseline in the middle of the paper and are especially useful in recording jitter on the SFEMG study. The continuous recording shows the changing potentials continuously on the paper as they occur. The raster recording mode displays several potentials in sequence from one side to the other. This mode is used mainly for recording the responses on the repetitive nerve stimulation test. In contrast to the slower speed of continuous recording, this mode has the advantage of recording the changing shape of the potential. Thus, artifacts are easily recognizable on the repetitive nerve stimulation test. The tape recording of potentials is achieved by connecting an analog magnetic tape recorder or a digital audiocassette to the output of the amplifier, thus permitting permanent recording of potentials on tape. One advantage of this sytem is that it simultaneously records the sounds of the potentials, making it useful for audiovisual teaching and for later analysis of the data for research purposes.

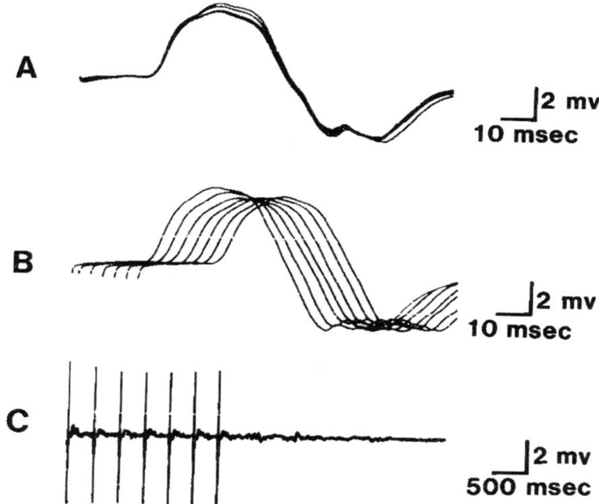

FIGURE 2.2. An 8% decremental response in the repetitive nerve stimulation test in a patient with myasthenia gravis recorded with varying recording modes. **A.** Superimposed mode. **B.** Raster mode. **C.** Continuous mode.

RECORDING ELECTRODES

There are two kinds of recording electrodes on the EMG machine: surface electrodes and needle electrodes. Regardless of the choices of electrodes, it is important to connect the active and reference electrodes accurately to the amplifier so that the upward deflection of the potential becomes negative and the downward deflection positive. If the active and reference recording electrodes are switched when connected to the amplifier, the negative and positive deflections are reversed. The consequences of such a mistake can be imagined. In most EMG machines, the cathode is assigned as the active electrode.

Surface Electrodes

Surface electrodes can record potentials from muscles or nerves. They are available as disposable or reusable electrodes (Fig. 2.3). The most commonly used electrodes are round, flat plates 1.0 cm in diameter. When surface electrodes are used, the impedance between them and the skin must be reduced to obtain a technically satisfactory recording. This can usually be achieved by applying electrode gel under the electrodes. If this method does not provide low enough impedance for the test, the skin must be washed with acetone to remove surface grease and scraped with a fine needle or sandpaper to remove the superficial scaly layer. Surface electrodes are used predominantly in the study of nerve conduction and for repetitive nerve stimulation tests. Disposable "stick-up" electrodes are especially well suited for the repetitive nerve stimulation (RNS) test.

Needle Electrodes

Needle electrodes are used predominantly for the needle EMG study. The two most commonly used needles for this purpose are Teflon-coated monopolar needle electrodes and concentric needle electrodes (Fig. 2.4).

The monopolar needle electrode is usually constructed from a stainless steel needle that is insulated except at its tip. The diameter of the needle averages approximately 0.8 mm, and the length of the needle varies from 12 to 75 mm. These are available as disposable or reusable needles.

The Teflon-coated monopolar needle electrode is less painful, less expensive, and more sensitive in identifying fibrillation and positive sharp waves than the concentric needle elec-

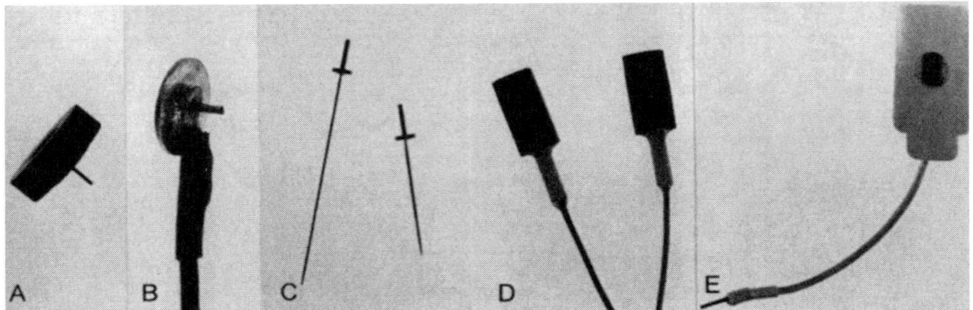

FIGURE 2.3. Various recording electrodes: **(A)** Dantec disc electrode, **(B)** TECA (Pleasantsville, NY) surface electrode, **(C)** Dantec near-nerve monopolar needle for the sensory or mixed CNAP, **(D)** Dantec surface electrode, **(E)** disposable Dantec "stick-up" surface electrode.

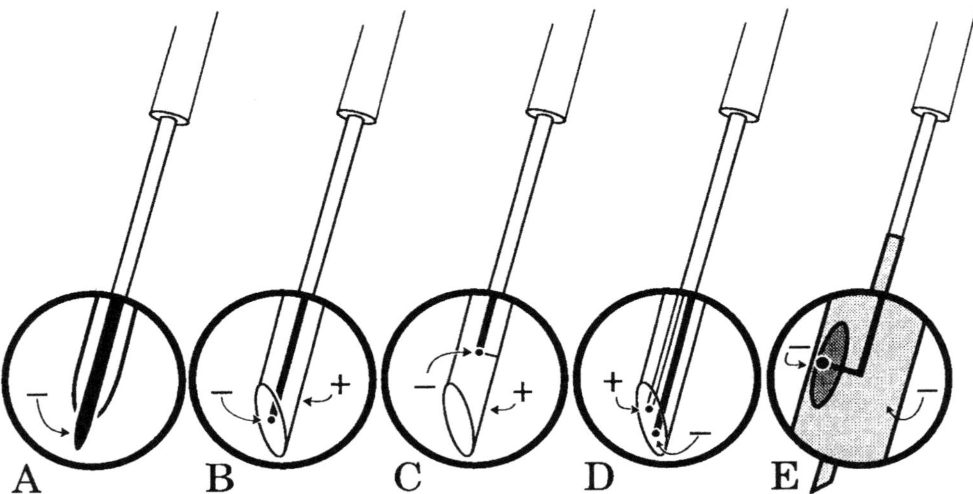

FIGURE 2.4. Needle electrodes: **(A)** monopolar needle electrode, **(B)** concentric needle electrode, **(C)** single-fiber needle electrode, **(D)** bipolar needle electrode, **(E)** macro needle. −, cathode; +, anode.

trodes, making it much more popular among electromyographers. For the needle EMG study, the monopolar needle electrode is used as the active electrode and the surface electrode nearby on the same muscle as the reference electrode. The concentric needle electrode consists of a platinum wire located centrally inside a hollow needle but completely insulated from it. The outside diameter of the needle varies from 0.3 to 1.0 mm, with a center wire of 0.1 mm diameter. The inside wire is the active electrode and the outside cannula is the reference electrode. When the concentric needle is connected to the connecting cable, caution should be used not to change the polarity of the electrodes.

Monopolar needle electrodes are used for the near-nerve needle nerve conduction. These electrodes are specially designed for leading off potentials from sensory nerves (Dantec 13R21-13R25, Dantec Medical, Inc., Allentown, NJ) (Fig. 2.4). Made of stainless steel, they are coated with Teflon in such a manner that only the tip is left uninsulated. The active electrode is inserted as close to the nerve as possible, and the reference electrode is placed 3 cm laterally from the active electrode. The near-nerve needle technique has several advantages over the surface electrode method. First, the signal–to–noise ratio can be diminished markedly by reducing the impedance. Second, very small nerve CNAPs that are not recordable by surface electrodes can be recorded. Also, the amplitude of the recording potential is much more reliable. Finally, the dispersion of the potential can be documented. Thus, the near-nerve needle is used in recording sensory and mixed CNAPs when the potentials cannot be recorded with surface electrodes even after signal averaging.

The subcutaneous needle electrode is used by some investigators as a recording electrode to record the CMAP from the belly of the muscle on the repetitive nerve stimulation test. Special SFEMG or macro EMG needle electrodes are used for the SFEMG or macro EMG, respectively.

STIMULATING ELECTRODES

Stimulating electrodes are usually surface electrodes, which commonly consist of two protruding metal or felt "buttons" fixed to a stimulator. Most EMG machines have the cathode as the active electrode and the anode as the reference electrode. In some EMG machines, one has a choice between using the cathode or the anode as the active electrode. Most surface electrodes are lightly covered with electrode gel before use, whereas the felt types are moistened with saline solution. Regardless of which electrode is the active electrode, it is important to remember that the active electrode should be closer to the recording electrode. If the active and reference electrodes are reversed, the distance and the latency become longer. The monopolar needle electrode is used to stimulate a deeply situated nerve (e.g., the sciatic nerve). To stimulate digital nerve fibers in the fingers and toes, a ring-shaped electrode or strap-type felt electrode is used (Fig. 2.5).

MACHINE SETTINGS FOR VARIOUS PROCEDURES

When adjusting the EMG machine for specific procedures, it is important to remember that the machine should be set to record the potentials accurately without any distortion and to permit reading of the latency and amplitude with the most accuracy. The recommended settings for the EMG machines are presented in Table 2.1.

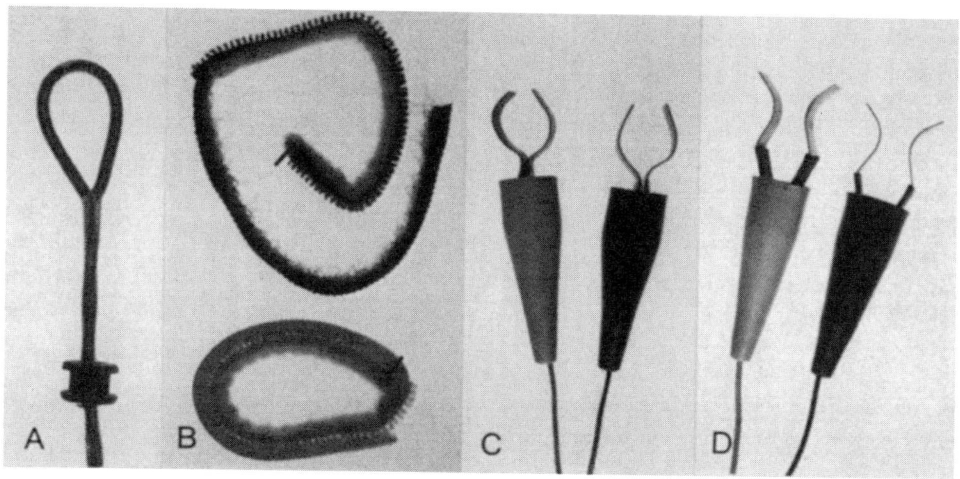

FIGURE 2.5. Various sensory stimulating electrodes: **(A)** TECA (Pleasantville, NY) ring electrode, **(B)** Dantec Velcro strap electrode, **(C)** neurodiagnostic surface electrode, **(D)** Oh's interdigital surface electrode.

CHAPTER 3

Nerve Conduction Study

The measurement of nerve conduction is an expression of the physiological or pathophysiological state of the nerves and an essential tool for the study of neuropathy. Although the first report of a conduction rate of 61.0 ± 5.1 m/s in a nerve-muscle preparation of the human median nerve was reported by Von Helmholtz in 1853, the modern technique of human nerve conduction in situ was not developed until the early 1900s. In 1909, Piper was the first to use the modern technique of recording the muscle action potential with surface electrodes instead of using the muscle twitch as a signal of the arrival of the nerve impulse at the muscle. However, little attention was paid to the measurement of nerve conduction in humans until 1948, when Hodes et al. introduced this as a diagnostic tool. Using present-day techniques, they measured the motor nerve conduction velocity (NCV) in median, ulnar, radial, peroneal, and tibial nerves in normal subjects and in patients with peripheral nerve injuries. They found in healthy subjects that the NCV varied from 46 to 67 m/s and the "residual latency" ranged from 1.4 to 3.8 ms. Since that time, the nerve conduction test has become the standard diagnostic test for neuropathy.

NERVE CONDUCTION AND LATE RESPONSES TESTS

Nerve Conduction Tests

There are three kinds of nerve conduction tests: the motor nerve conduction test, the sensory nerve conduction test, and the mixed nerve conduction test.

Motor Nerve Conduction. The motor nerve conduction of a peripheral nerve is tested by stimulating the nerve with a single supramaximal stimulus at each of two proximal points along the course of the peripheral nerve and then recording the compound muscle action potential (CMAP) with a surface electrode from a muscle innervated by that nerve (Fig. 3.1). For example, the median nerve may be stimulated at the elbow and again at the wrist, with the recording electrode placed over the belly of the abductor pollicis brevis muscle. The time required for this response with distal stimulation is called the terminal latency. To obtain the conduction time, the terminal latency is subtracted from the latency at the proximal point of stimulation. The distance from the proximal to the distal point of stimulation is measured. NCV is determined by dividing this distance by the conduction time. The CMAP amplitude and shape are also analyzed. The procedure is limited to nerves that are accessible to stimulation. In the upper extremities, these include the median, ulnar, and radial nerves; in the lower extremities, they are the sciatic, femoral, posterior tibial, and peroneal nerves.

Sensory Nerve Conduction. The sensory nerve conduction of a peripheral nerve is tested either orthodromically or antidromically (Fig. 3.2). In the orthodromic method, the sensory nerve conduction is tested by stimulating the distal part of the nerve and recording the compound nerve action potential (CNAP) directly over the proximal part of the nerve. For example, conduction along the sensory fibers of the median or ulnar nerve can be tested by stimulating the digital nerves at the fingers and recording the potential at the wrist. When the stimulating and recording electrodes are switched, this is called antidromic stimulation. The latency and conduction velocities are identical in the orthodromic and antidromic methods. Recorded with a surface electrode, the antidromic response is larger in amplitude than the orthodromic. As a rule, the diagnostic yield of the antidromic measurement is poorer than that of the orthodromic measurement. A major disadvantage of the antidromic method

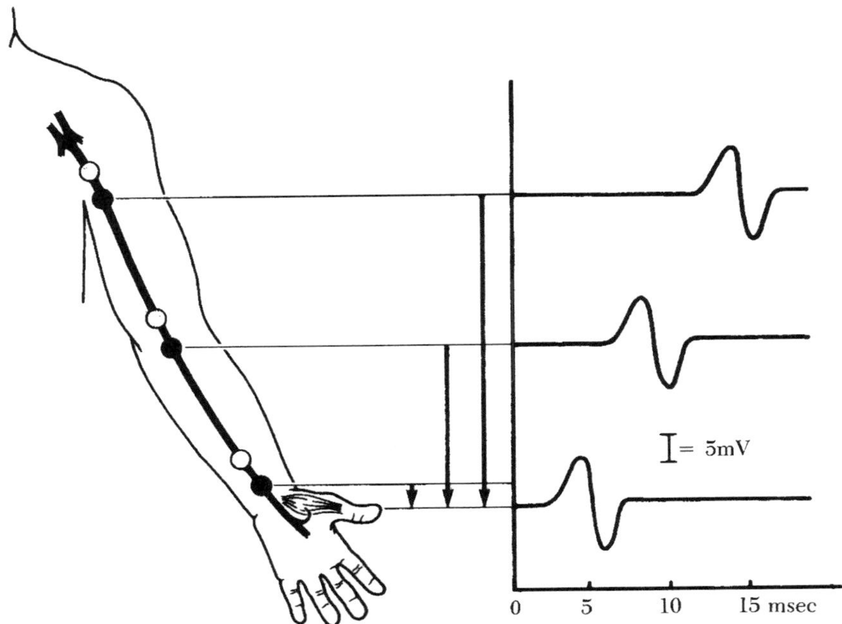

FIGURE 3.1. Motor nerve conduction study in the median nerve. The recording electrodes are placed over the belly of the abductor pollicis brevis. The median nerve is stimulated at the wrist, elbow, and axilla.

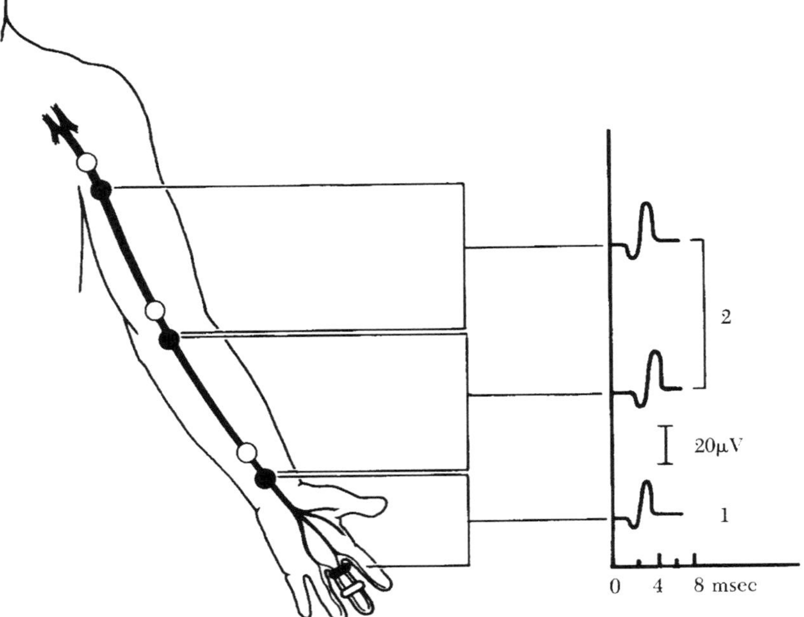

FIGURE 3.2. Sensory (*1*) and mixed (*2*) nerve conduction study in the median nerve. The recording electrodes are placed over the proximal part of the nerve and the stimulating electrodes are over the distal part of the nerve. A reference stimulating electrode is placed distal to the active stimulating electrode.

is that the antidromic sensory CNAPs are obscured by the muscle potential from a neighboring contracting muscle. Unlike motor nerve conduction, the sensory nerve conduction time is equal to the latency in sensory nerve conduction. Thus, the NCV is determined by dividing the distance by the conduction time or latency. The CNAP amplitude is measured from peak to peak. This procedure is used most often for studying the ulnar, median, sural, and radial nerves. Because a special technique is needed to obtain CNAP in the sciatic, posterior tibial, and peroneal nerves, this procedure is usually not used to study these nerves.

Mixed Nerve Conduction. The mixed nerve conduction of a peripheral nerve is tested by stimulating the distal part of the mixed nerve (sensory and motor fibers) and recording the CNAP directly over the proximal part of the nerve (Fig. 3.2). For example, conduction along the mixed fibers of the median and ulnar nerves can be tested by stimulating the mixed nerve at the wrist and recording the CNAP at the elbow. The methods of testing, measuring amplitude, and calculating velocity are identical to the orthodromic method of sensory nerve conduction. The only difference is that mixed (motor and sensory) nerve fibers are being stimulated. The clinical significance of mixed nerve conduction studies is also identical to that of the sensory nerve conduction studies.

Late Responses

There are two late responses commonly used in daily practice in the electromyography (EMG) laboratory: H-reflex and F-wave tests (Fig. 3.3).

H-Reflex. The H-reflex in the gastrocnemius-soleus muscle is the electrophysiological counterpart of the ankle reflex. The H-reflex is a late response with longer latency that has a threshold usually lower than that of direct CMAP (M-wave) in motor nerve conduction studies. In newborn infants, the H-reflex can be elicited from almost every muscle. However, in adults, it is obtained regularly only from the calf muscle after stimulation of the posterior tibial nerve. The H-reflex duration and amplitude are less clinically useful than the H-reflex latency. In peripheral neuropathy or S1 radiculopathy, the H-reflex in the gastrocnemius-soleus muscle is often absent or prolonged in latency because the ankle reflex is frequently absent. The H-reflex has been used mainly in studies of motor neuron excitability and has only limited value in the investigation of peripheral nerve disorders.

F-Wave. Another late response is the F-wave, which is evoked by supramaximal stimulation during the motor nerve conduction study. Originally considered to be a variant of the H-reflex, the F-wave is now considered to be caused mainly by antidromic volleys in the motor fibers. The F-wave is invariably evoked in a normal individual during the motor nerve conduction study by stimulating the distal portion of the nerves. In recent years, the F-wave has been used to measure the NCV of proximal motor fibers. Recent studies have shown that F-wave latency may be the sole abnormality in some patients with peripheral neuropathy when other nerve conductions are all normal. This is especially true in Guillain-Barré syndrome.

TERMINOLOGY OF NERVE CONDUCTION

Motor Nerve Conduction

CMAP. Action potential recorded in a muscle after stimulation of a motor nerve. Terms for the various components of the CMAP are defined in Figure 3.4.

Latency. Time (ms) from the stimulus onset to the beginning of the initial deflection of the CMAP.

Terminal (distal) Latency (ms). Latency obtained by stimulating at the most distal site possible along the nerve.

Conduction Time. Time (ms) for conduction of nerve impulse between two stimulation sites.

Nerve Conduction Velocity (NCV) (m/s). Distance between two stimulation sites (mm) divided by Conduction time (ms) between two stimulation sites.

Sensory or Mixed Nerve Conduction

CNAP. Action potential recorded in the nerve after the stimulation of sensory mixed nerves. Terms for the various components of the CNAP are defined in Figure 3.5.

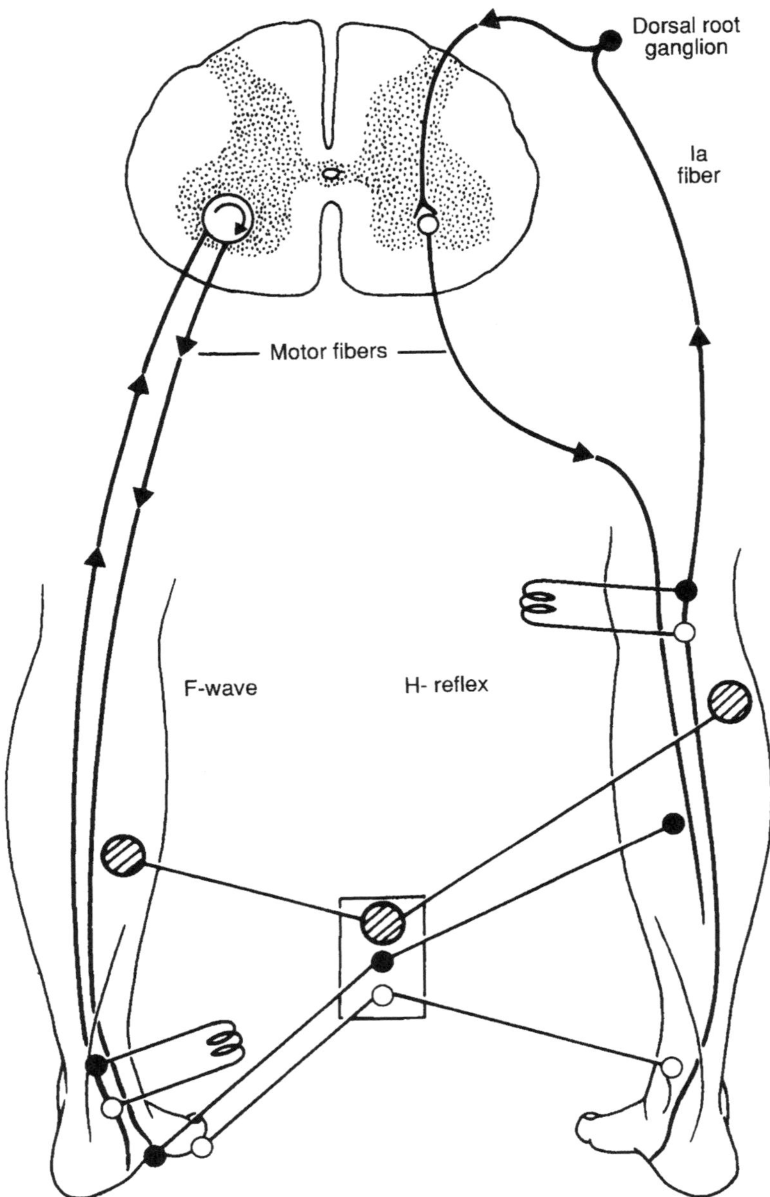

FIGURE 3.3. Anatomical pathways for the H-reflex and F-wave. For the H-reflex, the Ia fiber is the afferent pathway and the alpha motor fiber is the efferent pathway. For the F-wave, the alpha motor fiber is the efferent and the efferent pathway. Note also the monosynaptic reflex arc in the H-reflex pathway.

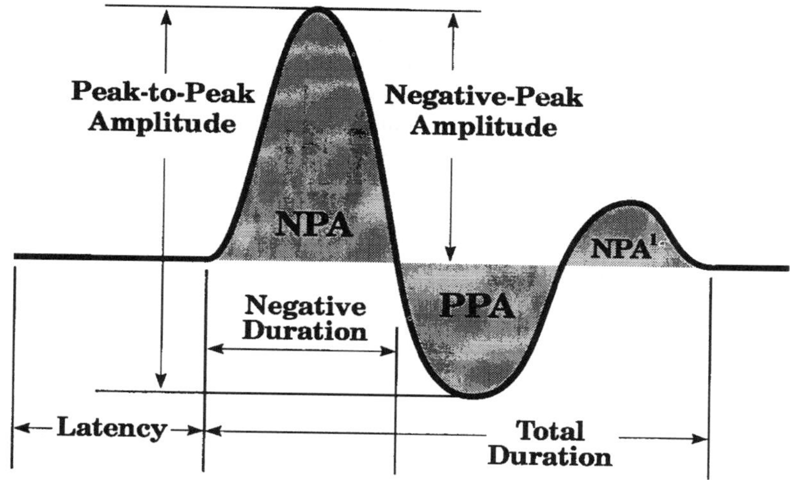

FIGURE 3.4. Components of the CMAP. *NPA*, negative-peak area; *PPA*, positive-peak area; *NPA*[1], additional negative-peak area. Total area = (NPA) + (PPA) + (NPA).

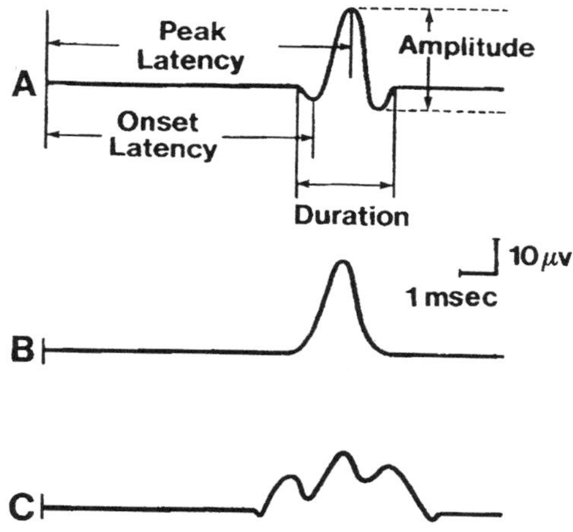

FIGURE 3.5. Components and shapes of the CNAP. **A.** Components of the sensory or mixed CNAP. **B.** Commonly observed CNAPs with the surface electrode. Initial positive deflection is not observed. **C.** CNAP with the abnormal temporal dispersion (dispersion phenomenon).

Conduction Time (latency). Time (ms) for conduction of nerve impulse from the stimulus onset to the initial positive peak with the near-nerve needle and to the onset of the negative peak or the negative peak of CNAP with the surface electrode, or between two stimulation sites if distal and proximal stimulations were done.

NCV (m/s). Distance between stimulation site and recording site (mm) divided by conduction time (ms).

PHYSIOLOGICAL PRINCIPLE OF THE NERVE CONDUCTION TESTS

Motor Nerve Conduction

Latency. Latency is a measure of the combined time for conduction of the nerve impulse from the point of stimulation to the axonal terminal, the neuromuscular transmission, and the depolarization of muscle fibers.

Amplitude. Amplitude is the rough estimation of the number of muscle fibers that are activated to nerve stimulation and subsequently of the number of nerve fibers that become excitable to nerve stimulation when neuromuscular transmission is normal. The CMAP, which is obtained with the surface recording electrode or subcutaneous needle from the belly of the muscle, represents the sum of muscle action potentials generated by all muscle fibers from the muscle and has a simple disphasic shape with an initial negative deflection. *The surface electrode is the only reliable method for documenting conduction block and volume conduction.* For these reasons, the surface recording electrode is essential in the motor nerve conduction. The motor nerve conduction study performed with a needle electrode is not recommended because the response is recorded from a more limited area of the muscle, the shape of the CMAP is more complex, and the initial deflection of the potential is not always negative. The amplitude of the CMAP is an insensitive measure of mild impairment because of its wide variation among normal subjects. Thus, a low CMAP amplitude represents a severe impairment of nerve conduction.

Duration. The duration reflects the synchrony of discharge of the individual muscle fibers. When the muscle fibers are activated in near synchrony, the duration of the CMAP becomes shorter. If the conduction velocities vary widely among different nerve fibers, some muscle fibers are activated earlier than others, producing a longer duration CMAP. Thus, the duration of the CMAP is related to the range of conduction velocities of the large-diameter motor nerve fibers. When the CMAP is split into numerous phases producing a long-duration abnormal temporal dispersion (dispersion phenomenon) (Fig. 3.6), this represents a wide range of conduction velocities of the large-diameter motor nerve fibers and thus demyelination.

Nerve Conduction Velocity. The NCV represents the maximum conduction velocity of the fastest nerve fibers. Almost all motor nerve fibers must be slowed for the NCV to be diminished. Thus, the presence of a few intact motor fibers may yield an entirely normal NCV in patients with neuropathy. According to Gillart, it is necessary for about 75% of the large-diameter, fast-conduction fibers to be lost before there is any noticeable effect on the supramaximal NCV of the nerve.

Sensory Nerve Conduction

Latency (conduction time). The latency is a measure of the time required for conduction of the nerve impulse from the point of stimulation to the point of recording. Latency to the initial positive peak with the near-nerve needle and to the onset of the negative peak (this is preferred because of the frequent absence of an initial positive peak) with the surface

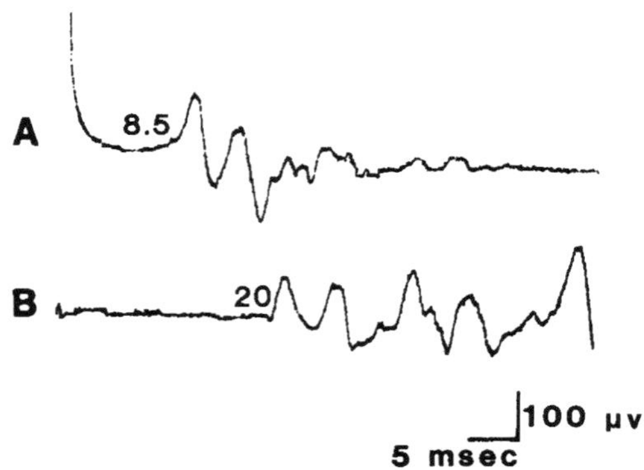

FIGURE 3.6. Dispersion phenomenon in the CMAP. This is from the posterior tibial nerve at the ankle **(A)** and the popliteal fossa **(B)** in a case of hypertrophic neuropathy. The reduced amplitude of the CMAP is due to a marked dispersion phenomenon (duration of the CMAP is 30 ms). Terminal latency is 8.5 ms. Motor NCV is 35.8 m/s.

electrode represents the time for the fastest sensory fibers. The negative peak latency includes the rise time of the action potential and may therefore give an additional indication of temporal dispersion, thus representing the average conduction of the group Ia fibers. The author prefers the negative peak latency measurement in the surface electrode recording because it gives more reliable and reproducible results than those obtained by measuring to the onset of the negative deflection.

Amplitude. The amplitude of the CNAP is the rough estimation of the number of large nerve fibers that are activated by nerve stimulation. With the surface electrode, the amplitude is heavily influenced by the distance of the recording electrode from the nerve. Thus, the amplitude is a less sensitive measure of mild impairment. With near-nerve electrodes, the amplitude is a more sensitive index of impairment. Low amplitude usually represents severe impairment of nerve conduction.

Duration. The duration is the range of NCVs of the various large-diameter sensory fibers. Thus, it is an index of temporal dispersion. Prolonged temporal dispersion is called abnormal temporal dispersion ("dispersion phenomenon"). Abnormal temporal dispersion is difficult or impossible to recognize with the surface electrode (Fig. 3.7) but is easily documented with the near-nerve needle and is typically observed in the presence of segmental demyelination (Fig. 3.8).

Nerve Conduction Velocity. The NCV represents the maximum conduction velocity of the fastest sensory fibers when the latency is measured to the first positive peak. When the latency is measured to the negative peak with the surface electrode technique, it provides an estimate of conduction of the slower fibers. When the latency is measured to the smallest recognizable component with the near-nerve needle technique, the slowest NCV can be calculated. In some diseased nerves, the minimum NCV is slowed, whereas other parameters are normal. With the surface electrode and without the aid of a signal averager, an NCV slower than 20 m/s is seldom seen because beyond this point the CNAP is too small to be registered.

Mixed Nerve Conduction

The physiological functions of the various parameters in mixed nerve conduction are similar to those in sensory nerve conduction, except that the CNAPs are generated from mixed motor and sensory fibers.

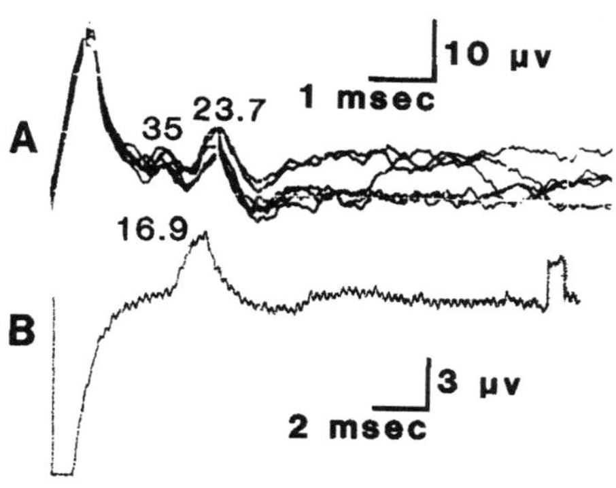

FIGURE 3.7. Dispersion phenomenon in the sensory CNAP recorded with a surface electrode in cases of carpal tunnel syndrome. **A.** Double-peaked CNAP over the palm-wrist segment. The first peak NCV is 35.0 m/s. The higher second peak NCV is 23.7 m/s. **B.** Note the long duration of the sensory CNAP (3.7 ms) over the finger-wrist segment. The NCV is 16.9 m/s.

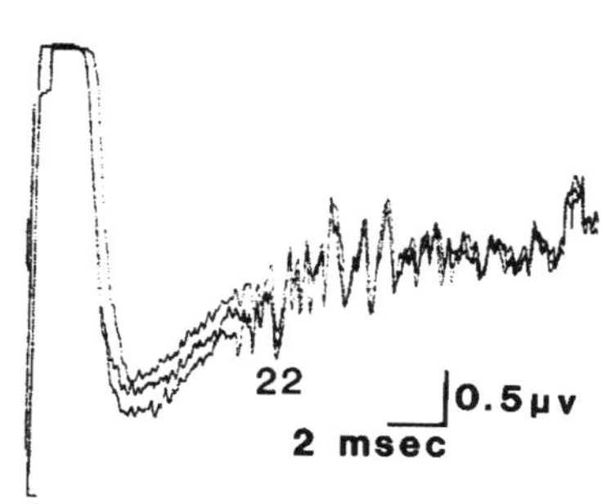

FIGURE 3.8. The sensory CNAP from the ankle with digits I to II interdigital nerve stimulation in a patient with tarsal tunnel syndrome. The maximum NCV is 22 m/s. The dispersion phenomenon is obvious.

FACTORS AFFECTING THE NERVE CONDUCTION TESTS

Among the various factors affecting the nerve conduction tests, four are important: skin temperature, age, height, and distance measurement.

Temperature

Among the various physiological factors, temperature is the most important factor affecting the nerve conduction test. This fact was recognized as early as 1867 by Von Helmholtz, and in 1948 Tasaki and Fujita observed that in frog nerve, the conduction time as related to temperature followed an almost straight line between 20 and 5 C. In 1956, Henricken was the first to study systematically this relationship in the human nerve; he reported an increase of 2.4 m/s per degree for motor NCV within the range of 29 to 38 C. Since then, various studies have shown that the NCV increases linearly with the temperature within the physiological range. In motor nerve conduction, the rate of increase ranges from 1.1 to 2.4 m/s. In sensory nerve conduction, this rate ranges from 0.76 to 2.3 m/s. Among the various correction formulae, the most commonly used is DeJesus's formula, which is based on the semilogarithmic relationship between NCV and temperature. His formula applies to motor and sensory fibers, offers a simple method of eliminating diagnostic error caused by temperature variation of the limbs, and requires only that the surface temperature be monitored. Thus, it is essential to measure skin temperature and adjust the NCV to the standard temperature if the skin temperature is below the desired level; otherwise, the surface of the area to be examined must be warmed to the standard temperature with a skin temperature control unit.

The distal motor latency is similarly influenced by changes in temperature: it increases by 0.2 ms per degree centigrade drop in temperature between 25 and 35 C. The amplitude of the CMAP and CNAP increases linearly with decreasing temperature. However, there is no reliable correction formula for the amplitude change with temperature.

Age

Age is an important variable in the study of nerve conduction. The changes in the nerve conduction are most important in the first 4 years of life and less marked in later years. Nerve conduction in motor, sensory, and mixed nerves is about 50% of the normal adult values in the full-term newborn, reaching about 75% of the adult value at 1 year of age and nears 100% at 4 years of age. The motor, sensory, and mixed NCVs increase in a logarithmic function. The increase in NCV during infancy and early childhood is most likely due to two factors: the increase in the number of large fibers between birth and 8 years of age, when the number is the same as in adult nerves, and the complete remyelination of nerve fibers by age 5. Thus, it is imperative to compare the NCV obtained in infants and babies with the normal values for that same age group.

In adults, the NCV of motor, sensory, or mixed nerve conduction decreases with age beginning in the 20s. The amplitudes of the CMAP and CNAP are also affected by age, showing a gradual decline. However, this decline is so minimal up to 60 years of age that there is no need for correction. After age 60, however, the decrease is more prominent with age. Thus, minor corrections are needed if the normal adult data were pooled from individuals between 20 and 60 years of age, as was the case in our laboratory. When interpreting the results in patients over age 60, a correction of 1 m per decade is allowed for the motor NCV and 2 m per decade for the sensory NCV measured with surface electrodes. For the amplitudes of CMAP and CNAP, the change in older individuals does not seem to be important in practice because of the wider range of CMAP and CNAP amplitudes in normal individuals.

Height

Height is not an important factor in the nerve conduction tests, but it is the most important factor in the study of F-waves, H-reflexes, and T-reflexes. Because the nerve impulse has to loop through the efferent fibers of nerves, the spinal cord, and the long afferent pathway of nerves in these long latency tests, their linear relationship with body height is obvious and well documented. Thus, it should be customary to compare the obtained values with normal values for a given height.

Distance Measurement

The distance is the second most important factor affecting the nerve conduction tests. Because distance is affected by the position of the limbs (e.g., flexion or extension of the elbow in the ulnar nerve conduction) and contour of the anatomical part (e.g., thoracic outlet segment), it is essential to follow the recommended position of the limb being tested and use the recommended devices (caliper versus flexible tape) for the distance measurement. Even when these obvious variables are followed, the possibility of examiner error is a serious problem in obtaining an accurate calculation of NCV. The shorter the distance, the more critical the examiner error becomes. To minimize this influence, 10 cm is recommended as the shortest acceptable distance for the segmental NCV. Certainly, the short-segment nerve conduction study (inching technique) violates this rule; thus, this factor has to be considered in interpretation. One study showed that examiners may differ by up to 1 cm when measuring the distance between two points on a limb if instructed to lay the tape along the course of a nerve. Distance error is primarily due to skin movement rather than to inaccurate reading of the tape measure. To reduce this error, it is best to measure the distance between the center of the stimulating cathode and the center of the active recording electrode using a flexible tape (unless stated otherwise) and adhering to the recommended position of the limb being tested.

TECHNICAL REQUIREMENTS

Supramaximal Stimulation: To obtain meaningful nerve conduction values, supramaximal stimulation is essential. A supramaximal stimulus can be achieved by increasing the intensity by 25 to 30% above maximal stimulation. The amplitude and latency of the potentials are affected by the intensity of the stimulus. With a gradual increase in the stimulus intensity, the amplitude of potentials increases continuously up to the maximum (the maximal stimulation) and then does not increase with further stimulation (supramaximal). This has been observed in motor and sensory nerve conduction with surface and needle recording electrodes. With a gradual increase of stimulus intensity, there is a continuous decrease in latency, which becomes still shorter after the CMAP has ceased to increase in amplitude.

Accurate Measurement of Distance: NCV is the most important parameter in the nerve conduction study. This can be influenced heavily by the distance measurement as discussed above. To obtain the most reliable distance measurement, it is important to follow the instructions for the position of the limbs and the measuring equipment.

Temperature Control and Correction for Temperature Difference: As discussed above, temperature control is essential for the proper interpretation of NCV. Without correction for temperature, NCVs obtained at lower temperatures can be interpreted as abnormal. Thus, it is important to control the skin temperature and correct the NCV to the standard temperature if required.

Surface Recording Electrodes and Belly-Tendon Placement of These Electrodes in the Motor Nerve Conduction: With surface electrodes, the amplitude of the CMAP gives a rough estimation of the number of muscle fibers that respond to nerve stimulation. If the electrodes are arranged in the belly-tendon position with one electrode overlying the end-plate region and the other over the tendon, the CMAP has a simple diphasic shape with an initial negative defection. Thus, the surface electrode is the only reliable method for documenting the conduction block and the decremental response in the repetitive nerve stimulation test and for the objective measurement of the progressive degeneration of motor nerves. It is also useful for identifying the volume-conducted potential by the initial positive deflection. With a needle electrode, the amplitude of the CMAP does not measure the entire number of muscle fibers responding to nerve stimulation but records the response from a more limited area of the muscle. Moreover, the shape of the CMAP is more complex than that obtained with surface electrodes, and the initial deflection of the potential is not always negative. The latency varies with the position of the needle electrode. If the needle is not inserted in the end-plate region, a slowing of nerve conduction may be simulated by the slow conduction in the muscle fibers (4 to 6 m/s). These factors make the needle electrode unsuitable for objective measurement of progressive degeneration of motor fibers, localization of a

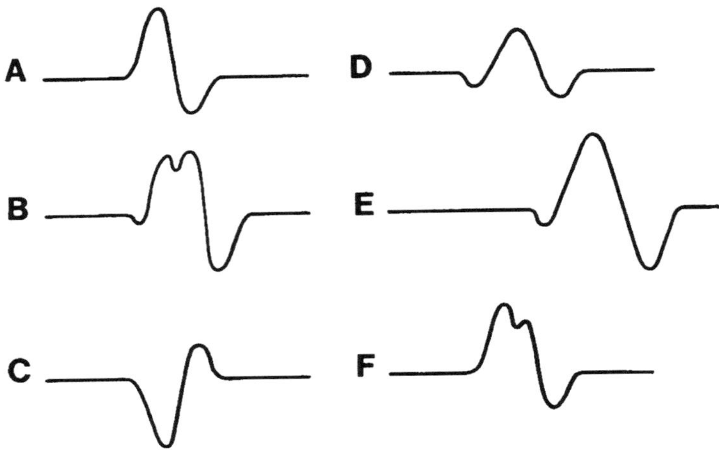

FIGURE 3.9. The various shapes of the CMAP. **A.** Normal CMAP is a diphasic wave with the initial negative deflection. **B.** Active recording electrode is away from the belly (motor point) and closer to the other muscle. **C.** The active and reference electrodes are reversed. **D.** Stimulation of the neighboring nerves either by misplacement of the stimulating electrodes or by stimulus spread when the stimulus is too strong. **E.** Conduction of the nerve impulse through anomalous innervation. **F.** An active recording electrode was placed on the bellies of the two muscles innervated by the same nerve.

conduction block, and testing of neuromuscular transmission. Clearly, surface electrodes have advantages over needle electrodes. Therefore, the author prefers the surface electrodes and placement of these electrodes following the belly-tendon method for motor nerve conduction studies.

With this method, the initial deflection of the CMAP is upward (negative). If the initial deflection is not negative, the following possibilities exist (Fig. 3.9):

a. Incorrect placement of the active and reference recording electrode on the desired muscle belly away from the motor point;
b. Transposition of the active and reference recording electrodes;
c. Stimulation of other neighboring nerves by misplacement of the stimulating electrodes;
d. Stimulation of other nerves by stimulus spread when the stimulus has increased in duration and intensity;
e. Conduction of the nerve impulse through anomalous innervation. This is observed in patients with carpal tunnel syndrome and Martin-Grüber anastomosis.

The first three possibilities can be easily checked. For confirmation of the last two possibilities, careful study by an experienced EMGer is needed.

TESTING OF NERVE CONDUCTION

General Guidelines for the Nerve Conduction Tests

1. Explain the procedure to the patient in the simplest terms. Remember that the electrical stimulation you apply is painful.
2. Place the limb to be tested in a relaxed and comfortable position for both the patient and the examiner. Nerve conduction is best carried out with the limb relaxed. Otherwise, movement or noise artifact produces unnecessary interference, especially for the sensory and mixed nerve conduction studies.
3. Measure the skin temperature on the part of the limb near the nerve to be tested. If the skin temperature is lower than the controlled temperature, the area to be tested should be warmed to the desired temperature with a temperature controlling unit or the NCV should be adjusted using the correction formula (Table 3.1).

TABLE 3.1. Conversion Factors for the Temperature Difference in NCV

Degree Difference (ΔT)	K
0.5	1.021
1.0	1.043
1.5	1.065
2.0	1.087
2.5	1.017
3.0	1.134
3.5	1.157
4.0	1.183
4.5	1.207
5.0	1.233
5.5	1.259
6.0	1.286
6.5	1.313
7.0	1.341
7.5	1.369
8.0	1.398
8.5	1.428
9.0	1.458
10.0	1.520

4. Lower the skin impedance. It is important to lower the skin impedance as much as possible to reduce any interference artifacts. This is usually achieved by applying electrode gel under the electrode. On rare occasions, the skin has to be cleaned with alcohol or acetone or gently scraped with a needle or sandpaper.
5. Attach a ground electrode on the limb being tested. This is ideally placed between the stimulating and recording electrodes.
6. Pediatric stimulating electrodes are recommended for infants and babies.
7. Perform motor nerve conduction studies first to locate nerves for the sensory and mixed nerve conduction studies.
8. Use the lowest adequate stimulus intensity to reduce the pain of stimulation as much as possible because the electrical stimulation is painful. A 1/s rate of stimulation is best tolerated by patients. Use the shortest stimulus duration (0.05 or 0.1 ms) on the EMG machine first. In normal individuals, 0.05 ms duration is long enough to produce the maximal response. In patients with neuropathy, a longer duration of stimulus is often needed to obtain the maximal response. For sensory and mixed nerve conduction studies, a further increase beyond 0.2 ms duration does not produce any increase in the amplitude of CNAPs. On the other hand, for motor nerve conduction studies, the stimulus duration may have to be increased to 1.0 ms to obtain a response.
9. Initially, follow the typical machine settings for the various nerve conduction tests but be ready to change the setting if necessary.

Motor Nerve Conduction

1. Place the recording electrode on the distal muscle that is innervated by the tested nerve, using the belly-tendon method (Figs. 3.10 to 3.14). This method specifies that the active (cathode) surface recording electrode be placed on the belly (theoretical motor point of muscle) and the reference (anode) surface recording electrode on the tendon of muscle. With this method, the initial deflection of the CMAP is upward (negative).
2. Inform the patient that you are about to stimulate, so that the patient is prepared for minor discomfort or pain.
3. At first, stimulate the distal site with the minimum stimulus intensity and gradually increase the stimulus intensity to achieve the supramaximal stimulation and record the CMAP.

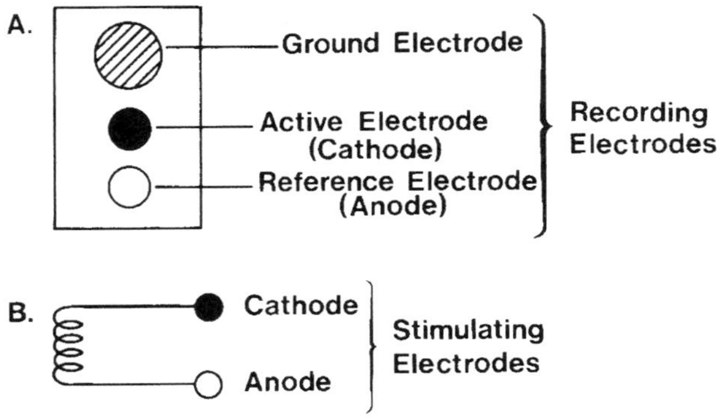

FIGURE 3.10. Symbols for electrodes. **A.** Recording electrodes. **B.** Stimulating electrodes.

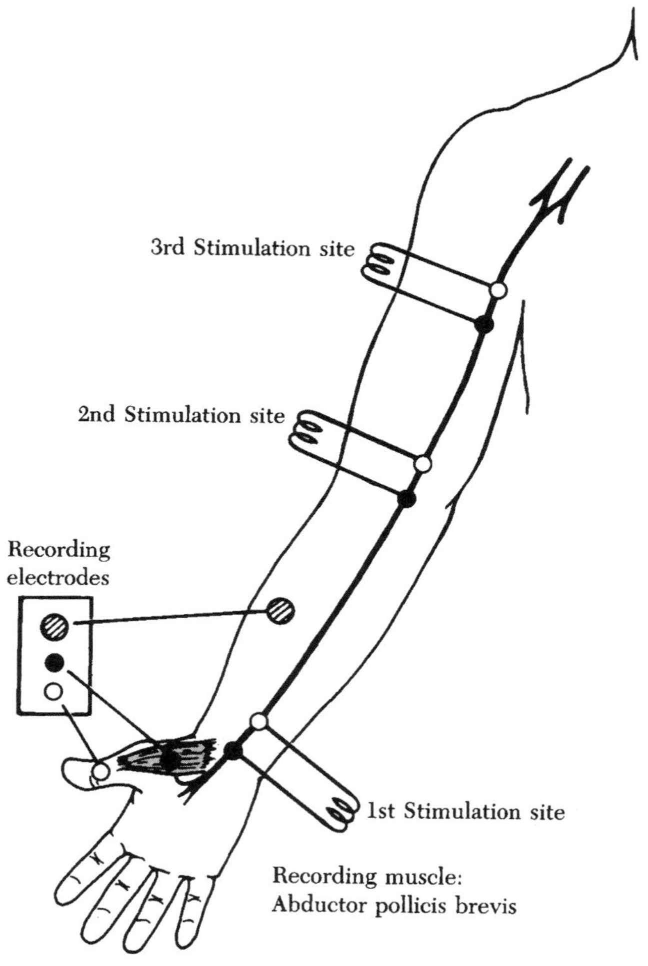

FIGURE 3.11. Motor nerve conduction study for the median nerve. Position: arm extended, palm up; Active Recording Electrode: midportion of the hyperthenar muscle (abductor pollicis brevis); Reference Recording Electrode: thumb; Ground Electrode: flexor surface of forearm; Instrument Setting: motor nerve conduction; Response: brisk movement of the thumb, index, and middle fingers. *1st Stimulation Site:* At the wrist, 5 cm proximal to the active electrode, between the two prominent middle tendons or on the midline along the crease between the hyper- and hypothenar muscles; *2nd Stimulation Site:* At the elbow crease, on the ulnar side of the pulsating brachial artery; *3rd Stimulation Site:* At the axilla, just forward of brachial artery.

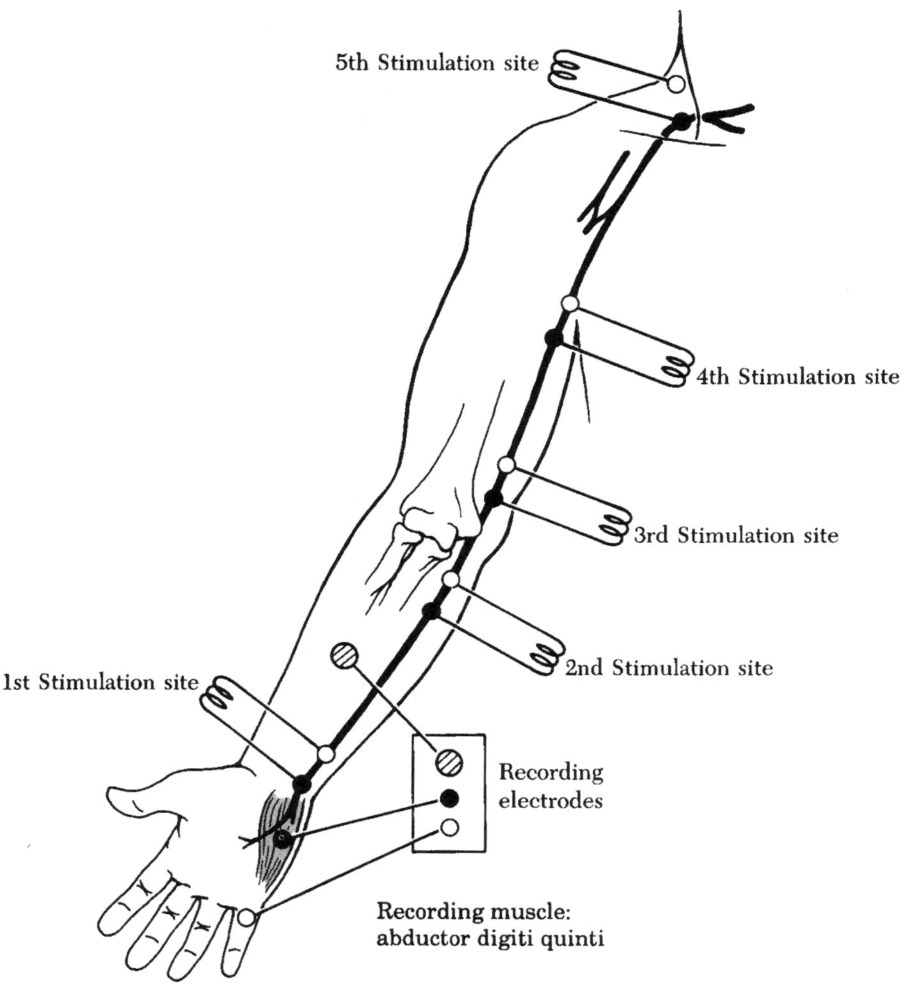

FIGURE 3.12. Motor nerve conduction study for the ulnar nerve. Position: arm extended, palm up; Active Recording Electrode: midportion of the hypothenar muscle (abductor digiti quinti); Reference Recording Electrode: little finger; Ground Electrode: flexor surface of the forearm; Instrument Setting: motor nerve conduction; Response: brisk movement of the little finger. *1st Stimulation Site*: At the wrist, 5 cm proximal to the active recording electrode, the radial side of the prominent tendon on the ulnar aspect (flexor carpi ulnaris tendon); *2nd Stimulation Site*: At 4 cm below the elbow sulcus (the distance across the elbow should be 9 to 10 cm); *3rd Stimulation Site*: At 5 to 6 cm above the elbow sulcus, between the biceps and triceps muscle; *4th Stimulation Site*: At the axilla, posterior to the pulsating brachial artery; *5th Stimulation Site*: At the supraclavicular fossa, lateral to the posterior border of the sternocleidomastoid and the superior margin of the clavicle. The distance between the Erb's point and axilla was measured with an obstetrical caliper with the arm 45 from the side.

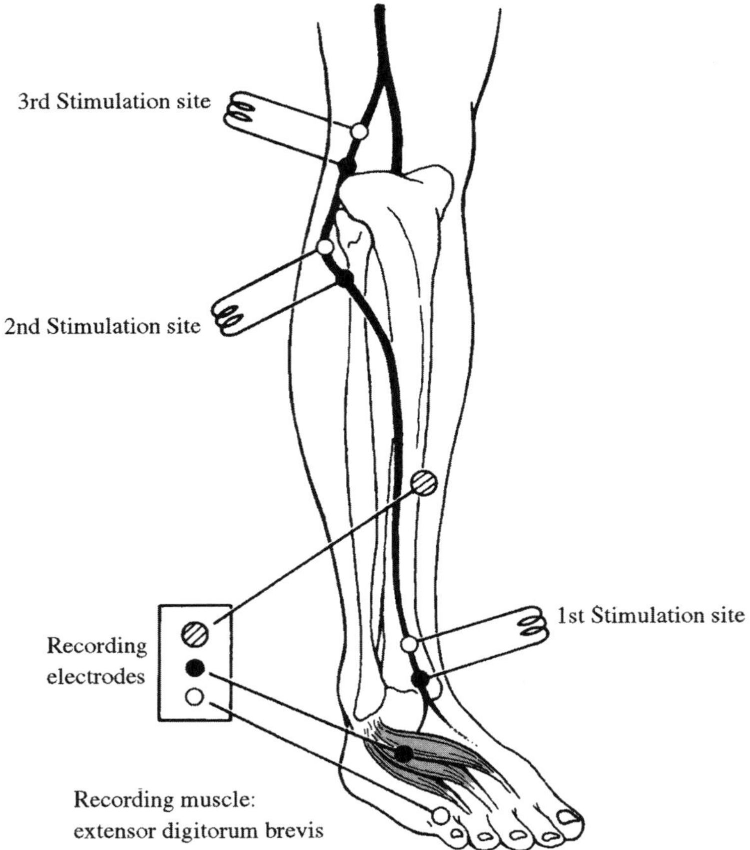

FIGURE 3.13. Motor nerve conduction study for the peroneal nerve. Position: patient lying on back; Active Recording Electrode: extensor digitorum brevis muscle (see above); Reference Recording Electrode: base of the little toe; Ground Electrode: anterior tibialis; Instrument Setting: motor nerve conduction; Response: upward movement of the great toe (toward the head). *1st Stimulation Site*: At the ankle, 8 cm proximal to the active recording electrode, at the midpoint between the medial and lateral malleoli at the top of the ankle; *2nd Stimulation Site*: At the knee, just below and anterior to the fibular head; *3rd Stimulation Site*: Just inside the lateral half of the popliteal space at the level of the midpatella.

4. Stimulate the proximal site again with the supramaximal stimulation and record the conduction time (ms) and amplitude (mV) of the CMAP (Fig. 3.15).
5. Measure the latency to the beginning of the initial deflection of the CMAPs and the amplitude (peak-to-peak or negative-peak amplitude) of the CMAPs from the distal and proximal sites. Note the duration and shape of the CMAPs at each site and compare them. *This is the only way to recognize abnormal temporal dispersion or dispersion phenomenon.*
6. Measure the distance in mm between the center of the active electrode and the center of the stimulation site.
7. Calculate the NCV following the formula:

$$NCV\ (m/s) = \frac{Distance\ between\ the\ proximal\ and\ distal\ site\ (mm)}{Conduction\ time\ to\ the\ proximal\ site\ -\ conduction\ time\ to\ the\ distal\ site\ (ms)}$$

8. Adjust the NCV to the standard temperature, if required, following the temperature correction formula (Table 3.1). Example:

The measured conduction velocity (Y_1) is 45.5 m/s when the skin temperature is 29 C. If the standard temperature is 31 C, then ΔT is 2. K in Table 3.1 is 1.087 at the 2 difference (ΔT). Then, the converted conduction velocity (Y_2) is calculated as follows:

$$Y_2 = 45.5\ (Y_2) \times 1.087 = 49.5\ m/s$$

9. Compare the measured NCV with the normal value. Also compare the amplitude, duration, and shape of the CMAPs with normal data.

Sensory Nerve Conduction

There are two methods of obtaining sensory CNAP: orthodromic and antidromic. In the author's laboratory, the orthodromic method is used for sensory nerve conduction studies of the median and ulnar nerves and the antidromic method is used for sural and radial nerve studies.

1. Place the recording electrodes on the correct sites following the anatomical guide (Figs. 3.16 to 3.18). With surface electrodes, the active and reference recording electrodes are placed along the nerve. With the near-nerve needle technique, the reference recording electrode is placed subcutaneously at the same level as the active electrode at a transverse distance of 3 to 4 cm.

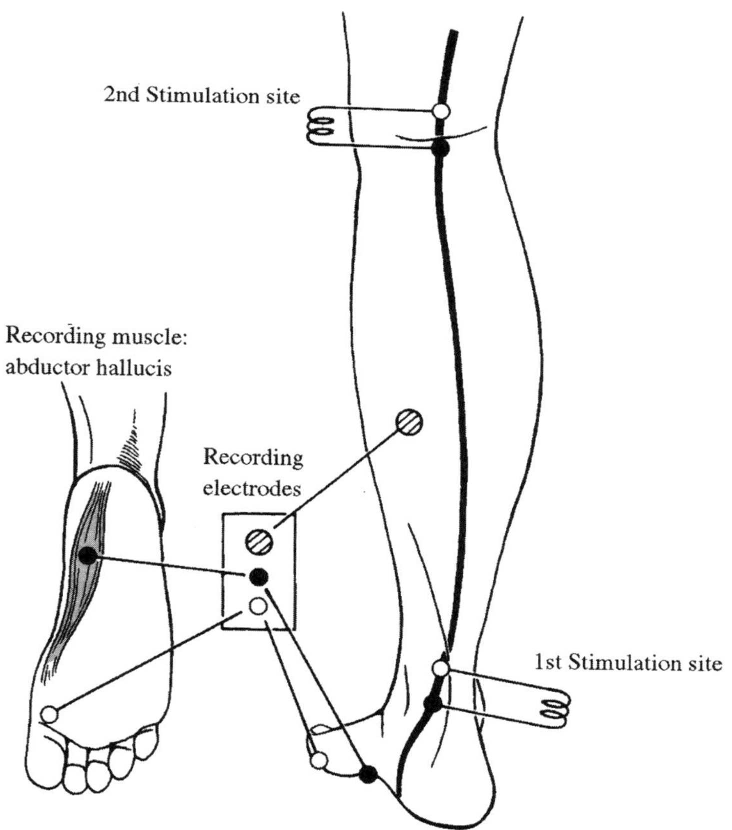

FIGURE 3.14. Motor nerve conduction study for the posterior tibial nerve. Position: patient lying on back; Active Recording Electrode: abductor hallucis muscle (see above); Reference Recording Electrode: base of the great toe; Ground Electrode: calf muscle; Instrument Setting: motor nerve conduction; Response: downward movement of the great toe (away from the head). *1st Stimulation Site*: At the ankle, just behind the medial malleolus, 10 cm proximal to the active recording electrode. *2nd Stimulation Site*: At the knee, just medial to the midpoint of the knee crease.

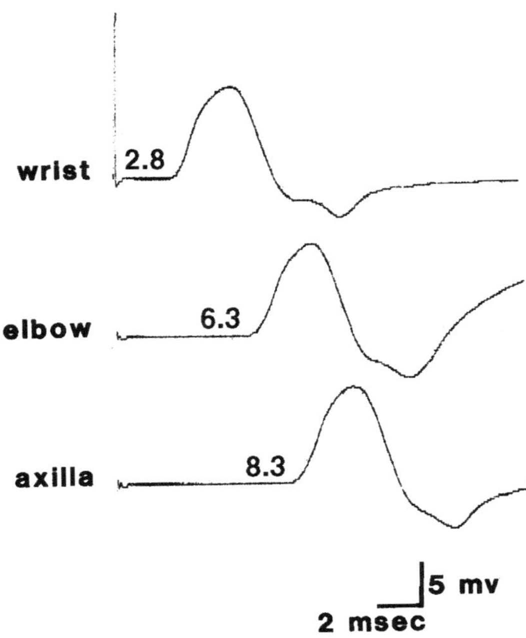

FIGURE 3.15. Example of the median motor nerve conduction study. The CMAP with wrist stimulation is 2.8 ms in latency, 17.5 mV in amplitude, and 11.5 ms in duration. The latency with elbow stimulation is 6.3 ms. The latency with axilla stimulation is 8.3 ms; the distance between the wrist and the elbow stimulation is 22 cm and between the elbow and axilla stimulation, 14 cm. Thus, terminal latency is 2.8 ms; the motor NCV over the forearm segment is 62.8 m/s (220 mm/(6.3 − 2.8)ms); the motor NCV over the elbow-axilla segment is 70 ms/s (140 mm/(8.3 − 6.3)ms). Skin temperature over the forearm is 32 C. No gross change in amplitude, shape, or duration of the CMAP is noted at the various stimulation sites.

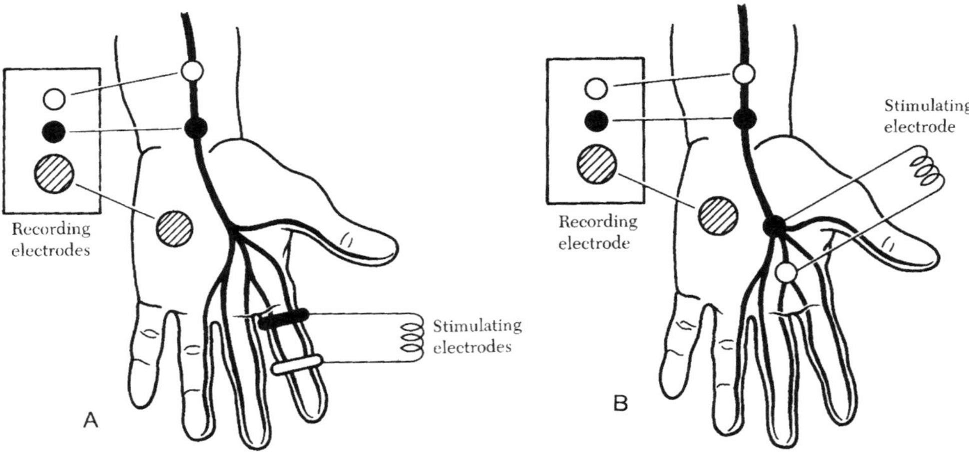

FIGURE 3.16. Sensory nerve conduction study for the median nerve. **A.** Finger-wrist segment. Position: palm up; Ground: palm; Instrument Setting: sensory nerve conduction; Response: no motor response; Recording Electrodes: at the wrist, between the two prominent middle tendons (site marked during motor nerve conduction study); Stimulating Electrodes: ring electrodes. **B.** Palm-wrist (carpal tunnel) segment. Active Stimulating Electrode: base of the index finger; Reference Electrode: about 3 cm distal to active electrode; Recording Electrodes: same as above; Stimulating Electrodes: 6 cm distal from the active recording electrode or at the midpoint between the base of the index finger and the active recording electrode, whichever is longer, along the line connecting the active recording electrode and the digit II to III interspace.

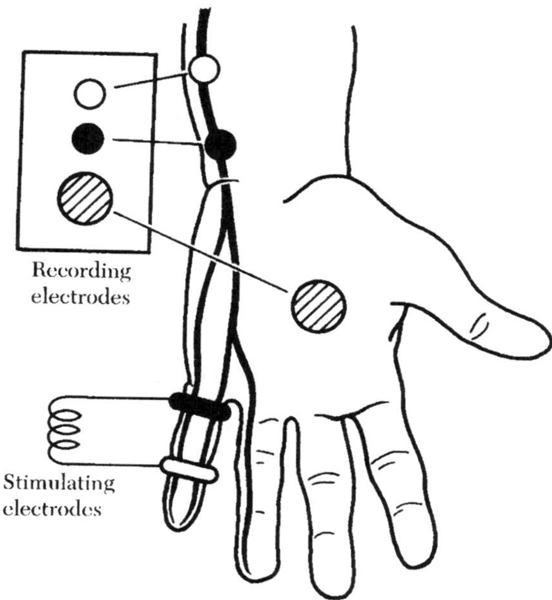

FIGURE 3.17. Sensory nerve conduction study for the ulnar nerve. Recording Electrodes: at the wrist, radial side of the prominent tendon on the ulnar side (already marked during the motor conduction study); Stimulating Electrodes: ring electrodes: Active Recording Electrode: at the base of the little finger; Reference Recording Electrode: about 3 cm distal to the active electrode; Position: palm up; Ground Electrode: palm; Instrument Setting: sensory nerve conduction; Response: no motor response.

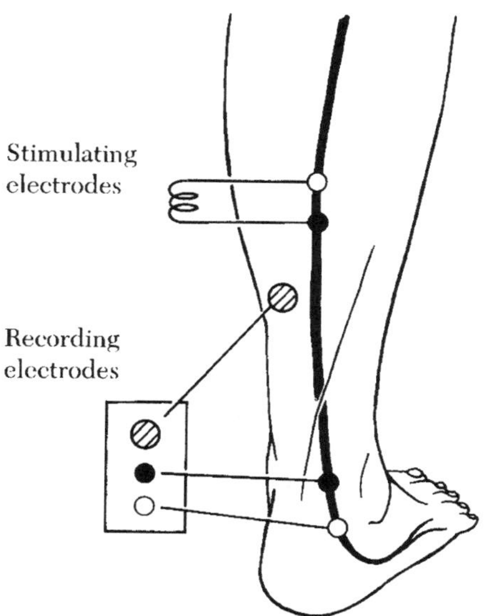

FIGURE 3.18. Sensory nerve conduction study for the sural nerve (antidromic sensory nerve conduction). Stimulating Electrodes: above 14 cm proximal to the recording electrode, just lateral to the midline of the width of the calf muscle; Recording Electrodes: just behind the lateral malleolus; Position: patient lying on side, knee resting on opposite knee, foot flexed back at a 45 angle; Ground Electrode: calf muscle; Instrument Setting: sensory nerve conduction; Response: pain radiating toward the little toe.

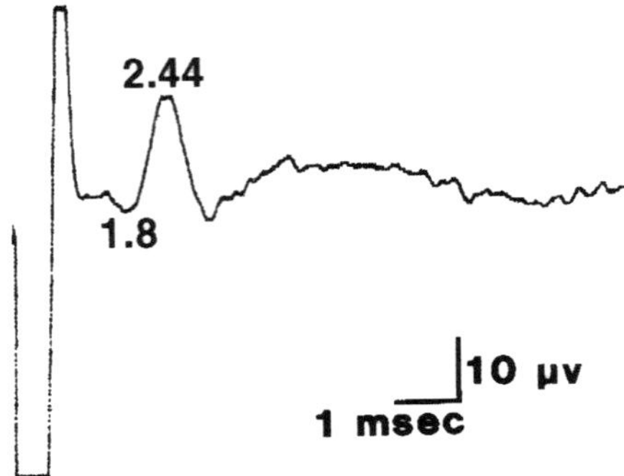

FIGURE 3.19. Example of the median sensory nerve conduction over the digit II-wrist segment. The positive peak (or onset) latency is 1.80 ms and the negative latency is 2.44 ms. The distance between the active stimulating and recording electrodes is 12.2 cm. The maximum sensory NCV is 67.7 m/s. The negative peak sensory NCV is 50.0 m/s. The amplitude and duration of the sensory CNAP are 21.5 μV and 1.05 ms, respectively. Skin temperature over the palm is 33 C.

2. Stimulate the distal sensory nerve fibers in the orthodromic sensory conduction test and the proximal sensory nerve fibers in the antidromic sensory conduction test using supramaximal stimulation. The active stimulating electrode (cathode) should be placed closer to the recording electrodes. Sometimes a large stimulus artifact may distort the CNAP because of baseline sway. This uninvited stimulus artifact can easily be eliminated by rotating the reference stimulating electrode around the active stimulating electrode.
3. Obtain and record the sensory CNAP (Fig. 3.19). When the CNAP is not easily obtainable with regular stimulation, then use the signal averager liberally. The CNAP is not obtainable when the sensory NCV is slower than 20 m/s with the surface electrode method. Thus, the absence of CNAP does not necessarily mean that the sensory NCV is zero.
3. Measure the latency from the onset of the stimulus to the initial positive peak or to the beginning of the major negative deflection. In the author's laboratory, we use the latency to the major negative peak.
4. Measure the peak-to-peak amplitude of the CNAP and observe the CNAP duration and shape. The dispersion phenomenon is indicative of segmental demyelination and may be the sole abnormality in some neuropathies.
5. The length of the nerve is measured by surface measurement from the center of the active stimulating electrode to the center of the active recording electrode. It is expressed in mm.
6. Calculate the NCV by dividing the conduction distance (mm) by the latency (ms):

$$NCV\ (m/s) = \frac{\textit{Distance between the active stimulating and recording electrodes (mm)}}{\textit{Latency over the same segment (ms)}}$$

7. Adjust the NCV to the standard temperature, if required. The same formula and table for the motor nerves are used to adjust the sensory NCV to the standard temperature.
8. Compare the measured NCV with the normal value. Also compare the amplitude, duration, and shape of the CNAPs with the normal data.

Mixed Nerve Conduction

Testing method and calculation of velocity are identical to those of the orthodromic method of sensory nerve conduction (Figs. 3.20 and 3.21). The clinical significance of the mixed nerve conduction is also identical to that of the sensory nerve conduction. The mixed nerve conduction study is usually performed over the wrist-elbow (Fig. 3.22) and elbow-axilla segments of the ulnar and median nerves and over the axilla-Erb's point segment of the ulnar nerve and, rarely, over the ankle-fibular head segment of the peroneal nerve.

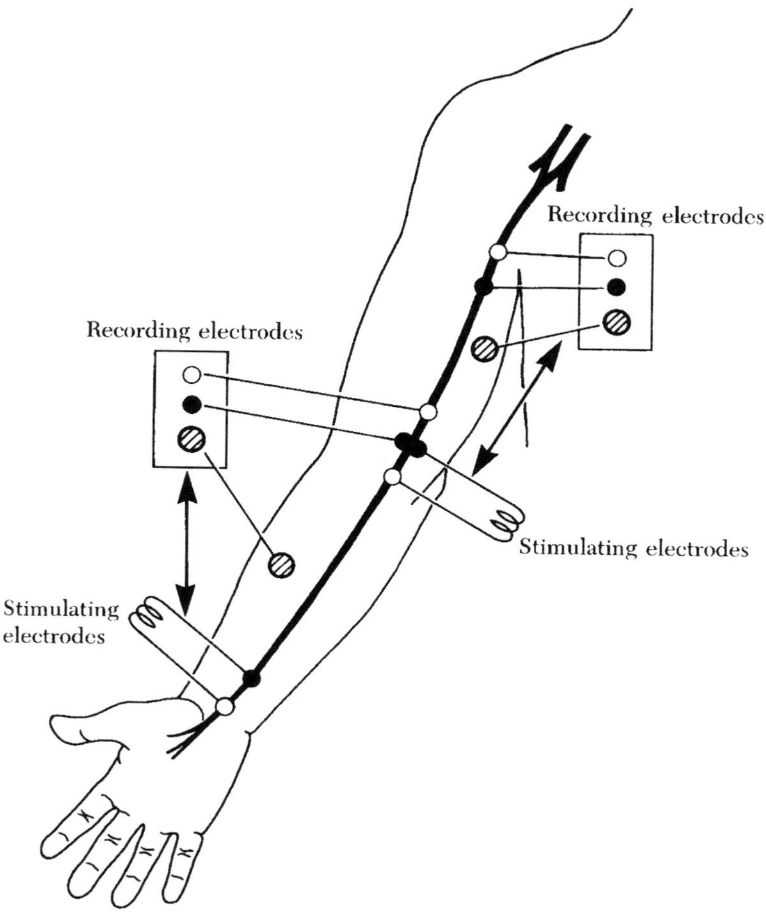

FIGURE 3.20. Mixed nerve conduction study for the median nerve. Position: arm extended, palm up; Ground Electrode: forearm; Instrument Setting: mixed nerve conduction; Response: brisk movement of the thumb, index, and middle fingers. (Sites for the recording and stimulating electrodes were marked at the wrist, elbow, and axilla during the motor conduction study.) Over the wrist-elbow segment—Recording Electrodes: just to the ulnar side of the pulsating brachial artery at the elbow; Stimulating Electrodes: between the two prominent middle tendons at the wrist. Over the elbow-axilla segment—Recording Electrodes: just forward of the pulsating brachial artery; Stimulating Electrodes: just to the ulnar side of the pulsating brachial artery at the elbow.

H-Reflex Study

The H-reflex study on the gastrocnemius-soleus muscle measures the latency over the monosynaptic reflex arc through the afferent Ia fibers and efferent alpha motor fibers of the S1 root (Fig. 3.3). The H-reflex is normally present at birth in the intrinsic hand and foot muscles but is present consistently only in the gastrocnemius-soleus muscle after 12 months of age. In other muscles, the facilitation technique is needed to obtain the H-reflex with some reliability. The H-reflex on the gastrocnemius-soleus muscle is best obtained when the patient is placed prone with the feet suspended over the edge of the table or with a pillow placed under the ankles. It is easily obtained with the motor conduction setup by changing the sweep velocity to 10 ms and the sensitivity to 500 μV.

1. Place the recording electrodes on the gastrocnemius muscle, as shown in the anatomical guide (Fig. 3.23).

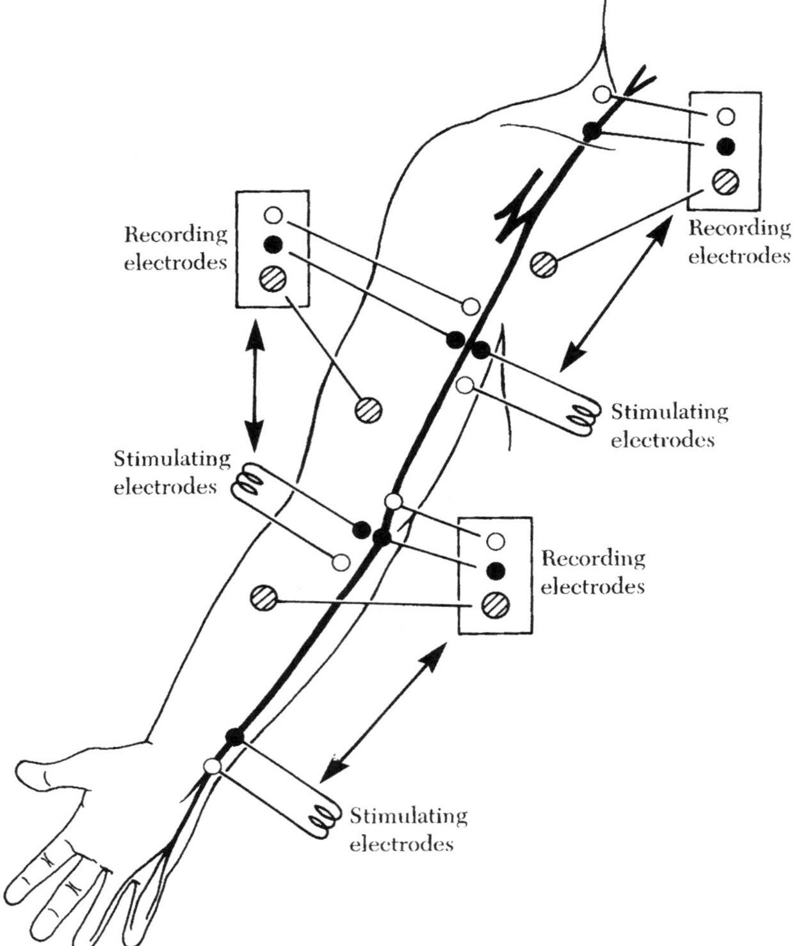

FIGURE 3.21. Mixed nerve conduction study for the ulnar nerve. Position: arm extended, palm up; Ground Electrode: forearm; Instrument Setting: mixed nerve conduction; Response: brisk movement of the little finger. (Sites for the recording and stimulating electrodes were marked at Erb's point, axilla, and wrist during the motor nerve conduction study.) Over the axilla-Erb's point segment (thoracic outlet segment)—Recording electrodes: lateral to the posterior border of sternocleidomastoid and the superior margin of the clavicle; Stimulating Electrodes: just behind the pulsating brachial artery. Over the elbow-axilla segment—Recording Electrodes: at the axilla, posterior to the pulsating brachial artery; Stimulating Electrodes: at the groove of the elbow. Over the wrist-elbow segment—Recording Electrodes: at the ulnar sulcus between two bony prominences; Stimulating Electrodes: just radial to the prominent tendon on the ulnar side of the wrist.

2. Stimulate the posterior tibial nerve at the popliteal fossa following the anatomical guide. The stimulus duration should be 0.5 or 1.0 ms, which makes it more selective for the afferent Ia fibers. Longer durations would favor the activation of motor axons. An active stimulating electrode should be placed closer to the spine (away from the recording electrodes). This location is marked when the motor conduction is performed.
3. Stimulate manually at the rate of once every 2 seconds (or longer) to avoid the blocking response. Increase the intensity gradually and observe the H-reflex and M-wave (CMAP from the gastrocnemius). The H-reflex is classically obtainable with an intensity that is

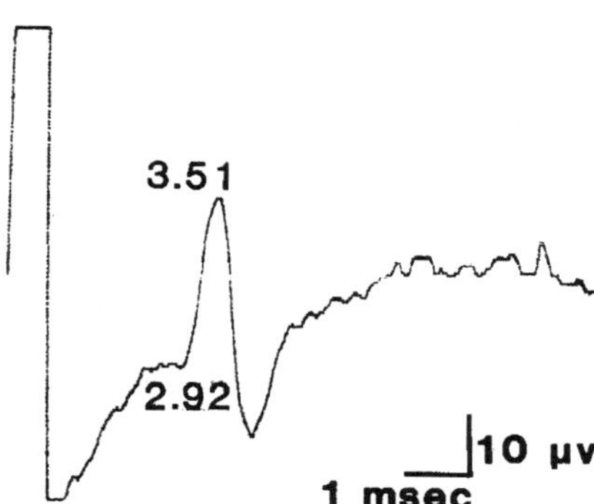

FIGURE 3.22. Example of the median mixed nerve conduction over the wrist-elbow segment. The onset latency is 2.92 ms and the negative peak latency 3.51 ms. The distance between the active stimulating and recording electrodes is 20.3 cm. The maximum mixed NCV is 69.5 m/s and the negative peak NCV 57.8 m/s. The amplitude and duration of the mixed CNAP are 40.8 μV and 1.71 ms, respectively.

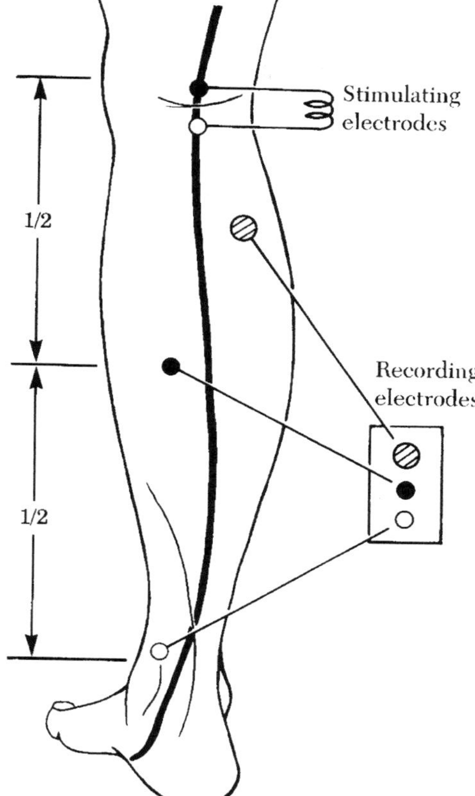

FIGURE 3.23. H-reflex study in the gastrocnemius-soleus muscle. Position: patient lying on belly (a towel or pillow under the ankle is helpful); Ground Electrode: calf muscle; Instrument Setting: H-reflex; Response: downward movement of the great toe (away from the head); Stimulating Electrode: just medial to the midpoint of the knee crease in the popliteal fossa (note that the active stimulating electrode is proximally located); Recording Electrode: halfway between the popliteal crease and the proximal medial malleolus over the medial gastrocnemius.

usually too low to produce the M-wave (Fig. 3.24). Thus, maximal amplitude of the H-reflex is often obtained with low intensity. With a gradual increase of intensity, the M-response increases in amplitude, while the H-reflex amplitude decreases. With supramaximal stimulation, the H-reflex is no longer obtainable and is sometimes replaced by an F-wave.

Differentiation between the H-reflex and F-wave is not always easy. The following guidelines are helpful in recognizing the H-reflex (Fig. 3.24). A late response is always the H-reflex when it meets one of the following criteria:

a. It is elicited by a subthreshold stimulus;
b. Its amplitude is higher than that of the M-wave at a given stimulus;
c. Its amplitude is more than 50% higher than the maximum M-wave amplitude.

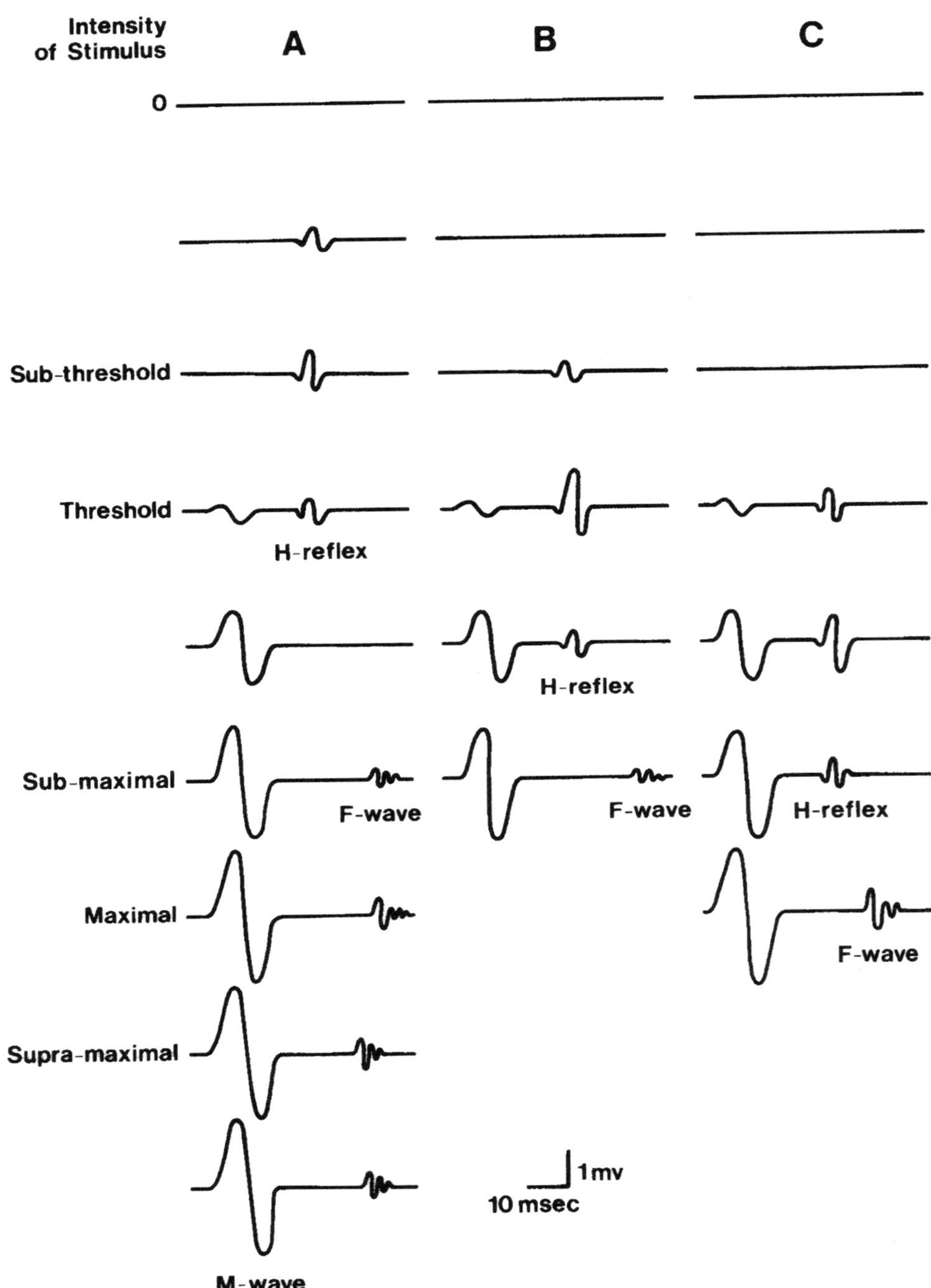

FIGURE 3.24. Differentiation between the H-reflex and F-wave. **A.** Any subthreshold late response is the H-reflex. The highest amplitude is noted with the subthreshold stimulus. **B.** Any subthreshold late response that becomes higher than the M-wave is the H-reflex. **C.** Any late response that is higher than M-wave in amplitude at a given stimulus is the H-reflex. Any supramaximal late response is the F-wave.

Conversely, a late response is always the F-wave when it is elicited with the supramaximal stimulus (Fig. 3.24). When the criteria are not met, the H-reflex should be differentiated from the F-wave by the classic change of amplitude of the H-wave in relation to the M-wave with a change in stimulus intensity and by the shape and latency of the late responses (Table 3.2). The H-wave is classically triphasic with an initial positive deflection and a large negative deflection in the gastrocnemius-soleus muscle. The H-reflex latency is shorter than the F-wave latency. The latency classically varies with each F-wave, whereas the latency of the H-reflex is relatively constant. The H-reflex recording is helped by the trace contraction of plantar flexors and by the Jendrassik maneuver, in which the patient hooks his or her hands together with flexed fingers and attempts to pull the hands apart as forcefully as possible.

4. Measure the latency from the start of stimulation to the onset of the initial deflection of the H-reflex (Fig. 3.25). The latency of the H-reflex is usually in the range of 25 to 35 ms in normal individuals.
5. Measure the body height (Table 3.3) or the length of the lower leg, both in centimeters, between the stimulating site and the medial malleolus. Because the H-reflex latency depends on the pathway traveled, the body height must be considered in judging the latency to be normal or abnormal. In those laboratories where the length of the lower leg is used to adjust the H-reflex latency, this length must be measured.
6. Compare the patient's H-reflex latency with the normal values (Fig. 3.26). The easiest comparison to make in the study of unilateral lumbosacral radiculopathy is to compare the involved and uninvolved sides. A difference of 1.5 ms between the H-reflex latencies in the right and left legs of the same patient has been considered objective evidence of S1 radiculopathy. Careful attention to technique and accurate measurement of leg length are prerequisites for this comparison to be meaningful.

TABLE 3.2. Differentiation Between H-reflex and F-response

Measurement	H-Reflex	F-Wave
Nature of response	Monosynaptic reflex; e.g., H-reflex on the gastrocnemius-soleus muscle is an electrophysiological counterpart of ankle reflex	Not a reflex; antidromic motor neuron discharge
Pathways		
Afferent arc	Ia sensory fibers	Alpha motor fibers
Efferent arc	Alpha motor fibers	Alpha motor fibers
Best stimulus to evoke the response relative to the M-response	Subthreshold; absent with the supramaximal stimulation	Supramaximal; absent with the subthreshold stimulation
Appearance and persistence of the response	Rather constant at low rates of stimulation (½–30 s)	Variable
Latency	Rather constant Latency shorter than the F-response latency	Variable
Highest amplitude	Can be up to 81% of the maximum M-wave; much bigger than the F-wave	Usually small, less than 5% of the maximum M-wave
The muscles to be tested without any facilitation[a]	Gastrocnemius-soleus muscle in adult; intrinsic hand and foot muscles in infants up to 1 yr	Almost every distal muscle

[a] In other muscles, H-reflex can be obtained with facilitation.

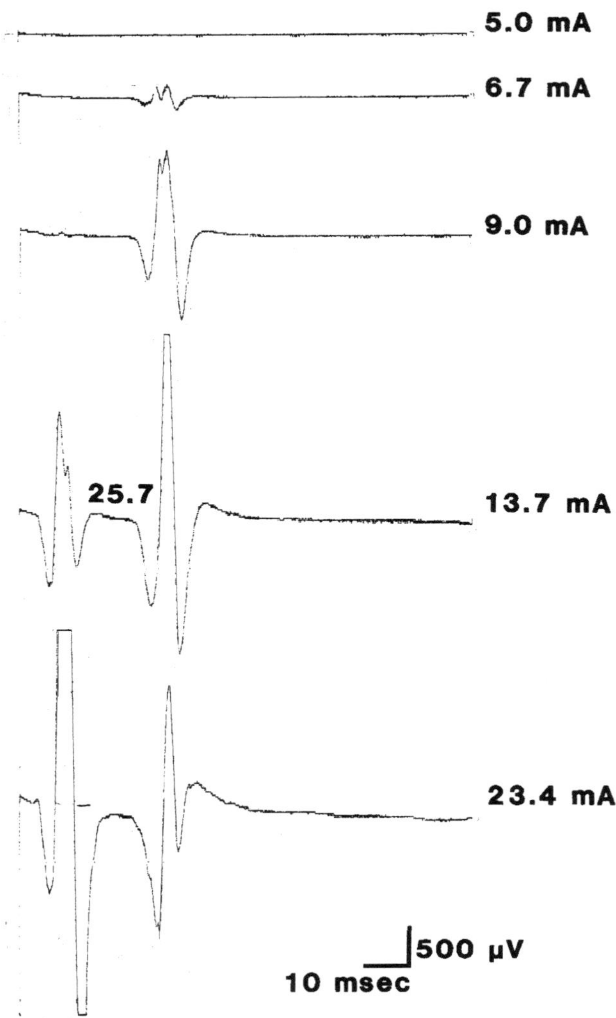

FIGURE 3.25. Example of the H-reflex from the medial gastrocnemius muscle. The numbers at the right show the stimulus intensities. The stimulus duration used for this test is 0.5 ms. The H-reflex shows the classic triphasic shape with 25.7-ms latency. The H-reflex amplitude is higher than the M-wave at 13.7-mA stimulus intensity. The 25.7-ms H-reflex latency is normal for a 45-year-old man with 167 cm height.

F-Wave Study

The F-wave study measures the latency over the afferent and efferent arcs of the motor fibers from the stimulating site and anterior horn cells (Fig. 3.3, Table 3.2). This response is evoked by supramaximal stimulation during the motor nerve conduction study. The F-wave is easily obtained by stimulating the distal portion of the median, ulnar, peroneal, and posterior tibial nerves using the motor nerve conduction setups and changing the sweep velocity to 10 ms and the sensitivity to 200 μV. If the F-wave is difficult to elicit, slight voluntary muscle contraction often enhances the response. The F-wave is easily obtained from the distal muscles after distal stimulation but is difficult to obtain after proximal stimulation because the latter yields an F-wave with a shorter latency, and the response is hidden in the CMAP (M-wave).

TABLE 3.3 Height Conversion Table[a]

Feet	Inches	Inches	Centimeter	Feet	Inches	Inches	Centimeter
3	0	36	91.4	5	0	60	152.4
3	1	37	94.0	5	1	61	154.9
3	2	38	96.5	5	2	62	157.5
3	3	39	99.1	5	3	63	160.0
3	4	40	101.6	5	4	64	162.6
3	5	41	104.1	5	5	65	165.1
3	6	42	106.7	5	6	66	167.6
3	7	43	109.2	5	7	67	170.2
3	8	44	111.8	5	8	68	172.7
3	9	45	114.3	5	9	69	175.3
3	10	46	116.8	5	10	70	177.8
3	11	47	119.4	5	11	71	180.3
4	0	48	121.9	6	0	72	182.9
4	1	49	124.5	6	1	73	185.4
4	2	50	127.0	6	2	74	188.0
4	3	51	129.5	6	3	75	190.5
4	4	52	132.1	6	4	76	193.0
4	5	53	134.6	6	5	77	194.6
4	6	54	137.2	6	6	78	198.1
4	7	55	139.7	6	7	79	200.7
4	8	56	142.2	6	8	80	203.2
4	9	57	144.8	6	9	81	205.7
4	10	58	147.3	6	10	82	208.3
4	11	59	149.9	6	11	83	210.8

[a] Conversion formula: 1 foot = 12 inches = 30.48 cm; 1 inch = 2.54 cm.

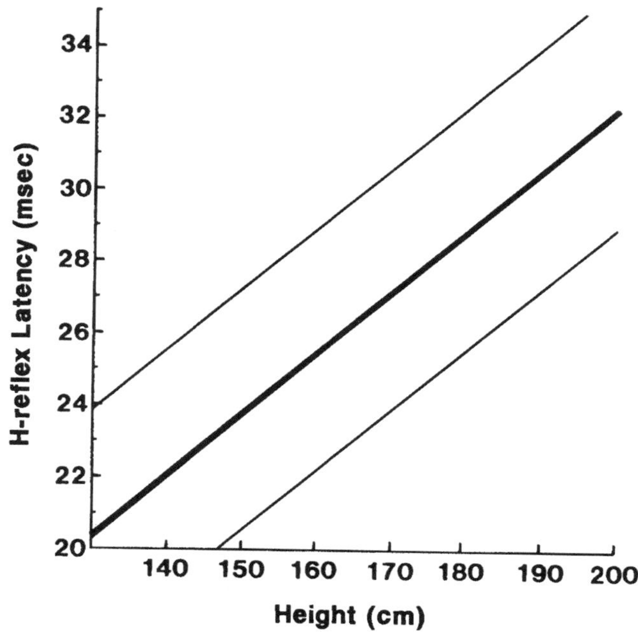

FIGURE 3.26. H-reflex from the gastrocnemius-soleus muscle.

1. Place the recording electrodes on the distal muscle that is innervated by the nerve being tested, using the belly-tendon method.
2. Stimulate the nerve in the distal portion, that is, the wrist for ulnar and median nerves and the ankle for peroneal and posterior tibial nerves. An active stimulating electrode (the cathode on most EMG machines) should be placed closer to the spine (away from the recording electrodes) (Fig. 3.27).
3. Stimulate manually at the rate of once every 2 seconds (or more) to avoid a blocking response. Stimulate the nerve with supramaximal intensity and observe the M-wave and the late F-wave.
4. Obtain F-waves at least 10 times and measure the latency from the start of the stimulus to the onset of the initial deflection of the F-wave with the shortest latency. The latency of the F-wave after distal stimulation is usually in the range of 23 to 33 ms for median and ulnar nerves and 50 to 60 ms for peroneal and posterior tibial nerves in normal individuals (Fig. 3.28).
5. Measure the body height in centimeters (Table 3.3). Because the F-wave is dependent on the traveling pathway of afferent and efferent motor fibers, body height is a major factor in judging the latency normal or abnormal. In some laboratories, the length of a leg or arm is used to obtain the F-wave NCVs, in which case the patient's arm or leg length must be measured.

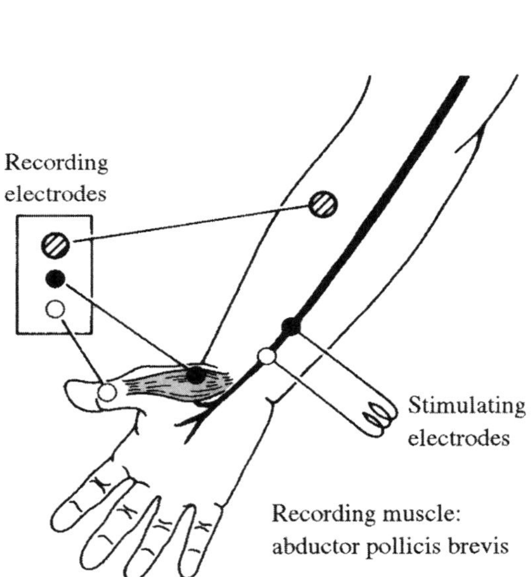

FIGURE 3.27. F-wave study for the median nerve. Position: arm extended, palm up; Active Electrode: midportion of the hyperthenar muscle (abductor pollicis brevis): Reference Electrode: thumb; Ground Electrode: flexor surface of the forearm; Instrument Setting: F-wave study; Response: brisk movement of the thumb; Stimulation Site: at the wrist; Active Stimulating Electrode: 5 cm proximal to the active recording electrode between the two prominent tendons or on midline following the crease between the hyper- and hypothenar muscles (note that the active stimulating electrode is proximally located); Reference Stimulating Electrodes: placed distally.

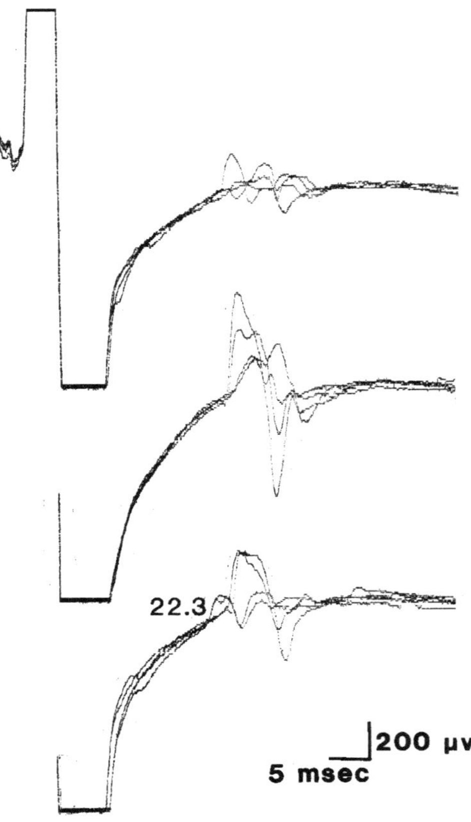

FIGURE 3.28. Example of the F-wave from the abductor pollicis brevis with wrist stimulation. The shortest latency among 12 F-waves is 22.3 ms, normal for a 45-year-old man with 167 cm height.

6. Compare the patient's F-wave latency with normal values (Fig. 3.29). The easiest comparison to make is the F-wave latencies between the right and left sides. If greater than 2 ms, the difference is considered significant. The F-wave latency is prolonged in patients with proximal peripheral neuropathy.

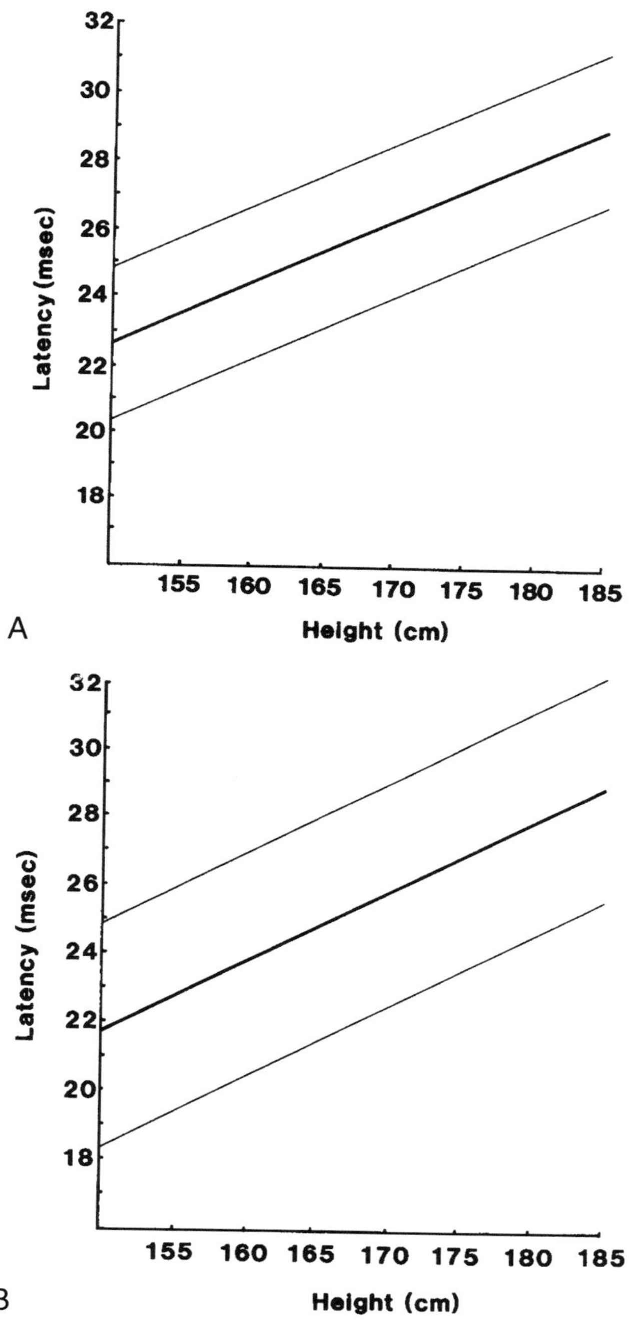

FIGURE 3.29. A. F-wave latencies in median nerves with distal stimulation. The thick line is the regression line; the thin lines indicate the normal limits (2 SD from the regression line). **B.** F-wave latencies in ulnar nerves with distal stimulation.

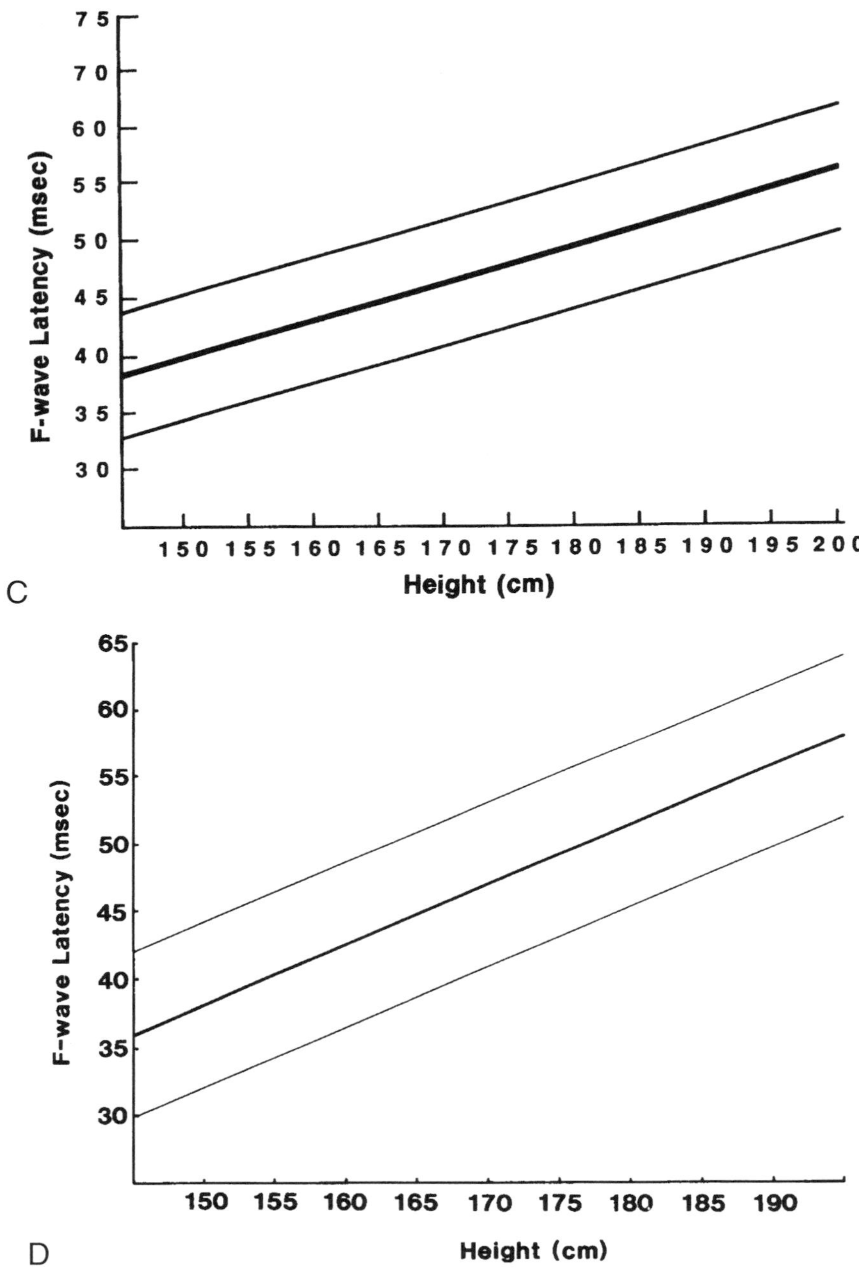

FIGURE 3.29. *(continued)* **C.** F-wave latencies in peroneal nerves with distal stimulation. **D.** F-wave latencies in posterior tibial nerves with distal stimulation.

ELECTROPHYSIOLOGICAL RESPONSES IN DISEASED NERVES

Electrophysiological responses in diseased nerves are limited to conduction slowing, conduction block, and reduced or absent excitability of the nerves. Nerve conduction slowing is the most important parameter in the nerve conduction study and is seen as prolonged latency or conduction time. This slowing may be attributed to segmental demyelination, loss of large-diameter fibers, and metabolic abnormalities. With segmental demyelination, nerve conduction slowing occurs because of the loss of saltatory conduction in the demyelinated fibers. Slowing of the NCV parallels the degree of demyelination. Because the NCV is proportional to the outer fiber diameter of myelinated fibers, the loss of large-diameter fibers slows the nerve conduction, usually not more than 20% below the normal mean. This is the pathological basis of the minimal slowing seen in axonal neuropathy.

Conduction block occurs with severe segmental demyelination. With mild segmental demyelination, slowing of conduction is a typical response. In more serious demyelination, many demyelinated fibers fail to conduct the nerve impulse, producing a conduction block. Conduction block is manifested by the reduction of amplitude of the CMAP and CNAP and is best recognized as a dramatic reduction of amplitude across the site of the block.

Reduced or absent excitability of the nerve is observed when conduction block or axonal degeneration becomes severe. This is measured by the need for an increase in duration and intensity of the stimulus to generate the muscle or nerve action potential. If the conduction block or axonal degeneration is complete, the nerve eventually becomes inexcitable. This is best observed in Wallerian degeneration, in which the nerve distal to the lesion becomes totally inexcitable 5 days after total separation.

NORMAL VALUES OF THE NERVE CONDUCTION

Normal values for the nerve conduction of the various nerves differ depending on the testing technique. If the patient's values are to be compared with normal values published in the literature, the tester must carefully follow the instructions for the measurement and techniques of the nerve conduction. For the most commonly tested nerves, the techniques are shown in the various figures in this chapter, and normal values are listed in Table 3.4. For less frequently examined nerves, *Oh's Clinical Electromyography Nerve Conduction Studies* (Williams & Wilkins 1993) is a valuable reference for the techniques of measurement and testing. When the values obtained vary by more than 2 SD from the mean values, they are considered abnormal with regard to the latency, NCV, and duration of the CMAP and CNAP. For the amplitude of the CMAP and CNAP, values below the lowest normal values are considered to be abnormal. For the benefit of readers, the values for demyelination are also given in Table 3.4. For the F-wave latency and H-reflex from the gastrocnemius-soleus muscle, the height-adjusted normal values are given in Figures 3.26 and 3.29.

INTERPRETATION OF NERVE CONDUCTION DATA

Electrophysiological Characteristics in Axonal Degeneration and Segmental Demyelination

There are two major components in peripheral nerves—axon and myelin—and it is logical to classify a peripheral neuropathy according to the predominant pathological involvement: axonal degeneration and segmental demyelination (Fig. 3.30). The pathophysiological differences between axonal degeneration and segmental demyelination are given in Table 3.5. Axonal degeneration or segmental demyelination can be recognized by the classic nerve conduction abnormalities (Table 3.6). In some diseased nerves, both processes may be present together.

Axonal Degeneration. The hallmark of nerve conduction abnormalities is the diminution of the amplitude of the CMAP in the motor nerve conduction and of the CNAP in the sensory and mixed nerve conduction in the presence of normal or near-normal maximal NCVs and of normal shape and duration of the CMAP or CNAP.

In the motor conduction, the following findings are typical of axonal degeneration:

1. Unequivocal reduction of the amplitude of the CMAP in proportion to severity of the axonal degeneration (Fig. 3.31);
2. Normal shape and duration of the CMAP;
3. Minimal prolongation of the terminal latency by not more than 50% of the normal mean (Fig. 3.32);
4. Normal or near-normal NCV (Fig. 3.33).

TABLE 3.4 Normal Nerve Conduction Data[a]: Electromyography Laboratory, The University of Alabama at Birmingham, May 1983

Anatomical Site	Terminal Latency (ms) and NCV (m/s)[b] Mean ± SD	Normal Limit	Amplitude, Normal Limit	Demyelination Criteria
Upper extremities				
Median nerve				
Sensory conduction				
Palm-wrist	41.85 ± 3.90	34.05	10 μV	25.1
Finger-wrist	49.54 ± 4.14	41.26	10 μV	29.7
Mixed conduction				
Wrist-elbow	55.99 ± 3.30	49.39	10 μV	33.6
Elbow-axilla	63.47 ± 4.76	53.95	10 μV	38.1
Motor conduction				
Terminal latency	2.78 ± 0.41	3.60	5 mV	4.2
Wrist-elbow	58.78 ± 4.41	49.96		35.3
Elbow-axilla	65.76 ± 4.90	55.96		39.5
F-wave latency	25.32 ± 2.19	29.70		38.0
Ulnar nerve				
Sensory conduction				
Finger-wrist	47.48 ± 4.11	39.26	8 μV	28.5
Mixed conduction				
Wrist-elbow	55.44 ± 3.99	47.46	10 μV	33.3
Elbow-axilla	57.14 ± 4.48	48.18	10 μV	34.3
Erb's point-axilla	64.09 ± 5.64	52.81	10 μV	38.5
Motor conduction				
Terminal latency	2.03 ± 0.24	2.51	5 mV	3.1
Wrist-elbow	61.15 ± 5.27	50.61		36.7
Across elbow	51.31 ± 4.25	42.81		30.8
Elbow-axilla	63.33 ± 5.47	52.69		38.0
Erb's point-axilla	68.36 ± 5.07	58.22		38.4
F-wave latency	25.68 ± 2.29	30.26		38.5
Radial nerve				
Sensory conduction (distal)	50.87 ± 3.28	44.31	10 μV	30.5
Lower extremities				
Peroneal nerve (motor)				
Terminal latency	3.72 ± 0.53	4.78	4 mV	5.6
Knee-ankle	49.51 ± 3.93	41.85		29.7
Knee-popliteal fossa	53.93 ± 7.11	39.11		32.4
F-wave latency	46.88 ± 4.25	55.38		70.3
Posterior tibial nerve (motor)				
Terminal latency	3.85 ± 0.63	5.11	5 mV	5.8
Knee-ankle	49.83 ± 4.60	40.63		29.9
F-wave latency	48.89 ± 4.19	57.27		73.3
H-reflex on the calf muscle	28.02 ± 1.95	31.93		42.0
Sural nerve (sensory)				
Mid-calf-lateral malleolus	43.26 ± 4.29	34.68	6 μV	26.0

[a] Skin temperature, above 31 C. Age range 20–60. Number of controls, 40.

[b] Terminal latency, F-wave latency, and H-reflex are expressed as ms. All other values represent NCV (m/s).

TABLE 3.5. Pathophysiology of Two Types of Peripheral Neuropathy

Type	Axonal Neuropathy	Demyelinating Neuropathy
Primary lesion	Axon	Myelin
Pathological process	Axonal degeneration	Demyelination
Pathology by teasing preparation	Myelin ovoids	Segmental demyelination
Regeneration		
Mechanism	Axonal sprouting	Remyelination
Speed	Slow	Rapid
Nerve conduction		
NCV	Mildly slow; above 30 m/s	Markedly slow; below 30 m/s
CMAP	Low amplitude	Dispersion; conduction block
Needle EMG		
Fibrillation & positive sharp wave	(+ + + +)	(−) or (±)
Fasciculation	Absent	Present in chronic form
Neuropathies[a]	Arsenic	Guillain-Barré syndrome
	Alcoholic	CIDP
	Nutritional	Hypertrophic
	Vasculitic	Metachromatic
	Giant axonal	Tomaculous
	Thallium	Leprosy
	Vitamin B_{12}	Hypothyroid
	Gold	Diphtheric

[a] Diabetic and uremic neuropathies are most likely due to the combined processes of axonal degeneration and demyelination. Recent studies suggest that axonal degeneration may be the predominant feature in diabetic neuropathy.

NCV, nerve conduction velocity; CMAP, compound muscle action potential; CIDP, chronic inflammatory demyelinating polyneuropathy.

TABLE 3.6. Electrophysiological Characteristics in Axonal Degeneration and Segmental Demyelination

Parameters	Axonal Degeneration	Segmental Demyelination
Motor nerve conduction (with surface electrodes)		
Amplitude	↓↓	N or ↓; conduction block
Duration	N	Dispersion phenomenon
Shape	N	N or multiphasic
Terminal latency	N or ↑ (<150%)	↑↑ (>150%)[a]
Conduction velocity	N or ↓ (>60%)	↓↓ (<60%)
Sensory nerve conduction		
With surface electrodes		
Amplitude	↓↓ or often absent	N, ↓, or absent
Duration	N	Rarely dispersion phenomenon
Shape	N	Rarely multiphasic
Conduction velocity	N or (>60%)	(<60%)
With near-nerve needle technique		
Amplitude	↓↓	N or ↓; conduction block
Duration	N	Prominent dispersion phenomenon
Shape	N	Multiphasic with many components
Conduction velocity	N or ↓ (>60%)	↓↓ (<60%)
F-wave	↑ <150% or absent	↑ >150% or absent
H-reflex	↑ <150% or absent	↑ >150% or absent

[a] Percentage of normal means.

↑, Increased; ↓, decreased; N, normal.

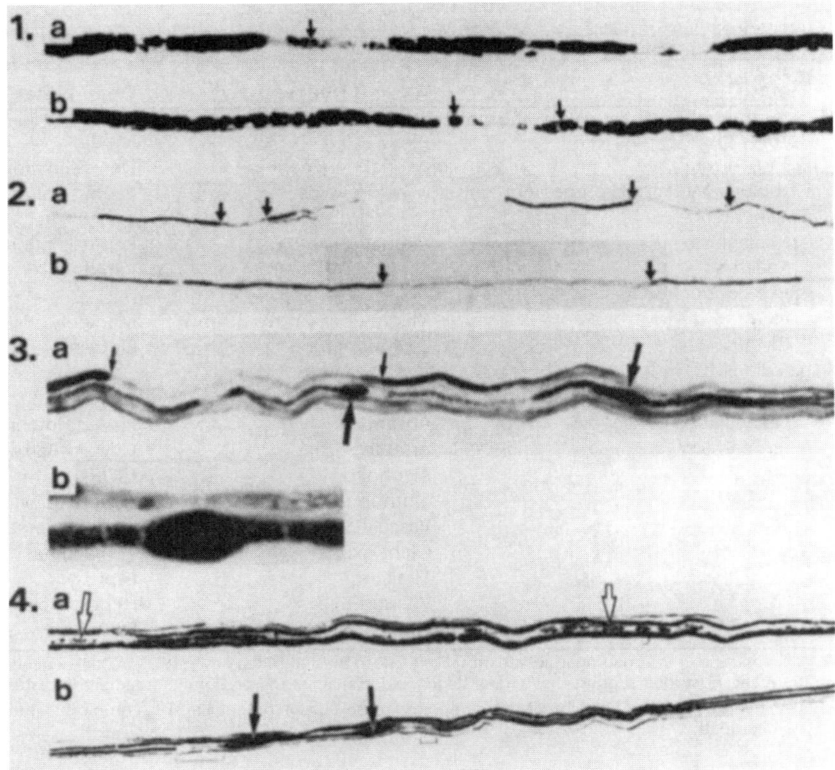

FIGURE 3.30. Teased nerve fibers. **1.** Axonal degeneration: arrows indicate row of myelin ovoids. **2.** Demyelination: arrows indicate demyelinated segments. **3.** Tomaculous change. **a.** Thin arrows indicate a demyelinated segment. Thick arrows indicate "tomaculous change." **b.** Enlarged tomaculous change. **4.** Giant axons. **a.** White arrows indicate rows of myelin ovoids. **b.** Arrows indicate giant axons. (Reproduced with permission from Oh SJ. Diagnostic usefulness and limitations of the sural nerve biopsy. Yonsei Med J 1990;31:16.)

NCV is normal or there is mild slowing in NCV, but not more than 40% below the normal mean. This slowing is due to marked loss of the large-diameter fibers because of axonal degeneration. The motor NCV in the median nerve is usually above 40 m/s and in the peroneal nerve above 35 m/s.

In the sensory conduction, the following findings are typical of axonal degeneration:

1. Unequivocal reduction of the amplitude of the CNAP (Fig. 3.31). With surface electrodes and without the use of signal averaging, the amplitude is so small that the CNAP is unrecordable. With the near-nerve needle electrode, the amplitude is significantly low in proportion to the severity of axonal degeneration.
2. Normal shape and duration of the CNAP.
3. Normal or near-normal NCV. Slowing of the NCV is less than 40% below the normal mean. The sensory NCV in the median nerve is usually above 35 m/s and in the peroneal nerve above 30 m/s using the negative peak latency method.
4. In cases of severe axonal degeneration, the nerve is inexcitable to obtain any CNAP, even with the near-nerve needle technique.

Segmental Demyelination. The hallmarks of nerve conduction abnormalities in segmental demyelination are:

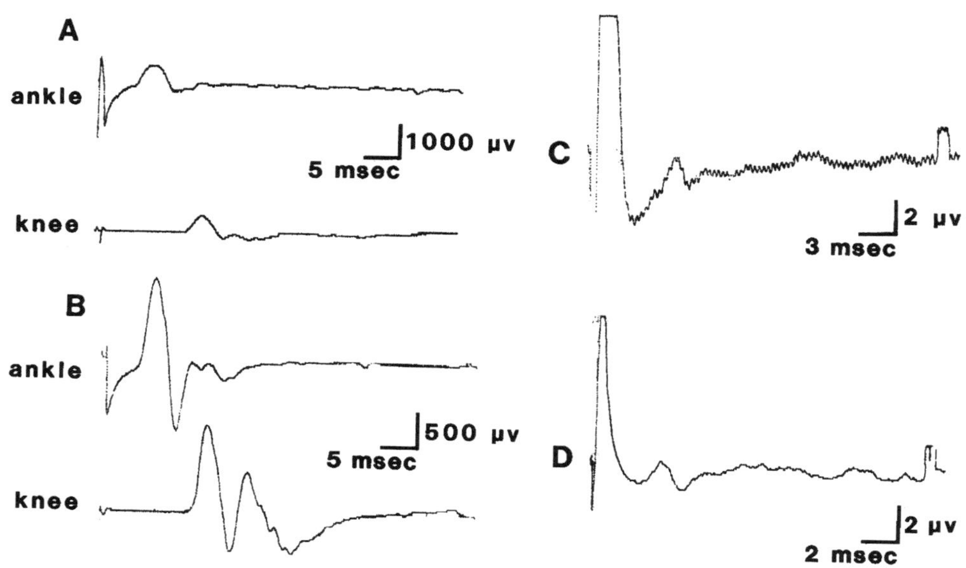

FIGURE 3.31. Motor and sensory nerve conduction in axonal degeneration (arsenic neuropathy). **A.** The amplitude of the CMAP in the peroneal nerve is markedly reduced. Terminal latency and motor NCV are minimally abnormal. **B.** Improved CMAP in the peroneal nerve 2 years later. **C.** Markedly reduced amplitude and mild slowing of the sensory NCV (34.3 m/s) over the finger-wrist segment of the median nerve. **D.** Reduced amplitude and mild slowing in the sensory NCV (33.3 m/s) over the finger-wrist segment of the ulnar nerve.

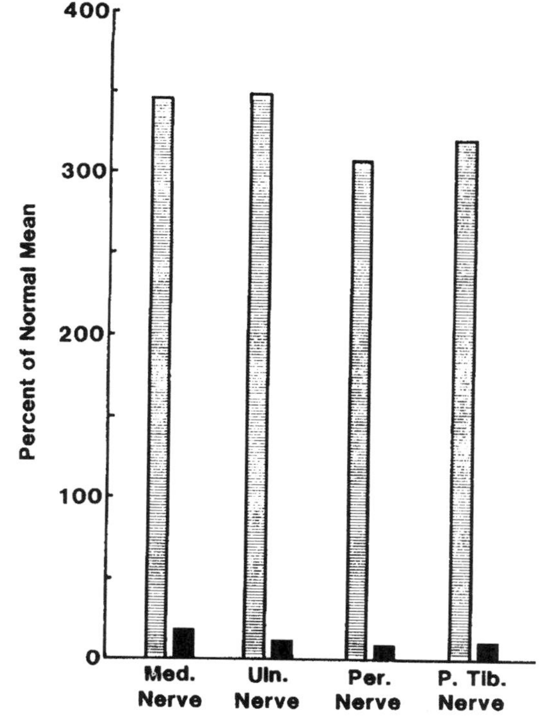

FIGURE 3.32. Comparison of the terminal latency of axonal degeneration (arsenic neuropathy) and segmental demyelination (chronic inflammatory demyelinating polyneuropathy [CIDP]). ▤, Mean terminal latencies from 18 cases of CIDP; ■, from 8 cases of arsenic neuropathy. The normal mean is at 0%. Markedly prolonged terminal latencies are noted in the presence of segmental demyelination, whereas with axonal degeneration terminal latencies are still within normal limits (30% of the mean).

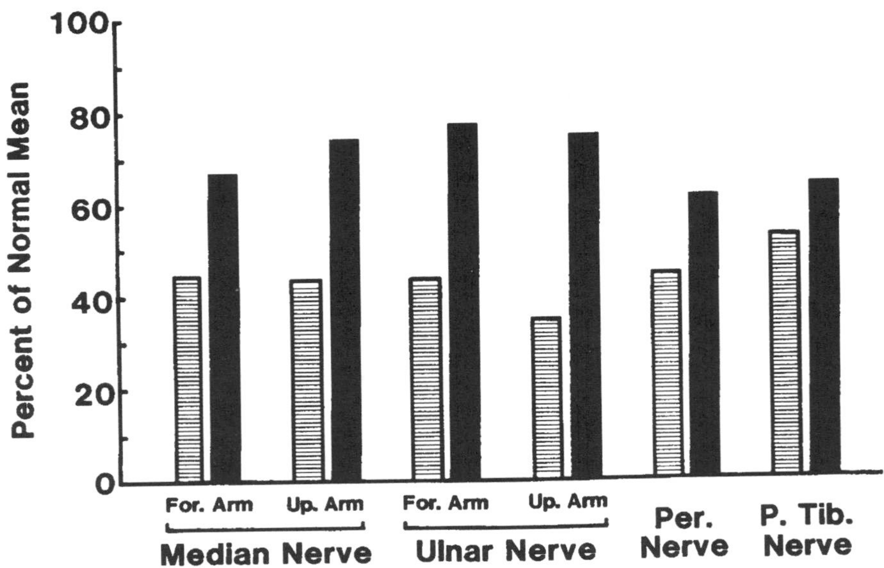

FIGURE 3.33. Comparison of the motor NCVs of axonal degeneration (arsenic neuropathy) and segmental demyelination (CIDP). ▤, segmental demyelination; ■, axonal degeneration. The normal mean is at 100%, and the lower normal limit at 80% of the mean. With segmental demyelination, the motor NCVs are below 60% of the normal mean, whereas with axonal degeneration they are above 60% of the normal mean.

1. Conduction block, usually applied to motor nerve conduction;
2. Abnormal temporal dispersion, usually applied to the CMAP in the motor nerve conduction and to the CNAP in the near-nerve sensory nerve conduction;
3. Marked slowing in the NCV.

In motor conduction, the following findings are typical of segmental demyelination:

1. Normal or reduced amplitude of the CMAP. Substantial slowing of the NCV in the presence of a normal amplitude is indicative of segmental demyelination. When the amplitude is reduced, this reduction is proportional to the degree of temporal dispersion of the CMAP and conduction block.
2. Abnormal temporal dispersion or "dispersion phenomenon" (abnormal CMAP with multiple phases and prolonged duration). This is judged in comparison either with the normal CMAP or with the CMAP at the distal site. We prefer the term "dispersion phenomenon" when comparing with the normal CMAP (Fig. 3.6) and the term "abnormal temporal dispersion" (Fig. 3.34) when comparing with the CMAP at the distal site. Abnormal temporal dispersion or dispersion phenomenon is typical of segmental demyelination.
3. Marked prolongation of the terminal latency (Fig. 3.32). The terminal latency is prolonged by more than 50% of the normal mean. Terminal latencies longer than 6 ms in the median nerve and longer than 10 ms in the peroneal nerve are indicative of segmental demyelination.
4. Markedly slow NCV (Fig. 3.33). Slowing of the NCV depends on the degree of segmental demyelination. NCV slowing by more than 40% below the normal mean is indicative of segmental demyelination. Motor NCVs below 35 m/s in the median nerve and below 30 m/s in the peroneal nerve are indicative of segmental demyelination.
5. Conduction block (Fig. 3.35). The amplitude is somewhat lower with stimulation at more proximal sites in normal subjects. Conduction block is defined as being present when there is a greater than 50% reduction of CMAP amplitude and area with normal duration with proximal stimulation as compared with distal stimulation.

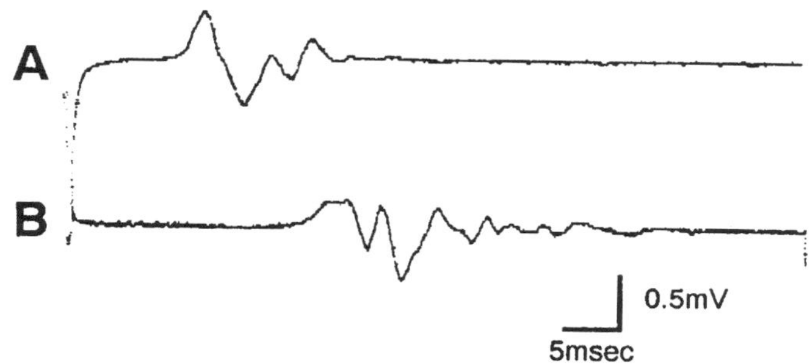

FIGURE 3.34. Abnormal temporal dispersion in the CMAP from the posterior tibial nerve at the popliteal fossa **(B)** compared with the CMAP at the ankle **(A)**. NCV in this segment was 40.0 m/s. No essential change is noted in the CMAP amplitude. There was a 35% increase in the negative duration and a 90% increase in the total duration in the proximal CMAP compared with the distal CMAP.

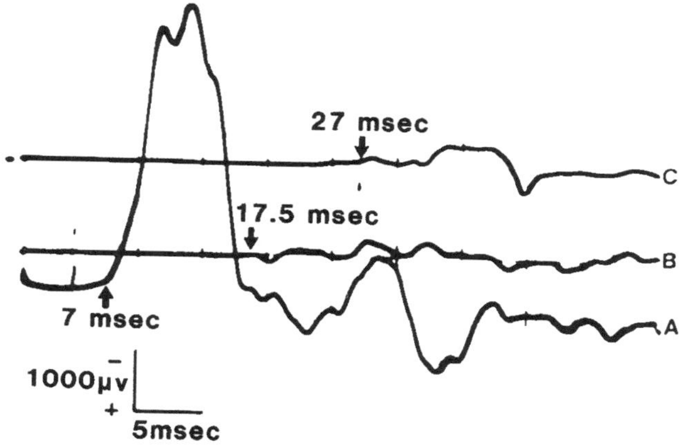

FIGURE 3.35. Conduction block in segmental demyelination. Median motor nerve conduction in a case of chronic demyelinating neuropathy. **A.** Normal amplitude of the CMAP with wrist stimulation. **B.** A dramatic reduction in amplitude of the CMAP with elbow stimulation. **C.** CMAP with axillary stimulation. Conduction block is clearly seen between wrist and elbow stimulation. The dispersion phenomenon is also observed. The motor NCV is 21.9 m/s over the wrist-elbow segment and 15.8 m/s over the elbow-axilla segment.

In the sensory nerve conduction, the following findings are indicative of segmental demyelination.

1. Normal or reduced amplitude of the sensory CNAP. Substantial slowing of the NCV in the presence of normal amplitude is indicative of segmental demyelination. When the amplitude is reduced, it is in proportion to the temporal dispersion and conduction block. With surface electrodes, the sensory CNAP is unobtainable in cases of severe segmental demyelination.
2. Dispersion phenomenon or abnormal temporal dispersion (Figs. 3.7 and 3.8). In the sensory nerve conduction, dispersion phenomenon is usually observed, because sensory nerve conduction is tested in one segment in the routine study. On very rare occasions, this phenomenon can be documented with the surface electrode, but it is best documented with the near-nerve needle electrode after signal averaging. When the sensory CNAP is markedly split and lengthened in duration with numerous smaller potential components

after the main component, this is termed dispersion phenomenon, which is indicative of segmental demyelination.

3. Marked slowing in NCV. Slowing of the sensory NCV depends on the severity of segmental demyelination. NCV slowing by more than 40% below the normal mean is indicative of segmental demyelination. Sensory NCV below 30 m/s in the median nerve and below 25 m/s in the sural nerve is indicative of segmental demyelination. It is rare to obtain an NCV below 20 m/s with surface electrodes in severe segmental demyelination because the sensory CNAP is unobtainable due to the smaller amplitude.
4. Conduction block. Because the sensory nerve conduction is tested in one segment in the routine nerve conduction study, conduction block cannot be documented by the routine sensory nerve conduction. This can only be demonstrated when the sensory fibers are orthodromically stimulated and the recording electrodes are placed in the short segment distal and proximal to the site of block, best seen with the near-nerve needle technique. In practice, because of these technical difficulties, it is almost impossible to demonstrate conduction block in the sensory nerve conduction.

Specific Patterns of Nerve Conduction Abnormalities

Although most peripheral neuropathies show mixed motor and sensory nerve conduction abnormalities in the nerve conduction study, there are certain patterns of abnormalities specific enough to be of value to clinicians in localizing the lesions to specific parts of the nerve axis and in suggesting the nature of a neuropathy (Table 3.7).

With a pure motor neuropathy, the motor nerve conduction is abnormal, whereas the sensory nerve conduction is completely normal. This neuropathy can be classified into two categories: axonal and demyelinating. Pure motor axonal neuropathy is characterized by a low CMAP amplitude and mild motor NCV slowing and normal sensory or mixed nerve conduction. This pattern is indicative of lesions in the anterior horn cells or ventral roots. The best examples of this pattern are seen in amyotrophic lateral sclerosis and in a few

TABLE 3.7. Characteristic Pattern in the Nerve Conduction

Motor NCS	Sensory NCS	Pathology	Typical Diseases
Pure motor neuropathy			
Axonal neuropathy	Normal	Anterior horn cell	Motor neuron disease (amytrophic lateral sclerosis)
		Polyradiculopathy	Axonal form of GBS
Demyelination	Normal	Pure motor neuropathy	Multifocal motor neuropathy
		Polyradiculoneuropathy	GBS (early stage)
Pure sensory neuronopathy			
Normal	Abnormal	Dorsal root ganglion	Friedreich's ataxia
			Sjögren' syndrome neuropathy
			Paraneoplastic subacute sensory neuropathy
Demyelinating mixed neuropathy			
Uniform demyelination	Abnormal	Hereditary neuropathy	HMSN type I
Nonuniform demyelination	Abnormal	Acquired demyelinating N	CIDP, GBS
Axonal mixed neuropathy			
Axonal	Abnormal	Axonal neuropathy	Alcoholic neuropathy, vasculitic neuropathy

NCS, nerve conduction study; HMSN, hereditary motor sensory neuropathy; CIDP, chronic inflammatory demyelinating polyneuropathy; GBS, Guillain-Barré syndrome.

cases of the axonal form of Guillain-Barré syndrome (GBS). A pure motor demyelinating neuropathy is characterized by nerve conduction abnormalities typical of demyelination confined to the motor fibers. This pattern is indicative of demyelinating neuropathy involving the motor fibers alone and is typically seen in multifocal motor neuropathy and in some cases of GBS, especially in the early phases. With a pure sensory neuropathy, the sensory nerve conduction is markedly abnormal, showing a pattern of axonal degeneration (extremely low or absent sensory CNAP with mild slowing of sensory NCV), whereas the motor nerve conduction is completely normal. This pattern is pathognomonic of a sensory neuronopathy involving the dorsal root sensory ganglia and is classically observed in Friedreich's ataxia, sensory neuropathy associated with Sjögren's syndrome, and paraneoplastic subacute sensory neuronopathy.

Uniform demyelinating neuropathy is a useful concept in differentiating between hereditary motor sensory neuropathy and acquired chronic demyelinating neuropathy. In uniform demyelinating neuropathy, the NCV is slowed "uniformly" to the same degree over all nerves and nerve segments. In addition, conduction block or abnormal temporal dispersion is absent because of the uniform demyelination of all fibers. This pattern is classically described in HMSN type I (CMT 1A) and familial neuropathies associated with metachromatic leukodystrophy, globoid leukodystrophy, and Cockayne's syndrome. In acquired demyelinating neuropathies, the nonuniform slowing of NCV over different nerves and nerve segments, conduction block, and abnormal temporal dispersion is typically observed.

Diagnostic Value of Motor and Sensory Nerve Conduction

Many studies have repeatedly shown that sensory conduction is a more sensitive indicator of a peripheral nerve lesion than motor conduction. The advantages of testing sensory nerve conduction are based on the following factors: sensory fibers are often affected earlier than motor nerves, severe loss of nerve fibers can be discriminated more precisely in sensory than in motor fibers, and a response from other than the fastest fibers can be recognized in sensory potentials.

The sensitivity of nerve conduction studies for identification of neuropathy is extremely high, being about 90% in most focal and diffuse neuropathies if the proper tests are selected for a given disorder and the tests are technically satisfactory.

The nerve conduction tests can identify axonal degeneration and segmental demyelination on the basis of nerve conduction characteristics (Table 3.6). This distinction is important because it helps in understanding the basic pathological process of disease without resorting to biopsy and in further identifying a definite etiology.

The nerve conduction study is helpful in identifying and localizing the site of individual nerve compression or entrapment. This information is crucial in the surgical management of many focal or entrapment neuropathies. A distinction can also be made by the nerve conduction study as to whether the neuropathy is multifocal (demyelinating or axonal) or diffuse. Multifocal demyelinating neuropathy is usually seen in multifocal motor neuropathy and multifocal axonal neuropathy in vasculitic neuropathy. Diffuse neuropathy is typical of polyneuropathy.

The nerve conduction study can identify the specific pattern of nerve conduction abnormalities on the basis of nerve conduction characteristics. This enables the clinician to localize a lesion to a specific part of the nerve and helps in identifying a definite etiology.

In summary, the nerve conduction data can provide the clinician with invaluable information about the diseased nerve, which cannot be obtained by any other means.

NERVE CONDUCTION ABNORMALITIES IN DISEASES

The discussion of nerve conduction abnormalities in each disease is beyond the scope of this chapter. Nerve conduction abnormalities in focal compression neuropathy and polyneuropathy in general are discussed here.

Focal Compression Neuropathy

Focal neuropathies present a common diagnostic problem for the clinical electromyographer. For the precise localization of a focal neuropathy, the nerve conduction study and needle EMG are essential. Among those with nontraumatic causes, the compression neuropathies, in which a nerve is compressed at an anatomically vulnerable site, are the most common. The basic pathological process in the focal compression neuropathy is focal segmental demyelination. In acute focal compression neuropathy, a mild focal demyelinating process is responsible for the conduction block that is the characteristic electrophysiological finding and explains the complete paralysis of the involved muscle. Abnormal temporal dispersion and nerve conduction slowing may be present. The best examples of acute focal compression neuropathies are "Saturday night palsy" (radial nerve palsy), "crossed leg palsy" (peroneal nerve palsy), and perioperative ulnar nerve palsy. In chronic focal compression neuropathy, focal demyelination by mechanical entrapment is responsible for the electrophysiological evidence of chronic focal demyelination: marked focal slowing of the NCV. The presence of conduction block is less often demonstrable by nerve stimulation in chronic entrapment neuropathies than in acute compression neuropathy. Secondary Wallerian degeneration is usually found in nerve segments distal to the site of compression.

To localize a focal demyelinating process, it is imperative to study the involved segment by means of the segmental nerve conduction study. In human entrapment neuropathy, it has been shown that the primary conduction abnormalities are confined to a short segment (often 5 to 10 cm) of the nerve. Most authorities regard 10 cm as the shortest acceptable distance for the segmental conduction study, as discussed above. This distance may be too generous to detect the segmental nerve conduction abnormality in some patients with focal neuropathy. Despite the inherent technical limitations of the short-distance technique, percutaneous stimulation at shorter intervals along the length of an involved nerve (the "inching technique") is especially useful in providing exact localization of the lesion by demonstrating the conduction block and conduction delay. This is used routinely in the authors laboratory in cases of ulnar neuropathy at the elbow to differentiate between an epicondylar sulcus lesion (tardy ulnar nerve palsy) and cubital tunnel syndrome.

In focal neuropathies, focal slowing of NCV, conduction block, and temporal dispersion across the compression site are the characteristic nerve conduction abnormalities. These nerve conduction abnormalities are seen in more than 90% of cases of focal neuropathy.

Polyneuropathy (Diffuse Peripheral Neuropathy)

The nerve conduction study is an essential part of the workup in patients with a peripheral neuropathy. This study helps in confirming peripheral neuropathy, determining the type of neuropathy, and following the course of the disease. The nerve conduction study identifies neuropathy in 76 to 80% of patients with diabetic neuropathy and in 81 to 100% of patients with GBS. To obtain a greater diagnostic yield in the nerve conduction investigation of patients with peripheral neuropathy, it is important to follow two important guidelines. First, testing should be performed on several nerves. McLeod et al. recommended several nerves in both upper and lower limbs. We recommend several nerves in one upper and both lower limbs. Second, the tests should include both sensory and mixed nerve conduction studies in addition to motor nerve conduction. Abnormalities in sensory conduction are a more sensitive indicator of impairment than the motor response, as discussed above. A specific pattern of motor and sensory nerve conduction abnormalities is specific enough to localize a lesion to specific parts of the nerve axis.

Nerve conduction abnormalities in peripheral neuropathy are usually diffuse. However, conduction abnormalities may not be observed in all nerves tested. When more than 50% of these nerves show evidence of abnormality, we interpret this as "indicative" of peripheral neuropathy. When less than 50% of nerves tested show abnormality, this is interpreted as "compatible" with peripheral neuropathy. The nerve conduction abnormalities in peripheral neuropathy depend on the nature of the pathological process (axonal versus segmental demyelination) and the site of the lesion, as discussed above.

CHAPTER 4

Repetitive Nerve Stimulation Test*

Neuromuscular transmission (NMT) disorders are classified into three distinct groups: postsynaptic disorders, presynaptic disorders, and combined presynaptic and postsynaptic disorders. Myasthenia gravis (MG), the most common and widely known postsynaptic disorder, is due to a decrease in the functioning acetylcholine (ACh) receptors induced by the acetylcholine receptor antibodies (AChR-ab). It produces the classic features of easy fatigability and oculobulbar limb muscle paresis. The best example of a presynaptic disorder is the Lambert-Eaton myasthenic syndrome (LEMS), which is commonly associated with carcinoma of the lung. The main defect in this disorder is the insufficient release of ACh at the presynaptic membrane induced by the antibodies against the voltage-gated calcium channels (VGCCs). The predominant symptoms of LEMS are easy fatigability and proximal leg weakness. Another well-known presynaptic disorder is botulism. Botulinum toxin is known to inhibit the release of ACh. Infant botulism has become the most common form of botulism in recent years. An example of a combined pre- and postsynaptic disorder is antibiotic-induced myasthenic syndrome, which is most commonly seen with aminoglycosides. These disorders can be diagnosed and differentiated from one another by the repetitive nerve stimulation (RNS) test and the single-fiber electromyography (SFEMG).

REPETITIVE NERVE STIMULATION TEST

The RNS test is the most commonly used technique for studying NMT disorders, because of the relative simplicity of technique and rapid results. In 1895, Jolly observed a progressive reduction in muscle response during faradic stimulation directly on the muscle, with recovery after rest, and published the first neurophysiological investigation of MG. A similar principle is used today in the performance of the RNS test, although nerve stimulation is used instead of stimulation on the muscle. For this reason, the RNS test is often called the Jolly test.

In 1941, Harvey and Masland published details of the first modern technique of the RNS test, using supramaximal stimulation of nerve to ensure that all excitable muscle fibers were activated. They found a progressive decline in the compound muscle action potential (CMAP) (decremental response) with stimulation at 3 to 50 Hz (per second) in patients with MG. Since then, the RNS test has become the standard diagnostic test for NMT disorders and still is the first-line test today, when the AChR-ab assay is available for the diagnosis of MG.

PHYSIOLOGICAL PRINCIPLES OF THE RNS TEST

The CMAP

The CMAP is the sum of muscle action potentials generated by muscle fibers and thus represents a rough estimation of the number of muscle fibers that are activated by nerve stimulation. This is the reason why supramaximal stimulation is an important technical requirement in the RNS test. The amplitude of the negative deflection of the CMAP is said to reflect a measure of the number of active muscle fibers. A more accurate measure would be calculation of the area under the negative portion of the CMAP. Almost all modern EMG machines are capable of measuring the area of the CMAP. Unfortunately, the normal value for the area change is undetermined at this time. We prefer to measure the peak-to-peak amplitude of

* This chapter is entirely quoted with permission from Oh SJ. Repetitive nerve stimulation test. Methods Clin Neurophysiol 1992:3:1. Dantec Medical A/S, Skovlunde, Denmark. A few minor modifications have been made.

the CMAP because it is easier and there is no significant difference between the negative amplitude and the peak-to-peak amplitude methods in calculation of decrement.

RNS Test

With the first stimulus, there is a relative decrease in the amount of immediately available ACh after release of a portion of the pool. Thus, a smaller number of ACh quanta are released by subsequent stimuli until the mobilization pool refills ACh in the immediately available pool. On the other hand, there is a relative increase in ACh release because of the accumulation of Ca^{++} in the axon terminal with each stimulus. Depending on the rate of stimulation, one of two processes becomes predominantly operative. At a low rate of stimulation (LRS) (less than 5 Hz stimulation), the depletion of immediately available quanta of ACh becomes more important. Thus, during LRS, presynaptic stores of immediately available quanta of ACh are depleted quickly and the number of quanta released declines, resulting in a gradual fall in amplitude of the end-plate potential (EPP). Due to a decreased quantal response because of the flattened postsynaptic folds in MG, a gradual fall in the EPP amplitude may lead to subsequent blocking of the contraction of some muscle fibers when the EPP falls below threshold, with eventual decremental response of the CMAP. In LEMS, the reduced quantal release of ACh by nerve stimulation is responsible for the failure of muscle fiber contraction, producing a decremental response. At a high rate of stimulation (HRS) (more than 10 Hz), an increase of ACh quantal release by Ca^{++} becomes more important. During HRS, an accumulation of Ca^{++} at the presynaptic terminal is increased, facilitating an increase of ACh release and subsequently an increase of EPP amplitude. In mild MG, the normal physiological events of an increased ACh quantal release at HRS can compensate for the diminished quantal response, producing a normal response. In severe MG, the NMT block is so severe that physiologically increased ACh release cannot compensate for the markedly diminished quantal response, thus still producing a decremental response. In LEMS, in which the basic defect is a reduced ACh release, the physiological increase in ACh release at HRS increases the EPP amplitude successively high enough to activate subthreshold muscle fibers, thus producing an incremental response.

TECHNIQUE OF THE RNS TEST

The RNS test can be performed by repetitive stimulation of any motor nerve with recording electrodes from its innervating muscles. Ideally, the testing should consist of recording the CMAP at rest, the CMAP after exercise, the response at LRS (1 to 5 Hz), the response at HRS (10 to 50 Hz), and post-tetanic or exercise responses. This ideal testing program can be easily applied in the distal muscles. However, because of the technical difficulty, proximal muscle testing usually consists of recording the CMAP at rest and the response at LRS.

The number of responses at LRS for analysis ranges from 4 to 15 according to the different EMG laboratories. At least the first six CMAPs are essential for adequate analysis because the decrement is noted within these six responses in most NMT diseases. For analysis of the response at HRS, a 1-second recording of the responses is usually satisfactory. One exception has been some cases of LEMS in which longer stimulation is necessary for a definite diagnosis.

The most popular and commonly described RNS test in EMG textbooks has been Lambert's method (Fig. 4.1). This method records the CMAP with a surface electrode from the abductor digiti quinti (ADQ) muscle with the stimulating electrodes at the ulnar nerve at the wrist. The nerve is stimulated at the rate of 3 Hz according to the testing program (Table 4.1). The amplitude of the negative phase of the first CMAP is compared with the lowest among the fourth through the eighth CMAPs (Fig. 4.2). For postexercise responses, the ratio of the CMAP amplitudes after and before exercise is compared and expressed as a percentage. For postexercise facilitation, the CMAP response immediately after exercise is compared with the pre-exercise response. For postexercise exhaustion, the response 2 minutes after exercise is compared with the pre-exercise response. When the values are outside the normal limit, they are considered abnormal. When the 2-minute postexercise CMAP amplitude is lower than the pre-exercise CMAP amplitude, postexercise exhaustion is said to be present. Unfortunately, skin temperature was not controlled and the normal values were not statistically expressed in Lambert's study.

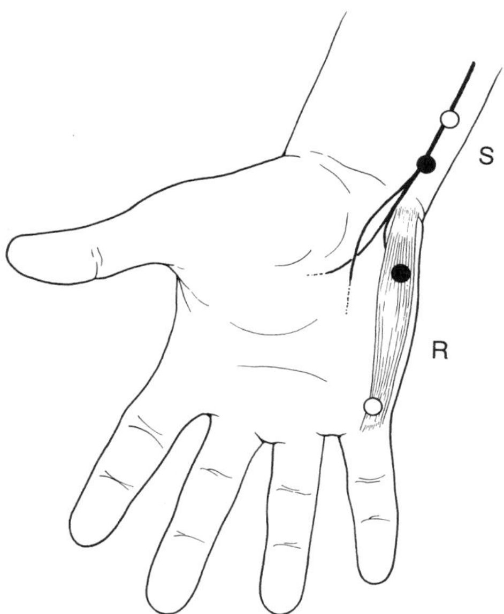

FIGURE 4.1. Lambert's methods of the RNS test on the abductor digiti quinti muscle. *S*, stimulating electrodes; *R*, recording electrodes. Black dot represents cathode and white anode.

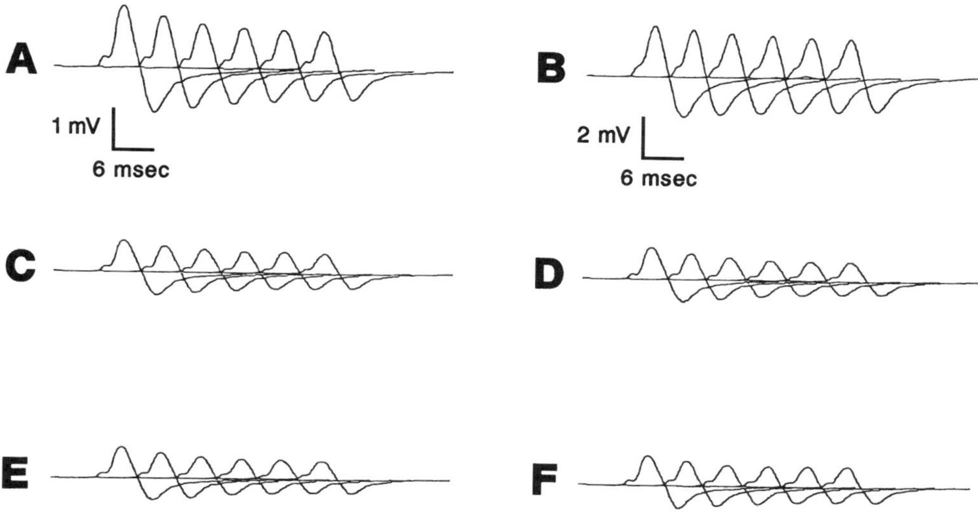

FIGURE 4.2. RNS responses in LEMS, following Lambert's method with the rate of 3-Hz stimulation. **A.** 36% decrement at rest. **B.** 19% decrement after exercise. **C.** 36% decrement 30 seconds after exercise. **D.** 40% decrement 1 minute after exercise. **E.** 40% decrement 2 minutes after exercise. **F.** 32% decrement 4 minutes after exercise. Note the postexercise facilitation by the amplitude (177% increase by ratio) and the decremental response. (Reprinted with permission from Oh SJ. The repetitive nerve stimulation test. Methods Clin Neurophysiol 1992;3:2.)

TABLE 4.1. Lambert's Method

Electrode placement
- Recording surface electrodes are placed in the ADQ muscle and stimulating surface electrodes are placed on the ulnar nerve at the wrist.

Testing program
- A single stimulation
- 3-Hz stimulation for 3 seconds
- Exercise of the ADQ for 10 seconds
- 3-Hz stimulation for 3 seconds (nine responses) at intervals of 3, 10, 30, and 60 seconds, and each minute thereafter for 5 minutes after exercise

Limits of normal values
- Negative peak CMAP (mV):[a] >5.6
- Decrement (%): <8[a]
- Postexercise facilitation (%):[b] <115

Skin temperature
- Not controlled

Measurement
- The negative peak amplitude of the first CMAP ($A1^a$) is compared with the lowest ($A2^a$) among the fourth through the eighth CMAPs. For postexercise facilitation, the ratio between the CMAP amplitudes before ($A1^b$) and immediately ($A2^b$) after exercise is compared and expressed as a percentage. For postexercise exhaustion, the response 2 minutes after exercise is compared with the pre-exercise response.

Interpretation
- When the values are outside the normal limit, they are considered abnormal. When 2-minute postexercise CMAP amplitude is lower than the pre-exercise CMAP amplitude, postexercise exhaustion is said to be present.

[a] $\frac{A1 - A2}{A1} \times 100$.

[b] Ratio percentage $= \frac{A2}{A1} \times 100$.

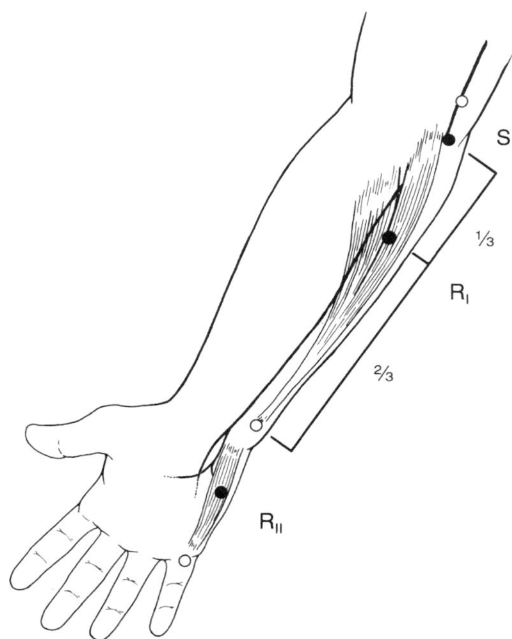

FIGURE 4.3. Oh's method of the RNS test on the flexor carpi ulnaris (R_I) and abductor digiti quinti muscles (R_{II}).

At the EMG Laboratory of the University of Alabama at Birmingham, we record the CMAPs with surface electrodes simultaneously from the ADQ and flexor carpi ulnaris (FCU) muscles with the stimulating electrodes on the ulnar nerve at the elbow. The CMAP is recorded at rest and after a 30-second exercise (Fig. 4.3). The nerve is stimulated at various low rates and at the high rate after the testing program (Table 4.2). The peak-to-peak amplitude is measured. The amplitude of the initial CMAP is compared with the postexercise CMAP to screen for LEMS. At LRS, the first response is compared with the lowest CMAP among the first five responses (Fig. 4.4). At 50 Hz, the first response is compared with the lowest or highest CMAP elicited in 1 second. One advantage of this method is that two muscles are tested simultaneously with one stimulation site. This increases the diagnostic sensitivity of MG by 5%. We use this testing program for three reasons. First, the LEMS will not be overlooked. There are two testing programs for screening for LEMS: post-exercise CMAP amplitude change and 50 Hz stimulation. Second, this test enables the investigator to judge the severity of NMT disease. Third, the diagnostic sensitivity of MG is higher compared with other methods.

TABLE 4.2. Oh's Method

Electrode placement
- Recording surface electrodes are placed in the ADQ and flexor carpi ulnaris muscles
- Stimulating surface electrodes are placed at the elbow sulcus of the ulnar nerve

Testing program
- A single stimulation to record the CMAP at rest
- Exercise of the ADQ muscle for 30 seconds
- Immediately after exercise, a single stimulation to record the CMAP to observe postexercise facilitation
- 2-Hz stimulation for 3 seconds (six responses)
- 3-Hz stimulation for 2 seconds (six responses)
- 5-Hz stimulation for 1 second (five responses)
- 50-Hz stimulation for 1 second (tetanic stimulation) (50 responses)
- 5-Hz stimulation for 1 second (five responses), immediately after tetanic stimulation to observe post-tetanic facilitation
- 5-Hz stimulation for 1 second (five responses), 4 minutes after tetanic stimulation to observe post-tetanic exhaustion

Measurements
- The peak-to-peak amplitude is measured. The amplitude of the initial CMAP is compared with the postexercise CMAP to screen for LEMS. At low rates of stimulation (2–5 Hz), the first response is compared with the lowest CMAP among the first five responses. At 50-Hz stimulation, the first response is compared with the lowest or highest CMAP elicited in 1 second.

Limits of normal values

	ADQ	FCU
CMAP (mV)	>4.8	>3.0
CMAP Ex (%)	<37	
2 Hz (%)	−7	−8
3 Hz (%)	−7	−9
5/second (%)	−5	−11
50/second (%)	−18	−19
	+42	+96
PTF/PTE (%)	−8	−11

Skin temperature
- >32 C

Interpretation
- Results are considered abnormal when the CMAP, CMAP response after exercise, and the decremental and incremental response are outside normal limits

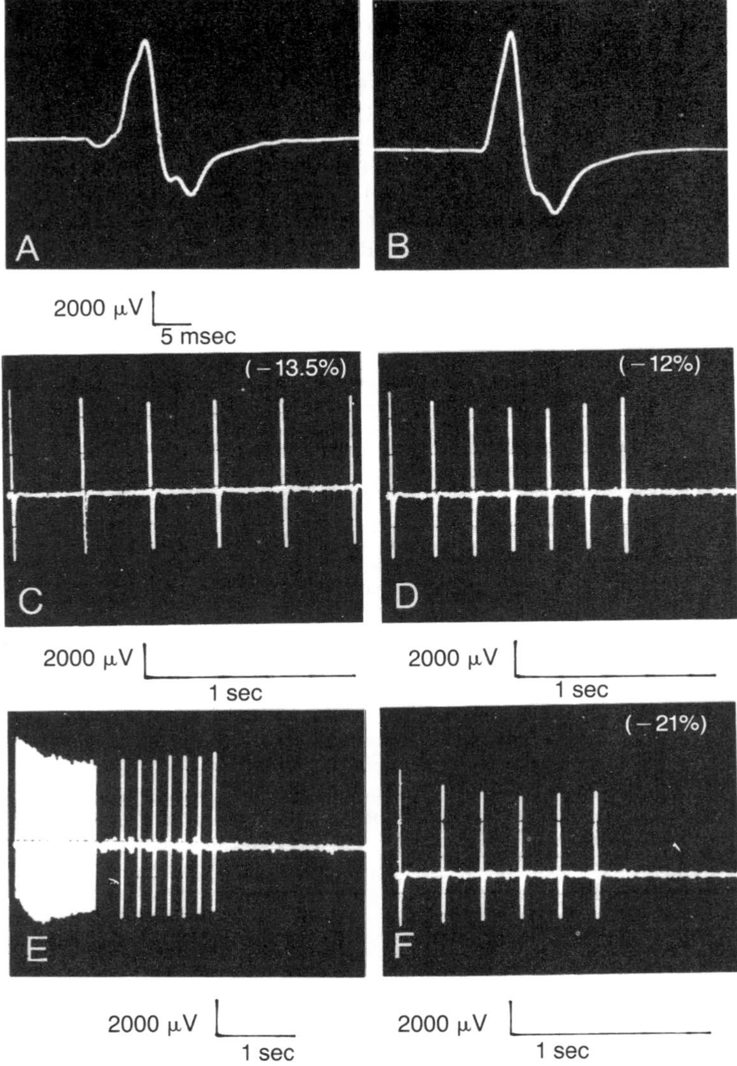

FIGURE 4.4. RNS responses in mild myasthenia gravis, following Oh's method. **A.** Normal amplitude (10 mV) of CMAP at rest. **B.** 10% increment of CMAP after exercise. **C.** decremental response at 3-Hz stimulation. **D.** Decremental response at 5 Hz. **E.** Normal response at 50 Hz followed by 5 Hz. **F.** Decremental response at 5 Hz 4 minutes after tetanic stimulation. Note the prominent post-tetanic facilitation and exhaustion phenomenon. (Reprinted with permission from Oh SJ, Eslami N, Nishihara T, et al. Electrophysiological and clinical correlation in myasthenia gravis. Ann Neurol 1982;12:352).

FACTORS AFFECTING THE RNS TESTS

Among the various factors affecting the RNS tests, temperature and recording electrodes are important.

Temperature

In 1973, Borenstein and Desmedt were the first to recognize the important effect of temperature on NMT block. Since then, many studies have confirmed this initial observation. With lowering of temperature, the CMAP amplitude increases but the decremental response de-

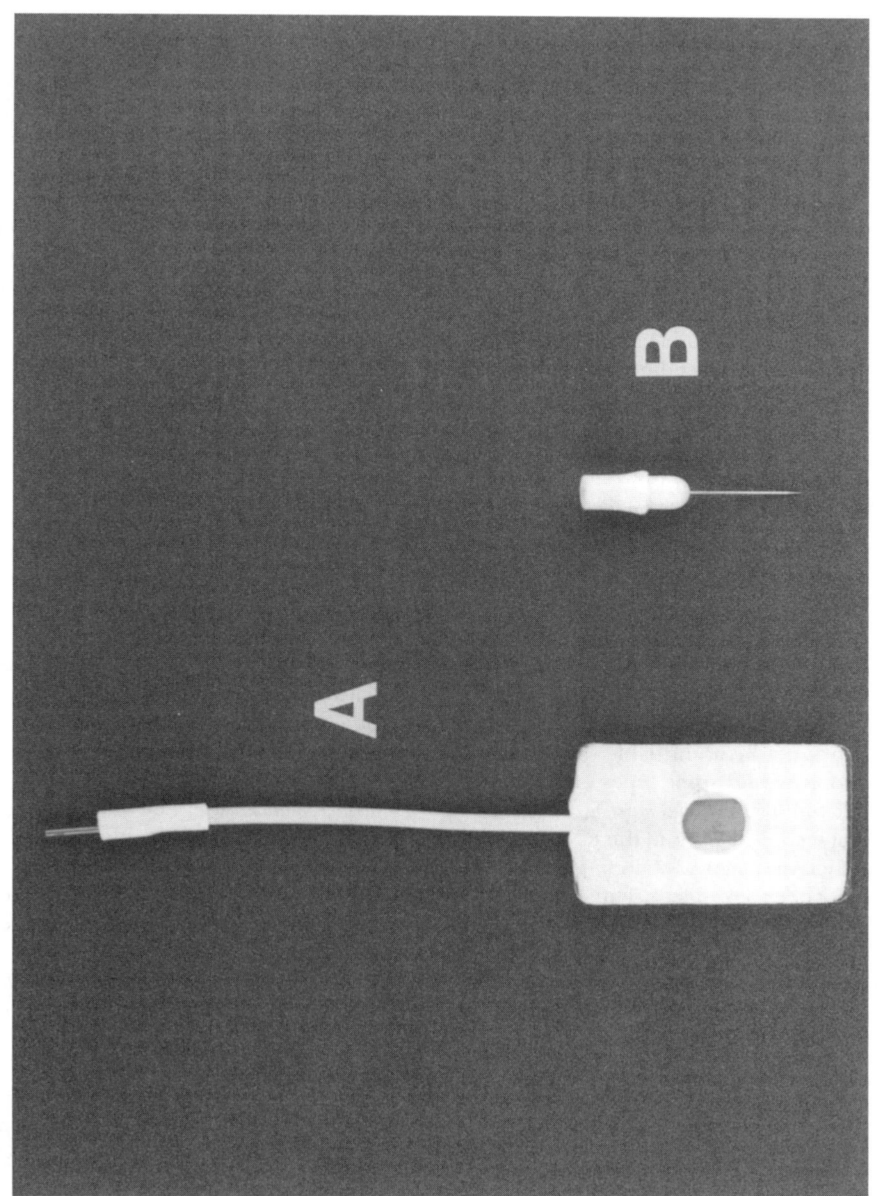

FIGURE 4.5. Recording electrodes best used for the repetitive nerve stimulation test. **A.** Disposable "stick-up surface electrode" (Dantec). **B.** Steel needle recording electrode (Dantec, Allendale, NJ). (Reprinted with permission from Oh SJ. The repetitive nerve stimulation test. Methods Clin Neurophysiol 1992;3:5.)

creases at LRS and HRS within the range of 25 to 40 C. Post-tetanic facilitation (PTF) and post-tetanic exhaustion (PTE) also improve with cooling. Thus, there is a danger that low skin temperature (27 to 31 C) may not demonstrate a decremental response at LRS in either MG or LEMS, especially in mild cases. Thus, it is clear that skin temperature should be routinely controlled during the RNS test. The standard temperature in many laboratories is 35 to 36 C. In our laboratory, the standard temperature is controlled above 32 C.

Recording Electrodes

On the RNS test, the CMAP amplitude should provide a rough estimation of the number of muscle fibers activated by a nerve stimulation. To achieve this goal, either surface electrodes or subcutaneous needle electrodes should be used as the recording electrodes. The intramuscular needle electrode is not suitable for the RNS test because it records the response from a more or less limited area of the muscle. Using a surface electrode as the recording electrode always presents the possibility of loosening of electrodes during the RNS test. This problem is resolved if "stick-up disposable electrodes" are used (Fig. 4.5). The subcutaneous needle has been used by some investigators as a recording electrode because the needle gave rise to fewer errors than did surface electrodes. The needle must be inserted subcutaneously into the belly of the muscle and firmly secured. The CMAP amplitude was 20 to 30% greater with a subcutaneous needle than with surface electrodes. We prefer surface stick-up recording electrodes because of their noninvasiveness and reduced risk of infection, particularly in patients with hepatitis, AIDS, or Jakob-Creuzfeldt disease.

TECHNICAL REQUIREMENTS

Because of the painful nature of the RNS test, it is not easy to obtain a technically adequate RNS study. Thus, the following technical requirements must be met.

1. *Stimulus intensity must be supramaximal.* The CMAP amplitude is one of the important parameters in differentiating postsynaptic NMT block from presynaptic block. Without supramaximal stimulation, the CMAP amplitude is meaningless for the RNS test.
2. *Recording electrodes should be placed using the belly-tendon method.* With this method, the initial deflection of the CMAP is upward, the CMAP is usually diphasic, and the highest amplitude of the CMAP is obtained. Without this method, the repetitive discharge in the CMAP may not be identifiable. Repetitive discharges are indicative of anti-cholinesterase (ChE) toxicity and some types of congenital MG.
3. *Recording electrodes must be firmly attached to the surface of the muscle.* The most common source of technical error in the RNS test is a loose recording electrode. To achieve this, disposable stick-up electrodes are a godsend. Since we have been using these, loose electrodes have not been a problem. Thus, disposable stick-up electrodes are essential items for the successful RNS test. When, because of profuse sweating in some patients, the electrodes do not adhere to the skin, subcutaneous needles are used as the recording electrodes.
4. *Stimulating electrodes must be firmly placed on the nerve so that supramaximal stimulus intensity is uniformly produced throughout the test.* Loose stimulating electrodes may result in submaximal nerve stimulation, producing a false decremental response. We secure the stimulating electrodes with a rubber band to achieve this when testing the distal muscles.
5. *Movement of muscles must be minimized.* Gross movement of contracting muscles is one source of loose recording electrodes. To reduce this artifact, we use a Jolly test board for the RNS test on the ADQ and FCU muscles and a hand-clamping device for the RNS test on the ADQ muscle (Fig. 4.6).
6. *Skin temperature should be controlled.* The reason for this requirement has already been discussed.
7. *The entire CMAP wave form should be monitored or recorded for analysis.* When there is a dramatic change in the shape of the CMAP, this is usually caused by loose electrodes. This artifact and "pseudofacilitation" (an increase in the CMAP amplitude due to narrowing of the duration) can be easily identified by analysis of the entire CMAP waveform. Unlike the older EMG machines, modern EMG machines are capable of recording the entire wave-

A
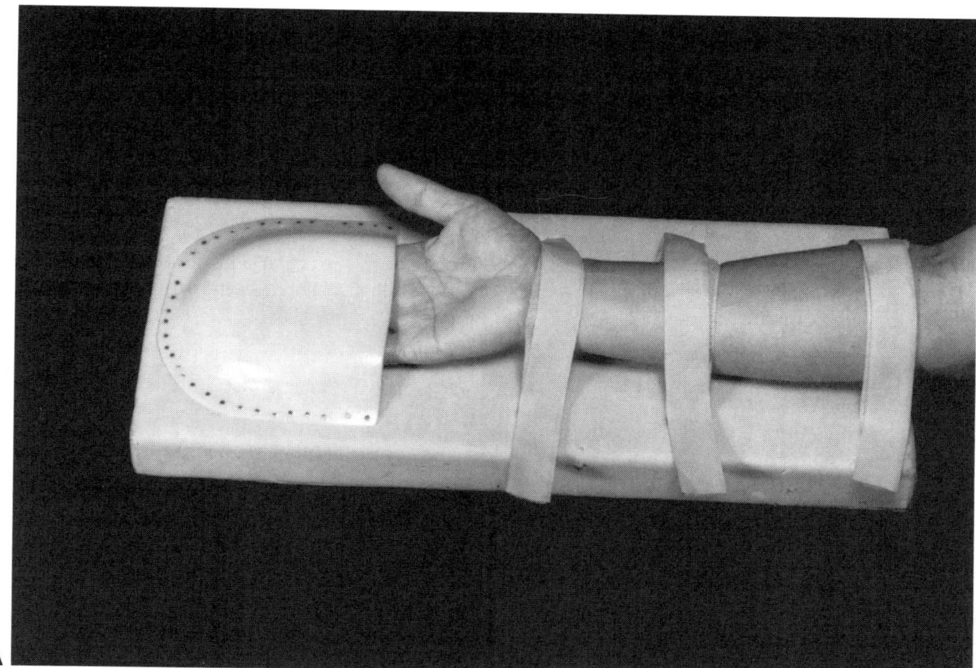

B
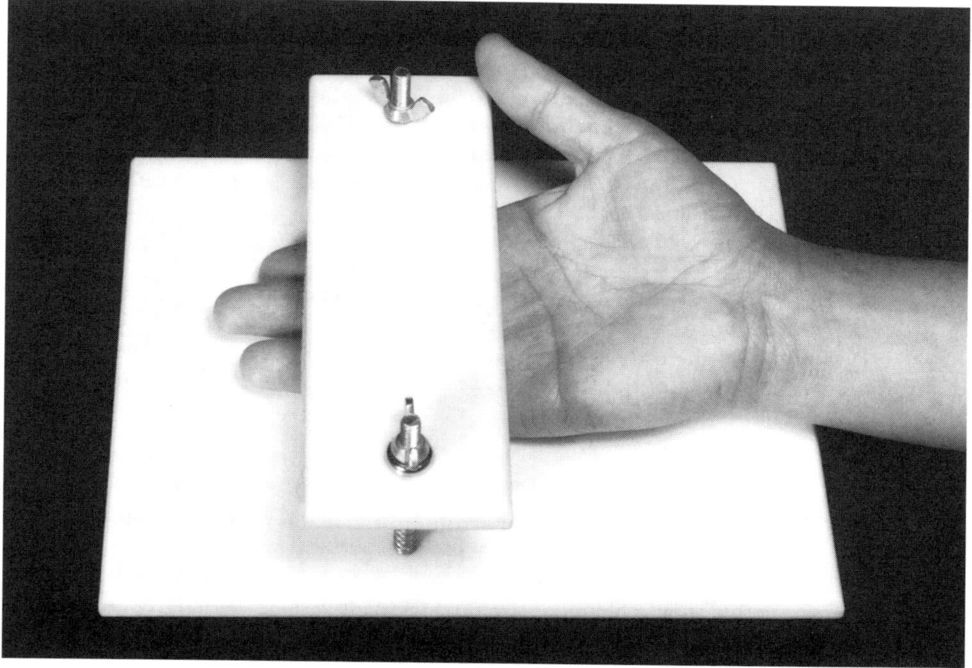

FIGURE 4.6. A. The Jolly board with hand and forearm. **B.** Hand-clamping device with hand. (Reprinted with permission from Oh SJ. The repetitive nerve stimulation test. Methods Clin Neurophysiol 1992;3:5.)

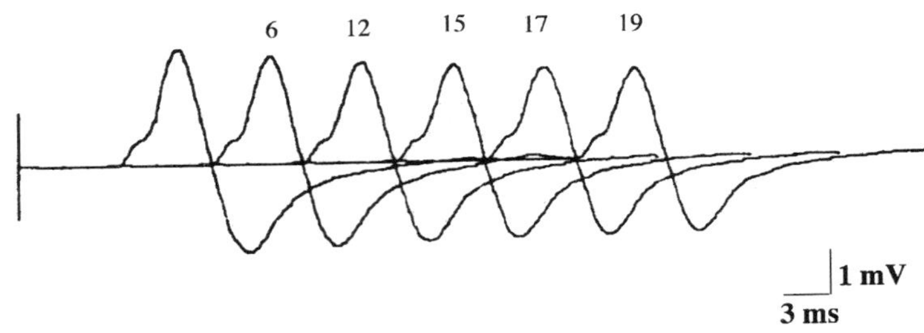

FIGURE 4.7. Genuine decremental response free from the artifacts in Lambert-Eaton myasthenic syndrome. Note the gradual decrement of the CMAP. Calculated decrements are shown above each response.

TABLE 4.3. Normal Values for the Decremental Response in the Facial and Trapezius Muscles[a]

Stimulating Nerve	Recording Muscle	Controlled Temperature (°C)	Rate of Stimulation (Hz)	Normal Limits (%)	Investigator
Facial	Orbiculari	32	2, 3, 5	−8	Oh
Accessory	Trapezius	32	5	−6	Schumm
	Trapezius	32	2, 3, 5	−5 for 2 Hz −8 for 3 and 5 Hz	Claussen

[a] Test is done with the surface electrodes as the recording and stimulation electrodes.

form in the raster form. If the continuous recording mode is used to record the response, the entire CMAP waveform should be carefully monitored on the oscilloscope.

8. *Genuine decremental or incremental response is characterized by a gradual and smooth change and by reproducibility.* A gradual and smooth change in the amplitude always represents a genuine decremental or incremental response (Fig. 4.7). Also, the genuine response should be reproducible on repeated testing. In contrast, a sudden or dramatic change in the shape or amplitude of the CMAP is usually due to artifacts. By the inherent nature, the response due to the artifacts are not reproducible.

NORMAL VALUES OF THE RNS TEST

A decrement greater than 8 to 10% has been universally accepted as abnormal. In fact, our study showed that an 8 to 10% decremental response is not the normal limit for all muscles. Depending on the rate of stimulation, the muscles, the techniques, and the activation tests, the normal values for the RNS tests are different (Tables 4.1 to 4.3). Next to the ulnar nerve stimulation, the facial and accessory nerve RNS tests are most commonly used and thus normal values are given in Table 4.3.

INTERPRETATION OF THE RNS DATA

All parameters of the RNS test are helpful in the diagnosis of NMT disorders.

The CMAP

The amplitude should be measured at rest and after exercise. The repetitive discharge must be recognized. A normal CMAP is indicative of a postsynaptic disorder, whereas a low CMAP indicates a presynaptic disorder. Repetitive discharges are indicative of one of the following disorders: excessive anti-ChE medications, organophosphate poisoning, or congenital MG type A or B (Fig. 4.8). Postexercise facilitation (a significant increase in the amplitude after exercise) is pathognomonic of a presynaptic disorder (Fig. 4.9). Postexercise depression (a significant decrease in the amplitude after exercise) is associated with excessive anti-ChE treatment, organophosphate poisoning, or myotonic syndrome.

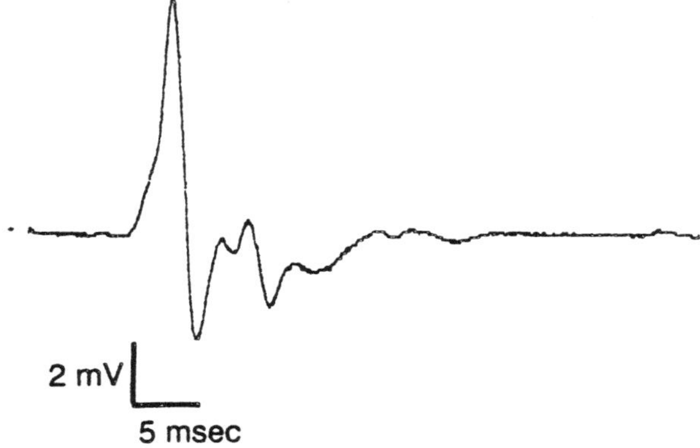

FIGURE 4.8. Simple repetitive CMAP in an MG patient overtreated with anticholinesterase medication.

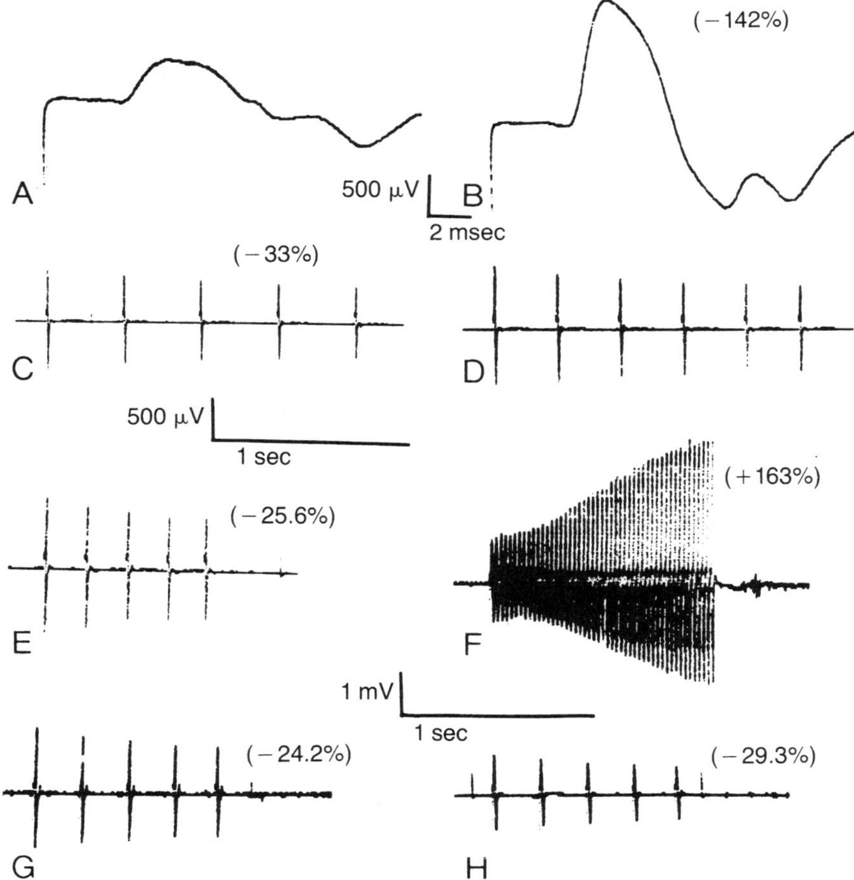

FIGURE 4.9. The classic RNS pattern in the flexor carpi ulnaris in LEMS. **A.** Low CMAP at rest. **B.** CMAP after exercise. Postexercise facilitation is obvious. **C.** Decrement at 2-Hz stimulation. **D.** Decrement at 3-Hz stimulation. **E, G, and H.** Decrements before, immediately after, and 4 minutes after 50-Hz stimulation. **F.** Note the marked incremental response at 50-Hz stimulation. The 0.5-mV calibration applies to **C, D,** and **E**; 1-mV calibration applies to **F, G,** and **H.**

The RNS Test at LRS

The decremental response is sought in this test because an abnormal decremental response at LRS is usually indicative of NMT block. Thus, the LRS is the most important parameter in the RNS test. In MG, the best diagnostic sensitivity is observed at LRS (Fig. 4.4). A dramatic improvement of the abnormal decremental response with edrophonium is typical of MG. A decrement at the second response with a gradual increment ("dip phenomenon") is pathognomonic of anti-ChE toxicity (Fig. 4.10).

The RNS Test at HRS

The HRS is crucial in the differentiation between presynaptic and postsynaptic disorders, because this is the single most important diagnostic test for LEMS. The decremental and incremental responses are sought in this test (Figs. 4.9 and 4.11). An abnormal decremental response is indicative of severe postsynaptic block. In mild postsynaptic block, the response

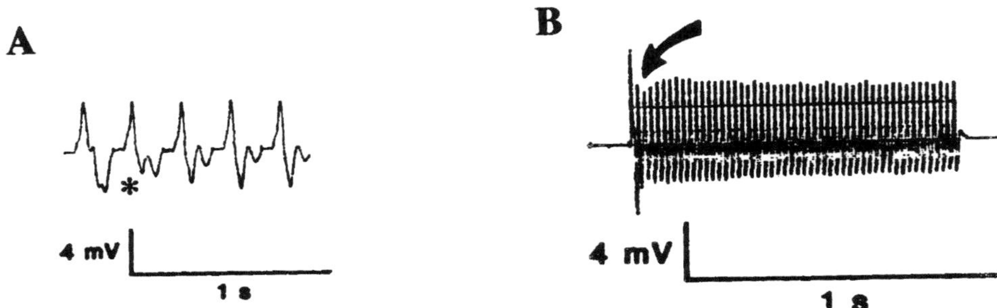

FIGURE 4.10. Dip phenomenon (decrement-increment response) indicative of anticholinesterase toxicity. **A.** Dip phenomenon (*) in 3-Hz stimulation. Notice also the repetitive discharge. **B.** Dip phenomenon (*arrow*) at 50-Hz stimulation.

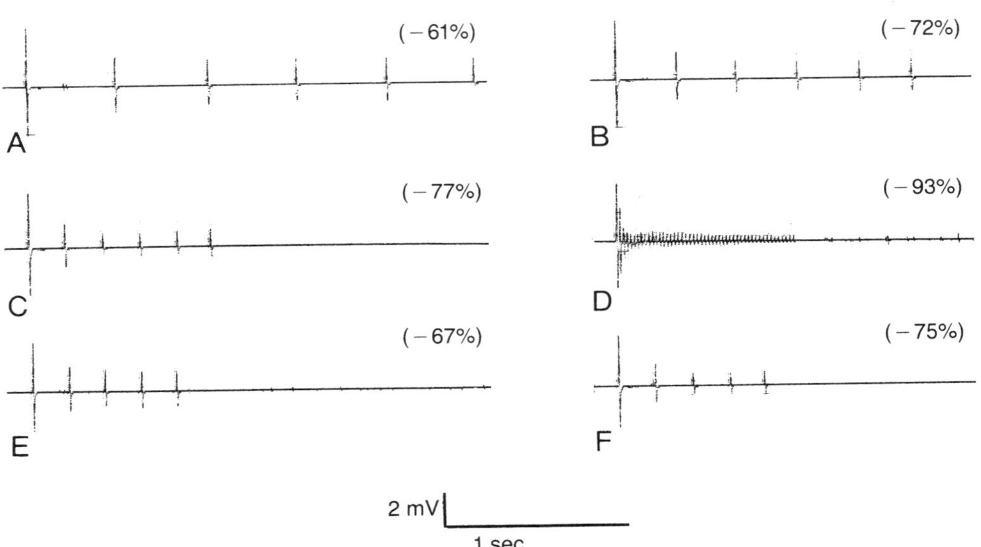

FIGURE 4.11. RNS responses in severe MG. **A.** Decremental response at 2-Hz stimulation. **B.** Decremental response at 3-Hz stimulation. **C, E,** and **F.** Decremental responses at 5-Hz stimulation before, immediately after, and 4 minutes after 50-Hz stimulation. **D.** Note the marked decremental response at 50-Hz stimulation.

TABLE 4.4. Typical RNS Patterns in the NMT Disorders

Defects	Postsynaptic	Presynaptic	Combined
CMAP at rest	Normal	Low	Low
CMAP Ex	No change	Increment	No change
LRS	Decrement	Decrement	Decrement
HRS	No change or decrement	Increment	Decrement
PTF/PTE	Present	Present	Absent

CMAP Ex, CMAP after exercise.

at HRS is normal. Markedly abnormal incremental response (more than 100%) is pathognomonic of the presynaptic disorders: LEMS, botulism, magnesium-induced weakness, or overlap myasthenic syndrome.

Post-tetanic Facilitation (PTF) and Post-tetanic Exhaustion (PTE)

After brief tetanic stimulation, there is a short-lived electrophysiological improvement in the decremental response (PTF) followed by a prolonged electrophysiological worsening (PTE) in MG (Fig. 4.4). The post-tetanic response is representative of a physiological change occurring at the synaptic cleft at HRS; PTF represents a short-lived increase of ACh available at the postsynaptic receptor, improving an NMT block, and PTE may be due to "receptor desensitization." PTF followed by PTE is observed in presynaptic and postsynaptic NMT disorders. Because this phenomenon represents a physiological change, technical artifact cannot reproduce this. Thus, PTF followed by PTE is pathognomonic of NMT disorders. On the basis of the patterns of abnormalities in the RNS test, one can differentiate between postsynaptic disorders, presynaptic disorders, and combined pre and postsynaptic disorders as noted in Table 4.4.

RNS ABNORMALITIES IN DISEASES

Myasthenia Gravis

MG is an autoimmune disease that is clinically characterized by exertional weakness. The primary abnormality is destruction of the ACh receptor by antibodies directed against the receptor protein. The best confirmatory diagnostic test for MG has been the time-honored intravenous edrophonium test, which shows positive results in 90 to 95% of patients. However, false-positive edrophonium tests have been reported in various diseases, including non-neuromuscular diseases. Thus, in recent years, the diagnosis of MG has been based on clinical features together with edrophonium responsiveness and other laboratory findings. The laboratory tests include serum AChR-ab assay, the RNS test, and the SFEMG (Table 4.5). The AChR-ab assay has been the single most useful test in MG because of its relatively high specificity. This test is positive in 70 to 87% of patients with MG. However, the test results may not be available for days or weeks. The RNS test offers the advantages of relative simplicity and rapid results. Although certain patterns of the RNS test are indicative of MG, it is less specific than the AChR-ab assay. Another advantage of the RNS test is good correlation between electrophysiological and clinical assessment of disease severity in MG. The SFEMG is the most sensitive test for MG as seen in our studies. However, this test has a drawback in that it requires fairly elaborate equipment and extensive training and patient cooperation. For this reason, this test is performed in only a limited number of EMG laboratories. Another drawback has been the nonspecificity of the SFEMG for MG because similar abnormalities may be observed in many neuromuscular diseases. Our study on the relative diagnostic sensitivities of these three tests in 120 MG patients showed that one of the tests is abnormal in 100% of cases and the SFEMG is needed in only 8% of cases. Thus, even in the era of AChR-ab assay, the RNS test has its place for the diagnosis and management of MG. Under the situations listed in Table 4.6, the RNS test offers the most effective objective means of evaluation that the other tests cannot offer.

TABLE 4.5. Specificity and Sensitivity of Laboratory Tests in MG

Test	Specificity	Sensitivity (%)
AChR-ab	High	70–87
RNS test	Moderate	55–77
SFEMG	Low	77–100

TABLE 4.6. Indications for the RNS Test

When the AChR-ab is negative
When a rapid, objective diagnosis of MG is needed
When objective improvement on the edrophonium test is needed
When an objective follow-up evaluation is needed
When an objective titration of anti-ChE is needed
When an objective evaluation of the severity of MG is needed

There are few practical considerations that clinicians or electromyographers must follow to maximize the usefulness of the RNS test:

1. The RNS test should be performed before any anti-ChE medication is administered, because it is well known that the anti-ChE can normalize the RNS abnormality in mild cases of MG;
2. Anti-ChE medications should be withdrawn, if possible, at least 12 hours before the test in patients who are taking these medications for the same reason given above;
3. To document electrophysiological improvement with edrophonium, the LRS should be given 2 minutes after the injection.

The diagnostic sensitivity of the RNS test for MG has been found to be about 55% in distal muscles and about 70% in proximal muscles. In our series, it was 62% in the ADQ and FCU muscles and 77% in proximal muscles. The higher diagnostic rates in our series are due to our five test parameters and testing of two muscles with a single stimulation site (Table 4.2). Because of its technical reliability, the RNS test on the distal hand muscles remains the most commonly used test and the first test of choice in our laboratory. When the distal muscles are normal, then the RNS test in the proximal muscles is recommended. This strategy increases the diagnostic sensitivity in MG by 15%. The test on the orbicularis oculi or the trapezius muscle is technically reliable as long as the stimulus is barely supramaximal and the rate of stimulation is less than 5 Hz. We do not recommend exercise in these muscles because it will invariably loosen the stimulating electrodes, inviting artifacts. The test on the deltoid muscle is inherently technically difficult to perform because it is impossible to immobilize the stimulating electrode at the Erb's point with confidence. We do recommend immobilizing the deltoid muscle with a Posey's strap and stimulating the axillary nerve at 2 and 3 Hz.

The most common types of RNS abnormalities are those typical of postsynaptic NMT blocks: normal CMAP amplitude, normal or minimal postexercise facilitation (PEF), decremental response at LRS, normal or decremental response at HRS, and PTF followed by PTE (Figs. 4.4 and 4.11). Among these, the decremental response at LRS is the most common and characteristic RNS finding in MG. This decremental response represents a progressive blocking at the neuromuscular junction of muscle fibers as transmitter depletion causes increasing numbers of EPPs to become subthreshold. In Oh's series, the LRS showed abnormality in 61% of cases. Normal CMAP amplitude has been reported in most patients. In 3 to 8% of cases, the CMAP was low. In MG, there is no increase or only a minimal increase in postexercise amplitude, thus providing a good contrast to the dramatic PEF seen in LEMS (Fig. 4.9). In many laboratories, HRS is not performed as a routine test because it is painful. We use HRS routinely for the RNS test and have found an increased diagnostic yield of

5% in MG. This test further ensures that LEMS has been ruled out completely. Abnormal decremental response at HRS was observed in 22% of cases in our series and in 47% in that of Slomic and coworkers. More typically in MG, postexercise or post-tetanic responses are better reflected in the decremental response than in the CMAP amplitude. In our series, PTF was observed in 40% of cases and PTE in 17% of cases. In 5% of our series, PTE was the only abnormality in the RNS test.

There is a good correlation between electrophysiological and clinical assessment of disease severity in MG. This is true regardless of the therapeutic mode and also true for serial tests in a given patient. In fact, the RNS test is the only objective test that can evaluate the severity of disease in MG. Two distinct patterns of the RNS test exist depending on the severity of disease: in mild MG, an abnormal decremental response at LRS, normal response at HRS, and prominent PTF and PTE phenomena (Fig. 4.4); in severe MG, an abnormal decremental response at LRS and HRS with less common PTF and rare PTE phenomena (Fig. 4.11). This difference can be reasonably explained by physiological changes in NMT during HRS. In mild MG, the normal mechanism of increase in ACh release during HRS can compensate for the minimally diminished safety factor, producing a normal response at HRS and subsequent PTF and PTE. In severe MG, however, the neuromuscular block is so severe that the normal mechanism of increased ACh release during HRS cannot compensate for the markedly diminished safety factor, thus producing a decremental response at HRS, less common PTF, and subsequent lack of PTE.

To increase the diagnostic value of the RNS test, various activation tests have been introduced in the past. Exercise, tetanic stimulation, and warming are now well incorporated into the routine study as discussed above. More sophisticated activation tests such as the exercise-ischemic test, regional curare test, and systemic curarization have been largely replaced by the SFEMG.

LEMS

LEMS is an autoimmune disease clinically characterized by easy fatigability, proximal leg weakness, paucity of oculobulbar symptoms, and hyporeflexia. The main defect in this disorder is the insufficient release of ACh at the presynaptic membrane induced by the antibodies against voltage-gated calcium channels (VGCCs). A recent study showed that this antibody was found in 52–90% of LEMS patients. Unfortunately, this assay is complicated and is not widely available as yet. Thus, the diagnosis of LEMS can only be confirmed by the RNS test. The RNS test is always abnormal in patients with this disorder. In LEMS, the RNS test on a distal muscle is sufficient to confirm the diagnosis in the majority of cases, and the most important test parameters are postexercise facilitation and response at HRS (Fig. 4.9). These two features are in good contrast to MG, in which the test on a distal muscle is not sufficient to confirm the diagnosis in a substantial number of cases, and the LRS is the most important test parameter.

The RNS test in LEMS is characterized by a presynaptic NMT block: low CMAP, dramatic PEF, decremental response at LRS, marked incremental response at HRS, and prominent PTF but less prominent PTE (Fig. 4.9). Low CMAP has been noted in 95% of cases in this disorder. In many patients, it is extremely low. The most dramatic increase in the CMAP amplitude after exercise (PEF) has been noted in this disease. Lambert et al. (1961) observed at 120 to 1800% increase of the CMAP amplitude in LEMS patients. This is in contrast to a 15% increase for normal individuals and a 94% increase for MG patients. Thus, a more than 100% increase in the CMAP amplitude after exercise is considered to be typical of LEMS. In our series, PEF was not observed in 27% of patients because of lack of cooperation or severe weakness of the hand muscles. Thus, although this test alone is not sufficient to rule out LEMS, this simple and relatively painless procedure should be performed in all suspected cases because it is abnormal in most LEMS patients. In almost all cases, a decremental response has been noted at LRS. In our series, decremental response was present in 93% of cases. The most dramatic facilitation at HRS was seen in this disease. In all cases, there was an incremental response at HRS, ranging from 100 to 4000%. In most cases, this incremental response can be documented at 50-Hz stimulation for 1 second. However, in a few cases, a prolonged HRS up to 10 seconds was needed to document an incremental response (Fig. 4.12). This was observed in one mild and two severe cases among 13 cases in our study. This

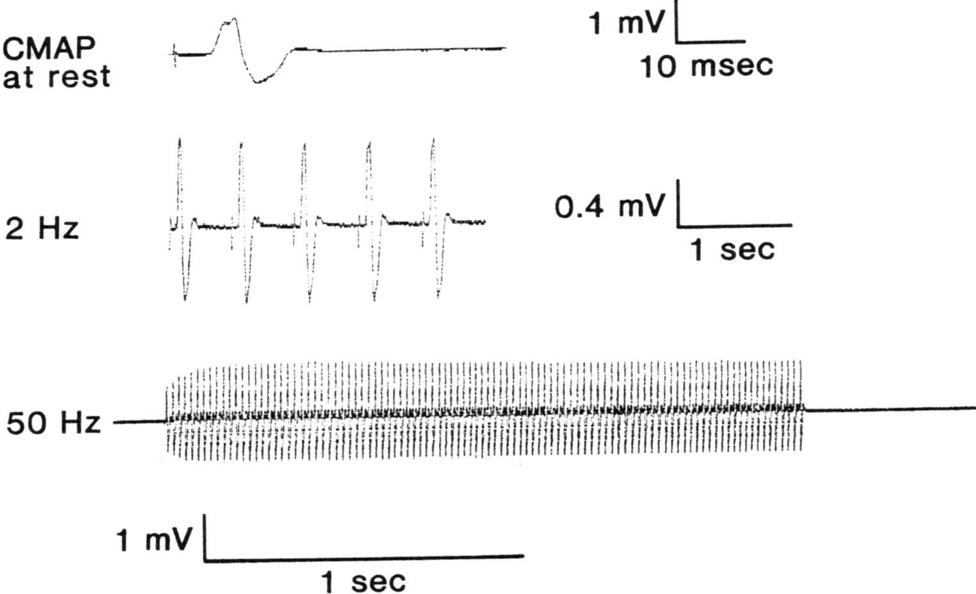

FIGURE 4.12. RNS pattern in infant botulism. Low CMAP amplitude at rest (1.4 mV). Decremental response (8%) at 2-Hz stimulation. Incremental response (122%) at 50-Hz stimulation for 2 seconds. (Reprinted with permission from Oh SJ. The repetitive nerve stimulation test. Methods Clin Neurophysiol 1992;3:11.)

observation indicates that a 10-second period of stimulation at 50 Hz should be tried before deciding that there is no incremental response in patients suspected of having LEMS.

There are two patterns of response at HRS in LEMS: a gradual incremental response from the first CMAP (Fig. 4.9) and an initial decremental response followed by a subsequent incremental response (see Chapter 13). The first pattern is more common. The second pattern represents a more severe presynaptic block; prolonged stimulation is required to increase the ACh quantal release by Ca^{++} sufficiently to compensate for the initial block and subsequently produce an incremental response. From a practical point of view, the second pattern mimics the RNS pattern observed in MG. Thus, when the second pattern occurs in patients suspected of having LEMS, a prolonged stimulation at HRS is essential in documenting an incremental response, making it possible to reach the diagnosis of LEMS. Just as there is dramatic PEF, PTF is also prominent in all cases of LEMS. On the other hand, PTE was observed in 69% of cases. In general, there is a correlation between the RNS abnormalities and the severity of disease. The best index of severity of disease is the CMAP amplitude, followed by facilitation at HRS in an inverse logarithmic scale. Thus, the RNS test can be used as an objective means of measuring severity during follow-up.

Overlap MG and LEMS

Overlap MG and LEMS refers to a combined syndrome of MG and LEMS in the same patient. AChR and VGCC antibodies were positive in all tested cases. The clinical features of these cases are best explained as a combination of MG and LEMS. Oculobulbar symptoms and a positive edrophonium test, two classic signs of MG, are common, as is areflexia, a classic feature of LEMS. The RNS test showed findings typical of LEMS in all cases.

Botulism

Botulism is an uncommon but often fatal NMT disease caused by *Clostridium botulinum*. Three distinct clinical syndrome have been described: food-borne botulism, wound botulism, and infant botulism. Among these, the most common type in the United States is infant botulism. Botulinum toxins interfere with the release of ACh at the cholinergic transmission sites of the peripheral nervous system. Botulism is characterized clinically by acute, areflexic, descending muscle weakness and dysautonomia (fixed pupils, ileus, and urinary retention). Diagnosis of botulism is made by the detection of botulinum toxin in the serum or organisms in the stool.

Because the RNS test provides the only relatively specific responses in botulism, this test has been found to be the most convincing objective evidence of botulism until microbiological confirmation is achieved. In all cases of botulism showing neuromuscular weakness, the RNS test shows some abnormalities. The most characteristic RNS abnormalities are those of presynaptic NMT blocks (Fig. 4.12). Although the RNS abnormalities in botulism are similar to those in LEMS, there are two important differences; in botulism, the abnormalities are seen in the more clinically affected muscles, and the RNS responses can change from day to day, with patients sometimes showing a normal response early in the disease. Thus, it is important to test several muscles with the RNS test if the first muscle does not show abnormality and to repeat the test on the following day if the initial test shows normal findings. The CMAP amplitude is not as low as in LEMS. The decremental response at LRS is absent or minimal in botulism, whereas the increment at HRs is less marked than in LEMS. In botulism, PTF is less notable and more prolonged than that seen in LEMS and PTE is absent.

There are two types of responses on the RNS test depending on the degree of severity of botulism. In mild forms, the RNS test is characterized by normal CMAP amplitude, a normal response at LRS, and a significant incremental response at HRS. In severe forms, the RNS abnormalities are characterized by a low CMAP amplitude, a normal or decremental response at LRS, and an insignificant incremental response at HRS. Because in botulism the correlation between a reduced CMAP and the clinical state has been a consistent finding, this test can be used as an objective measurement of the severity of disease in the follow-up evaluation.

Other Diseases

The pattern of abnormalities in other NMT diseases is summarized in Table 4.7.

TABLE 4.7. Classical Findings in the RNS Test in Neuromuscular Transmission Diseases

	CMAP					
Diseases	**Rest**	**Exercise**	**LRS**	**HRS**	**PTF**	**PTE**
Normal	N	Same	Same	Same	−	−
Postsynaptic disorders						
Myasthenia gravis	N	Same	↓	↓/same	±	±
Mild	N	Same	↓	Same	+	+
Severe	N	Same	↓	↓	−	−
Anticholinesterase toxicity[a]	RD**	Same	↓	↓	+	+
Presynaptic disorders						
Lambert-Eaton myasthenic syndrome	Low	↑↑	↓	↑↑	+ +	+
Botulism	N/low	↑	↓/same	↑/same	+	−
Mild	N	↑	Same	↑		
Severe	Low	Same	↓	Same		
Combined NMT disorders						
Antibiotic-induced myasthenic syndrome	Low		↓	↓	−	−
Procainamide-induced myasthenic syndrome	Low		↓	↓	−	−

[a] This includes organophosphate poisoning.

N, normal; −, absent; +, mildly present; + +, prominently present; ↓, decremental response; ↑, mild incremental response; ↑↑, marked incremental response; RD, repetitive discharge.

CHAPTER 5

Needle Electromyography Study

Needle electromyography (EMG) is designed to study the physiological and pathophysiological status of muscle function by means of a needle inserted into the muscle being tested. It records the action potentials generated from 5 to 12 muscles fibers in a 1-mm-diameter recording field of muscle through a 0.1-mm-diameter exposed needle tip, under the control of the firing motor unit during minimal and maximal voluntary movement. Thus, it records any change in action potentials due to irritable muscle fiber membrane or to the enlarging or shrinking motor unit territory.

MONOPOLAR AND CONCENTRIC NEEDLES

Two kinds of recording electrodes, concentric and monopolar, are available for the needle EMG study. The concentric needle has an active recording electrode at its center and a surrounding cannula as a reference electrode. The monopolar needle has an exposed Teflon-coated tip as an active recording electrode, with a separate reference electrode (usually a 0.5-mm-diameter surface electrode) being placed on the same muscle near the monopolar recording electrode. There are several differences in physical and physiological characteristics between concentric and monopolar needles (Table 5.1). In general, the monopolar needle is less painful and better tolerated by patients because of its Teflon coating. Less electrically stable, the monopolar needle has a sharper sound than the concentric needle. Because of this audio characteristic and its somewhat larger recording area due to the greater distance between active and reference electrodes, the monopolar needle is more sensitive in detecting fibrillations and positive sharp waves (PSWs).

The most important difference is in the motor unit potentials (MUPs); MUP amplitude is higher and MUP duration is longer with the monopolar needle. The amplitude of MUPs with monopolar needles is about 1.5 times higher than with concentric needles. For this reason, the sensitivity setting for the needle EMG study should be different for the two needles: 50 μV for the concentric needle and 100 μV for the monopolar needle to evaluate resting potentials and 200 μV for the concentric needle and 500 μV for the monopolar needle to evaluate MUP. Although the duration of MUPs with the monopolar needle is longer than with the concentric needle, this difference is not as great as that noted in the MUP amplitude. Thus, the same sweep velocity is used for both needles. The monopolar needle has a larger pickup area because of its larger recording surface (about two to three times larger than the concentric needle) and remote reference electrode. Thus, more distant motor units will contribute to the signal and give rise to a higher amplitude and longer duration than those recorded with the concentric needle. In general, the monopolar needle is popular in the United States, whereas the concentric needle is more commonly used in Europe. In our EMG Laboratory at the University of Alabama at Birmingham (UAB), we prefer the monopolar needle for the routine needle EMG study. There are, however, two specific situations when the concentric needle is mandatory for the needle EMG study. For the quantitative analysis of MUPs, we use a concentric needle because the most commonly used normal data were obtained with a concentric needle. When an isolated MUP from a small deep muscle is needed, we use a concentric needle to avoid any contamination of action potentials from neighboring muscles.

TABLE 5.1. Physical and Physiological Differences Between Monopolar and Concentric Needles

	Monopolar Needle	Concentric Needle
Pickup surface	2–3 times larger	Smaller
Recording area	Variable after repeated use[a]	Constant even after repeated use
Electrical stability	Less, hence noisier	
Sharpness	Sharper and less painful	Less sharp
Patient discomfort	Less painful	More painful
Sensitivity for recording spontaneous activity	Increased[b]	Decreased
CMAP		
Amplitude	1.5–2 times larger	Smaller
Area	1.5 times larger	Smaller
Duration	1.2 times longer	Shorter
Turns	1.2 times more	Fewer
Phases	1.2 times more	Fewer
Polyphasic MUPs (%)	1.5 times higher	Fewer

[a] This is due to the breakdown of Teflon coating.

[b] One study showed that the concentric needle identified more sites with spontaneous activity than did the monopolar needle.

CMAP, compound muscle action potential.

MOTOR UNIT POTENTIALS

The action potential recorded with concentric or monopolar needles is called a MUP or motor unit action potential. Recent studies have suggested that the spike component of MUPs recorded with a concentric needle having a 150 × 580-μm recording surface is generated from 5 to 12 muscle fibers within a radius of 1 mm. Thus, *the MUP represents the summated activity of the muscle fibers in a motor unit but does not represent the activity from all fibers of a motor unit.* Because MUPs are generated with minimal voluntary contraction in which low-threshold small motor neurons are preferentially activated (size principle), type 1 fibers are predominantly responsible for the generation of MUPs.

If the electrode is inside the motor unit territory and outside the end-plate zone, the MUP consists of positive initial and terminal parts with a central component, the main spike, between them (Fig. 5.1). According to Stålberg, the initial part is generated by the approaching volley of action potentials from a large proportion of fibers in the motor unit. The duration of the initial part increases linearly with the distance between the electrode and the end-plate zone. This is explained by the longer conduction time along the muscle fibers. The spike is the sum of the action potentials of muscle fibers closest to the electrode, probably resulting from fewer than 15 fibers in the normal motor unit. The spike usually has one negative peak but may have several peaks. The terminal part is generated by the volley of action potentials leaving the electrode.

Almost all parameters of MUPs are helpful in the diagnosis of neuromuscular disorders because each represents a particular physiological function (Fig. 5.2).

Amplitude

Amplitude is measured from peak to peak. The MUP amplitude (the spike) primarily reflects the summated activity from fibers nearest the tip of the recording electrode. Thus, this parameter is determined by the number and size of the closest fibers and the synchronicity of their action potentials. In normal individuals, the MUP amplitude is relatively constant with minimal variation. With a concentric needle, it ranges from 150 μV to 3 mV and with a monopolar needle, from 300 μV to 5 mV (Table 5.2). In myopathy, the amplitude of MUP is normal or smaller. The amplitude increases after reinnervation, particularly in late stages of disease. Thus, in chronic denervation, the amplitude of MUPs is larger than normal, representing a large motor unit territory.

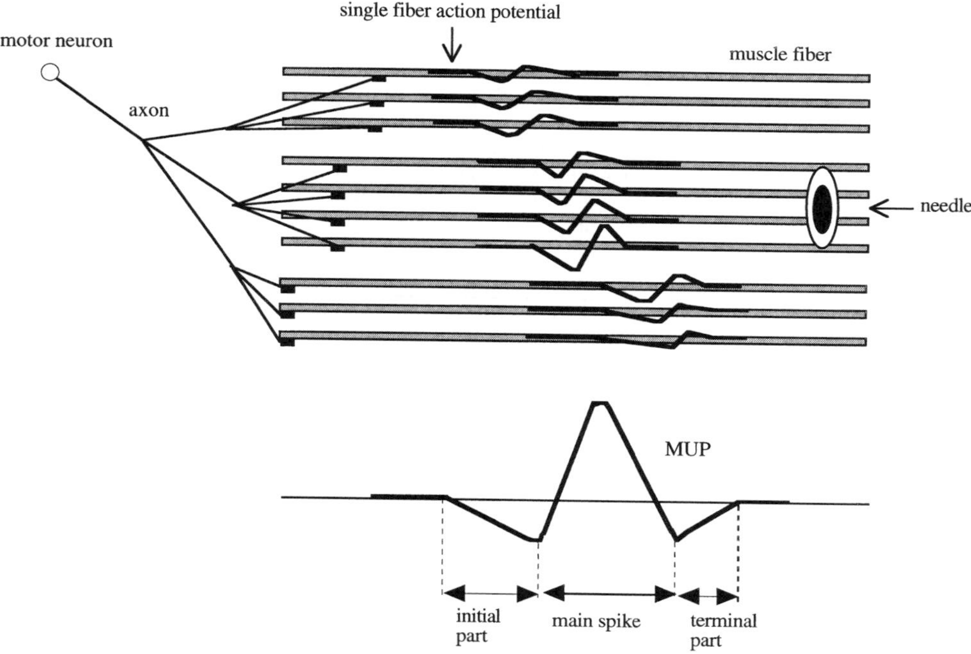

FIGURE 5.1. The contribution of single fiber action potentials to the various part of MUP recorded with a concentric needle electrode.

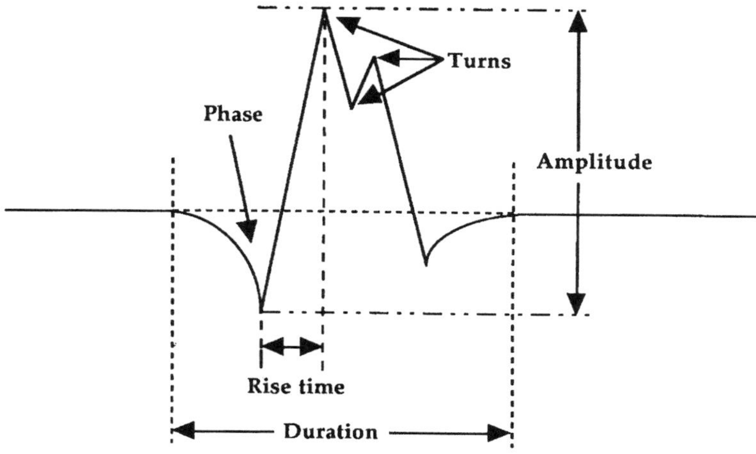

FIGURE 5.2. The various components of motor unit potentials.

Rise Time

This parameter is measured from the initial positive peak to the subsequent negative peak. It is an indicator of the distance between the recording tip of the electrode and the depolarizing muscle fibers: the shorter the rise time, the closer the unit. *The rise time should be less than 500 μs before a MUP is accepted as a genuine near-field MUP.* According to Stålberg, this recommendation is not based on any critical arguments, and MUPs with somewhat longer rise times are also acceptable. *A MUP with a short rise time is characterized by a sharp, crisp sound.*

TABLE 5.2. Normal MUPs[a]

Shape	Usually 2–3 phases; 4 phases are rare
Initial deflection	Any deflection
Duration	6–16 ms
Amplitude	0.5–5 mV with monopolar and 0.3–3.5 mV with concentric needle
Frequency	Depends on degree of effort; 4–5 Hz with minimal contraction to 20–50 Hz with maximal contraction
Sound	Sharp and crisp[b]
Key finding	Regular firing
Generator	Normal fibers near the tip of needle electrode
Significance	Normal

[a] Limb muscles. In facial muscles, MUPs are shorter in duration and smaller in amplitude.

[b] Near-field MUP. Sound of distant MUPs is dull.

Thus, sound characteristics can provide an important clue for recognition of MUPs with a short rise time. If the MUP is associated with a dull sound, the electrode should be adjusted until MUPs with sharp and crisp sounds are detected. The rise time is then measured to determine if the potential is acceptable for assessment of its amplitude and duration.

Duration

Duration is measured from the first deflection of MUPs from the baseline to the last return of MUPs to the baseline. Thus, we are measuring the total duration: the duration of the initial part, the main spike, and the terminal part of a potential. This value depends on the depolarization of many muscle fibers away from and close to the tip of the needle (Fig. 5.1). Most muscle fibers in the motor unit, at least within a radius of 2.5 mm from the electrode, contribute almost equally to the initial and terminal parts despite the fact that the spike of a normal MUP is generated by one to eight muscle fibers closest to the electrode. Thus, unlike the amplitude, the duration of the MUP is significantly affected by distant muscle fibers. According to Stålberg, this value would be more dependent on the number of depolarizing muscle fibers within a restricted area of the motor unit. In normal subjects, the MUP duration is relatively constant with some variation with consecutive firing. Thus, it is important to try to capture the constant MUP duration before measurement. This can be achieved by superimposing the MUPs with a delay line. Some EMG machines have the capability of averaging the duration of 10 to 20 MUPs. This is the most important MUP parameter in differentiation between myopathy and denervation process. The duration of MUPs is shorter in myopathy than in denervation process. In myopathy, some fibers within a motor unit are nonfunctional because of muscle fiber necrosis, and thus the electrode is less likely to record activity from distant fibers. As a consequence, the initial and terminal portions of MUPs are simply not recorded, producing a short-duration MUP. In denervation process, the denervated muscle fibers are reinnervated by surviving motor neurons and a greater number of fibers are activated in a motor unit. The total duration and amplitude of the MUP are also increased.

Phase

Phase refers to the number of potential peaks crossing the baseline (the number of baseline crossings plus one). The shape of the MUP reflects the synchronization (or temporal dispersion) of the individual single-fiber action potentials that are influenced by variability in fiber diameter and fiber density per motor unit. The number of phases in the MUP depends largely on the synchrony of depolarization of the muscle fibers. In normal motor units, the arrival times of the single-fiber potentials at the electrode will be evenly distributed, thus producing a smooth bi- or triphasic MUP. An even distribution of the single-fiber potentials into separate groups and an increased temporal dispersion of the single-fiber potentials can result in an increased number of phases. MUPs with five or more phases are called polyphasic. Up to 12% polyphasic MUPs have been described in normal muscles. We use 20% of MUPs as the criterion for "increased polyphasic MUPs" in a semiquantitative analysis. The percentage of polyphasic MUPs is increased in denervation process and myopathy. An increase in the number of phases has proved to be a good indicator of early reinnervation or myopathy. In myopathy, polyphasic MUPs are short in duration and small in amplitude, whereas in denervation, polyphasic MUPs are long in duration and high in amplitude.

Turns

A turn is defined as a change in the sign of the slope (derivative) of the signal, provided that the amplitude difference between two successive peaks is more than 50 μV. Thus, there could be many turns in a single phase. The concept of phase in the EMG is different from that in EEG, in which phase refers to a "turn." If a MUP has more than five turns, it is called "complex." The physiological and pathophysiological significance of turns is similar to that of phases. Turns are not ordinarily used for routine MUP analysis but are more commonly used in the automated interference analysis of MUPs.

Variability

In normal muscles, the shape of consecutive MUPs from one motor unit is relatively stable. In the routine EMG study, only a large variability of amplitude can be detected. Variability in shape can be seen by means of a triggered and delayed display of the MUPs, but it is difficult to quantify. In 1994, Stålberg et al. introduced the computer technique of quantitative analysis of MUP variability that showed that in normal subjects, the change in absolute amplitude within 3 seconds ranged from 0 to 28% (average 5.8 ± 7.4%). In neuromuscular transmission disorders such as myasthenia gravis (MG), there is a great variability in MUP shape because of "jitter" and "blocking" between individual single-fiber potentials. Not uncommonly, this variability can be detected by visual inspection. The MUPs are more unstable in early reinnervation than in chronic neurogenic conditions, producing MUP variability. Variability can be observed in amyotrophic lateral sclerosis and early reinnervation after nerve injury.

NONPHYSIOLOGICAL FACTORS INFLUENCING MUP PARAMETERS

Type of Needle

This has already been discussed above. The most important difference between the monopolar and concentric needle is the amplitude of MUP, which is 1.5 times larger with a monopolar needle than with a concentric needle. The difference in the MUP duration is not significant between the two kinds of electrodes.

Needle Position

In the MUP analysis, it is important to recognize the MUPs generated from the muscle fibers very near the tip of the needle. Distant MUPs are characterized by their dull sound and slow rise time, whereas nearby MUPs have a crisp and sharp sound and a rise time shorter than 500 μs. A minimal change in needle position can greatly affect the amplitude of MUPs. At a distance of 0.12 mm from the depolarized fibers, the amplitude is decreased by as much as 50% and at 1 mm by an astounding 90%. Therefore, to precisely determine the MUP amplitude, maximum amplitude should be achieved by careful manipulation of needle position.

PHYSIOLOGICAL FACTORS INFLUENCING MUP PARAMETERS AND OTHER EMG POTENTIALS

Temperature

The duration and amplitude of the MUPs increase with decreasing temperatures. The duration of MUPs was found to increase by 5 to 10%/ C decrease in temperature. The MUP amplitude is also known to increase with decreasing temperature. Buchthal et al. also found an increased number of polyphasic MUPs at lower temperatures. On the basis of these findings, Stålberg et al. recommended that the intramuscular temperature should be controlled, if possible. This may be critical if the MUP parameters are compared quantitatively in serial tests. However, in everyday practice, temperature control is not recommended because the changes in the MUP parameters are too minimal to be of clinical significance and most EMG interpretation is based on semiquantitative data. More important in this connection is that fibrillations and PSWs are less easily recordable in severe cold. Thus, it is important to perform the needle EMG at a comfortable room temperature to ensure the adequate recording of fibrillations and PSWs. Unlike fibrillations and PSWs that decrease or disappear altogether with cold, myotonic discharges may be enhanced by lower temperature.

Muscle

The duration of MUPs in normal individuals varies depending on which muscle is tested and on the innervation ratio. In general, smaller muscles have a shorter MUP duration and larger muscles, a longer duration (e.g., 1 to 2 ms for the ocular muscles and 8 to 14 ms for the quadriceps muscle). Thus, one has to be extremely careful in judging myopathy on the basis of MUPs from ocular or facial muscles, because they appear "short" when compared with the MUPs from the limb muscles. For muscles in the lower extremities, the MUP duration tends to be slightly longer than in the upper extremities.

Age

The most important physiological factor for the MUP parameter is age. The duration and amplitude of MUPs increase with age. In general, the duration of MUPs in all muscles increases by 60% from birth to the eighth decade of life, with the most prominent increase occurring in the first decade. From the second decade onward, there is a steady increase in duration up to the eighth decade. On the other hand, Bishoff et al. reported no marked increase of mean duration between ages 20 and 55 years and a slight tendency toward increased MUP duration in subjects older than 55. The amplitude of MUPs increased by 33% between ages 3 months and 20 years but remained constant after age 20. In children from birth to age 3 years, the normal MUP amplitude varied from 100 to 700 μV, and MUPs with an amplitude greater than 1000 μV were rare with a concentric needle. The incidence of polyphasic MUPs increased between infancy and adulthood: from 0.6% in infants to 2.5% in adults in the abductor digiti quinti and biceps muscles. The patient's age must be considered in assessing the incidence of fibrillations in certain muscles. In the intrinsic foot muscles, fibrillations or PSWs were observed in 15 to 29% of control subjects in the 16- to 70-year-old groups, and age was not a significant factor in the frequency of either. However, in the paraspinal muscles, age was clearly a factor. None of the controls under 30 years of age had fibrillations or PSWs in the L4, L5, and S1 paraspinal muscles, but 32% of those over age 40 had fibrillations or PSWs.

REQUIREMENTS OF THE NEEDLE EMG TEST

Patient Cooperation

The most important requirement of a successful needle EMG study is the patient's cooperation, which is needed from the beginning to the end of testing. To observe abnormal spontaneous potentials at rest, the muscles have to be completely relaxed. To ascertain the various parameters of MUPs, each MUP should be isolated from others. To obtain a genuine interference pattern, the full maximal contraction is needed. Because of its invasiveness, the needle EMG test is painful and the patient's full cooperation is not always guaranteed. However, in general, this test is well tolerated by adults, but it is usually not possible to do a completely satisfactory EMG study in young children because of pain. This is a definite but inherent limitation in pediatric EMG. To secure the best possible cooperation of the patient, it is important to explain the procedure in very simple terms before the test begins.

Accurate Clinical Assessment of the Patient's Problem

The second most important requirement for a successful needle EMG is the examiner's accurate clinical assessment of the patient's problem. For the nerve conduction study (NCS) and repetitive nerve stimulation (RNS) tests, the standard methods and normal values are relatively well established. However, with the needle EMG, the results depend heavily on the electromyographer's clinical and technical expertise. By means of the patient's history and examination, the examiner must form a tentative working diagnosis and consider the possibility of differential diagnoses before proceeding with the actual needle examination. Only then can the physician choose which muscles to test and what to look for during the test. In general, we recommend the following guidelines in this regard: the muscle with the greatest probability of abnormality and crucial diagnostic information should be studied first, (e.g., the paraspinal muscles for radiculopathy and the proximal muscles for myopathy) and the most clinically involved muscles should be studied first, followed by the most affected muscles. This is done because the most clinically involved muscles have the best chance of showing abnormality. One exception to this rule is muscles showing end-stage atrophy. In these muscles, because of extensive fibrosis, it is often impossible to obtain EMG abnormalities representative of disease. During the test, the electromyographer should always be prepared to change the test strategy depending on the findings. Once the test is performed, the EMG findings must be interpreted in light of the clinical findings because no EMG results are pathognomonic of a specific disease entity. For these reasons, it is essential that the clinical problem is assessed thoroughly and that a careful neurological examination is performed before the electrophysiological study.

Delay Line and Duration Measurement

The various parameters of the MUPs are important in assessing abnormality of the needle EMG findings. To measure these, it is essential to isolate a single MUP from other MUPs and confirm the consistency of the shape. For this purpose, the delay line on the EMG machine is used. In this way, the entire MUP can be recorded every time it appears and in the same position on the oscilloscope screen by delaying each MUP after it has triggered the sweep. This permits accumulation of the desired number of potentials and measurement of the MUP parameters in a short time. Thus, the delay line is an essential component for the quantitative analysis of MUPs in the needle EMG and is a desirable tool for the semiquantitative analysis of MUPs. Once a single MUP is isolated, there must be either an automatic or a manual capability for electronic measurement of duration on the EMG machine.

NEEDLE EMG TECHNIQUE

1. Explain the procedure to the patient using the simplest language. Because the needle EMG requires painful needling and the full cooperation of the patient for all phases of the test, it is important to explain the procedure using the simplest language. In our laboratory at the UAB, we usually describe the needle EMG test as follows: "We will cleanse the skin with alcohol and insert a very fine needle directly into the muscle being tested. The EMG test shows how the muscles react to commands. Upon insertion of the needle you may feel some pain, depending on the sensitivity of the area being tested." Especially with the paraspinal EMG, it is important to explain to the patient that the needle does not go into the spinal canal but into the muscle. Also, be sure that the patient understands that nothing is being injected into the muscle through the needle.
2. Place the patient in a relaxed and comfortable position both for the patient and the examiner. Usually, the needle EMG is best done with the patient lying down. Depending on the part of the body being tested, the patient is positioned so as to achieve maximal relaxation of the tested muscles. There are no set rules for this, but the techniques must be learned from an experienced electromyographer or gained from experience. For the lumbar and cervical paraspinal EMG, for example, it is best for the patient to be lying in the "fetal position" on one side with the side to be tested uppermost.
3. Once the EMG procedure has been explained and the patient is positioned comfortably, the EMG needle is inserted through the skin briskly with one quick thrust into the muscle to be tested. This technique usually produces the least pain. Several handy references are available for anatomical guidance in performing the needle EMG. It is usually a good idea to consult these references when in doubt about the location of a specific muscle. However, it is always important to verify the exact location of EMG needle. To do this,

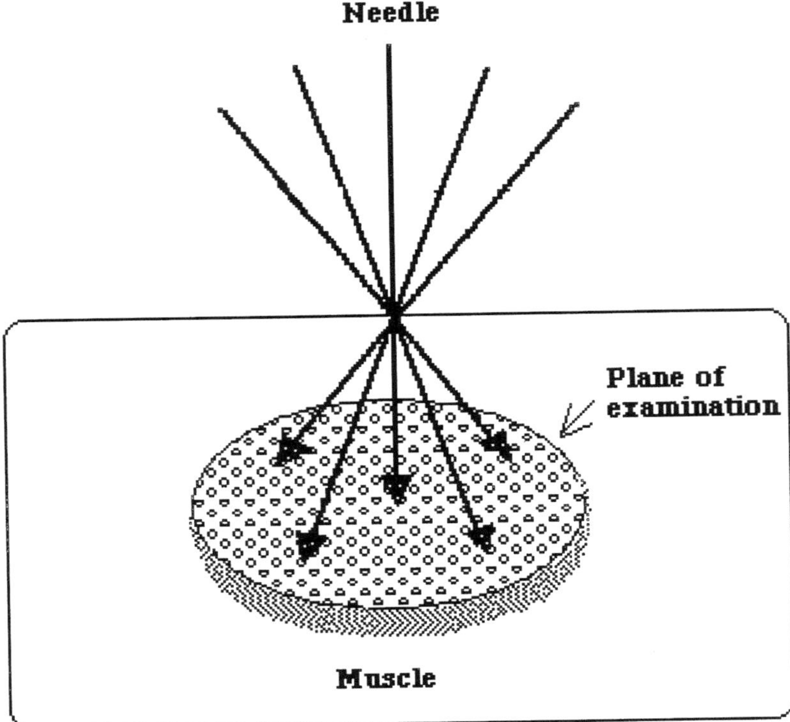

FIGURE 5.3. Recommended position of the needle position during the EMG needle examination at the single puncture site.

the examiner asks the patient to move the tested muscle minimally. If crisp-sounding MUPs are produced, one can be assured that the EMG needle is in the right muscle.

4. Once the needle is inserted into a muscle, four different quadrants of the muscle sphere must be studied at various depths (Fig. 5.3). This guarantees a random selection of various MUPs from the muscle. Depending on the muscle size and the degree of EMG abnormality, the electromyographer must decide how many needlings must be done in a single muscle. At least two needling sites in the same muscle are recommended before the EMG is considered "normal."

NEEDLE EMG STUDY

The needle EMG study consists of three parts: observation at rest, MUP on minimal voluntary contraction, and the recruitment pattern of MUPs on maximal contraction. Machine settings for each part of needle EMG study are different (Table 5.3). This is to obtain the various EMG potentials as best as one can.

Muscle Activity at Rest

Normal muscle is quiet because no MUP is generated. To study spontaneous potentials adequately, the muscle has to be completely relaxed. Sometimes, complete relaxation of muscles is not easily achieved because of pain caused by the EMG needle. An experienced electromyographer develops his or her own tricks over the years to achieve complete relaxation of certain muscles. In general, the first rule is that the patient has to be placed in the most comfortable position for the test. For example, for the lumbar needle EMG, the patient lies on the side opposite that is to be tested, assuming the lumbar puncture position. The second rule is to give the patient specific instructions about relaxation, rather than simply telling him or her

TABLE 5.3. Typical Machine Settings for the Needle EMG

	At Rest	Minimal Contraction	Maximal Contraction	Quantitative MUP Analysis[a]
Sweep velocity (ms)	10	10	100	10
Sensitivity (μV)				
Monopolar	100	500–1000	1000	
Concentric	50	200–500	500	100
Filter				
High (kHz)	10	10	10	10
Low (Hz)	2–20	2–20	2–20	2
Audio	On	On	On	On
Delay line	Off	On	Off	On

[a] Buchthal's method.

to "relax." For example, for the lumbar EMG, the examiner may tell the patient. "Push your belly back toward me," placing his or her hand on the belly to promote relaxation of the lumbar paraspinal muscles. Relaxation may also be achieved by gentle manipulation or passive positioning of the extremities. Occasionally, it can be obtained by gentle activation of an antagonistic muscle; for example, to test the cervical paraspinal muscles, the examiner may ask the patient to rest his or her head gently on the examiner's fist, which is placed under the chin. Sometimes, for anxious adults and children, pharmacological intervention is needed. For adults, we recommend Valium 5 mg by mouth 30 minutes before the test. For children, we recommend chloral hydrate at a dose of 60 to 70 mg/kg/body weight, 30 minutes before the test. The needle EMG should be performed after the nerve conduction study, so that MUPs can be evaluated at the end of the study when the child is more aroused. When the needle EMG is to be performed in the tongue muscle, local xylocaine gel is applied locally to induce a local anesthetic effect.

Insertion activity and spontaneous potentials are studied at rest. Insertion activity is the electrical response of muscle membrane to the insertion of the EMG needle. In normal individuals, insertion activity disappears as soon as the needle movement stops. When the insertion activity persists beyond the cessation of needle movement, it is described as increased. Thus, insertion activity is usually increased when abnormal spontaneous activity is present. Sometimes, insertion activity may be increased, but not long enough to clearly record abnormal spontaneous activity. An increase in insertion activity is usually the first EMG clue to suggest the presence of abnormal spontaneous potentials in the muscle (Table 5.4). Thus, when increased insertion activity is encountered, the examiner must spend more time and examine more sites before determining no abnormal spontaneous potentials. When insertion activity is not elicited on needle movement, as if the EMG were going through fatty or connective tissue rather than muscle, it is described as decreased. Before confirming decreased insertion activity, however, the examiner must be sure that the EMG needle is indeed in the muscle and not in the subcutaneous fatty tissue. Increased insertion activity alone without fibrillations, PSWs, or myotonic potentials is not clinically important. On the other hand, decreased insertion activity is clinically significant because it is indicative of fibrosis or fatty replacement of muscle. Electrical silence of muscles is seen in periodic paralysis during paralysis and in McArdle's disease during contracture. One has to remember that rare fibrillations or PSWs may be observed even in an area of decreased insertion activity. Thus, one is not exclusive of the other.

Spontaneous potentials are defined as any activity that persists beyond the cessation of needle insertion long enough to be recorded without undue difficulty. There are two normal spontaneous potentials: end-plate noise and end-plate spikes (nerve potentials) occurring at the end plate. Often the patient feels "tingling" or "pain" when these normal spontaneous potentials are observed, especially with end-plate spikes. Their sounds and shapes are characteristic enough to be easily and clearly recognizable. End-plate noise is the irregular continu-

TABLE 5.4. Insertion Activity

Increased insertion activity (hyperexcitable muscle membrane)
- Abnormal spontaneous potentials (fibrillation, positive sharp waves, myotonic potentials, or complex repetitive discharges) are present

Decreased insertion activity (decreased muscle membrane irritability)
- Fibrosis of muscle
- Fatty replacement of muscle
- Periodic paralysis during paralysis[a]
- McArdle's disease during contracture[a]
- Rippling myopathy during "rippling"[a]

[a] "Silent MUPs": MUPs are not generated.

TABLE 5.5. End-Plate Noise (Monophasic End-Plate Activity)

Shape	Monophasic low-amplitude potentials with initial negative deflection in a dense steady pattern
Initial deflection	Negative
Duration	0.5–1 ms
Amplitude	10–20 μV (may go up to 100 μV)
Frequency	Continuous irregular noise; difficult to distinguish each potential
Sound	Sound of seashell held to the ear; "seashell roar" or "noise"
Key finding	Irregular low amplitude "seashell" noise localized to the end-plate area; the patient sometimes feels pain
Generator	Extracellular recording of spontaneous miniature end-plate potentials
Significance	Normal

TABLE 5.6. End-Plate Spike (Nerve Potential; Biphasic End-Plate Activity)

Shape	Biphasic potential with initial negative deflection
Initial deflection	Negative
Duration	2–4 ms
Amplitude	100–300 μV
Frequency	Rapid irregular firing at 50–100 Hz
Sound	"Sputtering fat in a frying pan"
Key finding	Biphasic potentials with initial negative deflection and a distinct sound localized to the end-plate area; the patient usually feels distinct pain
Generator	Mechanical activation of an intramuscular nerve terminal with secondary discharge of muscle fibers
Significance	Normal

ous low-voltage short-duration waves with "sea-shell sounds" and "thickened baseline appearance," representing spontaneous miniature end-plate potentials (Table 5.5 and Fig. 5.4). End-plate spikes (nerve potential) are irregularly firing brief spikes with a sound like the "sputtering of fat in a frying pan." (Table 5.6 and Fig. 5.5). The most important criterion for recognition of these normal spontaneous potentials is the initial negative deflection, because almost all pathological spontaneous potentials have an initial positive deflection. Thus, *one rule to remember is that any spontaneous potential with an initial negative deflection should not be regarded as "abnormal."*

There are six abnormal spontaneous potentials to look for at rest: fibrillations, PSWs, fasciculations, myokymic potentials, complex repetitive discharges, and myotonic potentials. *It is important to allow sufficient pause between each needle movement to observe abnormal spontaneous potentials*—a pause of 1 to 2 seconds for fibrillations and PSWs. For fasciculations, this time is less than adequate and a longer time lapse is usually needed—sometimes 10 to 15 seconds for adequate documentation of fasciculations. A shorter pause between needle movements

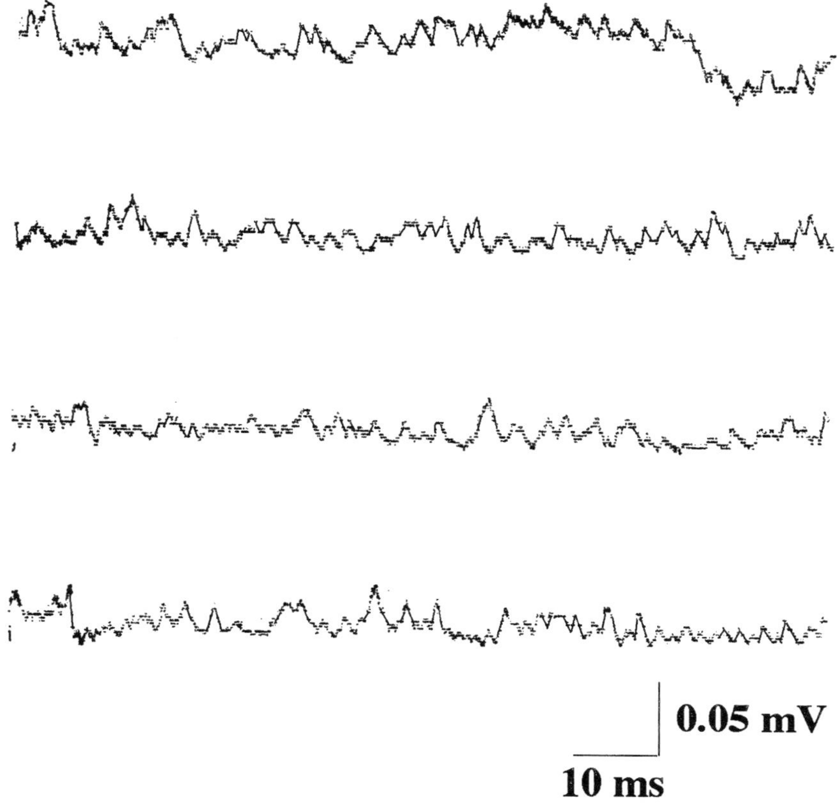

FIGURE 5.4. End-plate noise characterized by monophasic low-amplitude irregular potentials with initial deflection.

is the most common technical source of error for missing fibrillations, PSWs, and fasciculations by the inexperienced electromyographer. Abnormal spontaneous potentials are present at rest but also may be induced or accentuated by needle movement or tapping with the finger. In milder cases, abnormal spontaneous potentials are caused only by needle movement or tapping the muscle. Thus, it is important to "wiggle" and move the needle around the insertion site and to tap the muscle to activate fibrillation or PSWs. Abnormal spontaneous potentials are often more easily generated in some areas than in others, especially in milder cases. This means that the examiner must test more than one site before making a final judgment.

MUP on Minimal Voluntary Contraction

Voluntary activity of muscles is assessed during three stages of contraction: mild, moderate, and maximal or full contraction. With mild contraction, only a few MUPs are observed, usually firing at 4 to 5 Hz. These are of relatively smaller amplitude because these units are recruited first, as discussed previously.

Not all MUPs are adequate for the needle EMG study. Once the EMG needle is inserted into the muscle, it is necessary to position the needle tip as closely as possible to the fiber generating the MUPs being studied. These must be genuine near-field MUPs that are generated at the tip of the needle because distant MUPs have different parameters, especially amplitude. As the "firing" muscle fibers are approached, the sounds of the MUPs become sharper and crisper, and as the amplitude increases, the duration decreases with a shorter rise time. *Genuine near-field MUPs can be recognized by their sharp, crisp sound and short rise time (usually*

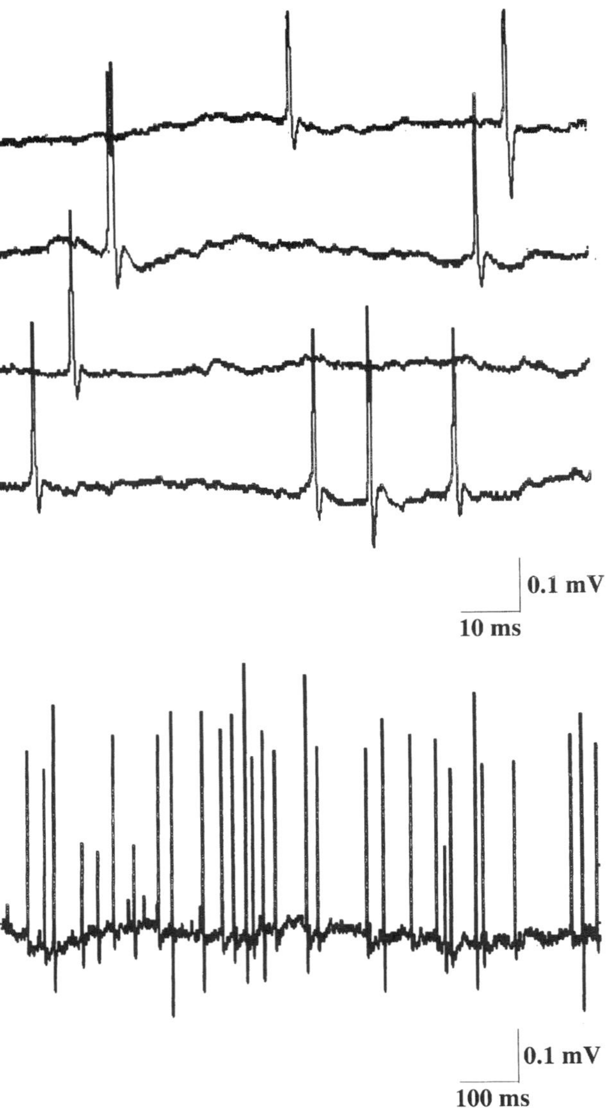

FIGURE 5.5. End-plate spike with initial negative deflection and irregular firing. Notice also the end-plate noise as the baseline.

<500 μs) (Fig. 5.6). On the other hand, more distant MUPs produce a characteristically dull sound and have a longer duration and slower rise time (usually >500 μs).

Because the various parameters of the MUP are important in assessing abnormality, it is important to isolate a single MUP from other MUPs. This is not always easy. However, delicate manipulation of the electrode and a carefully controlled volitional effort by the subject will usually produce success in the isolation of a single MUP, even without a delay line. With the additional help of the delay line, which is commonly available on modern EMG machines, this task is easier. Once a MUP is isolated, it is useful to "freeze" or store the MUPs on the screen so that their rise time, phase, amplitude, and duration can be analyzed. Some EMG machines have the capability of automatic MUP analysis of MUP. However, this automatic

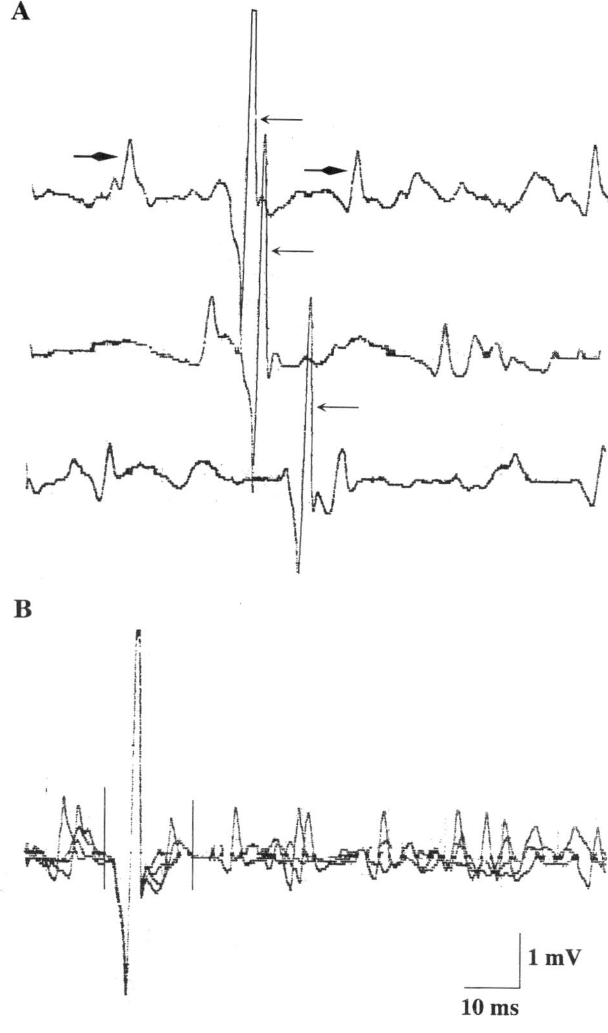

FIGURE 5.6. Near-field MUP and distant MUPs. **A.** Thin arrows indicate near-field MUPs. Notice the rapid rise time. Thick arrows indicate distant MUPs. **B.** A near-field MUP is isolated with triggering point. Duration is indicated by two vertical lines. Notice a random firing of distant MUPs.

analysis is not always accurate, and it is always safer to assess its accuracy and be ready to adjust the measurement if necessary.

An adequate number of MUPs must be obtained to answer specific clinical questions. Thus, depending on the clinical assessment of the patient, the electromyographer must decide how many MUPs to examine in each muscle. In obvious cases of myopathy or chronic denervation, not too many MUPs may be needed to reach a final clinical conclusion. However, many MUPs may have to be obtained when there is a mixed pattern of myopathy and denervation or in mild cases of myopathy and denervation.

For the quantitative MUP analysis, at least 20 MUPs should be analyzed in each muscle for an adequate needle EMG study (see below). This is not practical for the routine needle EMG test. The most commonly used method of interpreting the needle EMG findings is by qualitative visual assessment (qualitative MUP analysis). The qualitative MUP analysis is based primarily on the detection of a few MUPs of definitely abnormal duration, amplitude, or number of phases.

For the routine EMG study, we generally recommend obtaining at least 10 MUPs in one muscle and measuring the shortest and longest duration and the smallest and highest amplitude of MUPs. Visual scanning of 10 MUPs in one muscle is not difficult and can be achieved in a short time. The measurement of duration and amplitude of two extreme values is a reasonable compromise and gives the examiner the range of MUP duration and amplitude. We have found this practice useful and practical in most routine EMG studies. Stålberg proposed the use of "outlier MUPs" (the value of a parameter that was never exceeded by more than two values in a healthy muscle) as the criterion of MUP abnormality. He found that no normal muscles had more than two outlier MUPs and that "outliers" were as sensitive as mean values in neuropathies and even more sensitive in myopathies. According to this criterion, if at least three "outliers" (definitely short-duration or long-duration MUPs) are observed, one can conclude that the MUPs are abnormal. Thus, if an increased number of outliers is detected after only a few MUPs have been obtained, it is not necessary to obtain all 20 MUPs before reaching a conclusion. This method decreases the investigator's time as well as the patient's discomfort, and we recommend the three-outlier method as a practical means of MUP analysis.

Recruitment Pattern of MUPs on Moderate and Maximal Contractions The next step of the needle EMG is to check the firing rate of MUPs on moderate contraction and the interference pattern on maximal contraction of muscles. To do this, the sweep velocity should be set to 100 ms per division and the "envelope" of MUPs is measured from peak to peak. Then it is possible to determine the firing rate of an individual MUP and whether the interference pattern is reduced or normal.

In normal muscles, increasing voluntary contraction increases the firing rate of single MUPs and recruits additional new MUPs. The average motor unit begins firing at a rate of about 5 Hz (200-ms inter-MUP interval). This rate increases to 25 to 50 Hz with increased effort. In practice, it is often difficult to estimate the firing rate of a single MUP when it exceeds 10 to 15 Hz because an additional motor unit is recruited. With moderate contraction, the firing rate of MUPs goes up and more MUPs are recruited. The MUPs seen at this stage are higher in amplitude than those seen with minimal contraction, and they fire at higher frequencies, usually at 10 to 15 Hz. An individual MUP can be still recognized, however. Thus, it is best to assess the firing rate and recruitment of MUPs with moderate contraction. With maximal contraction, the firing rate of MUPs increases further, reaching 40 to 50 Hz, and many MUPs fire together, rendering it impossible to evaluate a single MUP in isolation because of the overlapping of MUPs. Instead, many MUPs are meshed together to form an "envelope." In normal subjects, the entire screen is filled with MUPs to show a thick envelope of uniform amplitude. This is termed "full or complete interference pattern" (Fig. 5.7). When there is a loss of MUPs in any disease process, the number of recruited MUPs is reduced, producing a gap in the envelope of MUPs. This is termed "reduced interference pattern" (Fig. 5.8). A single MUP firing in the extreme loss of MUPs is termed a "discrete pattern" and shows a typical "picket-fence appearance" (Fig. 5.8). In the denervation process, to maintain a certain force, the existing MUPs fire at an inappropriately rapid rate (<20 Hz for onset firing rate and <30 Hz for recruitment firing rate) to compensate for the reduced number of motor units. In practice, the firing rate has to be assessed for a single MUP on minimal contraction. There are two ways to measure the firing rate of MUP: onset and recruitment firing rates. Onset firing rate refers to firing rate of a single MUP at onset of firing and recruitment firing rate to firing rate of the initial MUP at the time of recruitment of a second MUP. Onset and recruitment firing rates vary from muscle to muscle. The average onset firing rate is 7.5 Hz and the average recruitment firing rate 11 Hz. Thus, when the firing rate of a single MUP exceeds 20 Hz for onset firing rate and 30 Hz for the recruitment firing rate, then it is strongly indicative of the denervation process (Fig. 5.9).

In assessing a reduced interference pattern, the electromyographer must assess the various factors involved in producing maximal effort. Even in normal individuals with good coopera-

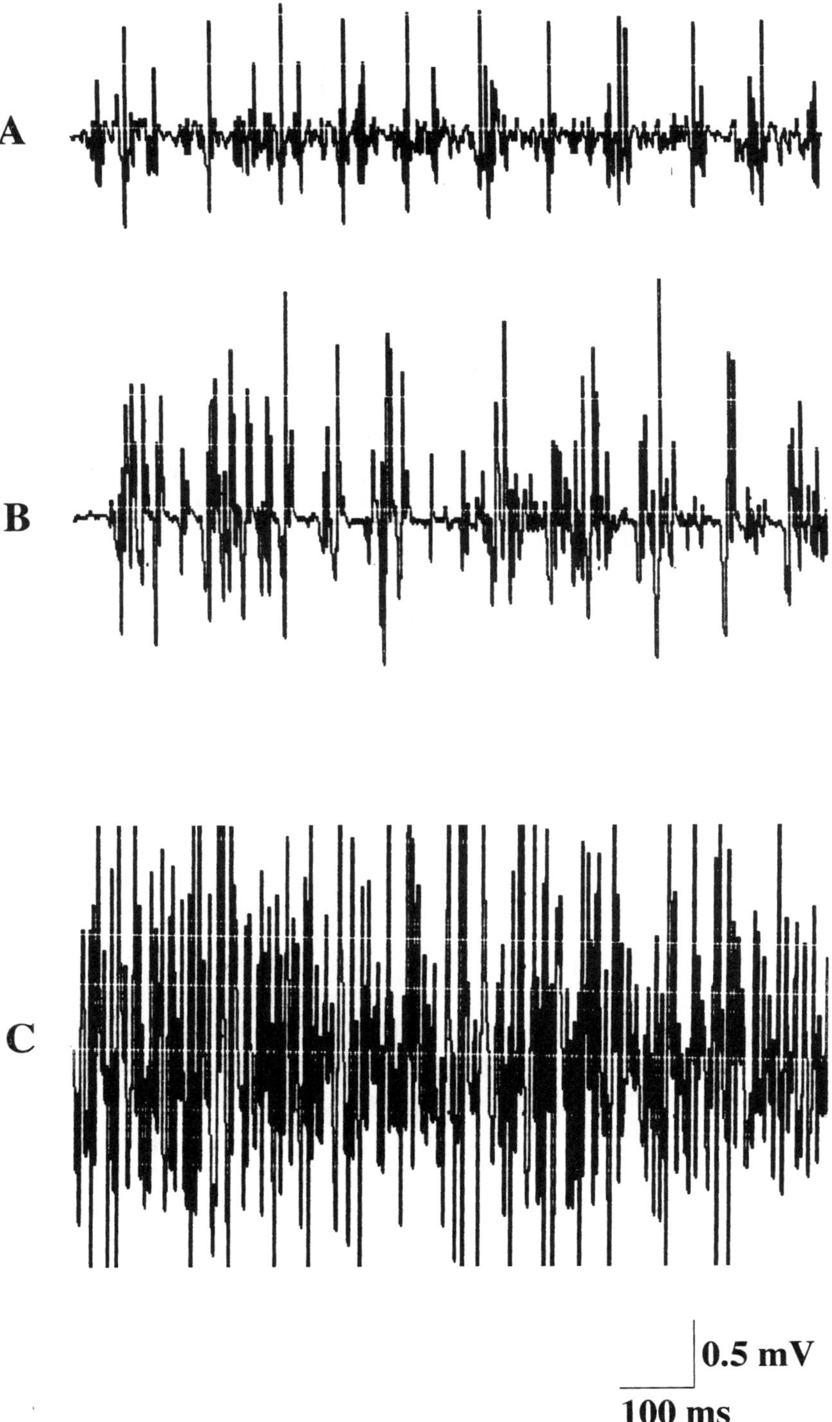

FIGURE 5.7. Gradual recruitment of MUPs during muscle contraction in normal subject from minimal contraction (**A**) to the maximal contraction (**C**) through moderate contraction (**B**). Notice recruitment of higher amplitude MUPs with stronger contraction.

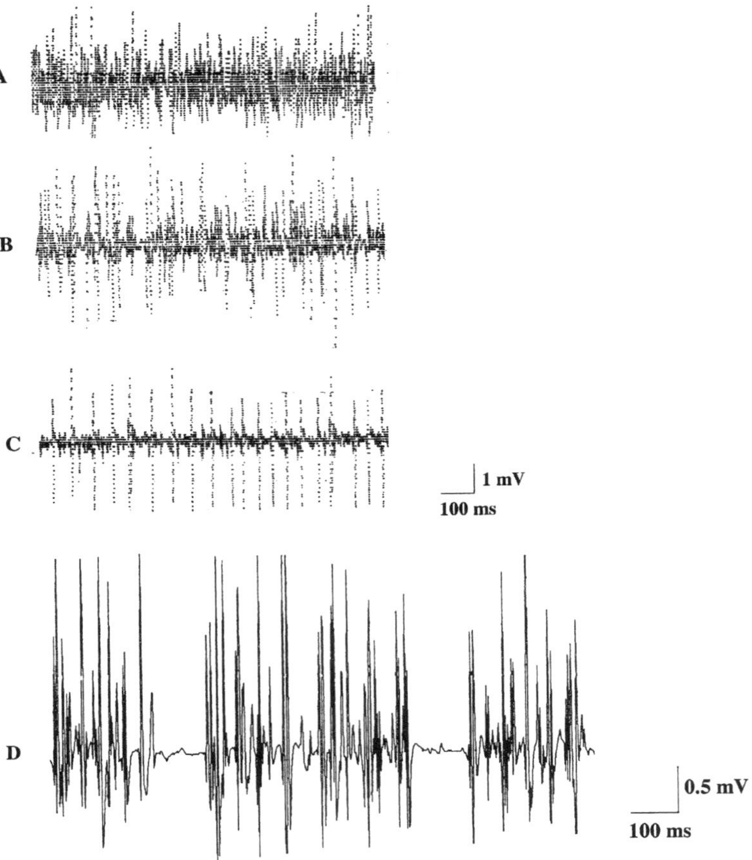

FIGURE 5.8. Different patterns of interference pattern. **A.** Full interference pattern. **B.** Reduced interference pattern. **C.** Discrete activity. **D.** Jerky interference pattern in hysterical weakness.

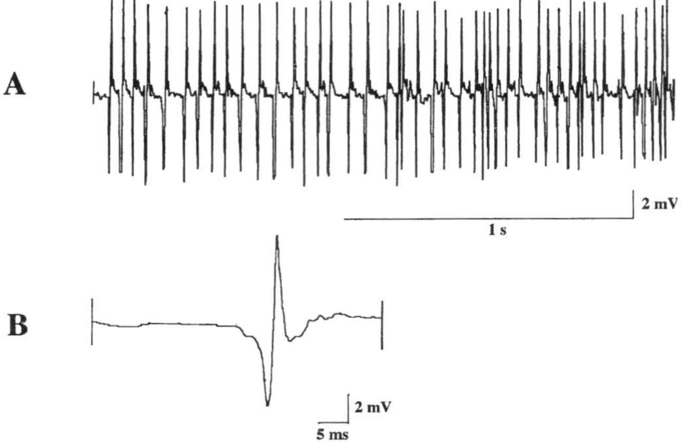

FIGURE 5.9. **A.** Rapid-onset firing (23 Hz) of a high-amplitude MUP (**B**) in a case with multifocal motor neuropathy.

tion, a full interference pattern is not observed in certain muscles (e.g., the gluteus muscles, the quadriceps muscles in the supine position, and the gastrocnemius and soleus muscles). The most common cause of reduced interference pattern in our experience is poor effort by the patient because of pain or lack of cooperation. Another rare cause of reduced interference pattern is "functional weakness" associated with a conversion reaction or malingering (Fig. 5.8). Thus, it is important to consider the degree of patient cooperation before judging the significance of the interference pattern. In upper motor neuron disorders, interference pattern is also reduced. A helpful distinction between denervation process and nondenervation processes that produce a reduced interference pattern is the firing rate of a single MUP; in denervation, the firing rate is fast, whereas in an upper motor neuron lesion or functional weakness, it is slow. However, in practice, it is not easy to distinguish between these two. Because of these limitations, the interference pattern is regarded as the least helpful needle EMG finding and a reduced interference pattern alone should not be regarded as pathognomonic of denervation. A reduced interference pattern together with other evidence of denervation is meaningful.

Classically, in all denervation disorders, the interference pattern is reduced or discrete because of the reduced recruitment of MUPs on maximal contraction. The degree of reduced interference pattern is supposed to correlate with the degree of muscle weakness, assuming that the patient is genuinely making a maximal effort. On the other hand, the examiner may encounter situations where a reduced interference pattern is the only EMG abnormality (e.g., in early denervation in which fibrillations or PSWs have not developed or in pure demyelinating neuropathy in which axonal degeneration is lacking). As a rule, in chronic denervation, high-amplitude MUPs are recruited earlier than normal MUPs and usually fire at a faster rate. Thus, on minimal or moderate contraction, fast-firing high-amplitude MUPs are easily recruited in chronic denervation. In myopathy, the interference pattern is normal and of low amplitude, because of the excessive or early recruitment of MUPs. In such cases, many motor units must fire to generate minimal power because of scattered loss of individual muscle fibers and relative preservation of the motor units. Thus, the classic pattern in myopathy is a full interference pattern with minimal or moderate effort due to the early recruitment of MUPs.

In the clinical setting, there are only two situations when an interference pattern is helpful: the early recruitment of small MUPs indicative of myopathy and the early recruitment and faster firing rate of high-amplitude MUPs indicative of chronic denervation.

EMG POTENTIALS

Fibrillations

Fibrillations are the most important potentials in the needle EMG (Fig. 5.10). Fibrillations are biphasic or triphasic, short-duration (<2 ms), low-amplitude (<100 μV) potentials with an initial positive sharp deflection (Table 5.7). Fibrillations, which are usually detectable by a needle EMG study in the muscle 2 weeks after denervation, represent the action potentials of single muscle fibers that are spontaneously twitching in the absence of innervation as an expression of denervation hypersensitivity. The most important criteria for recognition of fibrillations are the initial positive deflection and regular firing. There is also a characteristic sound like "rain drops on a tin roof." Two other potentials showing an initial positive deflection are end-plate spikes (nerve potentials) with initial positive deflection and "artifact potentials" from "time-locked pacemakers" or stimulators that produce potentials with an initial positive deflection (see below). End-plate spikes classically have an initial negative deflection, but on rare occasions end-plate spikes with an initial positive deflection are observed (Fig. 5.11). Regardless of the initial deflection, they have the characteristic sound of "sputtering fat in a frying pan." Thus, end-plate spikes with initial positive deflections can be differentiated from fibrillations by their characteristic sound and irregular firing. A potential with an initial negative deflection is not fibrillation. Another important point to remember is that although each single fibrillation fires at a regular rate, many fibrillations firing at the same time sound like irregular firing because their firing rates are different. Rarely, fibrillations

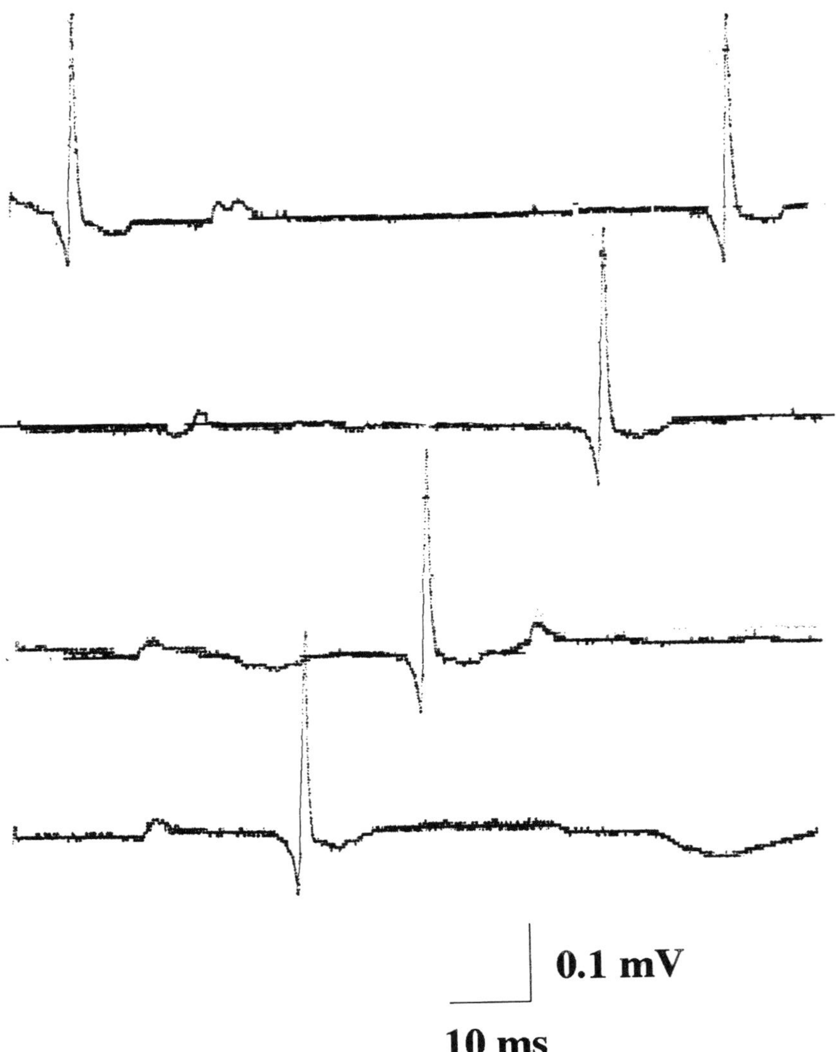

FIGURE 5.10. Fibrillations. Notice an initial positive deflection and regular firing.

may have an amplitude greater than 1 mV. These have been called "giant fibrillations" and are only observed in chronic denervation, according to our experience (Fig. 5.12).

For fibrillations and PSWs to be considered clinically significant, two criteria must be met. First, spontaneous activity must be recorded away from the end-plate region. This is necessary because end-plate spikes with an initial positive deflection may be mistaken for fibrillations if the characteristic sound is not heeded. Second, spontaneous activity must be recorded in at least two muscle sites because fibrillations in one site have been found in 4% of normal muscles.

Fibrillations and PSWs are the cardinal signs of denervation process, representing axonal degeneration. The degree of fibrillations and PSWs is a rough estimate of the number of denervated muscle fibers. However, they are not pathognomonic of denervation because they are also observed in active myopathy and myotonia. One may argue that myopathy may represent "denervation" when muscle fibers are sectioned transversely or divided longitudi-

TABLE 5.7. Fibrillation

Shape	Biphasic or triphasic with initial sharp positive wave followed by sharp negative wave
Initial deflection	Positive
Duration	1–5 ms (usually closer to 1–2 ms)
Amplitude	10–200 μV with concentric needle 20–600 μV with monopolar needle (usually under 100 μV)
Frequency	Regular, 1–50 Hz (usually close to 10 Hz)
Sound	"Raindrops on tin roof"
Key finding	Initial positive deflection with regular firing at rest
Generator	Fibrillating single muscle fiber
Significance	Hyperirritable membrane; usually means active denervation and myotonia but can occur in active myopathy
Diseases (essential)[a]	Amyotrophic lateral sclerosis, axonal neuropathy, and active myopathy
Diseases (common)[b]	Radiculopathy, plexopathy, mononeuropathy Myotonic syndromes, inclusion body myopathy, polymyositis, acid maltase deficiency, botulism, myotubular myopathy

[a] Diseases in which this potential is essential for diagnosis.
[b] Diseases with which this potential is commonly associated.

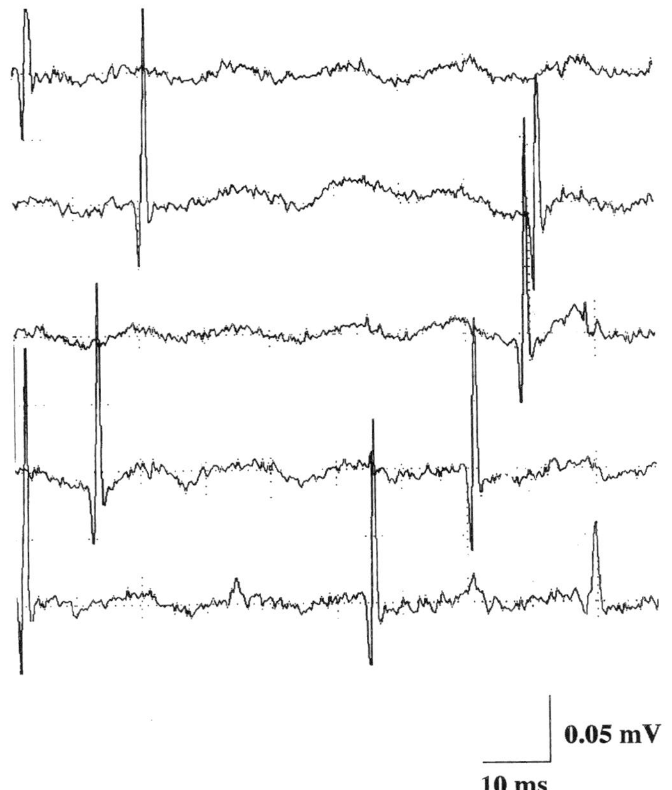

FIGURE 5.11. End-plate spike (nerve potential) with initial positive deflection. The sound of these potentials is the same with the classic end-plate spike with initial negative deflection. Notice also the end plate noise as the baseline.

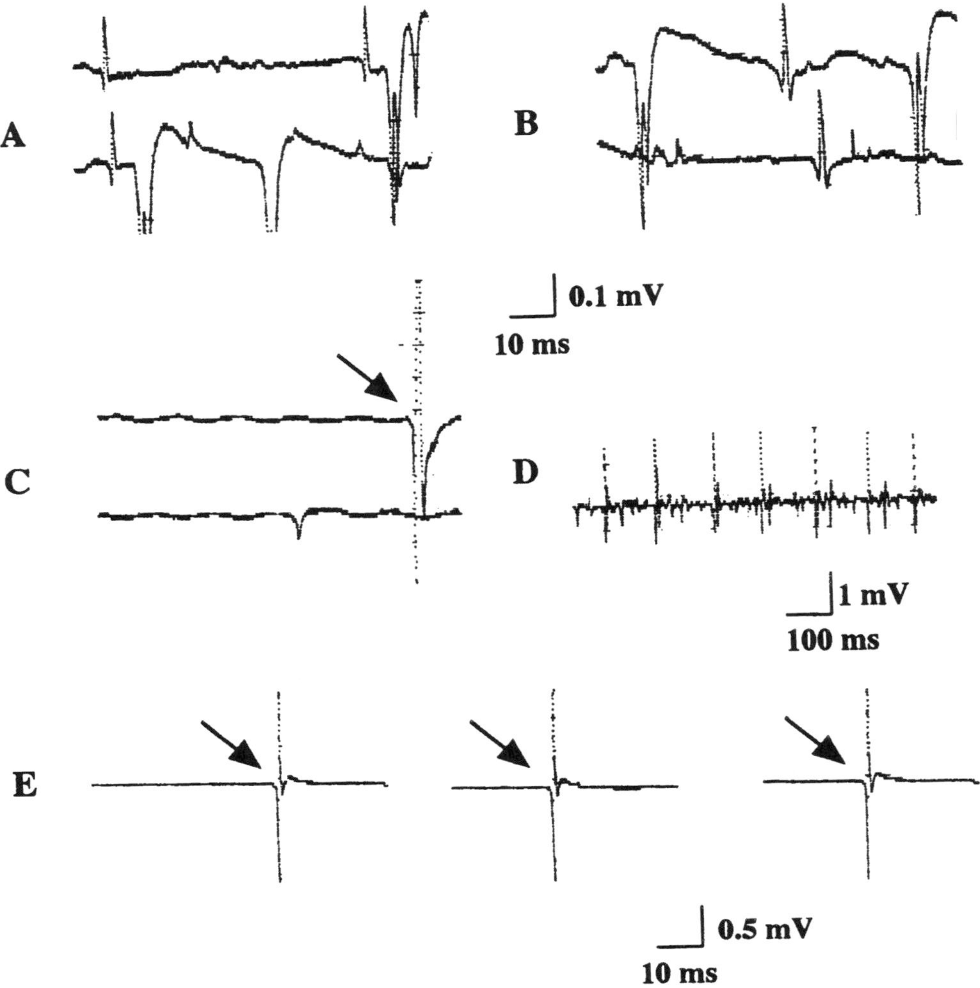

FIGURE 5.12. Giant fibrillations in a case of chronic inflammatory demyelinating polyneuropathy (CIDP). **A–C.** Fibrillations and positive sharp waves. **C.** A giant fibrillation (*arrow*). **D.** Regular firing of a giant fibrillation. **E.** Giant fibrillations (*arrows*).

nally in myopathy. However, it is more likely that fibrillations and PSWs in active myopathy and myotonia represent "hyperexcitable membrane." This conclusion is based on the observation that fibrillations and PSWs are detectable early in rhabdomyolysis, long before the required 10 to 14 days for denervation.

In cases of nerve injury, time and distance are two important factors for fibrillations and PSWs. The earliest significant objective evidence of denervation is the transient appearance of PSWs after insertion or movement of the needle electrode. Positive sharp waves appear 8 to 14 days after injury and spontaneous fibrillations within 2 to 4 weeks after injury, occurring first in the muscles just distal to the injury.

Fibrillations and PSWs are not always present, even in denervation process. Lambert described five circumstances under which they may be absent: insufficient time (2 to 4 weeks) having elapsed for degeneration of the nerve to appear, primarily demyelinating neuropathy (conduction block) without secondary axonal degeneration, too low temperature of the muscle or poor circulation, severe atrophy or degeneration of the muscle fibers, and reinnervation already in progress.

In grading fibrillations and PSWs, every authority agrees on four grading scales, from + to + + + +, although their specific criteria may be different (Table 5.8 and Fig. 5.13). However, in general, the criteria are based on the frequency of potentials by site and by firing rate and thus reflect quite well the severity of the lesion.

Another important point to remember with regard to fibrillations and PSWs is that they are present in certain muscles in a substantial number of asymptomatic subjects. In the intrinsic foot muscles, fibrillations and PSWs were reported in 6 to 29% of normal subjects. In the lumbar paraspinal muscles, fibrillations and PSWs were detected in 15% of normal subjects and in about 30% of an older group above 40 years of age. Thus, fibrillations and PSWs in these muscles are not necessarily indicative of denervation process. Therefore, their presence should be interpreted in the clinical context. Because of the difficulty of interpretation, in practice it is best to avoid the needle EMG in the intrinsic muscles of the foot if possible.

In recent years, there has been an increasing number of patients who use cardiac pacemakers, spinal cord epidural stimulators, and transcutaneous nerve stimulators (Fig. 5.14). These devices have become a major source of artifacts mimicking fibrillations and PSWs. These

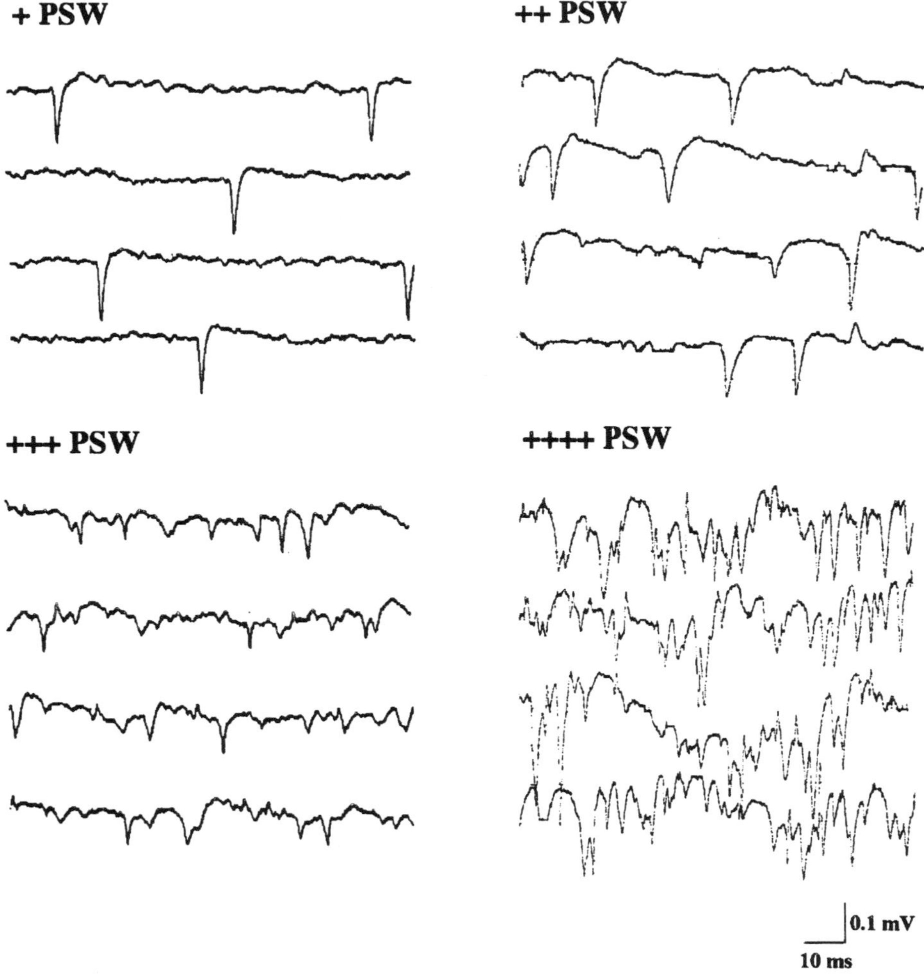

FIGURE 5.13. Grading of abnormal spontaneous potentials (PSWs here).

TABLE 5.8. Grading of Abnormal Spontaneous Potentials

Grade	Description
–	No abnormal spontaneous potentials observed.
+	One abnormal spontaneous potential persisting for at least 400 ms in at least two sampling sites. Alternatively, one abnormal spontaneous potential should persist long enough to be captured manually on the screen without any difficulty.
+ +	Two or more spontaneous potentials continuously active, filling one-third of the screen noted in three or more sampling sites.
+ + +	Continuously active abnormal spontaneous potentials filling half the screen and easily found in most sampling sites.
+ + + +	Many continuously active abnormal spontaneous potentials nearly filling the entire screen in all sampling sites.

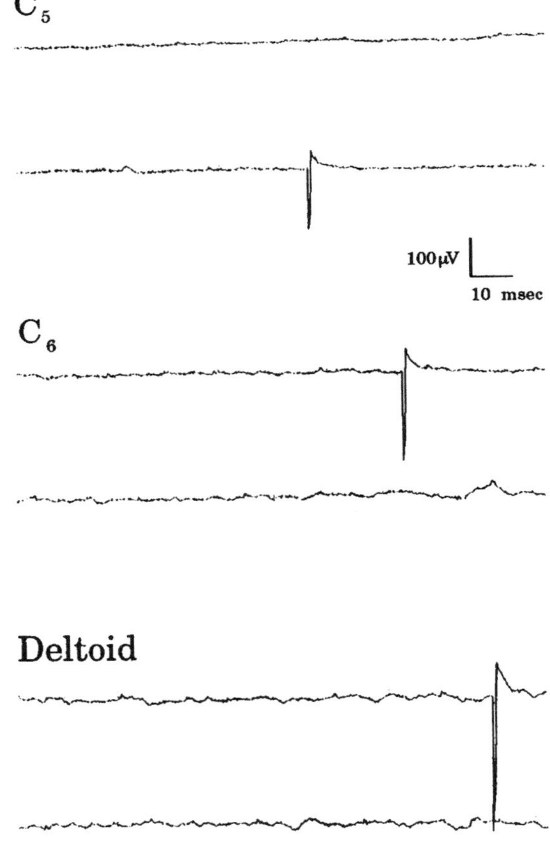

FIGURE 5.14. Artifacts in the cervical paraspinal and deltoid muscles, mimicking positive sharp waves. Notice that the amplitude of artifact increases as the EMG needle is placed closer to the heart.

artifacts can meet two criteria of fibrillations and PSWs: regular firing and initial positive deflection. The most important distinction between them is the sharp turn of potentials in the artifacts in contrast to the smooth turn in genuine fibrillations and PSWs. Usually, their sound is much louder and sharper. A high index of suspicion is needed to recognize this artifact, which may otherwise be interpreted as fibrillations or PSWs. Thus, whenever confronted with unexplainable regular tiny artifacts, it is wise to ask the patient whether he or she has any such implanted pacing device. If possible, turning off the pacemaker will eliminate the source of artifacts.

PSW

PSW, the second most important EMG finding, are characterized by a sharp initial positive deflection followed by a relatively prolonged negative slope and typical "thumping" sound (Table 5.9 and Fig. 5.15). Although some authorities regard PSWs as a kind of fibrillation, most regard these potentials as separate because of their distinct shape and sound. Although a few electromyographers consider PSWs as abnormal insertional activity, we take the view that these are spontaneous abnormal potentials because they are not always induced by the insertion or movement of the EMG needle. PSWs, like fibrillations, are considered to originate from a single fibrillating muscle fiber. The only difference from fibrillations is that they are

TABLE 5.9. Positive Sharp Waves

Shape	Biphasic with initial sharp positive wave followed by long negative wave Usually initiated by needle movement
Initial deflection	Positive
Duration	10–100 ms (usually 30 ms)
Amplitude	Usually 20–200 μV with concentric needle 50 μV to 1 mV with monopolar needle
Frequency	Regular, 2–50 Hz (may go up to 100 Hz)
Sound	Dull thud or ticking of clock
Key finding	Initial positive deflection with regular firing spontaneous potential at rest
Generator	Fibrillating single muscle fibers
Significance	Same as fibrillations
Diseases (essential)	Same as fibrillations
Diseases (common)	Same as fibrillations

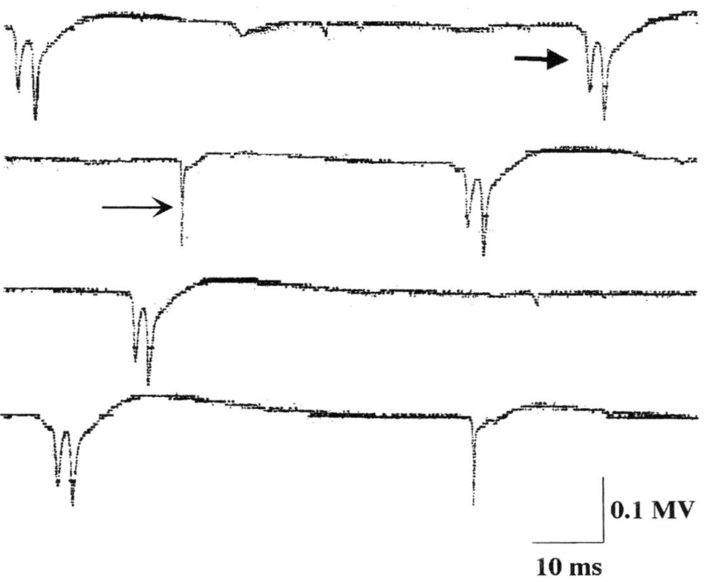

FIGURE 5.15. Two different positive sharp waves. Classic positive sharp waves (*thin arrow*) and positive sharp waves with double positive peaks (*thick arrow*).

recorded from an injured area of the fiber and represent "injury potentials." Certainly, this is obvious in practice in that PSWs are much more easily evoked by EMG needle movement than are fibrillations. In essence, the electrophysiological characteristics and clinical significance of PSWs are identical with those of fibrillations. One major difference is the fact that PSWs appear earlier than fibrillations after nerve injury: within 8 to 14 days for PSWs compared with 2 to 4 weeks for fibrillations. The major component of myotonic potentials is positive potentials, and they are nearly identical to PSWs. However, myotonic potentials are easily differentiated from PSWs in that they are always triggered by needle insertion or mild voluntary contraction, characteristically wax and wane in frequency and amplitude, and have a characteristic "dive-bomber sound."

Fasciculation Potentials

Clinically, fasciculation refers to the visible twitching of muscles. It is usually "fleeting" but can be continuous, simulating a "bag of worms." Continuous fasciculations (vermicular movement of muscles) are referred to clinically as myokymia (the EMG term "myokymic potentials" is different). Fasciculation is recorded as fasciculation potentials by the EMG needle. These are characterized by the irregular firing of single MUPs and are usually accompanied by visible needle movement (Table 5.10 and Fig. 5.16). Fasciculation potentials may mimic normal or abnormal MUPs. Depending on the closeness of the needle to the origin of the fasciculation, the sound can be crisp, representing "nearby fasciculation potentials," or dull, indicating "distant MUPs." In the former case, fasciculation potentials are invariably accompanied by tiny visible needle movements, an important distinguishing feature from other spontaneous potentials. Fasciculation potentials are spontaneous discharges of a group of muscle fibers representing a whole or possibly part of a motor unit, and are thought to originate from the ephatic firing of MUPs from a lesion in the anterior horn cells or entire axis of the peripheral nerves. Sometimes, a single fasciculation can be continuous, firing at an almost regular rate and mimicking a regular single MUP. In this instance, it is important to ascertain that the muscle is completely relaxed and to recognize the tiny visible movement of needle. Careful, prolonged analysis of the recording shows that the firing rate is not always regular. It is likely that this continuous fasciculation is what Buchthal et al. call "spontaneous MUP discharges," which have been described in infantile spinal muscular atrophy (Fig. 5.17).

According to our experience, fasciculation potentials are one of the most difficult needle EMG potentials for inexperienced electromyographers to recognize. To such examiners, fasciculation potentials are nothing more than random MUPs from nonrelaxed muscles. To recognize fasciculation potentials reliably, there must be an ample pause between the needle movements (sometimes, a 10 to 20-second interval is needed to document irregularly firing fasciculations) and the muscle must be fully relaxed. Because fasciculation potentials are

TABLE 5.10. Fasciculation

Shape	Any MUPs
Initial deflection	Same as MUPs
Duration	Same as MUP duration
Amplitude	Same as MUP amplitude
Frequency	Random irregular, 1–50/m
Sound	Irregular thumping thud or "large rain drops on a roof"[a]
Key finding	Needle moves together with irregular firing "fasciculation"
Generator	Ephatic firing of MUPs from anterior horn cell and any portion of peripheral nerve
Significance	Together with other EMG findings of "denervation"; this finding alone is not pathological
Diseases (essential)	Fasciculation-cramp syndrome, benign fasciculation (normal observation)
Diseases (common)	Amyotrophic lateral sclerosis, Isaacs' syndrome, myokymia-cramp syndrome, radiation plexopathy, demyelinating neuropathy, radiculopathy

[a] Daube's description.

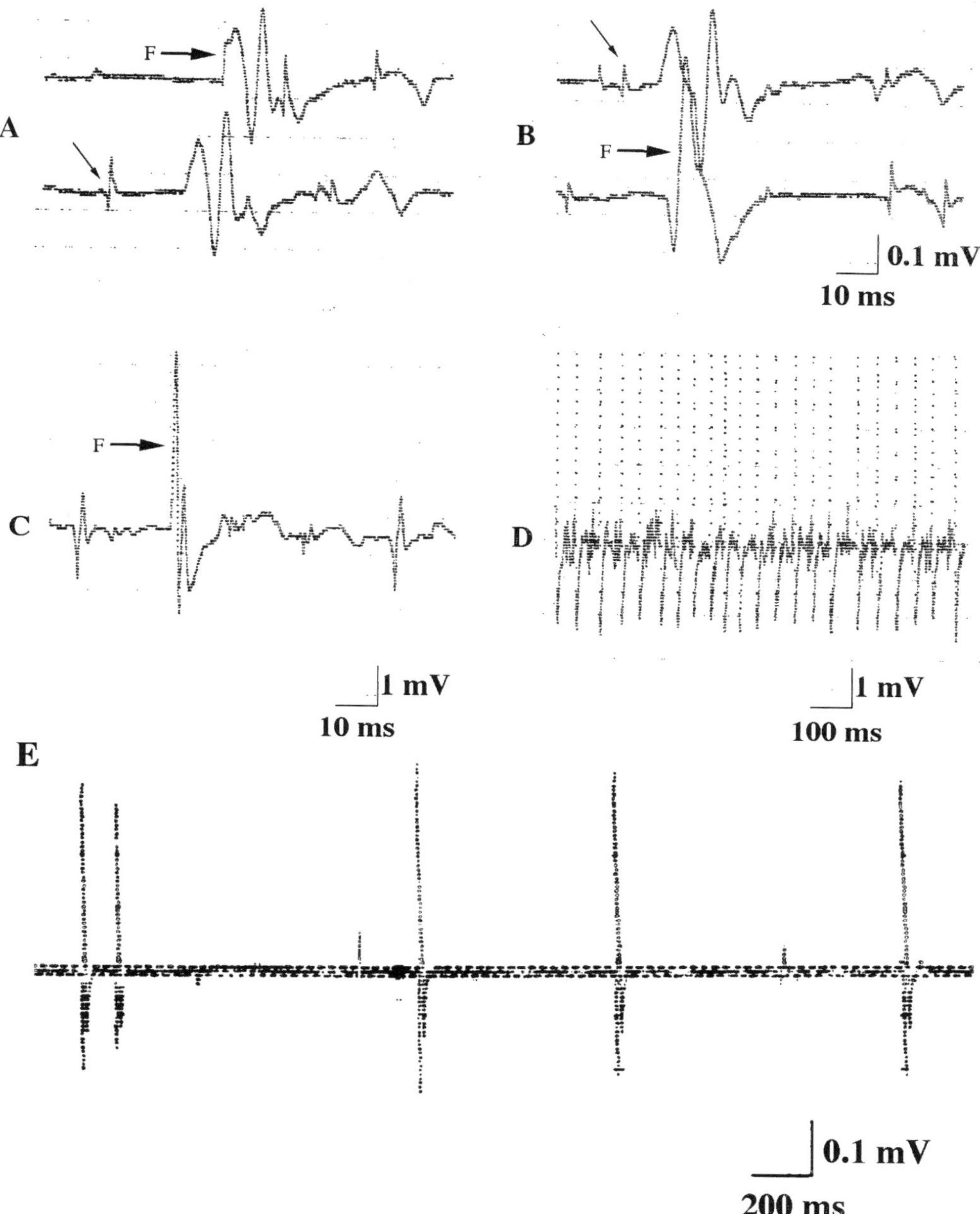

FIGURE 5.16. Fasciculations. **A–C.** Thin arrows indicate some of the fibrillations. *F* arrows indicate fasciculations. **D.** Continuous fasciculation. **E.** Classic irregular firing of fasciculation. These are from a patient with amyotrophic lateral sclerosis.

spontaneous potentials in the muscle at rest, there is no way to recognize them in an unrelaxed muscle. As long as the above requirements are followed, it is not difficult to recognize fasciculation potentials. Fasciculation may be induced by percussion. The needle EMG, in contrast to the clinical examination, has the definite advantage of detecting fasciculation from a muscle depth that would otherwise remain unrecognized visually.

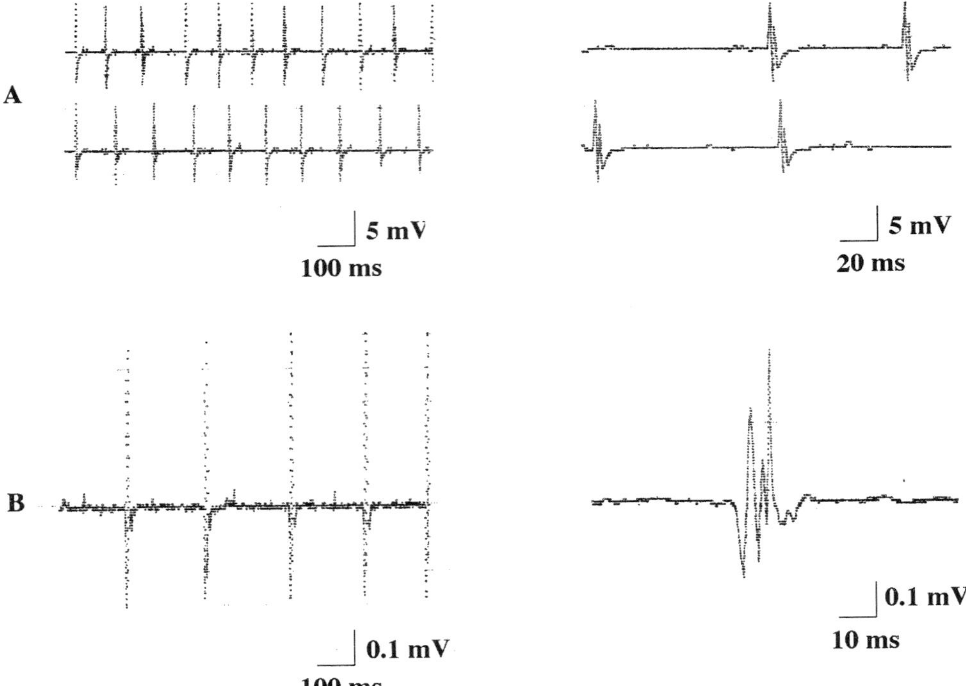

FIGURE 5.17. Spontaneous MUP discharges. **A** and **B.** Continuous firing of spontaneous MUP discharge at almost regular firing rate. Spontaneous MUP discharge may be confused with single MUP firing. Be sure that these discharges are originating from muscle at rest.

Fasciculation potentials are observed in normal muscle and in anterior horn cell diseases, cervical spondylotic myelopathy, radiculopathy, and demyelinating neuropathy. Fasciculations occur in about 15% of the normal population and are experienced by 70% of healthy medical personnel. Fasciculations in normal subjects are termed "benign" fasciculations. Several studies have attempted to differentiate between benign fasciculations and fasciculations in the disease state. Trojaborg et al. reported that fasciculations occur more rapidly in benign conditions than in anterior horn cell diseases, but our experience has shown that this rule is not reliable. Two conclusions may be drawn. There is no reliable method of differentiating between benign fasciculations and fasciculations in disease states on the basis of fasciculation potentials alone. Also, fasciculation potentials are abnormal when associated with other EMG abnormalities of denervation, such as fibrillations, PSWs, and high-amplitude long-duration MUPs. In benign fasciculations, the MUPs are normal.

Myokymic Potentials

Myokymic potentials refer to specific spontaneous potentials in the needle EMG that are characterized by the rhythmical firing of "grouped MUPs" (Table 5.11 and Fig. 5.18). The most important distinction from fasciculations is that instead of a single MUP, fixed groups of MUPs are firing in bursts, usually at a regular rate, in myokymia. Myokymic potentials occur in bursts of group of 2 to 10 potentials and are characterized by the typical sounds of "marching soldiers." They are not affected by voluntary movement, sleep, or needle movement. Certainly, they can be induced by percussion on the muscle. Unlike myotonic potentials, myokymic potentials do not wax or wane. Some have maintained that myokymic potentials may be regarded as "grouped fasciculations." These should be differentiated on the basis of their distinct patterns and sounds and because of different clinical implications. Depending

TABLE 5.11. Myokymic Potentials

Shape	Rhythmic bursts of groups of normal MUPs (2–10 MUPs in one group) that fire with a fixed pattern and rhythm; this is unaffected by voluntary activity
Initial deflection	Same as MUPs
Duration	Same as MUPs
Amplitude	Same as MUPs
Frequency	Bursts of 2–10 potentials that fire at 2–60 Hz; the bursts may recur at regular intervals of 0.1–10 s
Sound	Footstep from marching soldiers
Key finding	Regular rhythmic bursts of groups of MUPs (more than one MUP in one group)
Generator	Ephatic firing of MUPs from anterior horn cell and any portion of peripheral nerve
Significance	Severe form of fasciculation; myokymia alone is pathological
Disease (essential)	Myokymia-cramp syndrome
Disease (common)	Radiation-induced plexopathy, rattlesnake bite poisoning, demyelinating neuropathy; multiple sclerosis and brainstem glioma for facial myokymia

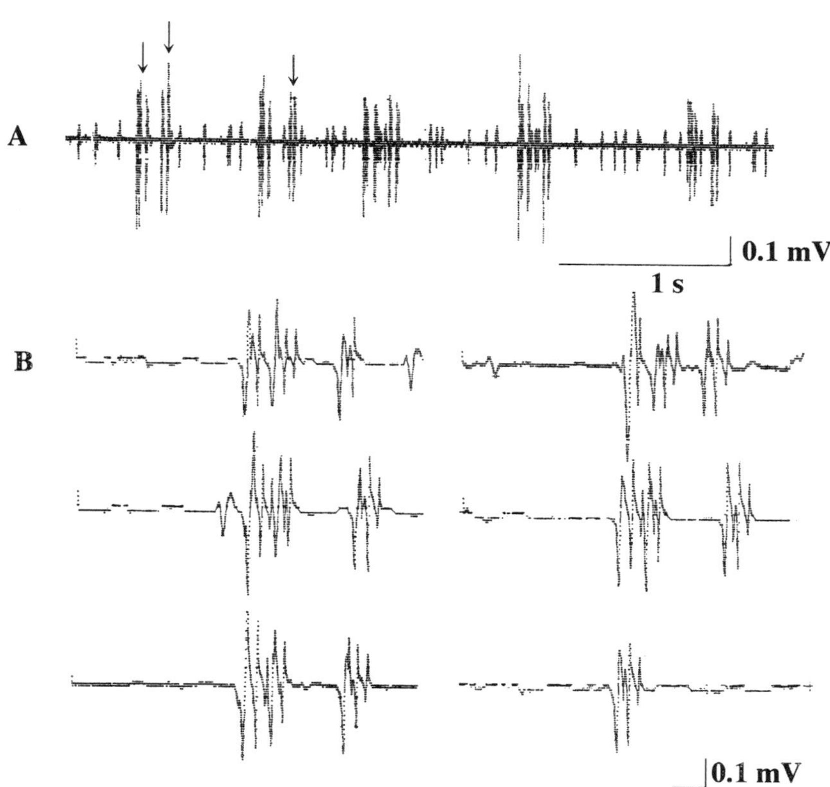

FIGURE 5.18. Myokymic discharges in a case of amyotrophic lateral sclerosis. **A.** Myokymic discharges (a few of them are indicated by *arrows*) are intermixed with fasciculation. **B.** Two polyphasic potentials representing grouped discharges (myokymic discharge).

on the site of the "generator," the peripheral nerve or axonal terminal block reduces or eliminates myokymic potentials.

Myokymic potentials are typically seen but are not a sine qua non in clinical myokymia. The reason for this is that in clinical myokymia, other EMG potentials can be observed: continuous fasciculation and continuous muscle fiber activity (neuromyotonia). Myokymic potentials are essential findings in myokymia-cramp syndrome. Myokymia is most frequently seen in Guillain-Barré syndrome, multiple sclerosis, radiation plexopathy, and timber rattlesnake envenomation. Depending on the nature of the disorder, fibrillations or PSWs may be associated with myokymic potentials. In pure hyperexcitable neuronal and peripheral nerve disorders, neither fibrillations nor PSWs are seen. On the other hand, in anterior horn cell or peripheral nerve diseases, other evidence of denervation is present together with myokymic potentials. In myokymia-cramp syndrome, fibrillations or PSWs have not been observed. Multiple sclerosis and pontine glioma are well-known causes of facial myokymia, which has also been reported in Guillain-Barré syndrome, timber rattlesnake envenomation, and facial palsy. In facial myokymia, two EMG patterns have been observed. In the continuous type, rhythmic single or paired discharges of one or a few MUPs recur with striking regularity at 5 to 10 Hz. In the discontinuous type, bursts of MUPs at 30 to 40 impulses per second last for 100 to 900 ms and repeat at regular intervals of 100 ms to 10 seconds. In the limb muscles, myokymic potentials arise focally at the site of a chronic peripheral nerve lesion. The most classic disease associated with limb myokymia is radiation-induced plexopathy; of 38 patients with limb myokymia, radiation plexopathy accounted for 27 cases in Albers' study.

Complex Repetitive Discharge (Bizarre High-Frequency Waves)

Complex repetitive discharge (CRD) refers to the repetitive discharge of complex potentials with sudden onset and cessation and the characteristic sound of a "motor boat" or "motor cycle" (Table 5.12 and Fig. 5.19). The waveform of a single CRD is typically polyphasic, complex, and uniform from one discharge to another. During discharge, there may be abrupt changes in their shape, amplitude, and frequency. The most important criteria of CRD is a lack of waxing or waning of amplitude or frequency of potentials. Another term for CRD is "bizarre high-frequency waves." In the past, the term "pseudomyotonia" was used because of a similarity in the sound produced, but this term is not recommended to avoid any possible reference to myotonia. There is a distinct difference between CRDs and myotonic potentials. In CRDs, there is no waxing and waning of amplitude or frequency of the potentials, whereas waxing and waning of potentials is a sine qua non in myotonia and is responsible for the classic divebomber sound. This distinction is important because myotonic potentials have a more specific connotation. CRD is usually an expression of hyperexcitable muscle membrane.

TABLE 5.12. Complex Repetitive Discharges (Bizarre High-Frequency Wave; Pseudomyotonic Discharge)

Shape	Repetitive discharge of polyphasic or serrated action potentials characterized by uniform frequency, shape, and amplitude with abrupt onset, cessation, or change in configuration
Initial deflection	Any deflection
Duration	Up to 50 ms
Amplitude	100 μV to 1 mV; uniform
Frequency	5–100 Hz; uniform
Sound	Motor bike or motor boat engine
Key finding	Repetitive discharges with uniform amplitude and frequency with abrupt onset, cessation, or change in configuration
Generator	Hyperirritable muscle membrane; a group of muscle fibers firing in near synchrony
Significance	Active denervation and active myopathy
Diseases (essential)	Schwartz-Jampfel syndrome
Diseases (common)	Myotonic syndromes, acid maltase deficiency, polymyositis, IBM amyotrophic lateral sclerosis, spinal muscular atrophy, HMSN I and II

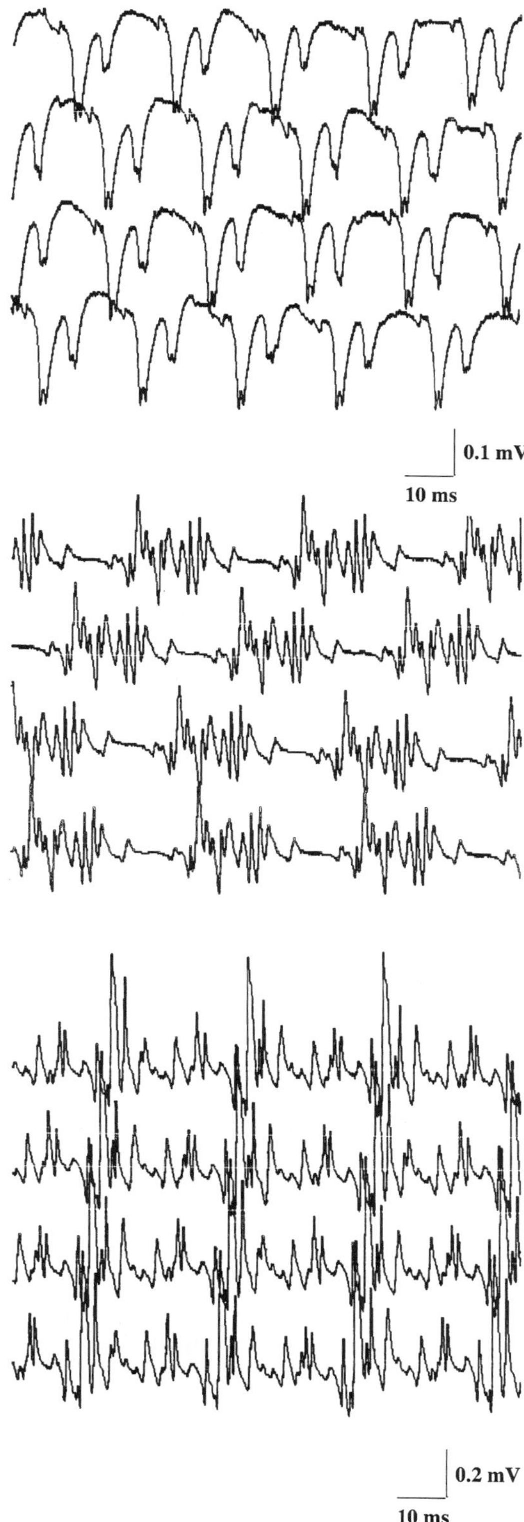

FIGURE 5.19. Three examples of complex repetitive discharge. Notice no change in frequency or amplitude of discharge.

In contrast to myokymic potentials, CRDs are not grouped but are the regular recurrence of complex waves that begin and terminate abruptly. A recent study suggests that CRD is the result of ephatic activation of groups of adjacent muscle fibers. CRD, although impressive in the needle EMG, is not associated with any clinical counterpart.

On rare occasions, CRDs may be observed in isolation in normal paraspinal, iliopsoas, and sphincter muscles. They are usually short-lasting and not associated with any other EMG abnormality, such as fibrillations or PSWs. Thus, transient CRDs without any other EMG abnormality in these muscles are not clinically significant.

In pathological states, CRDs are usually associated with profuse fibrillations and PSWs, making clinical correlation easy and supporting the theory that CRDs are EMG evidence of hyperexcitable membrane. CRDs have been reported in spinal muscular atrophy, Charcot-Marie-Tooth disease, amyotrophic lateralis sclerosis, inclusion body myositis, acid maltase deficiency, polymyositis, and Schwartz-Jampel syndrome. On many occasions, the generator can be accurately pinpointed, because with minimal needle movement from the generator, CRDs will cease firing. This phenomenon is especially true in denervation states.

Neuromyotonic Discharges

Neuromyotonic (or neurotonic) discharges refer to the continuous muscle fiber activity (motor unit potentials) firing at 100 to 300 Hz (Table 5.13 and Fig. 5.20). These potentials may

TABLE 5.13. Neuromyotonic Discharges (Neurotonic Discharges)

Shape	Bursts of MUPs firing at more than 150 Hz for 0.5 to 2 s, unaffected by voluntary movement
Initial deflection	Any deflection
Duration	Same as any MUP
Amplitude	Typically wanes
Frequency	100–300 Hz; may be continuous for long intervals or recur in bursts
Sound	"Ping",[a] popcorn sounds,[b] or "bomber potentials"[b]
Key finding	Continuous MUP discharges
Generator	Hyperexcitable peripheral nerve disorders; probably from the distal axon
Significance	Continuous muscle fiber activity (Isaacs' syndrome); irritated exposed nerve

[a] Lambert's description when short-lasting.

[b] Prass's description of a train of neuromyotonic discharges in response to mechanical or metabolic irritation of the nerve innervating muscle during the surgery is described as "bomber potentials" or "popcorn sounds."

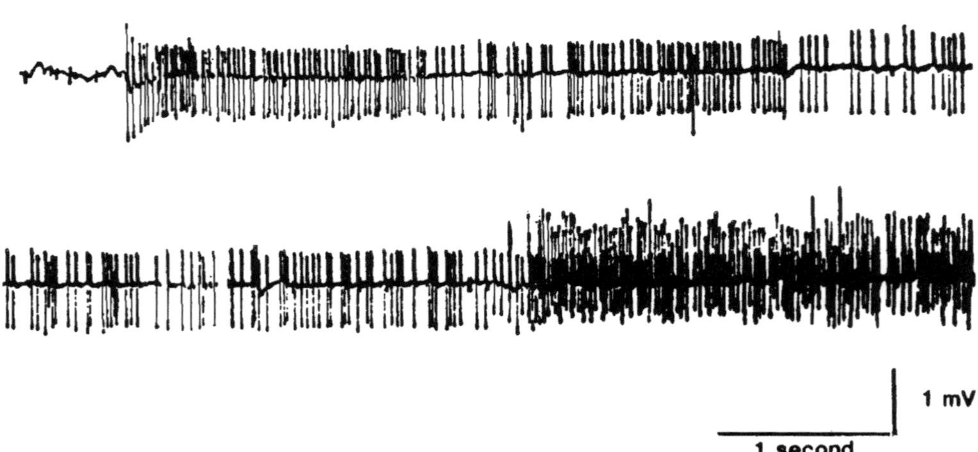

FIGURE 5.20. Neuromytonic potentials. Continuous MUP discharge from abductor pollicis brevis muscle in a case of Isaacs' syndrome.

decrease in amplitude during continuous muscle fiber activity. This high-frequency decrementing discharge produces a unique musical sound, or "ping," that differs from those of other spontaneous discharges including myotonic discharges; neuromyotonic discharges are unaffected by voluntary activity. Artificially induced ischemia or electrical stimulation of the nerve or tapping of the nerve may abruptly initiate a spontaneous discharge. This phenomenon is only seen in neuromyotonic discharges. Classically, neuromyotonic discharges persist during sleep and under general or spinal anesthesia. During voluntary contraction, many motor units fire successively with overlap. Depending on the site of generation, a peripheral nerve block may or may not block neuromyotonic discharges. Local administration of curare abolishes these potentials. These findings suggest that neuromyotonic discharges are generated from the hyperexcitable peripheral nerve anywhere from the proximal segment to the axon terminal. Diphenylhydantoin and carbamazepine were reported to be effective in relieving neuromyotonic discharges in some patients with continuous muscle fiber activity.

The clinical counterpart of neuromyotonic discharges is continuous muscle contraction that may be painful in severe forms and give rise to an abnormal posture, difficulty relaxing the muscles, or clinical myokymia in milder forms. Neuromyotonic potentials are a sine qua non for a diagnosis of Isaacs' syndrome and familial continuous muscle fiber activity syndrome. Neuromyotonic potentials are also reported with spinal muscular atrophy, peripheral neuropathy, and tetany. Neuromyotonic potentials with tetany may be distinguished by their precipitation or augmentation with ischemia. Neuromyotonic potentials also occur intraoperatively when cranial or peripheral nerves are mechanically irritated and are thus valuable in alerting surgeons to possible nerve damage.

Myotonic Potentials

Myotonic potentials are the most specific potentials in needle EMG. If they are recognized by the needle EMG test, the patient is considered to have myotonic syndrome until proven otherwise. Only a few other diseases show myotonic potentials on the needle EMG in a substantial percentage of cases. Myotonic potentials are spontaneous potentials with waxing and waning amplitudes and frequencies and that produce the classic "dive-bomber sound" (Table 5.14 and Fig. 5.21). They are easily induced by needle insertion and movement, muscle tapping, or minimal voluntary contraction of the muscle. Myotonic potentials are characterized by an initial positive deflection, either in the form of PSWs or fibrillations, depending on the relationship of the needle to the muscle fibers. Usually, myotonic potentials assume the form of PSWs when initiated by insertion of the needle and that of fibrillations when initiated by voluntary contraction. If a single myotonic potential fires at a slower rate, this may sound and look like fibrillations or PSWs. Until waxing and waning of amplitude and frequency are documented with additional discharges of potentials, it is impossible to

TABLE 5.14. Myotonic Potentials

Shape	Repetitive discharge of monophasic or biphasic potentials, usually triggered by insertion of needle or tapping on muscle
Initial deflection	Positive
Duration	2–20 ms
Amplitude	Waxing and waning in amplitude
Frequency	20–50 Hz with waxing and waning rate
Sound	"Dive-bomber" sound
Key finding	Abnormal spontaneous potentials with waxing and waning amplitude and frequently accompanied by dive-bomber sound
Generator	Myotonic muscle membrane
Significance	Myotonic disorder
Diseases (essential)	Myotonic dystrophy, proximal myotonic myopathy, myotonia congenita (Thomsen's disease), generalized myotonic syndrome (Becker's disease), paramyotonia congenita
Diseases (common)	Acid maltase deficiency, hyperkalemic periodic paralysis

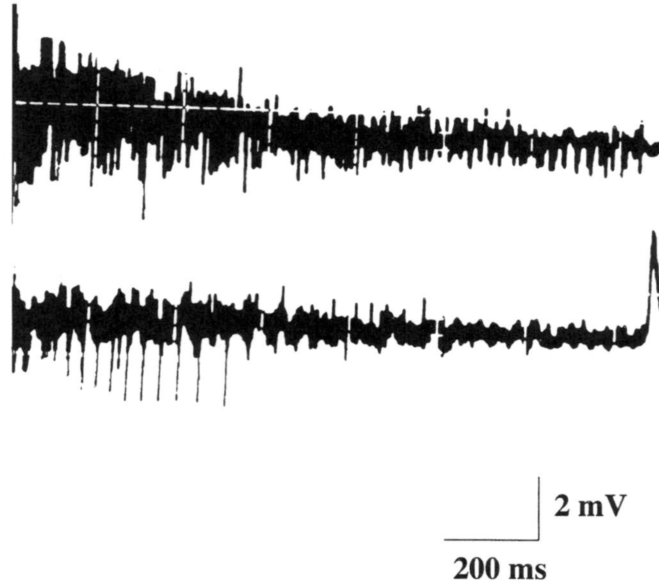

FIGURE 5.21. Myotonic potentials. Notice waxing and waning of amplitude and frequency of MUPs.

distinguish fibrillations or PSWs from myotonic potentials. Myotonic potentials are generated by the spontaneous (constant) depolarization of the muscle membrane.

Myotonic potentials are the EMG hallmark of myotonia and are invariably associated with clinical myotonia, such as grasp or percussion myotonia. Without myotonic potentials, the diagnosis of clinical myotonia is not justifiable. A delayed relaxation of muscles on percussion or grasping is documented by the clinical examination in rare cases of Isaacs' syndrome, stiff-man syndrome, or McArdle's disease during the attacks. In these cases, myotonic potentials are absent, confirming that the delayed relaxation of muscles is not due to myotonia. When myotonic potentials are documented in the needle EMG, it is important to check for clinical myotonia in patients, because a simple clinical test will confirm the diagnosis of myotonic syndrome in many unsuspected cases. There is one disease that has consistently shown myotonic potentials in a substantial number of cases—acid maltase deficiency. In this disease, genuine myotonic potentials were observed in all 10 patients with no clinical signs of myotonia in one study. Thus, if genuine myotonic potentials are observed without clinical myotonia, acid-maltase deficiency should be ruled out by appropriate tests. Polymyositis is listed as a disease with myotonic potentials as is inclusion body myositis. According to our experience, it is extremely rare to record myotonic potentials in these disorders. Usually, CRDs in these diseases are mistaken for myotonic potentials. Thus, it is important to record the abnormal spontaneous potentials to differentiate between CRDs and myotonic potentials by documenting the waxing and waning of amplitude and frequency of myotonic potentials. In paramyotonia, in which muscle stiffness increases with exposure to cold, myotonic potentials disappear with cooling.

Short-Duration MUPs

Short-duration MUPs are the EMG hallmarks of myopathy (Table 5.15 and Fig. 5.22). Short-duration MUPs refer to MUPs with a duration below the normal lower limit. As discussed above, the duration of MUPs is different for different ages and different muscles. In adult limb muscles, MUPs of less than 6 ms are considered to be short in duration. In the quantitative MUP analysis, the mean duration of 20 MUPs should be lower than the "mean minus 20% of the mean" for the patient's age and the specific muscle to be significant for myopathy. Short-duration MUPs are usually also low in amplitude (<500 μV) and recruited early with minimal voluntary contraction of muscles. Thus, small-amplitude short-duration (SASD)

TABLE 5.15. Small-Amplitude Short-Duration (SASD) MUPs

Shape	SASD monophasic or diphasic MUPs, often with many SASD polyphasic MUPs
Initial deflection	Any deflection
Duration	0.5–4 ms; up to 6 ms in small-polyphasic MUPs
Amplitude	50–300 μs with monopolar and 25–200 μs with concentric needle
Frequency	Early recruitment
Sound	Sharp rasping scratchy sound from "newspaper rubbing between two fingers"[a]
Key finding	SASD MUPs with early recruitment
Generator	Either histological or physiological functional loss of random muscle fibers
Significance	Myopathy and neuromuscular transmission disorders
Diseases (essential)	Myopathy
Diseases (common)	Myotonic dystrophy, MG, Lambert-Eaton myasthenic syndrome, botulism, periodic paralysis (during attack)

[a] One of the author's former residents compared this sound with that of a needle on "a cracked old 48 gramophone slow-play record." The problem with this is that few modern-day physicians have ever heard this sound.

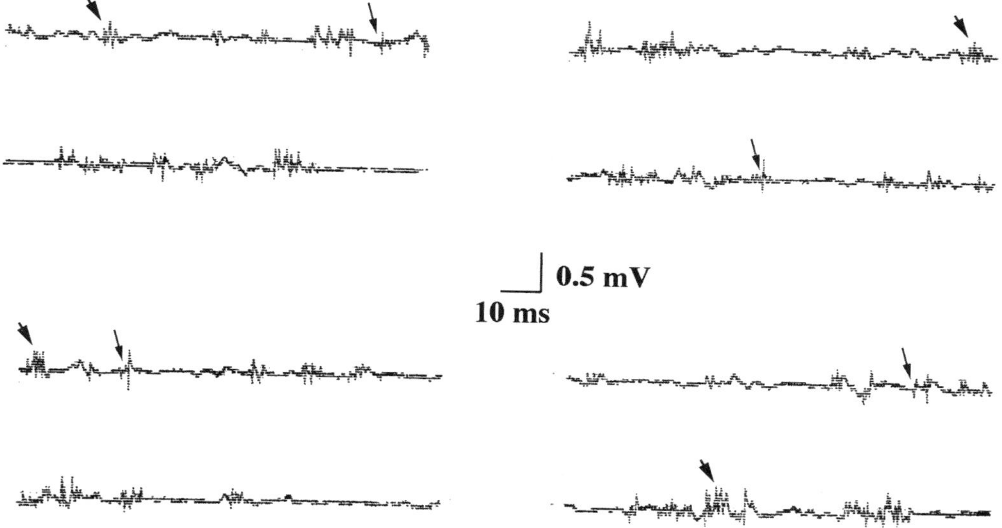

FIGURE 5.22. Many SASD MUPs and SASD polyphasic MUPs in mitochondrial myopathy. Thin arrows represent some of SASD MUPs and thick arrows, some of SASD polyphasic MUPs.

MUPs (brief small action potentials) are typically observed in myopathy. In myopathy, the polyphasic MUPs are also short (<6 ms) and small (<500 μV) (Fig. 5.21). These SASD simple and polyphasic MUPs produce extremely characteristic sounds like a "scratchy" recording on an old 48 gramophone plate (it is extremely difficult to describe this sound). Once the electromyographer is familiar with the typical sound, however, he or she can recognize it. Thus, experience is necessary in learning to recognize short-duration MUPs. In myopathy, some of the fibers within a motor unit are nonfunctional because of muscle fiber necrosis, so that the electrode is less likely to record activity from distant fibers. Thus, the initial and terminal portions of MUPs are simply not recorded, producing short-duration MUPs.

In severe myopathy, it is not difficult to detect short-duration MUPs, but in milder cases, short-duration MUPs can be focal. Thus, it is important to search for a spot that induces short-duration MUPs. A short-duration MUP may be as short as a fibrillation potential, and when fibrillations are also present, distinguishing between them can be difficult. In this situation, it is important to observe the potentials in the completely relaxed muscle. Short-duration MUPs disappear when the muscle is relaxed, whereas fibrillations persist in the relaxed muscle.

It is also important to know that short-duration MUPs can be seen in neuromuscular transmission disorders: MG, Lambert-Eaton myasthenic syndrome, and botulism.

Long-Duration MUPs

Long-duration MUPs are the EMG hallmarks of chronic denervation (Table 5.16 and Fig. 5.23). Long-duration MUPs refer to MUPs with a duration longer than the normal upper limit. As discussed above, the duration of MUPs differs according to age and muscle. In the adult limb muscles, MUPs lasting longer than 17 ms are considered to be long in duration. In the quantitative MUP analysis, the mean duration of 20 MUPs should be higher than the "mean plus 20% of the mean" for age and muscle to be significant for chronic denervation.

TABLE 5.16. High-Amplitude Long-Duration (HALD) MUPs

Shape	HALD monophasic or diphasic MUPs, often with HALD polyphasic MUPs
Initial deflection	Any deflection
Duration	>17 ms; >20 ms in polyphasic MUPs
Amplitude	>5mV with monopolar and 3mV with concentric needle
Frequency	>15Hz
Sound	No special sound characteristic
Key finding	HALD MUPs with reduced recruitment
Generator	Large motor unit territory; type grouping
Significance	Chronic denervation
Diseases (essential)	Chronic denervation
Diseases (common)	Amyotrophic lateral sclerosis, spinal muscular atrophy, chronic myelopathy involving anterior horn cells, radiculopathy, chronic peripheral neuropathy, chronic mononeuropathy, IBM

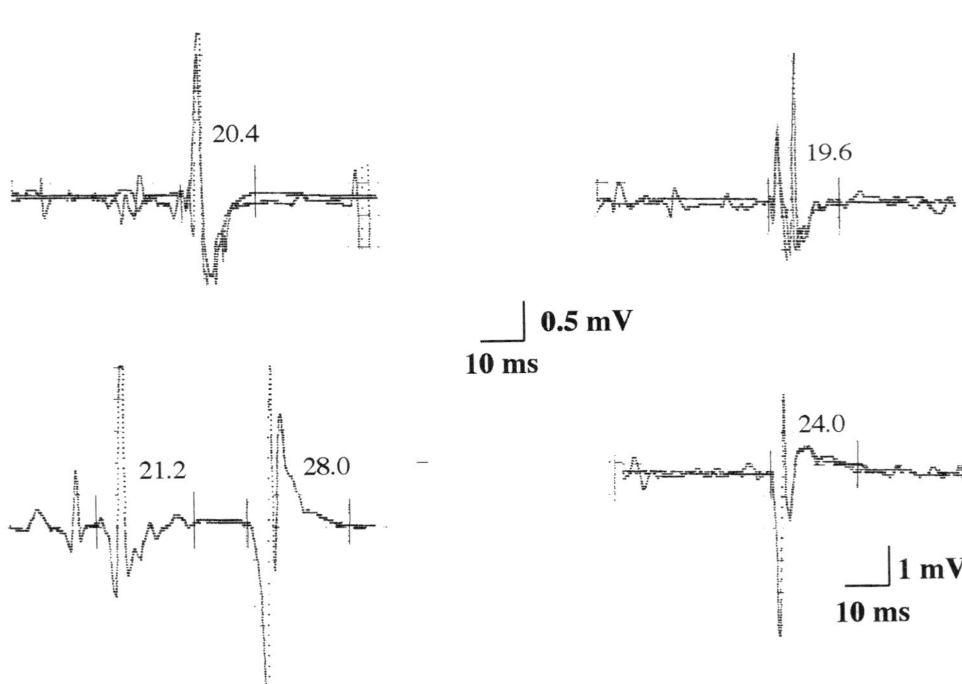

FIGURE 5.23. High-amplitude-long-duration MUPs indicative of chronic denervation. Numbers above each MUP represents the MUP duration.

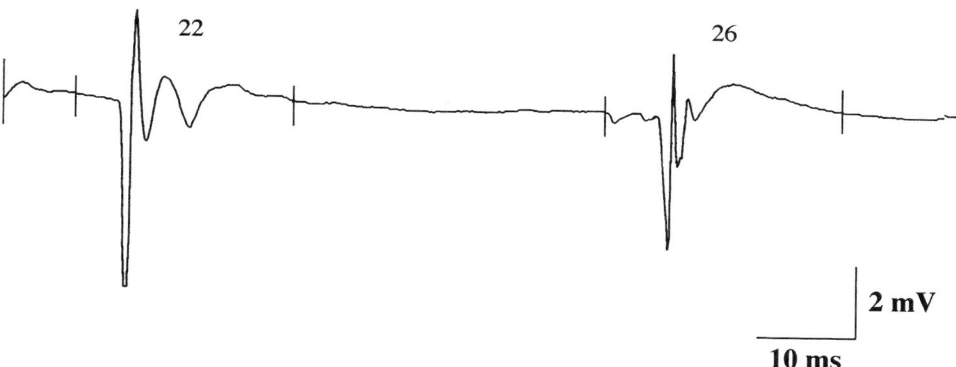

FIGURE 5.24. Two HALD polyphasic MUP (six phases) indicative of chronic denervation in amyotrophic lateral sclerosis.

TABLE 5.17. Diseases with Mixed SASD MUPs and HALD MUPs

Diseases in which this potential is commonly observed
Anterior horn cells diseases
Rapidly progressing motor neuron diseases
Spinal muscular atrophy
HMSN type II
Myopathy
Inclusion body myopathy

HMSN, hereditary motor sensory neuropathy.

Long-duration MUPs are commonly also high in amplitude (>3.5 mV) and fire at a faster rate (>15 Hz) with minimal voluntary contraction, but they are poor in recruitment. Polyphasic MUPs are also high in amplitude and long in duration in chronic denervation (Fig. 5.24). In practice, the presence of high-amplitude MUPs (HA MUP; "giant MUPs," >5 mV) has become an extremely useful EMG marker for chronic denervation because it is usually associated with long-duration MUPs. Thus, high-amplitude long-duration (HALD) MUPs are typically observed in chronic denervation and indicative of denervation process. When measuring the duration of MUPs with satellite potentials, one has to measure the duration of the main MUP. Otherwise, the MUP duration would be long, giving a false impression of long-duration MUPs.

Long-duration MUPs are due to the enlargement of the motor unit territory in a motor unit due to reinnervation of denervated muscles. Thus, it takes at least several months before long-duration MUPs become obvious in the needle EMG after nerve injury. Until that point, MUP duration is not helpful in diagnosing denervation. A combination of poor recruitment, increased polyphasic MUPs, fibrillations, and PSWs is indicative of denervation process.

Mixed Short-Duration and Long-Duration MUPs

Although rare, this combination may occur in the same muscle. This is one instance where the quantitative analysis of MUPs is not helpful because the mean duration of MUPs could well be normal due to the effect of averaging short- and long-duration MUPs (Fig. 5.25). When this combination is observed, inclusion body myositis (IBM) should be ruled out because it has been observed in one-third of patients with IBM (Table 5.17). This combination is also rarely seen in patients with rapidly progressing anterior horn cell diseases and in Kugelberg-Welander disease.

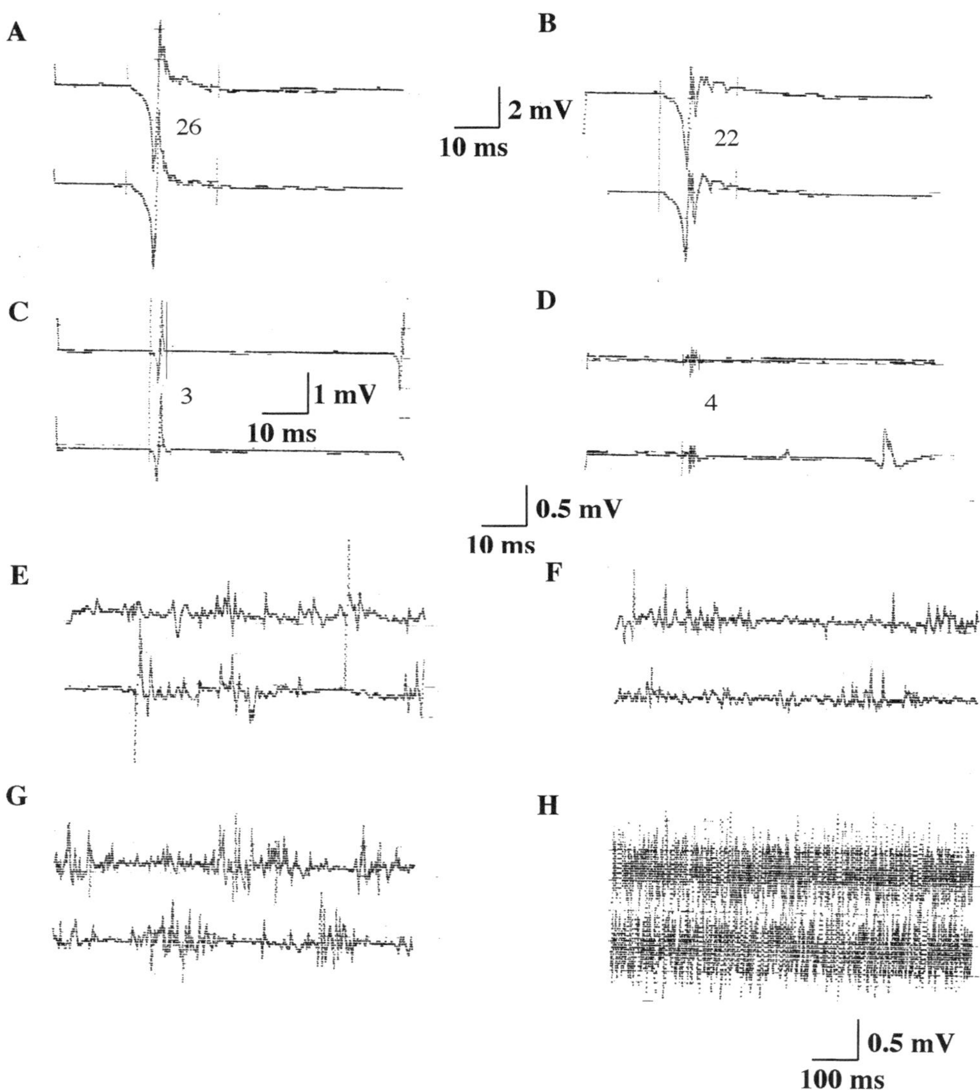

FIGURE 5.25. Mixed MUPs in a same muscle in inclusion body myositis. **A.** and **B.** HALD MUPs. **C.** Short-duration MUP. **D.** SASD polyphasic MUP. **E.** and **F.** Many SASDs. **G.** SASD polyphasic or normal amplitude polyphasic MUPs. **H.** Full interference pattern.

Polyphasic MUPs

Polyphasic MUPs refer to MUPs with five or more phases (Table 5.18). When more than 20% of MUPs are polyphasic, the number is considered to be "increased." Polyphasic MUPs are increased in myopathy and denervation processes. However, an increased number of polyphasic MUPs alone is of dubious significance and should thus not be regarded as a definite EMG abnormality. When increased polyphasic MUPs are associated with other abnormal EMG potentials, then they become clinically meaningful. On the other hand, the duration of polyphasic MUPs is an important EMG index of abnormality. Short duration (<6 ms) is indicative of myopathy (Fig. 5.22) and long duration, of denervation process (Fig. 5.24). Short-duration polyphasic MUPs are usually associated with a small amplitude, whereas long-

TABLE 5.18. Polyphasic MUPs

Shape	MUPs with 5 or more phases
Initial deflection	Any deflection
Duration	2–25 ms
Amplitude	0.2–10 mV
Frequency	Variable
Sound	Cracking; rough, rasping, or rattling[a]
Key finding	MUPs with 5 or more phases with cracking sound
Generator	Muscle fiber firing in asynchronous pattern in a single motor unit
Significance	Depending on the amplitude and duration of polyphasic MUPs, myopathy or denervation: SASD polyphasic MUPs, myopathy; HALD MUPs, chronic denervation; and small-amplitude polyphasic MUPs with normal or long duration, regeneration; Increased number of polyphasic MUPs with normal duration and amplitude alone is not clinically significant

[a] Rodriques description.

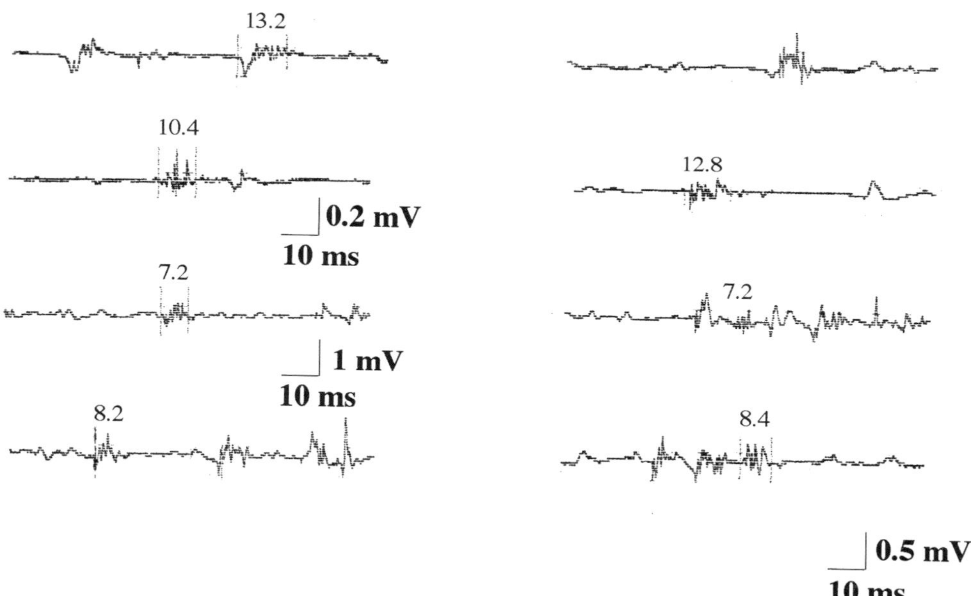

FIGURE 5.26. Small polyphasic MUPs during regeneration after nerve injury. Notice the duration of MUP ranged from 7.2 to 13.2 ms (number above the MUPs).

duration polyphasic MUPs generally have a high amplitude. During the reinnervation period after nerve injury, small polyphasic MUPs appear as the first sign of reinnervation. In the past, these small polyphasic MUPs were termed "nascent motor unit potentials," but this term is not recommended at this time. Because of their small amplitude, these potentials are often mistaken for myopathic potentials. For the most part, however, these potentials have a normal or long duration (Fig. 5.26). If long-duration and short-duration MUPs are present in the same muscle, then IBM must be ruled out.

Varying Amplitude of MUPs

In normal muscles, when an individual MUP fires in isolation, its amplitude, duration, and shape are relatively constant. When the amplitude of the MUP changes by more than 30%, it is termed "varying amplitude" (Table 5.19 and Fig. 5.27). Varying amplitude of MUPs is

TABLE 5.19. Diseases with MUPs with Varying Amplitude[a]

Diseases in which this potential is typically observed
- Neuromuscular transmission disorders
  - Myasthenia gravis
  - LEMS
  - Botulism

Diseases in which this potential is commonly observed
- Rapidly progressing axonal degenerations
- Reinnervation after nerve injury

[a] Single-fiber EMG shows prominent blocking.

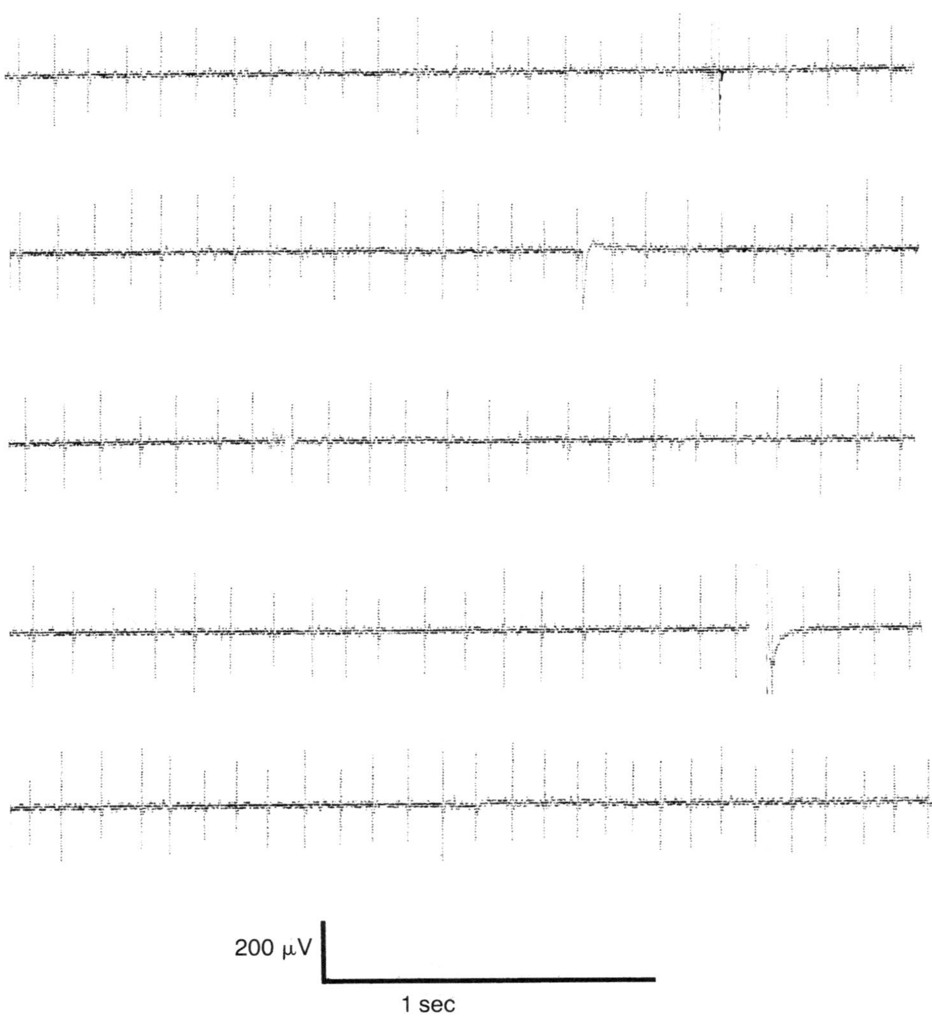

FIGURE 5.27. Varying amplitude of a same MUP in a patient with myasthenia gravis.

typical of neuromuscular transmission disorder. Because some end-plate potentials become subthreshold, some muscle fibers will fire intermittently due to "blocking" and the MUPs will vary in amplitude and configuration. This phenomenon was first described in MG and later in Lambert-Eaton myasthenic syndrome. No one as yet has reported how often this phenomenon is observed in MG or Lambert-Eaton myasthenic syndrome. Although the varying amplitude of MUPs is characteristic of neuromuscular transmission disorders, it can also be seen in neurogenic disorder (Fig. 5.28). The best examples are reinnervation after nerve injury and rapidly progressing amyotrophic lateral sclerosis. In all these disorders, the single-fiber EMG shows prominent blocking, supporting the theory that blocking is responsible for the fluctuating single-fiber MUP amplitude. It has been reported that in MG, the amplitude of MUPs is normal or nearly so on initiation of contraction but that it rapidly declines as fewer and fewer muscle fibers respond. This is in contrast to Lambert-Eaton myasthenic syndrome, in which the MUPs are small at the onset of contraction but gradually increase

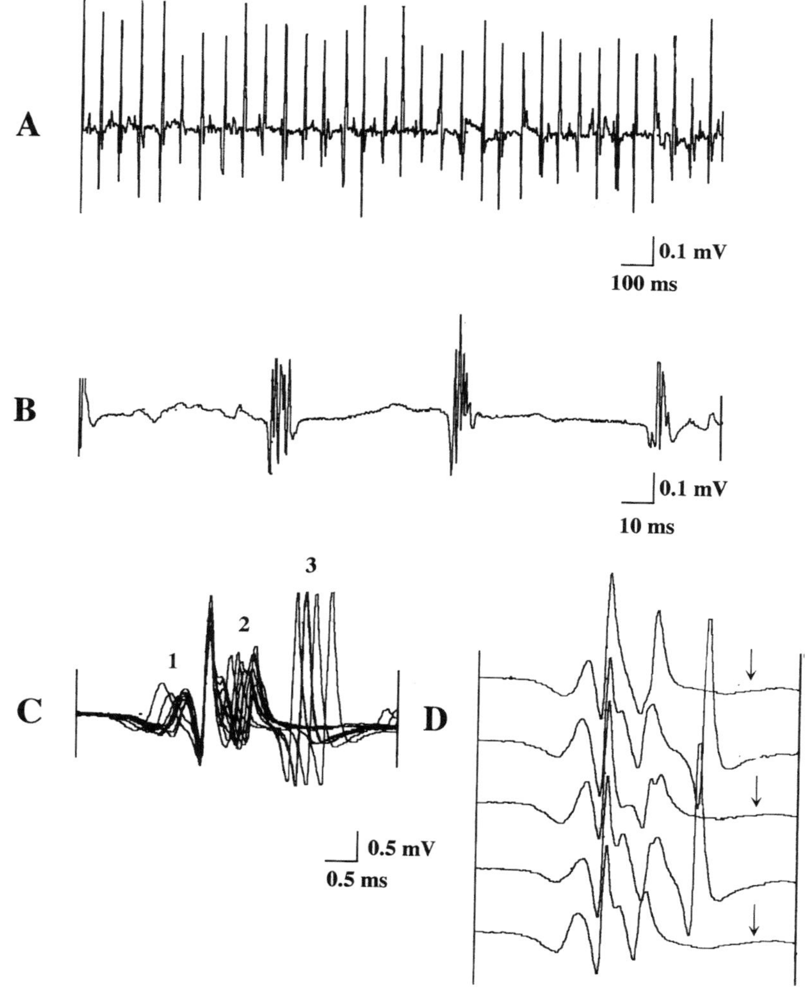

FIGURE 5.28. Varying amplitude of MUPs in a case with multifocal motor neuropathy. **A.** Varying amplitude of a same MUP. **B.** This MUP represents polyphasic MUP. **C.** Ten superimposed tracings of single fiber potentials in the same muscle. Notice abnormal jitter in all three (traces *1*, *2*, and *3*) slave potentials and blocking in three potential. **D.** Five tracings of single fiber potentials. Arrows indicate blocking of three slave potential.

in amplitude as contraction continues. However, such classic observations are extremely rare according to our experience.

MUP Doublets and Triplets

Normally, MUP fires as a single potential on minimal contraction. In patients with tetany and hyperventilation, each potential fires two or three times at short intervals of 2 to 20 ms. These MUPs are called doublets or triplets and represent the repetitive firing of a motor unit at very short intervals, probably due to hyperexcitability of the motor neuron pool. This phenomenon is observed on rare occasions in poliomyelitis, motor neuron disease, Gullian-Barré syndrome, other neuropathies, radiculopathy, and myotonic dystrophy. These MUPs should be differentiated from polyphasic MUPs, which are not repetitive discharges.

QUANTITATIVE MUP ANALYSIS IN NORMAL SUBJECTS

Although various computer-aided methods of quantitative MUP analysis have been developed to make this process easier and faster, one major problem has been the lack of normative data for the various muscles and different age groups, based on a particular method. Without normative data, the quantitative MUP data obtained by faster and easier computer programs are meaningless. In that sense, there is nothing that can surpass the value of the time-honored normative data of MUP duration developed by Buchthal et al. in the 1960s. In our laboratory, regardless of the computer program used, the duration of individual MUPs is checked for accuracy and the quantitative MUP data are compared with the normal MUP parameters from the Laboratory of Clinical Neurophysiology, Rigshospitalet, Copenhagen. The most important requirement is to follow the recommended methods of testing, machine setup, and measurement parameters.

NORMAL DATA FOR MUPS WITH A CONCENTRIC NEEDLE

The normal parameters for MUPs obtained with a concentric needle were most extensively studied by Buchthal et al. at the Laboratory of Clinical Neurophysiology, Rigshospitalet, Copenhagen. These normal data follow.

Test Methodology

1. Following the standard method, the MUPs are obtained with a concentric needle during weak voluntary effort.
2. MUPs are captured on the oscilloscope with the help of the delay-line.
3. At least 20 (20 to 40) different MUPs are obtained from at least 20 (20 to 40) different points within the same muscle.

Machine Setup

Filters, 2 Hz to 10 kHz
Sensitivity, 100 to 300 μV/cm
Sweep velocity, 10 ms/1 cm (rarely 5 ms or 20 ms/cm)

Measurement

1. Duration (total duration) is measured at a sensitivity of 100 μV from the initial deviation from the baseline to the final return to it.
2. Amplitude is measured from peak to peak routinely at a sensitivity of 100 or 300 μV.
3. Phase is measured by the number of deflections above and below the baseline. MUPs with five or more phases are designated polyphasic MUPs.
4. These are first manually measured from the recordings.

Normal data

Table 5.20

Interpretation

When a value deviates by more than 20% from the mean value for MUP duration, it is considered abnormal. If a value is lower than the mean minus 20%, it considered to be indicative of myopathy. If the value is higher than the mean plus 20%, it is indicative of denervation process.

Table 5.20. Mean MUP Duration (ms) in Various Muscles at Different Ages (Concentric Electrodes)[a]

	Arm Muscles						Leg Muscles					Facial Muscles
Age (yr)	Deltoideus	Biceps Brachii	Triceps Brachii	Extensor Digitorum Communis	Opponens Pollicis; Interosseus	Abductor Digiti Quinti	Biceps Femoris; Quadriceps	Gastrocnemius	Tibialis Anterior	Peroneus Longus	Extensor Digitorum Brevis	Orbicularis Oris superior: Triangularis: Frontalis
0	8.8	7.1	8.1	6.6	7.9	9.2	8.0	7.1	8.9	6.5	7.0	4.2
3	9.0	7.3	8.3	6.8	8.1	9.5	8.2	7.3	9.2	6.7	7.2	4.3
5	9.2	7.5	8.5	6.9	8.3	9.7	8.4	7.5	9.4	6.8	7.4	4.4
8	9.4	7.7	8.6	7.1	8.5	9.9	8.6	7.7	9.6	6.9	7.6	4.5
10	9.6	7.8	8.7	7.2	8.6	10.0	8.7	7.8	9.7	7.0	7.7	4.6
13	9.9	8.0	9.0	7.4	8.9	10.3	9.0	8.0	10.0	7.2	7.9	4.7
15	10.1	8.2	9.2	7.5	9.1	10.5	9.2	8.2	10.2	7.4	8.1	4.8
18	10.4	8.5	9.6	7.8	9.4	10.9	9.5	8.5	10.5	7.6	8.4	5.0
20	10.7	8.7	9.9	8.1	9.7	11.2	9.8	8.7	10.8	7.8	8.6	5.1
25	11.4	9.2	10.4	8.5	10.2	11.9	10.3	9.2	11.5	8.3	9.1	5.4
30	12.2	9.9	11.2	9.2	11.0	12.8	11.1	9.9	12.3	8.9	9.8	5.8
35	13.0	10.6	12.0	9.8	11.7	13.6	11.8	10.6	13.2	9.5	10.5	6.2
40	13.4	10.9	12.4	10.1	12.1	14.1	12.2	10.9	13.6	9.8	10.8	6.4
45	13.8	11.2	12.7	10.3	12.5	14.5	12.5	11.2	13.9	10.1	11.1	6.6
50	14.3	11.6	13.2	10.7	12.9	15.0	13.0	11.6	14.4	10.5	11.5	6.8
55	14.8	12.0	13.6	11.1	13.3	15.5	13.4	12.0	14.9	10.8	11.9	7.0
60	15.1	12.3	13.9	11.3	13.6	15.8	13.7	12.3	15.2	11.0	12.2	7.1
65	15.3	12.5	14.1	11.5	13.9	16.1	14.0	12.5	15.5	11.2	12.4	7.3
70	15.5	12.6	14.3	11.6	14.0	16.3	14.1	12.6	15.7	11.4	12.5	7.4
75	15.7	12.8	14.4	11.8	14.2	16.5	14.3	12.8	15.9	11.5	12.7	7.5

[a] Values are mean values from different subjects without evidence of neuromuscular disease. The standard deviation of each value is 15% (20 potentials for each muscle). Therefore, deviations up to 20% are considered within the normal range when comparing measurements in a given muscle with the values of the table.
From Buchthal E. Introduction to electromyography. Copenhagen: Scandinavian University Books, 1957.

INTERPRETATION OF NEEDLE EMG ABNORMALITIES

All needle EMG parameters are useful for the diagnosis of neuromuscular diseases. Previous studies showed a concordance between the clinical and EMG findings in 80 to 95% of patients with myopathy and nearly all patients with denervation process. Needle EMG is most helpful in detection of myotonia and in differentiating between denervation process and myopathy. This is because needle EMG is the only way to detect the specific EMG patterns indicative of these disorders. On the other hand, peripheral neuropathy can be more specifically diagnosed by the nerve conduction study, and neuromuscular transmission disorders are best studied by the repetitive nerve stimulation test.

Among the various EMG potentials, myotonic potentials are most specific because they are almost pathognomonic of myotonic disorders and are usually associated with clinical myotonia. The next most specific EMG parameter is probably the duration of MUPs: a short duration is indicative of myopathy and a long-duration of denervation process (Fig. 5.29).

1. The needle EMG can differentiate myopathy from denervation. The constellation of specific EMG potentials, MUP parameters, and recruitment of MUPs is indicative of the specific diagnostic patterns of myopathy and denervation (Table 5.21 and Fig. 5.29). Among the various parameters, the most important in differentiation between myopathy and denervation process is the MUP duration. With these criteria, it is usually possible to differentiate myopathy from chronic denervation process. However, in cases of acute (relatively short-duration) denervation, these criteria have definite limitations because there has not been enough time for the appearance of reinnervation, which is responsible for long-duration and high-amplitude MUPs. Fibrillations and PSWs, when present, are definitely more helpful in the diagnosis of acute denervation.
2. The needle EMG can predict "activity" of the disease process, either in myopathy or denervation (Table 5.22). Activity is heavily judged on the basis of fibrillations and PSWs. In active myopathy, fibrillation and PSWs are invariably present along with a shorter MUP duration. For example, in untreated polymyositis, fibrillations and PSWs are prominent, but they are the first to disappear with treatment. In inactive (often chronic) myopathy,

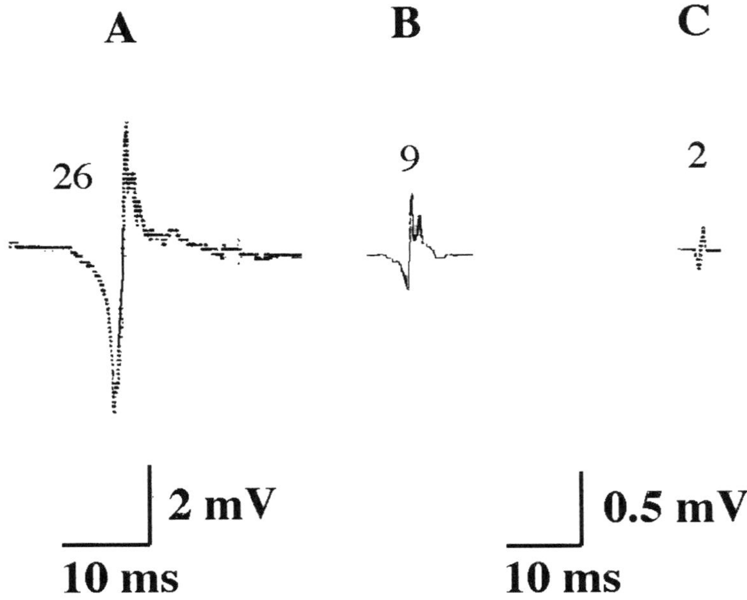

FIGURE 5.29. Typical MUPs in myopathy and denervation. **A.** HALD MUP in denervation. **B.** Normal MUP. **C.** SASD MUP in myopathy. Numbers above MUP represents the duration of MUP.

TABLE 5.21. MUP Parameter Criteria for Myopathy and Denervation Process

	MUP Parameters			
	Duration	**Amplitude (mV)**	**Polyphasic MUP**	**Interference Pattern**
Normal	6–16 ms[a]	0.5–5 (M)[a]	Normal duration	FIP with maximal contraction
		0.3–3.5 (C)[a]	Normal amplitude <20% of MUPs	
	Mean ± 20% of mean[b]			
Myopathy	<6 ms	<0.5 (M) <0.3 (C)	Small amplitude Short duration	Early recruitment FIP with minimal or moderate contraction
	<Mean −20% of mean		Increased	
Denervation	>16 ms	>5 (M) >3.5 (C)	High amplitude Long duration	Rapid firing rate RIP or DA with maximal contraction
	>Mean +20% of mean		Rarely increased	

[a] Limb muscles.
[b] Quantitative MUP duration.
M, monopolar needle; C, concentric or coaxial needle; FIP, full interference pattern; RIP, reduced interference pattern; DA, discrete pattern.

TABLE 5.22. Characteristic Needle EMG Pattern

Fibrillation and PSW	**MUP**	**Interference**	**Pathology**	**Typical Diseases**
Active (subacute or ongoing) denervation pattern				
Profuse	Markedly polyphasic MUPs; amplitude and duration usually normal	Moderately or highly reduced	Axonal degeneration	Nerve injury Amyotrophic lateral sclerosis, Werdnig-Hoffman disease Axonal neuropathy Plexopathy
Chronic (inactive) denervation pattern				
No or little	HALD MUP with relatively unremarkable polyphasic MUPs	Greatly reduced; rapid firing	Reinnervation Type grouping	Spinal muscular atrophy Kugelberg-Welander disease CIDP HMSN type I
Active myopathy pattern				
Profuse	SASD MUP; markedly polyphasic	Normal or excessive	Profuse myopathy	Polymyositis Alcoholic myopathy Inclusion body myopathy[a]
Inactive myopathy pattern				
No	SASD MUP with less polyphasic MUP	Normal or excessive	Minimal myopathy	Benign congenital myopathy

[a] In one-third of cases, HALD MUPs are mixed with active myopathy pattern.

fibrillations and PSWs are absent and a shorter MUP duration is the sole finding. In active (ongoing) denervation, fibrillations and PSWs are prominent with increased polyphasic MUPs and reduced MUP recruitment. On the other hand, in inactive (usually chronic) denervation, fibrillations and PSWs are minimal and the MUP amplitude and duration are high and long.

3. Needle EMG is helpful in distinguishing axonal neuropathy from demyelinating neuropathy. Fibrillations and PSWs, electrophysiological hallmarks of axonal degeneration, are prominent in axonal neuropathy but absent or scarce in demylinating neuropathy. Their presence in demyelinating neuropathy is due to a secondary axonal degeneration. On the other hand, in demyelinating neuropathy, fasciculation or myokymia is a more prominent finding. The final distinction between demyelinating neuropathy and axonal degeneration depends on the nerve conduction data.

In general, the needle EMG provides extremely helpful information for the diagnosis of almost all neuromuscular diseases when properly performed and interpreted. Unlike the nerve conduction studies and RNS tests, which are relatively standardized, however, the quality of the needle EMG depends heavily on the ability of the electromyographer to search for, recognize, and interpret the specific EMG potentials and to synthesize these into a meaningful clinical context. In this sense, the needle EMG is truly an extension of the clinical evaluation where the knowledgeable and experienced clinician stands out.

CHAPTER 6

Single-Fiber Electromyography

The single-fiber electromyography (SFEMG), a relatively new test, is a selective recording technique in which a single-fiber EMG needle is used to identify and record action potentials from individual muscle fibers. This technique has already proven to be of value in the diagnosis of myasthenia gravis and other neuromuscular transmission (NMT) disorders.

DIFFERENCES BETWEEN SFEMG AND CONVENTIONAL EMG

Because the SFEMG needle records action potentials from individual muscle fibers, the SFEMG is the test used to study the microphysiology of the motor unit and end plate. Thus, the SFEMG has the following advantages over the conventional EMG test:

1. The SFEMG can generate quantitative data about NMT and motor unit topography: the jitter in NMT and the fiber density (FD) in motor unit topography;
2. The SFEMG is extremely sensitive in detection of a disturbed microphysiology of the motor unit and end plate;
3. The SFEMG can detect abnormalities in NMT and reinnervation status earlier than conventional electrophysiological tests;
4. The SFEMG is better tolerated by most patients than the repetitive nerve stimulation (RNS) test for the study of NMT;

On the other hand, there are some disadvantages of the SFEMG in comparison with the conventional EMG study:

1. The SFEMG is more difficult to learn and to perform than the conventional needle EMG test, a major obstacle to the popularity and availability of this test.
2. The SFEMG requires the cooperation of the patient more so than does the conventional voluntary EMG study. Although most adults are able to cooperate well enough to permit adequate SFEMG studies, it is impossible to make satisfactory recordings from muscles during voluntary activation if the patient is uncooperative or has a tremor. In such a case, recordings of jitter can be made with the stimulation SFEMG.
3. The SFEMG cannot be performed using basic EMG machines. Special SFEMG needles and sophisticated EMG equipment are needed. Many commercially available EMG machines now do have these capabilities, including automated jitter analysis.
4. In most neuromuscular disease, the SFEMG shows the same nonspecific abnormalities, i.e., abnormal jitter and increased FD. Because of their nonspecificity, SFEMG data must be interpreted along with the clinical and other electrophysiological data. Thus, this test is extremely sensitive but not specific. It cannot be used to differentiate between myopathy and denervation process.

SINGLE-FIBER ACTION POTENTIALS

Using a tiny SFEMG needle with a recording diameter of 25 μm (smaller than the average normal muscle fiber) that is exposed at a port on the side of the electrode, the action potential of a single muscle fiber is obtainable. This potential is called a single-fiber muscle action potential (SFAP).

To obtain the SFAP, the EMG machine should have a delay line, superimposition capability, low filter up to 500 Hz, and sweep velocity of 2.0 to 1 ms (Fig. 6.1). For the SFEMG, the low filter must be set at 500 Hz to stabilize the baseline of the oscilloscope and to exclude signals from distant fibers.

The most important criterion of an SFAP is a stable shape for consecutive discharges. An SFAP is typically biphasic and produces a high-pitched crisp sound. It has a rise time of less than 300 μs, a duration of less than 1 ms, and an amplitude higher than 1 mV (Fig. 6.2).

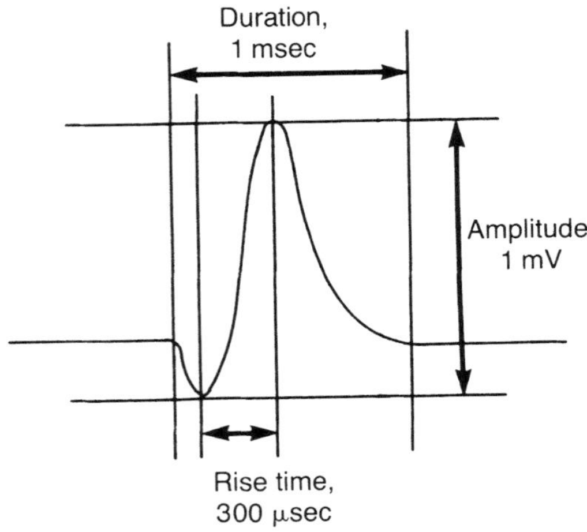

FIGURE 6.1. Characteristics of the single-fiber action potential.

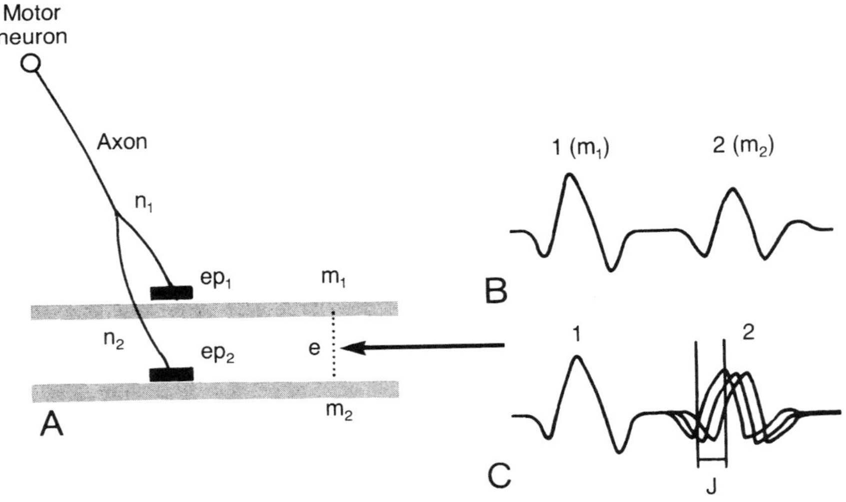

FIGURE 6.2. Anatomical basis for the single-fiber potential pair. **A.** Single-fiber EMG needle *e* is located midway between muscle fibers m_1 and m_2. These two muscle fibers are innervated by two branches, n_1 and n_2, from the same motor neuron. **B.** A single-fiber potential pair: one single-fiber action potential is generated from m_1 and another single-fiber action potential from m_2. **C.** Jitter *J* represents variation in the interpotential intervals, which is mainly due to the variability in transmission time in the motor end-plates, ep_1 and ep_2.

SFEMG PARAMETERS

There are three parameters that are essential in the SFEMG: jitter, blocking, and FD.

Jitter

When recording the SFMAP from two single muscle fibers belonging to the same motor unit by inserting the electrode between the two fibers, there is always a slight variability in the time interval between the two potentials in such "potential pairs." This variability is called the "jitter" and is expressed as mean consecutive discharge (MCD). Typically, the MCD is of the order of 20 μs (less than 55 μs for the EDC). The main cause of the jitter is probably the variability in synaptic delay between the two motor end plates.

Blocking

When one potential of a potential pair is missing, this is referred to as blocking. Blocking is usually seen in cases of markedly abnormal jitter and typically begins when jitter values exceed 80 to 100 μs. Blocking is due to a total failure of NMT to one muscle fiber of a potential pair with the same motor unit. Thus, blocking represents the most extreme abnormality of the jitter. There are two kinds of blocking: *neuromuscular blocking and neurogenic blocking*. When one potential of the potential pair is missing, this simple blocking is referred to as neuromuscular blocking and is characteristically seen in myasthenia gravis (MG) and other NMT disorders (Fig. 6.3). Neuromuscular blocking occurs when neuromuscular transmission is sufficiently impaired and end-plate potentials intermittently fail to reach the threshold needed to generate action potentials in the muscle fibers. When two or more of the components block together rather than independently, this is called neurogenic blocking and is invariably observed in neurogenic conditions (Fig. 6.4). The neurogenic block is probably localized in a terminal nerve twig, perhaps in newly formed sprouts. It is due to an intermittent conduction block at the proximal portion of the common axon twig from which the final two or three terminal twigs originate and innervate two or three muscle fibers from which blocking components are recorded. This block, however, is distal to the point of nerve branching to other muscle fibers recorded in the complex.

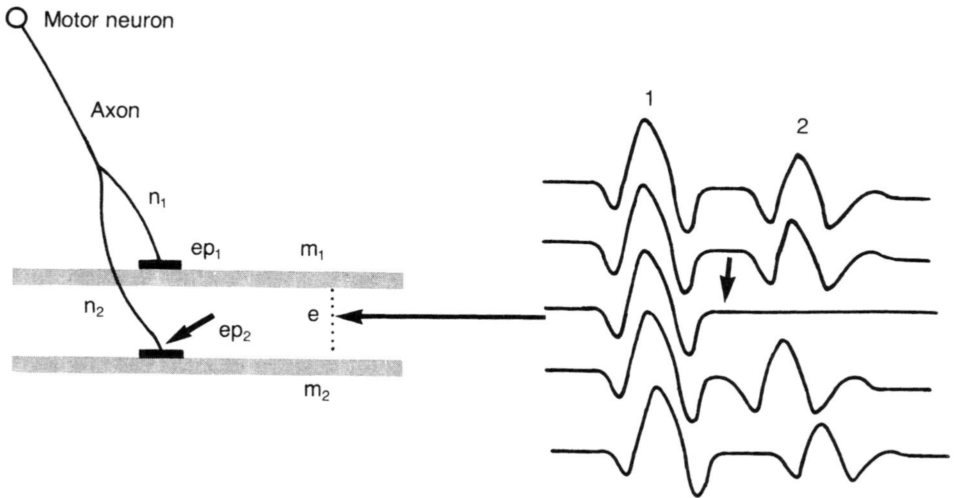

FIGURE 6.3. Anatomical basis for neuromuscular blocking. Blocking occurred at end-plate 2 (*ep_2; arrow*), resulting in blocking of potential 2 in the third tracing. n_1, n_2 branches of the same motor neuron; m_1, m_2, muscle fibers; *e*, single-fiber EMG needle.

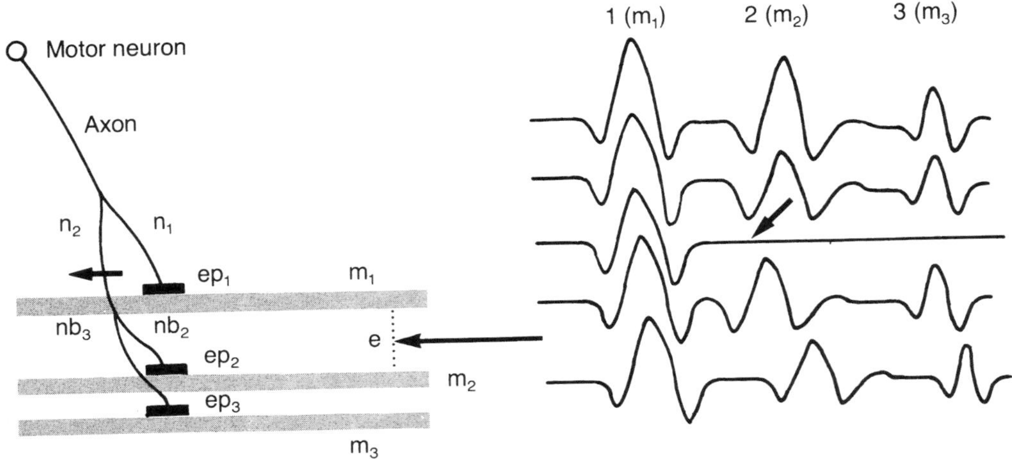

FIGURE 6.4. Anatomical basis for neurogenic blocking. Blocking occurred at an axon n_2 that has two axonal sprouts, nb_2 and nb_3, resulting in concomitant blocking of potentials 2 and 3 in the third tracing (*arrow*). Other abbreviations explained in Figure 6.3.

Fiber Density

The FD measures the number of muscle fibers in a motor unit that lie within 200 μm of the active recording surface of the SFEMG electrode. The mean FD can be calculated by counting the number of single muscle fibers from one motor unit in each of many electrode positions. After reinnervation, the FD is increased due to collateral sprouting, and often 3 to 10 fibers from the same motor unit are recorded with one electrode surface (Fig. 6.5). Increased FD thus indicates an increased number of muscle fibers belonging to the same motor unit within the uptake area and is usually a sign of reinnervation. However, the FD is also increased in myopathies but normal in NMT disorders (Fig. 6.6). In short, FD quantitates the local organization of the motor unit, providing information that is analogous to type grouping in muscle biopsies. Thus, FD is the most sensitive means of detecting and quantitating reinnervation. The most important variable in FD is age. The FD is relatively constant up to 65 years of age, after which it increases sharply. The increase in FD with advancing years is a result of compensatory reinnervation associated with normal Wallerian degeneration of aging nerves.

SFEMG TESTING

Jitter is measured from SFEMG recordings performed during voluntary activation of the tested muscle (conventional SFEMG) or during electrical stimulation of the nerve twig (stimulation SFEMG). The conventional SFEMG test can be performed in all muscles usually studied with conventional EMG needles. However, the most commonly tested muscle is the extensor digitorum communis (EDC) muscle in the forearm (Fig. 6.7).

FD can be measured in any muscle. The electrode is randomly inserted into the muscle to be tested. At least 20 SFAPs should be recorded from different recording sites. The number of "spikes" with amplitude $> 200\ \mu$V and rise time $< 300\ \mu$s are counted.

NORMAL VALUES AND CRITERIA FOR JITTER ABNORMALITIES

At least 50 consecutive discharges are recorded for each pair, and 10 or more potential pairs are analyzed for jitter. Jitter is expressed as the MCD, which is calculated by means of the automatic analyzer in the EMG machine equipped with SFEMG capability. Ideally, the MCD should be calculated on the basis of 20 potential pairs, but in practice, this is often difficult. Thus, for the voluntary SFEMG, we prefer the Duke University approach that accommodates fewer than 10 potential pairs.

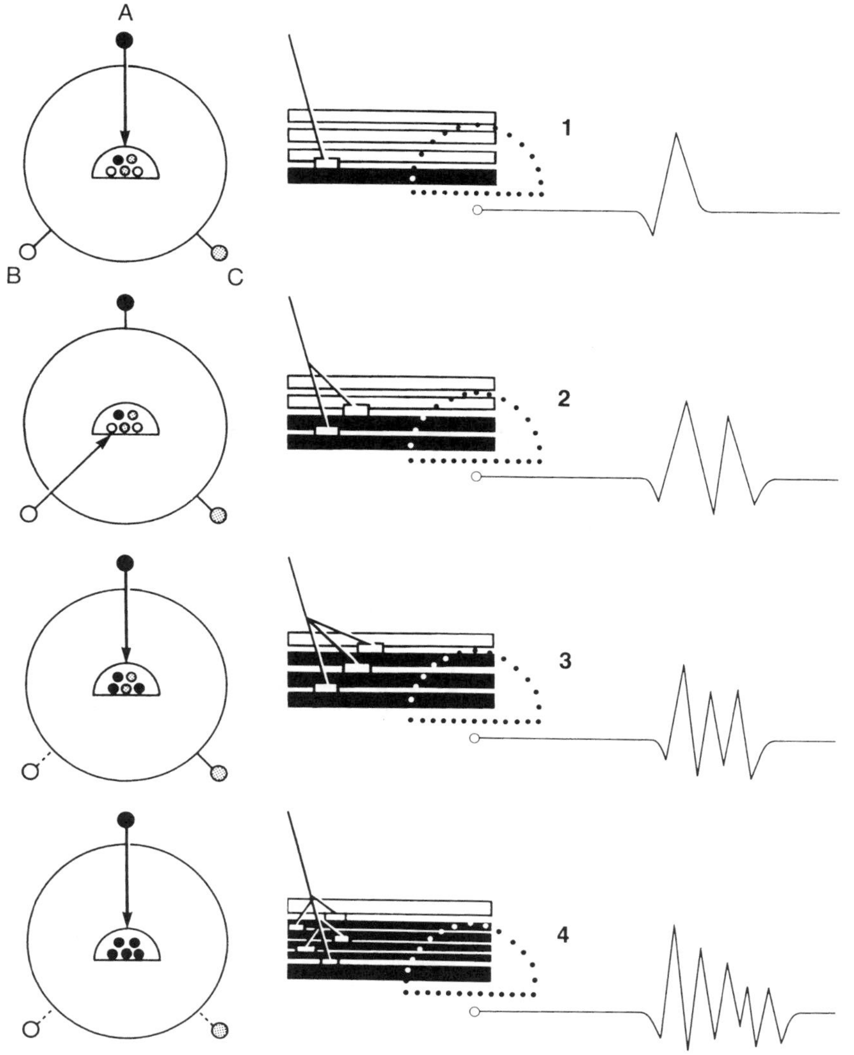

FIGURE 6.5. Anatomical basis of fiber density. **1.** One fiber is due to one muscle fiber activated by *axon A.* **2.** Two fibers are due to two muscle fibers activated by *axon B.* **3.** Three fibers are due to three muscle fibers activated by *axon A. Axon A* has axonal sprouts to two muscle fibers that were originally innervated by a completely denervated *axon B.* **4.** Five fibers are due to four activated muscle fibers by *axon A. Axon A* has axonal sprouts to four muscle fibers that were originally innervated by dead *axons B* and *C.*

The SFEMG is considered abnormal when one of the following three criteria is met (Table 6.5):

1. If the mean MCD value exceeds the normal limit (40 μs for the EDC muscle);
2. If more than 10% of potential pairs (more than two potential pairs if fewer than 10 are recorded) have blocking or jitter greater than the upper limit of an individual MCD (53 μs for the EDC muscle);
3. When blocking is frequently seen in most fiber pairs in a muscle, so that it is impossible to calculate the MCD.

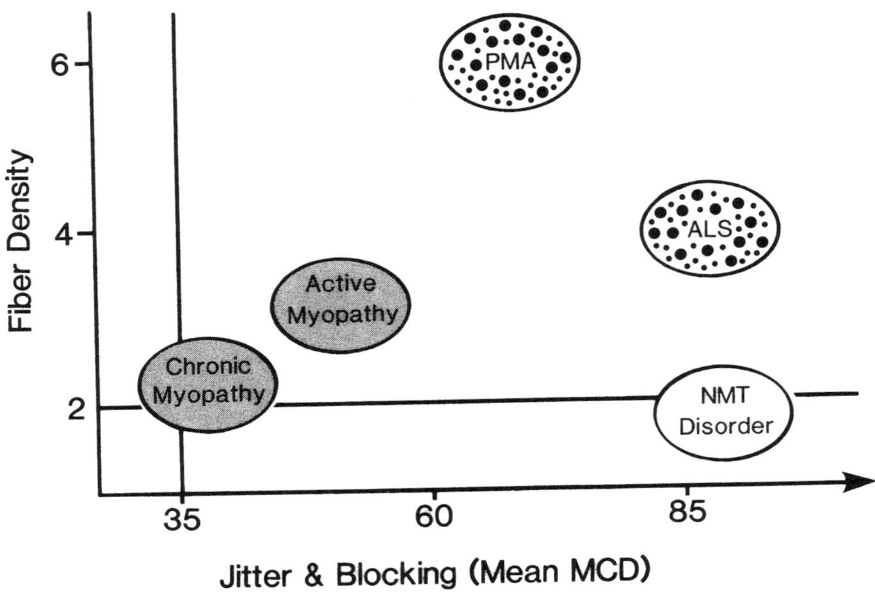

FIGURE 6.6. Relationship of fiber density to jitter and blocking in the various disorders. *Dotted circles* represent denervation disorders; *gray circles*, myopathies; *open circle*, NMT disorders. Percentage of abnormal jitter among single-fiber action potentials is also increasing in the direction of the arrow. *PMA*, progressive muscular atrophy; *ALS*, amyotrophic lateral sclerosis.

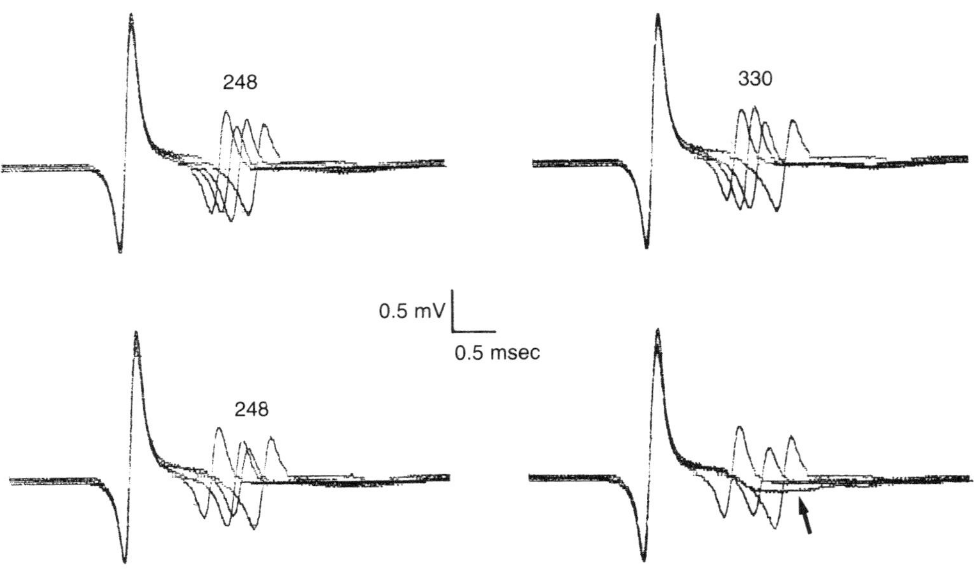

FIGURE 6.7. Markedly abnormal jitter in the EDC muscle in a patient with moderately severe MG. Numbers above the jitter represent MCD values. Neuromuscular blocking (*arrow*) is noted in one of the recordings.

The above criteria are applicable when 10 or more potential pairs are obtained. When fewer than 10 are obtained, the last two criteria are used.

To determine if a muscle is normal, jitter should be measured in up to 20 potential pairs. This means that the SFEMG test is much more difficult to ascertain as "normal" in a given muscle.

Jitter measured during axonal stimulation is less than the jitter measured during voluntary activation, because only jitter from a single end-plate is assessed. The normal values for jitter during axonal stimulation in the EDC are 47 μs for the upper limit of individual MCD and 25 μs for the mean MCD.

The FD is considered abnormal when it is above the normal limit (mean $\pm$ 3SD) for age in a given muscle. In general, FD more than 2.0 is definitely abnormal in subjects below 65 years of age.

INTERPRETATION OF SFEMG DATA

The SFEMG is extremely sensitive in identifying subclinical or clinical NMT disturbances. Thus, jitter is abnormal in many neuromuscular diseases, such as peripheral neuropathy, myopathy, and denervation process, thereby making *the SFEMG notoriously nonspecific*. However, if jitter is considered together with FD and the nature of the blocking, a certain pattern of SFEMG abnormality emerges that is typical of three distinctive categories of neuromuscular disease (Fig. 10.4 and Table 6.1).

Because of nonspecificity of SFEMG, it is always important to interpret SFEMG abnormalities in the context of clinical and other EMG and nerve conduction data.

SFEMG ABNORMALITIES IN NMT DISORDERS

The SFEMG is the most sensitive diagnostic test in all NMT disorders and, thus, best clinically indicated in diagnosis of these disorders.

The characteristic SFEMG findings in NMT disorders in which this test is most useful are a definite increase in jitter, neuromuscular blocking, and normal FD.

SFEMG in MG

In MG, the EDC muscle is usually tested first and the frontalis muscle is tested as the second muscle if the EDC muscle is normal. This guideline has been found to give the best diagnostic yield. One advantage of the SFEMG is that jitter is usually abnormal even when the patient is taking anticholinesterase medications. This is not the case for the RNS test in which a 12-hour anticholinesterase-off period is essential before the test. In rare patients, abnormal jitter has been demonstrated only after anticholinesterase was discontinued. Thus, we prefer to do the SFEMG test before anticholinesterase is started or after it has been discontinued for 12 hours.

The SFEMG is extremely sensitive in MG, being positive in an average 95% of cases, if the above guideline is followed, and in an average 85% of cases if only the EDC is tested. The test is so sensitive that Stalberg and Trontelj concluded that the diagnosis of MG can be abandoned if abnormal jitter is not found in a weak muscle. The classic SFEMG pattern in MG is characterized by a definitely increased jitter with or without neuromuscular blocking and normal FD. In MG there is typically a spectrum of jitter observations: normal jitter,

TABLE 6.1. Differentiation Among NMT Disorders, Myopathy, and Denervation Process by SFEMG Findings

Parameters	NMT Disorders	Myopathies	Denervation Processes
Fiber density	Normal	+ +	+ + +
Abnormal jitter	+ + +	+ +	+ +
Blocking			
Neuromuscular	+ +	–	+
Neurogenic	–	–	+

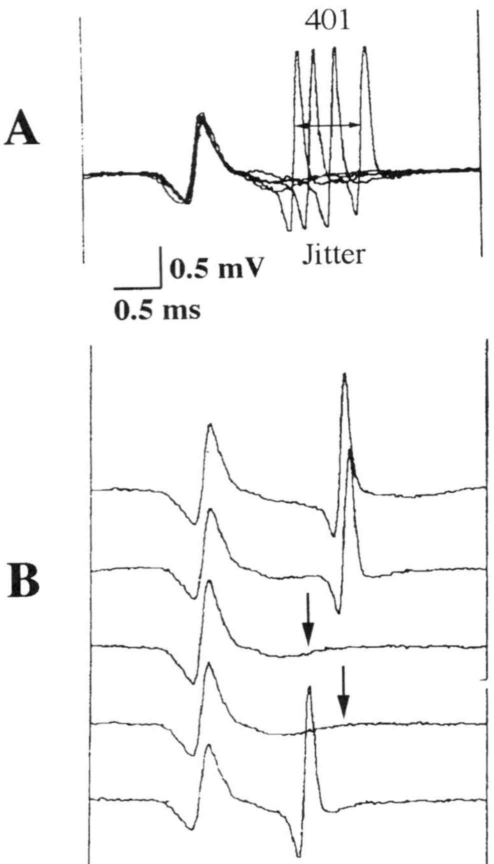

FIGURE 6.8. Neuromuscular blocking in a case of MG. **A.** Markedly abnormal jitter (MCD, 401 μs with neuromuscular blocking of one tracing). **B.** Neuromuscular blocking in two tracings.

increased jitter, and increased jitter with blocking (Fig. 6.8). Classically, in the case of initially abnormal jitter, the jitter and the frequency of blocking increase with an increasing discharge rate (Fig. 6.8). This is comparable with clinically observed exertional weakness in MG. However, this effect cannot be demonstrated in all potential pairs.

The 95% sensitivity of the SFEMG in MG contrasts with an average 80% sensitivity for the AChR antibody and 75% for the RNS tests. Although its sensitivity is highest, unfortunately the SFEMG is the least specific of the three diagnostic tests because it is abnormal in many other neuromuscular diseases. Thus, the SFEMG is best indicated in patients with MG in whom the AChR antibody and RNS tests are normal (9% in our study) because it is the crucial objective test for the diagnosis of MG. The SFEMG is also most helpful in confirmation of diagnosis in patients with mild MG (ocular and mild generalized), negative RNS tests, and negative AChR-ab titers. In these groups, the SFEMG is the most sensitive test, showing abnormality in more than 89% of cases. In mild MG, the RNS test and the AChR-ab are often negative.

In general, there is a good correlation between SFEMG abnormalities and the clinical severity of disease. The mean MCD and the number of potential pairs showing blocking are correlated with the patient's clinical symptoms and with the degree of decrement on the RNS test. Thus, the SFEMG may be used to monitor the effects of treatment. However, in this context, the RNS test is simpler and better.

Thus, the SFEMG study is the most sensitive diagnostic test in MG and is best indicated in patients with negative AChR-ab and RNS tests. It is also helpful in those with the milder form of MG and pure ocular MG in which the AChR-ab and/or the RNS test often show normal results. Unfortunately, the SFEMG is least specific among the three objective MG tests. The FD is normal in 75% of cases and slightly increased in others.

SFEMG in Lambert-Eaton Myasthenic Syndrome

The Lambert-Eaton myasthenic syndrome (LEMS) is a voltage-gated calcium-channel antibody-induced presynaptic disorder with resultant presynaptic block of acetylcholine release. LEMS is often associated with small-cell lung carcinoma. According to our studies, FD is normal. Jitter is markedly abnormal in all tested cases of LEMS, frequently out of proportion to the severity of weakness, usually with neuromuscular blocking (Fig. 6.9). It is not unusual to have difficulty obtaining a single-fiber potential pair because of extreme blocking. In some cases, we find it easier to perform the test in a less affected muscle, such as the frontalis, rather than the EDC, or to postpone testing to a later date when the patient shows clinical improvement. These findings are in good contrast to those in MG in which the SFEMG was abnormal in the EDC muscle in 95% of cases. As expected in a presynaptic NMT disorder, decreasing jitter abnormality and blocking were observed with a higher discharge rate in many end plates (Fig. 6.10). However, the absence of this relationship does not rule out such an abnormality because it is not observed in all end plates in LEMS patients. Tjontelj and Sanders agreed that a "dramatic decrease in jitter or blocking at higher rate, especially when starting from highly abnormal values at the lowest rates, strongly suggests presynaptic abnormality." Our study showed a good correlation between mean MCDs and clinical severity of disease as well as the compound muscle action potential amplitude and the incremental response (on a logarithmic scale) at HRS in the abductor digiti quinti and flexor carpi ulnaris muscles. Although the SFEMG is extremely sensitive in LEMS, it has a limited diagnostic value because of its lack of specificity. In LEMS, the RNS test is specific and sensitive.

SFEMG in Overlap MG/LEMS

There are some patients with a combination of MG and LEMS clinically. In these cases, the RNS test showed the classic pattern of LEMS. In four cases of overlap MG/LEMS, the SFEMG

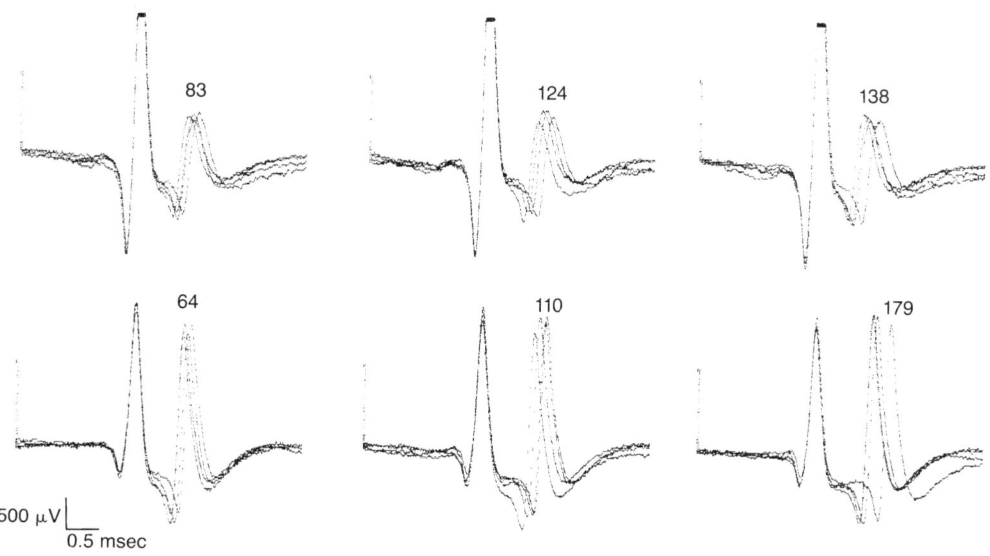

FIGURE 6.9. Abnormal MCD values in two potential pairs in a case of LEMS.

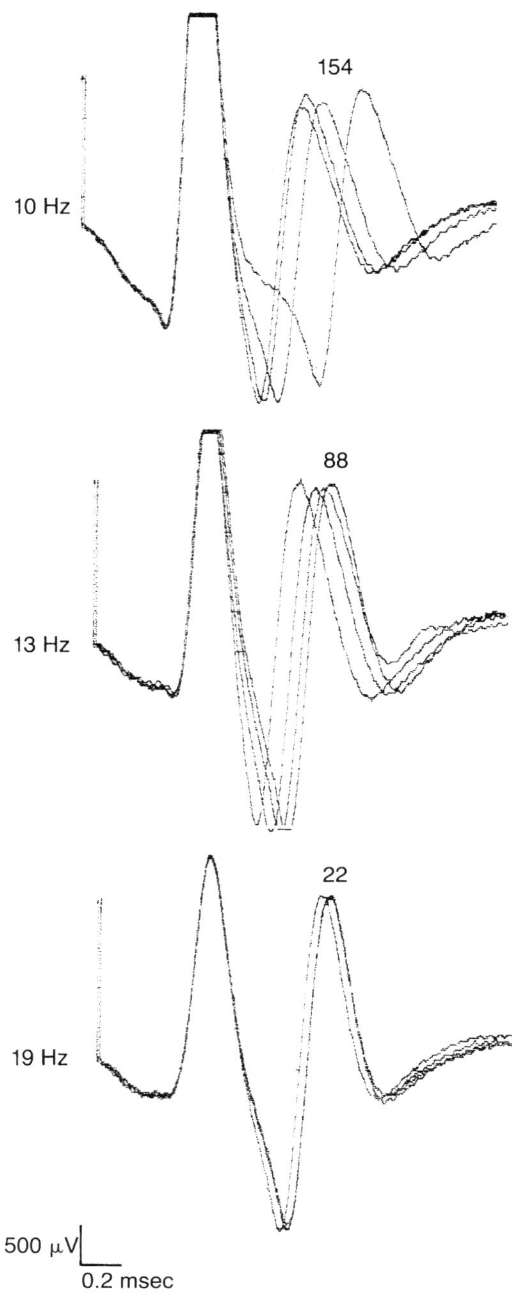

FIGURE 6.10. Decreasing MCD values with increasing discharge rates from 10 to 19 Hz in a case of LEMS.

was abnormal, showing markedly abnormal jitter with frequent neuromuscular blocking. Decreasing jitter was documented with a higher discharge rate in one tested case.

SFEMG in Botulism

Botulism is caused by a presynaptic block of acetylcholine release by *Clostridium botulinum*. The SFEMG was found to be abnormal in 95% of 15 tested cases and was abnormal in all patients who showed clinical weakness. This is in contrast to a 50% abnormality (7 of 14 tested cases) on the RNS test in the same series. The classic SFEMG pattern is characterized by a definite increase in jitter with or without neuromuscular blocking, decreasing jitter abnormality with a higher discharge rate, and normal FD. The SFEMG findings improved with clinical recovery. Thus, the SFEMG test is extremely sensitive in identifying the NMT abnormalities in botulism, especially in milder cases in which the RNS test is normal, and is also helpful in the follow-up of patients.

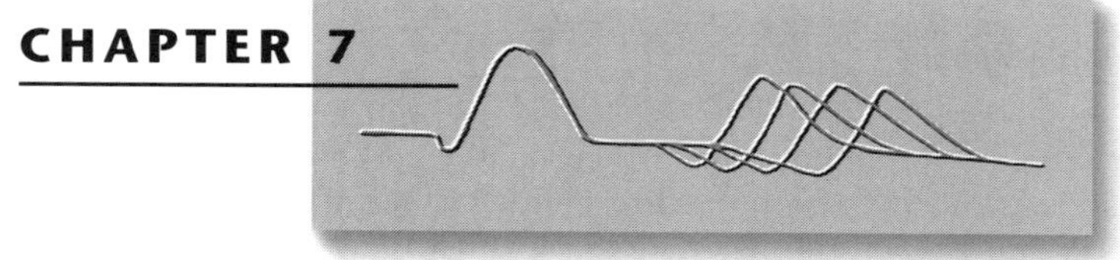

CHAPTER 7

Focal Neuropathy

Focal neuropathies are common diagnostic problems for the clinical electromyographer. Nerve conduction study (NCS) and needle electromyography (EMG) are essential for the precise localization of a focal neuropathy. The electrophysiological changes revealed by NCS in these disorders vary according to the rapidity with which the neuropathy develops, the duration and severity of the lesions, and the underlying causes. The characteristic nerve conduction abnormalities in a focal neuropathy are focal slowing of NCV, conduction block, and temporal dispersion across the compression site. These abnormalities are seen in more than 90% of cases of focal neuropathy.

Compression neuropathy refers to a focal neuropathy that is induced by compression of a nerve at an anatomically vulnerable site and is the most common form of focal neuropathies among nontraumatic causes. The ulnar, common peroneal, and radial nerves, respectively, are those most commonly compressed by external pressure. The median nerve is most frequently affected by constriction by a fascial band at the carpal tunnel. The axillary nerve is commonly affected in an allergic reaction to injection of serum and the sciatic nerve by direct injection of drugs.

ACUTE COMPRESSION NEUROPATHY

Acute compression neuropathy is characterized by the acute onset of neuropathy after a prolonged period of pressure compression on the nerve. The classic example is "Saturday night palsy," so called because of the number of cases attributable to prolonged resting of the head on the upper arm while the patient is in an alcoholic stupor. In the past, acute compression neuropathy was thought to be the result of neurapraxia, or conduction block, without any structural damage. However, studies with animals have revealed mild focal demyelination of large-diameter fibers as the pathological basis for this disorder. In severe cases, Wallerian degeneration is also present. This mild focal demyelinating process is responsible for the conduction block that is the characteristic electrophysiological finding in this disorder and explains the complete paralysis of the involved muscles. Abnormal temporal dispersion and nerve conduction slowing may be present. Acute compression neuropathies includes touniquet paralysis, Saturday night palsy, crossed-leg palsy, and perioperative ulnar nerve palsy.

Acute compression neuropathies have some common features: their symptoms are acute and predominantly motor, focal conduction block is common in the NCS, fibrillations and PSWs are rare, the prognosis is good, and thus surgical decompression is not indicated. These clinical and electrophysiological features are compatible with focal demyelination.

CHRONIC COMPRESSION (ENTRAPMENT) NEUROPATHY

Entrapment neuropathy refers to a mononeuropathy produced by chronic mechanical impingement of a nerve in normally narrow anatomical sites. The best example of this neuropathy is carpal tunnel syndrome. Regardless of the nerve involved in the entrapment process, there are common features in all entrapment neuropathies.

1. The most prominent symptom of an entrapment neuropathy is sensory, ranging from pain to numbness. Pain is usually present in the distribution of the peripheral nerve. The pain may be more severe at night and can occur at rest or with activity. In advanced cases, motor weakness and muscle wasting are present. Classically, the symptoms and signs are confined to the territory of the involved nerve.
2. Retrograde pain radiating proximal to the entrapment site (Valleix phenomenon) is common. This may cause confusion with such entities as radiculopathy.
3. Nerve trunk tenderness and Tinel's sign are common when the nerve is tested at the affected site.
4. Electrodiagnostic studies are essential in localizing the exact site of entrapment.
5. Many cases require surgical intervention, although some may respond favorably to local steroid injection.

Pathologically, entrapment neuropathies are characterized by paranodal demyelination in the early stages, complete segmental demyelination in the full-blown stage, and complete degeneration of fibers in the later stage. Wallerian degeneration in the nerve distal to the entrapment is a natural consequence of the late stage. NCS has been the means of definite diagnosis of entrapment neuropathies. The focal demyelinating process caused by mechanical entrapment is responsible for the electrophysiological evidence of chronic focal demyelination, marked focal slowing of the NCV. The presence of conduction block is less often demonstrable by nerve stimulation in chronic entrapment neuropathies than in acute compression neuropathies. To localize the focal demyelinating process, it is imperative to study the involved segment by means of the segmental NCS.

There are a few technical problems to be addressed in this connection. In human entrapment neuropathies, it has been shown that the primary abnormalities in conduction are confined to the short segments (often 5 to 10 mm) of the nerve. The consequence of the discrete nature of these lesions is that when nerve conduction is measured over long segments (8 to 10 cm), the NCVs could become less abnormal or even normal because of the inclusion of longer normal or near-normal segments in the calculation. Most authorities regard 10 cm as the shortest acceptable distance for the segmental NCV. This distance may be too generous to detect the segmental nerve conduction abnormality in some patients with focal neuropathy. Despite the inherent technical limitations of the short distance technique, the shorter distance has been used by several investigators in studies of sensory nerve conduction in the palm-wrist segment and in precise localization of the lesion in ulnar and peroneal compression neuropathies. In all these studies, the authors were able to pinpoint the lesion better with the shorter distance technique as long as the technique was carefully controlled. Percutaneous stimulation at short intervals along the length of an involved nerve (the "inching" technique) is especially useful in providing exact localization of the lesion by demonstrating conduction block and conduction delay. This is used as a routine test in our laboratory in patients with ulnar neuropathy at the elbow. The common entrapment neuropathies and their characteristic features are summarized in Table 7.1.

TESTS FOR CARPAL TUNNEL SYNDROME

The test for carpal tunnel syndrome should include motor, sensory, and mixed NCS in the median and ulnar nerves in the symptomatic arm. If carpal tunnel syndrome is confirmed in the symptomatic arm, the terminal latency and sensory nerve conduction should be checked over the finger-wrist and palm-wrist segments in the opposite median nerve. Special attention should be given to the finger-wrist and palm-wrist segments of the median nerve. It is very important to standardize the distance (5 cm) between the active recording electrode and the stimulating electrode at the wrist in the terminal latency study. If the sensory NCS in the II digit-wrist and palm-wrist segments are normal, the sensory nerve conduction should also be tested in the I digit-wrist and III digit-wrist segments before concluding that there is no electrophysiological evidence of carpal tunnel syndrome. The needle EMG test in the abductor pollicis brevis or opponens pollicis muscle is recommended to document any secondary axonal degeneration.

TABLE 7.1. Compression Site and Typical Clinical Features of the Common Compression Neuropathies

Compression Syndrome	Entrapment Site	Typical Clinical Features
Median nerve		
Carpal tunnel syndrome	Carpal tunnel	Tinel's sign at the wrist; sensory impairment over the first 3.5 fingers; motor deficits on thenar muscles
Anterior interosseous syndrome	At its origin from the median nerve	Pure motor weakness of the flexion of the middle phalanx of the first three fingers
Pronator syndrome	At the level of pronator teres	Entire motor and sensory neuropathy with pronator teres spared; pronator muscle tenderness and Tinel's sign on it
Ulnar nerve		
Tardy ulnar palsy Cubital tunnel syndrome	Elbow	"Claw hand," motor deficit on hypothenar muscles; sensory impairment over the dorsal and palmar aspects of the last 1.5 fingers
Guyon's canal	Wrist	Same as above except sensory impairment over palmar aspects of the last 1.5 fingers
Thoracic outlet syndrome	Thoracic outlet	Sensory impairment over the ulnar side of the entire arm and hand; motor deficits of the intrinsic hand muscles
Radial nerve		
Saturday night palsy	Spiral groove	Wrist drop
Posterior interosseous syndrome	The tendinous arcade of Frohse	Finger drop
Suprascapular nerve	Suprascapular foramen	Motor deficits of the supra- and infrascapular muscles
Long thoracic nerve		Scapular winging
Peroneal nerve		
Crossed-leg palsy	Fibular head	Foot drop
Posterior tibial nerve		
Tarsal tunnel syndrome	Tarsal tunnel	Sensory impairment over the palmar aspect of the foot; Tinel's sign at the ankle
Morton's neuroma	III–IV interdigital nerve	Sensory impairment over the V-shaped area between the III and IV toes
Laternal femoral cutaneous nerve		
Meralgia paresthesica	Anterior iliac crest	Sensory impairment over the lateral thigh
Femoral nerve	Inguinal ligament	Weak knee extension; absent knee jerk
Saphenous nerve	Hunter's canal	Sensory impairment in the medial aspect of knee and leg
Sural nerve		Sensory impairment over lateral aspect of the foot

Because carpal tunnel syndrome is caused by compression of the median nerve at the carpal tunnel (the wrist), typical findings are absent sensory nerve potentials or slow sensory NCV over the finger-wrist segment and prolonged terminal latency. In mild cases, the abnormalities in sensory NCV over the finger-wrist and palm-wrist (carpal tunnel) segments are the sole abnormalities; the terminal latency is usually normal. Carpal tunnel syndrome is bilateral in 32% of the cases. For this reason, the opposite median nerve must be tested when carpal tunnel syndrome is confirmed on one side.

TESTS FOR ULNAR COMPRESSION NEUROPATHY AT THE ELBOW (TARDY ULNAR NERVE PALSY OR CUBITAL TUNNEL SYNDROME)

The tests for ulnar compression neuropathy at the elbow should include motor, sensory, and mixed NCS in the median and ulnar nerves in the symptomatic arm. Special attention should be paid to the motor NCV across the elbow. The distance across the elbow in the extended arm should be 9 to 10 cm. In some EMG laboratories, a distance of 10 cm with the arm flexed is recommended. If the latter method is used, the values obtained must be compared with the normal NCV values for that method. If an ulnar neuropathy is confirmed on one side, the opposite extremity must be tested because ulnar neuropathy is bilateral in 39% of cases. To distinguish tardy ulnar nerve palsy (transsulcal compression) from cubital tunnel syndrome, the ulnar nerve should be studied across the elbow segment by the short-segmental incremental method (inching technique). For the needle EMG, the test in the abductor digiti quinti or first dorsal interosseous muscle and the flexor carpi ulnar muscle is recommended to document whether there is any secondary axonal degeneration.

Tardy ulnar nerve palsy is caused by compression of the ulnar nerve at the elbow sulcus. Typical findings are slow motor NCV across the elbow and slow NCV or absent nerve potential in mixed nerve conduction over the elbow-wrist segment and in sensory nerve conduction over the finger-wrist segment. In mild cases, abnormalities in the mixed and sensory NCS may be the sole findings. In cubital tunnel syndrome, the most prominent nerve conduction abnormalities are noted in the segment 2 cm distal to the epicondylar line, whereas in tardy ulnar nerve palsy, the most prominent nerve conduction abnormalities are noted in the segment 2 cm distal or proximal to the epicondylar line.

TESTS FOR PERONEAL NERVE PALSY

The tests for peroneal nerve palsy should include motor NCS in the peroneal and posterior tibial nerves in the symptomatic leg and sensory NCS in the superficial peroneal nerve. The segmental NCS across the fibular head (below the fibular head-popliteal fossa) should always be included. The needle EMG test in the anterior tibialis, peroneus longus, and extensor digitorum brevis muscles is recommended to document the extent of denervation and the presence of a secondary axonal degeneration.

Because the compression is usually across the fibular head, slow motor NCV across the fibular head and abnormal sensory nerve conduction in the superficial peroneal nerve are typical findings. When the peroneal nerve is stimulated at the popliteal fossa, the movement of the great toe should be observed. If it moves toward the head, the peroneal nerve is being stimulated. When the posterior tibial nerve is being stimulated, the toe moves away from the head.

TESTS FOR OTHER FOCAL NEUROPATHIES

Nerve conduction techniques have been well described for most nerves in the body. Thus, to confirm a focal neuropathy of a particular nerve, one has to use the technique described and refer to the normal data for that particular nerve in the interpretation of findings. However, there are still a few nerves in which the nerve conduction technique has not yet been described. To confirm a focal neuropathy in such nerves, one has to compare the findings with the unaffected side.

CASE 1

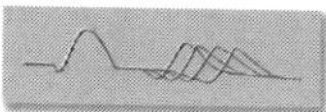

ACUTE ONSET OF BULBAR PALSY

CASE PRESENTATION

A 55-year-old man experienced acute onset of swallowing difficulty followed by slurring of speech and chewing difficulty for 7 days. These symptoms were constant and did not worsen with exertion or improve with rest. Abnormal neurological findings were dysphonia, soft palate paralysis, weak hypoglossal muscles, and absent gag reflexes. Limb muscles were neurologically normal and there was no myasthenic weakness in his speech. There was no history of antecedent event or infection.

CASE ANALYSIS

This patient developed acute bulbar palsy. Three diagnostic possibilities should be considered: MG, cranial polyneuropathy (cranial form of Guillain-Barré syndrome), and botulism. MG and the cranial form of GBS are certainly more common than botulism. MG was the first disease to rule out in this situation. The absence of fluctuating symptoms and myasthenic weakness were against the possibility of MG. On the other hand, there was no finding indicative of GBS. Thus, until proven otherwise, we had to assume that the patient has MG. If his pupils had been affected, clearly MG would have to be ruled out automatically.

PLAN OF TESTING

1. RNS test: To confirm or rule out MG and botulism.
2. Needle EMG: To find whether there is any denervation process in hypoglossal or masseter muscles.
3. NCS: To confirm or rule out GBS. This should include facial and hypoglossal nerves (1).
4. Blink reflex: To check the proximal pathways of facial nerves.
5. Other tests: Tensilon test. AChR antibody test. Spinal fluid.

ELECTROPHYSIOLOGICAL TESTS AND FINDINGS

`NCS Findings` (Fig. 7.1)

1. Normal motor and sensory NCS in median, ulnar, peroneal, and posterior tibial nerves.
2. Normal latency and CMAPs in the right and left facial and accessory nerves.
3. Prolonged terminal latency and low CMAP amplitudes in the left and right hypoglossal nerves.

`Blink Reflex` (Fig. 7.1)

1. Normal R1 and R2 latencies in the right OO muscle with right-side stimulation.
2. Low amplitude response in the left OO muscle with right-side stimulation.
3. Markedly prolonged R1 and R2 latencies and low amplitude response in the left OO muscle with the left stimulation.
4. Markedly prolonged R2 latency and low amplitude response in the right OO muscle with left-side stimulation.

`Masseter Reflex` (Fig. 7.1). Absent reflex in the right and left masserter reflex.

`Needle EMG`

1. A few but definite PSWs and normal MUPs in the genioglossal and masseter muscles.
2. Normal EMG findings in the FDI, triceps, anterior tibialis, and vastus lateralis muscles.

`RNS Test Findings`. Normal in the ADQ, FCU, orbicularis oris, and trapezius muscles.

ELECTROPHYSIOLOGICAL INTERPRETATION

1. No evidence of neuromuscular transmission disorder or systemic neuropathy.
2. Cranial polyneuropathy involving facial, trigeminal, and hypoglossal nerves.

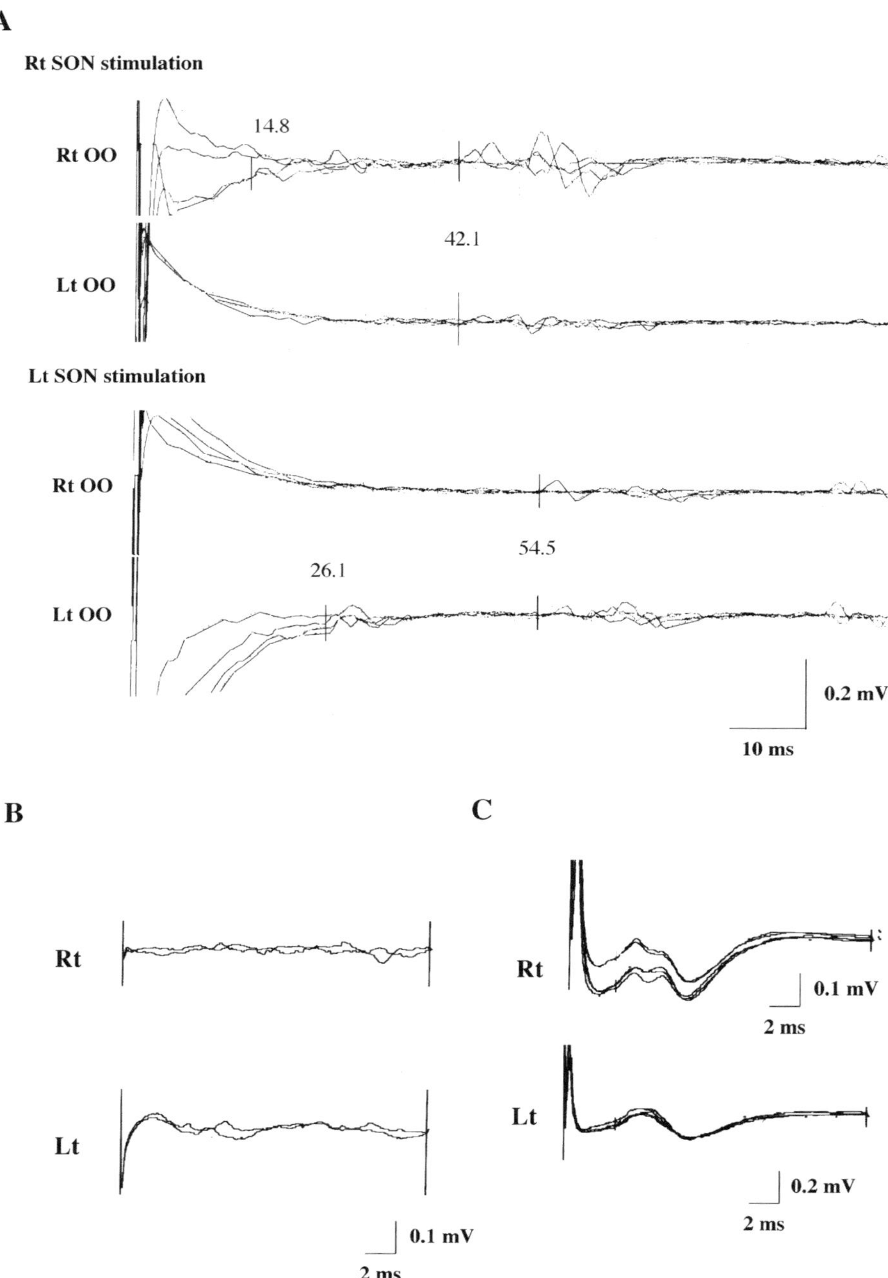

FIGURE 7.1. **A.** Blink reflex. **B.** Masseter reflex: no response on either side. **C.** Hypoglossal nerve motor conduction. *OO*, orbicularis oculi; *SON*, supraorbital nerve. Numbers represent latencies in ms.

OTHER TEST FINDINGS

CSF protein was 96 mg/dL. No cells in the CSF. Negative Tensilon and AChR antibody tests. Normal chest x-ray.

FINAL DIAGNOSIS

Cranial polyneuropathy, most likely the cranial form of GBS

TREATMENT AND FOLLOW-UP

Because of swallowing difficulty, the patient was fed through a nasogastric tube and treated with one course of IVIg therapy without any improvement. One course of plasma exchange was added. There was a slow but definite improvement noted.

COMMENTS

The low amplitude response from the left OO in the blink reflex was suggestive of left facial neuropathy. Prolonged latency of all responses with left-side stimulation clearly was indicative of left trigeminal neuropathy. Hypoglossal nerve stimulation, which is a relatively new test, identified bilateral hypoglossal neuropathy. Absent masseter reflex is indicative of trigeminal neuropathy.

The term cranial polyneuropathy has been reserved for an acute disorder characterized by multiple cranial nerve involvements in which no other known diseases are found. Infiltrative tumors or carcinomatous meningitis have to be ruled out. In this case, MG and botulism were well ruled out. The diagnosis of cranial polyneuropathy was made by electrodiagnostic tests. The high CSF protein suggested the possibility of a cranial form of GBS in this case. Sarcoidosis may also cause cranial polyneuropathy, but in this case there was no sign of sarcoidosis.

The blink reflex is an electrically induced glabellar response that has long been used in clinical neurology. The blink reflex is a polysynaptic reflex with an afferent arc through sensory fibers of the trigeminal nerve and with an efferent arc through the motor fibers of the facial nerve. There are R1 and R2 responses from the OO ipsilateral to the stimulation and R2 response from the side opposite to the stimulation. R1 is mediated via the main sensory nucleus of cranial nerve V in the pons, whereas R2 is mediated via the spinal nucleus and tract of nerve V in the medulla oblongata. The blink reflex is most useful in the evaluation of lesions of the trigeminal nerve and facial nerve, especially in patients with hemifacial spasm (see Chapter 14). To detect a lesion in the first division of the trigeminal nerve, the blink reflex is the only physiological test available at this time. The classic findings indicative of such a lesion are an "afferent defect," a prolonged latency of both ipsilateral R1 and R12 and contralateral R2, as seen in the left-side stimulation in our case. In the facial nerve lesion, there is a delay in the reflex latency only on the affected side, regardless of the side of stimulation ("efferent defect"). In hemifacial spasm, a synkinetic response has been observed in the OO muscle, whereas no synkinetic response is observed in this muscle in normal individuals.

MAXIMS

1. The blink reflex is the only physiological test for the first division of trigeminal nerve and can identify the lesion in the first division of trigeminal nerve.
2. Cranial polyneuropathy can be seen as a cranial form of GBS or in sarcoidosis.

REFERENCES

1. Oh SJ. Clinical electromyography. Nerve conduction studies. Baltimore, MD: Williams and Wilkins, 1993; Blink reflex, pp. 389. Facial nerve, pp. 151–155. Hypoglossal nerve, pp. 161–163. Masseter reflex, pp. 391–393.

CASE 2

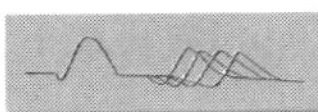

ACUTE ONSET OF HOARSENESS AND SWALLOWING DIFFICULTY: SIGNS OF MG?

CASE PRESENTATION

A 75-year-old woman was sent for evaluation of MG. About 3 months before, she had a throat infection followed by hoarseness and difficulty swallowing. She was very sick and had a lot of stridor to the degree that a tracheostomy was considered at one point. Her swallowing difficulty was such that food tended to come out through her nose. With intravenous antibiotics, her condition improved. Since then, her hoarseness and swallowing also gradually improved, especially in the 2 to 3 weeks preceding our evaluation. She reported no limb weakness or diplopia. The only abnormal neurological finding was hoarseness. The patient had no weakness of the soft palate, nasal dysphonia, or sensory abnormality in the mouth or pharynx. Gag reflex was normal. MRI of the head showed ischemic vasculopathy. Acetylcholine receptor antibody was negative.

CASE ANALYSIS

The history strongly suggested the possibility of diphtheria. Apparently, there was no diphtheric membrane in the pharynx and the diagnosis of diphtheria was never made. Whatever the etiology of her throat infection, she developed rather acute swallowing difficulty and hoarseness. Her description of the swallowing difficulty clearly suggested soft-palate paresis, and her lingering hoarseness could represent vocal cord paralysis.

PLAN OF TESTING

1. Needle EMG: Thyroarytenoid muscle through the cricothyroid notch (1, 2).
2. RNS test: To rule out MG.

ELECTROPHYSIOLOGICAL TESTS AND FINDINGS

Needle EMG (Fig. 7.2)

1. Fibrillation and PSWs and reduced MUP recruitment in the right thyroarytenoid muscle.
2. Normal needle EMG findings in the left thyroarytenoid and right cricothyroid muscles.

RNS Test Findings. Normal RNS test on the ADQ, FCU, OO, and trapezius muscles.

ELECTROPHYSIOLOGICAL INTERPRETATION

Recurrent right laryngeal neuropathy.

FINAL DIAGNOSIS

Recurrent right laryngeal neuropathy, postinfectious

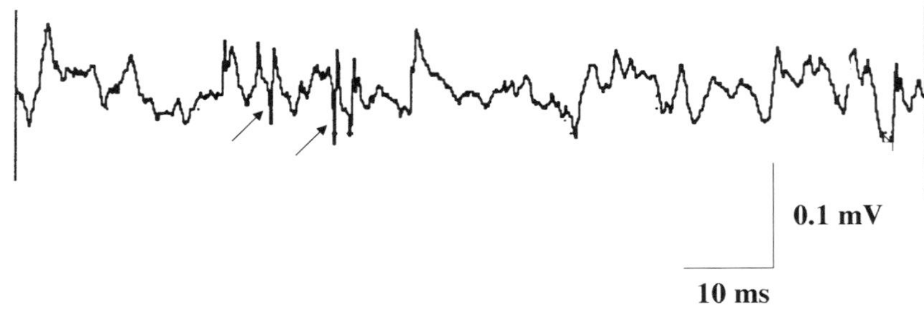

FIGURE 7.2. Fibrillations *(arrows)* in the right thyroarytenoid muscle. Other discharges are distant MUPs from nonrelaxed neighboring muscles.

TREATMENT AND FOLLOW-UP

MG was well ruled out by the negative AChR antibody and negative RNS tests. Needle EMG in the laryngeal muscles confirmed neuropathy in the right recurrent laryngeal nerve. There has been gradual improvement in the patient's hoarseness.

COMMENTS

Two branches of the vagal nerve innervate three laryngeal muscles. The recurrent laryngeal nerve innervates the thyroarytenoid (adductor) and posterior cricoarytenoid (abductor) muscles. The superior laryngeal nerve innervates the cricothyroid muscle. Thus, the needle EMG can differentiate between recurrent laryngeal neuropathy and superior laryngeal neuropathy.

The most frequent cause of vocal cord paralysis is unilateral laryngeal neuropathy, producing hoarseness as the chief complaint. In bilateral vocal cord paralysis, patients complain of hoarseness and shortness of breath.

The needle EMG in the thyroarytenoid muscle can be performed by inserting a "Botox" EMG needle through the cricothyroid notch and the needle EMG in the cricothyroid muscle, by inserting the needle lateral to the cricothyroid notch. A description of the method for the needle EMG is found in detail in the listed references. One cardinal rule in the diagnosis of MG is that hoarseness, whispering, or loss of voice, whether at rest or induced by exertion, is not a sign of MG. These are common symptoms in pseudo-MG patients.

MAXIMS

1. The thyroarytenoid muscle is innervated by the recurrent laryngeal branch of the vagal nerve, whereas the cricothyroid muscle is innervated by the superior laryngeal nerve.
2. Hoarseness, whispering, or loss of voice, whether at rest or induced by exertion, is not a clinical feature of MG.

REFERENCES

1. Simpson D, Sternman D, Graves-Wright J, Sanders I. Vocal cord paralysis: clinical and electrophysiological features. Muscle Nerve 1993;16:952–957.
2. Rodriquez A, Myers B, Ford C. Laryngeal electromyography in the diagnosis of laryngeal nerve injuries. Arch Phys Med Rehabil 1990;71:587–590.

CASE 3

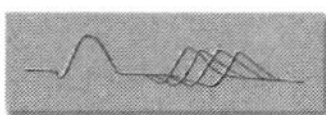

WEAKNESS AND PAIN IN THE SHOULDER AREA AFTER REMOVAL OF A BRAINSTEM MENINGIOMA

CASE PRESENTATION

A 52-year-old woman had removal of a meningioma in the medullocervical junction 7 months previously and had pain and weakness in the right shoulder without any improvement since then. The neurosurgeon made a diagnosis of long thoracic nerve palsy on the basis of scapular winging and wanted to know the exact location of the injury because of his interest in exploration of the lesion. Our examination showed upper scapular winging and a scaphoid line in the upper border of the right trapezius muscle.

CASE ANALYSIS

The upper scapular winging, which was accentuated by arm abduction at the shoulder level, was pathognomonic of accessory nerve palsy. Atrophy of the upper border of the trapezius is also usually prominent. The main question was whether this was an intracranial or extracranial lesion. If it was an extracranial lesion, the surgeon wanted to surgically explore the lesion because it was not improving. To determine this, the SCM muscle should be included in the testing and nerve conduction should be performed with stimulation proximal to the SCM muscle.

PLAN OF TESTING

1. NCS: Right accessory nerve test with stimulation proximal to the SCM muscle (1).
2. Needle EMG: Right SCM and trapezius muscles.

ELECTROPHYSIOLOGICAL TESTS AND FINDINGS

NCS Findings ***(Fig. 7.3)***

1. Normal latency to the right SCM muscle (3.1 ms with 1.5-mV CMAP).
2. Prolonged latency to the right trapezius muscle (5.7 ms with 0.5-mV CMAP).

Needle EMG. Fibrillations and PSW, some long-duration MUPs, and RIP in the right SCM and trapezius muscles.

ELECTROPHYSIOLOGICAL INTERPRETATION

Incomplete right proximal accessory neuropathy.

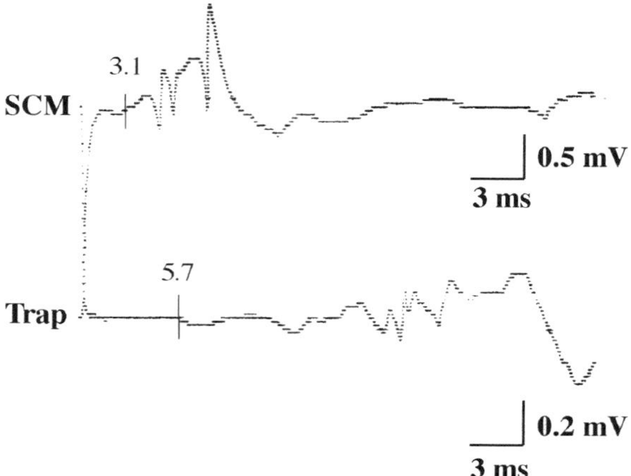

FIGURE 7.3. Accessory nerve conduction. *Trap*, trapezius muscle; *SCM*, sternocleidomastoid muscle. Notice multiphasic CMAP due to concentric-needle recording. This does not necessarily represent dispersion phenomenon. Numbers above the responses represent latencies in ms.

FINAL DIAGNOSIS

Right proximal accessory neuropathy due to intracranial injury during surgical excision of a meningioma

TREATMENT AND FOLLOW-UP

No surgical exploration was done, and slow but gradual improvement was noted.

COMMENTS

The accessory nerve, the 11th cranial nerve, arises from the C1-4 spinal roots and ascends into the intracranial cavity through the foramen magnum, leaves the intracranial cavity through the jugular foramen accompanied by the glossopharyngeal and vagus nerves, and descends into the neck to supply the SCM first. The distal branch appears at the posterior border of the SCM at the upper edge of the thyroid cartilage and runs obliquely downward and backward toward the posterior cervical triangle to supply the upper third or upper half of the trapezius muscle. If the intracranial portion of the nerve is injured, the SCM muscle is affected.

The most common cause of accessory nerve palsy is surgery on the posterior triangle of the neck. In accessory nerve palsy, the trapezius muscle is always involved. Accessory nerve palsy may mimic long thoracic nerve palsy because of the scapular winging. In long thoracic neuropathy, the scapular winging is localized to the lower part of the scapular and accentuated by forward elevation and pushing with outstretched arms, a maneuver that further displaces the inferior angle of the scapula from the midline. However, the scapular winging in trapezius paralysis is localized to the upper part of the scapula and accentuated by arm abduction to the shoulder level, which displaces the inferior angle of the scapula closer to the midline. Thus, differentiation can easily be made by careful evaluation. It is also important to remember that the trapezius muscle covers the deeper muscles in the neck and scapular area. Thus, if the EMG needle is not inserted deeply (at least 3 cm), fibrillation and PSW in the superficial cervical paraspinal muscles can be mistaken for signs of cervical radiculopathy.

MAXIMS

1. If involvement of the intracranial accessory nerve is suspected, the SCM muscle should be examined because it is the most proximal muscle innervated by the accessory nerve.
2. Scapular winging due to accessory nerve palsy is characterized by winging of the upper part of the scapula and is accentuated by arm abduction to the shoulder level.

REFERENCES

1. Oh SJ. Clinical Electromyography. Nerve conduction studies. Baltimore, MD: Williams and Wilkins, 1993:170–171.
2. Saeed MA, Gatens PF Jr, Singh S. Winging of the scapula. Am Fam Physician 1981:24:139–143.

CASE 4

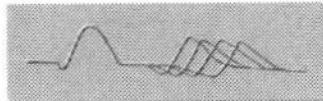

WEAKNESS OF SHOULDER ABDUCTION AFTER A FALL

CASE PRESENTATION

A 44-year-old man fell out of a "rolling chair" and injured his left arm 4 months previously. He fell backward on his buttocks and back with his arm extended behind him, taking the force of the blow and stretching his shoulder. Since then, he had shoulder pain and bruising on his shoulder area. X-ray was normal. About 2 weeks later he began to notice weakness in his left arm, particularly in the deltoid muscle, which progressed for 2 weeks and then stabilized. Two months ago, a needle EMG was done and a diagnosis of C6 radiculopathy was made. CT/myelogram showed a large herniated disc at the C4–5 level. An anterior discectomy was performed without any improvement in his weakness. Abnormal neurological findings were 0 MRC strength and atrophy in the deltoid, infraspinatus, and supraspinatus muscles, and decreased pin-prick sensation over the left deltoid. No reflex change was noted.

CASE ANALYSIS

Clinically, this patient had weakness and atrophy of the left supraspinatus, infraspinatus, and deltoid muscles and sensory loss over the axillary nerve territory. The main question was localization of the lesion: C5 radiculopathy, upper trunk plexopathy, or individual neuropathies. Certainly, a large herniated disc at the C4–5 level involving the C5 root fit quite well with his clinical findings. However, a herniated disc at the C5 level is extremely rare. If this was a pure C5 radiculopathy, it would have been extremely unusual that the rhomboid was not clinically involved. Because the biceps muscle was spared, an upper trunk lesion was less likely. With the history of a fall, it was possible that multiple individual nerves were affected. It was critical to do a needle EMG in the paraspinal muscles to distinguish radiculopathy from brachial plexopathy.

PLAN OF TESTING

1. NCS: Latency test for the deltoid, biceps, triceps, and supra- and infraspinatus muscles.
2. Needle EMG: Cervical paraspinal, rhomboid, supra- and infraspinatus, deltoid, biceps, and triceps muscles.

ELECTROPHYSIOLOGICAL TESTS AND FINDINGS

NCS Findings (Table 7.2; Fig. 7.4)

1. Prolonged terminal latency and slow-sensory NCV over the finger-wrist segment in the left median nerve.
2. No CMAP in the left deltoid with stimulation at Erb's point.
3. Prolonged terminal latencies to the left supra- and infraspinatus muscles.

Needle EMG (Table 7.3)

1. Prominent fibrillation and PSW and no MUP on maximal contraction in the left supra- and infraspinatus muscles.
2. Prominent fibrillation and PSW and some HALD MUPs in the left deltoid muscle.

ELECTROPHYSIOLOGICAL INTERPRETATION

1. Left suprascapular and axillary neuropathy.
2. Left carpal tunnel syndrome (asymptomatic).

FINAL DIAGNOSIS

Posttraumatic severe left suprascapular and partial axillary neuropathies

TREATMENT AND FOLLOW-UP

We repeated the tests after 1 month. There was no evidence of improvement whatsoever. Thus, surgical exploration of the left suprascapular and axillary nerves was done (Fig. 7.5). The axillary nerve looked intact. Intraoperative NCS was performed across the suprascapular

TABLE 7.2. Nerve Conduction Data in Case 4

	Latent/NCV (ms/m/s)	Amplitude (mV/μV)		Latent/NCV (ms/m/s)	Amplitude (mV/μV)
Left	**Median**	**Motor N**		**Ulnar**	**Motor N**
TL	4.0	14	F-W	45.7	10
E-W	58.3	13	W-E	48.6	30
AX-E	60.7	13	E-AX	56.8	20
F-wave	29.2				
	Ulnar	**Motor N**		**Brachial plexus**	**Motor N**
TL	2.4	10	Deltoid	NP	Initial positive
BE-W	59.2	8	Biceps	5.6	4.1
AE-BE	50.0	8	Triceps	5.4	5.3
AX-AE	61.1	8	Supraspinatus*	3.8	1.6
F-wave	30.8		Infraspinatus*	4.8	2.4
	Median	**Sens/Mixed N**		**Musc cut**	**Sensory N**
F-W	39	30		48.2	16.4
W-E	51.5	35			
E-AX	56.4	50			

Height: 185 cm.

* Recording with concentric needle.

TL, terminal latency; E, elbow; W, wrist; AX, axilla; BE, below elbow; AE, above elbow; F, finger; NP, no potential.

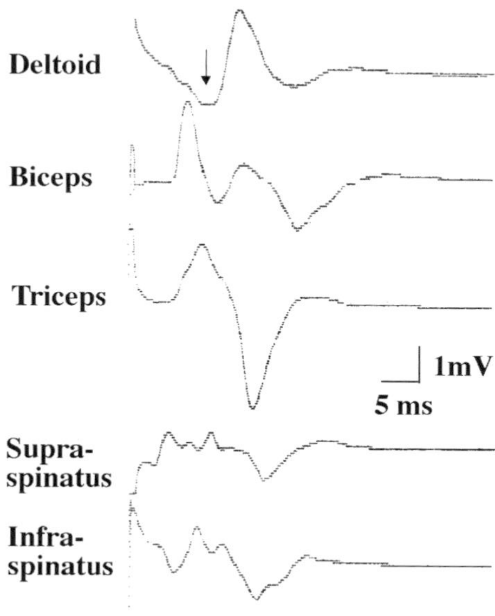

FIGURE 7.4. Brachial plexus latency study. Recording of response was made with surface electrodes in the deltoids, biceps, and triceps muscles and with a concentric needle in the supraspinatus and infraspinatus muscles. *Arrow* indicates a positive deflection showing a volume conduction response in the deltoid muscle.

TABLE 7.3. Needle EMG Data in Case 4

				Spontaneous Potentials				Motor Unit Potential				Interference	
Muscle	**Root**	**Nerve**	**Insertion Activity**	**Fib**	**PSW**	**Fasc**	**Myotonia CRD**	**Amplitude (K)**	**Duration (ms)**	**Polyphasic Potential**	**HA MUP**	**Pattern**	**Mean Amplitude (K)**
Lt C5-8 paraspinal	C5-8		N	–	–	–	–						
Rhomboids	C5	Dorsal scapular	N	–	–	–	–	0.5–2	6–10	N	0	FIP	1.0
Supraspinatus	C5,6	Suprascapular	+	+++	+++	–	–	No	MUP				
Infraspinatus	C5,6	Suprascapular	+	+++	+++	–	–	No	MUP				
Deltoid	C5,6	Axilla	+	+++	+++	–	–	0.5–8.5	9–26	+	+	RIP	1.5
Biceps	C6	Musc cut	N	–	–	–	–	0.5–2	8–12	–	–	FIP	2.0
Triceps	C7	Radial	N	–	–	–	–	1–3	6–12	–	–	FIP	1.5

Fib, fibrillation; PSW, positive sharp waves; Fasc, fasciculation; HA MUP, high-amplitude MUP; N, normal; FIP, full interference pattern; RIP, reduced interference pattern; +, present or increased; –, absent.

A

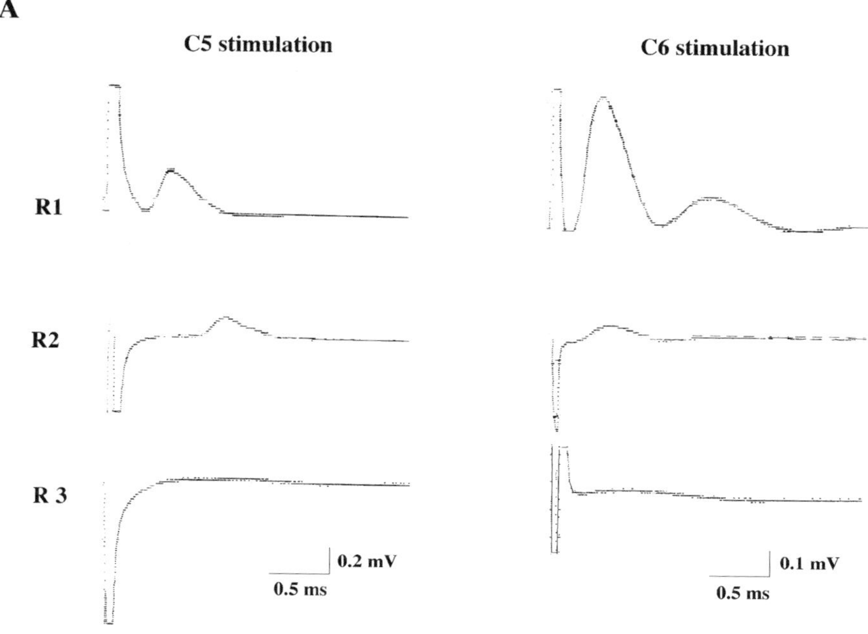

B

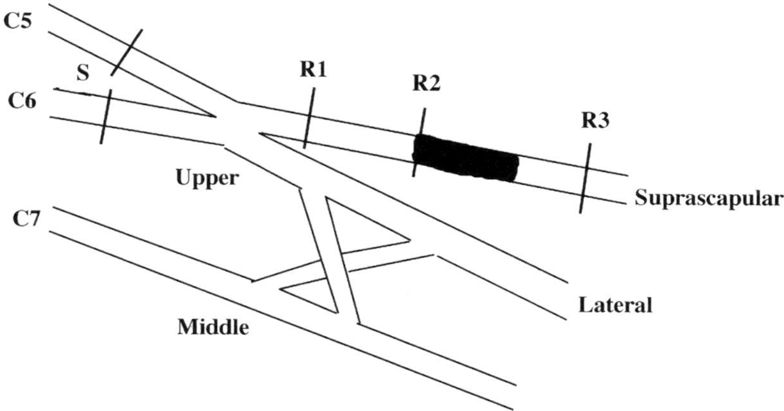

FIGURE 7.5. Intraoperative nerve conduction. **A.** CNAP with C5 and C6 root stimulation. Stimulation was done at 2.9 and 9.3 mA with stimulus duration of 0.05 ms. R1, R2, and R3 indicate the recording sites. Notice more than 200 μ V CNAP amplitudes at R1 site and no response at R3 site. **B.** Anatomical location of lesion (*darkened area*) in the suprascapular nerve. *S*, stimulation site; *R*, recording site; *Upper*, upper trunk; *Middle*, middle trunk; *Lateral*, lateral cord; C5,6,7, roots.

nerve lesion. Because no CNAP was recorded across the lesion, the lesion was resected and the sural nerve was grafted. The first sign of recovery was documented on the needle EMG 6 months after the surgery.

COMMENTS

During surgical exploration, NCS directly on the exposed nerve can render valuable help to the surgeon. A nerve that is completely cut presents no question in surgical management and must be sutured. On the other hand, nerves that have been crushed, stretched, contused, or partially lacerated present a real problem. The management of these lesions in continuity has been improved by the in vivo recording of CNAPs from the surface of the peripheral nerve. In general, if a CNAP can be evoked through the area of injury and recorded distally, careful neurolysis is carried out, leaving the nerve intact. However, if a CNAP cannot be recorded distal to an area of injury, the lesion is resected and neurorrhaphy is done. Thus, recording a CNAP provides an objective measurement of injury and identifies the area of injury. This in vivo technique provides objective, early evaluation of "reinnervation" before maturation (which is shown by the EMG study) and makes possible earlier surgical exploration without potential damage to the surviving or regenerating nerve fibers.

MAXIMS

1. The rhomboid muscle is innervated by the C5 root alone.
2. If no CNAP can be recorded across the lesion in an in vivo recording, neurorrhaphy is recommended.

REFERENCES

1. Oh SJ. Clinical electromyography. Nerve conduction studies. Baltimore, MD: Williams and Wilkins, 1993; Intraoperative nerve conduction, pp. 340–355.
2. Nelson K. Uses of peripheral nerve action potentials for intraoperative monitoring. Neurol Clin 1988; 6:917–933.

CASE 5

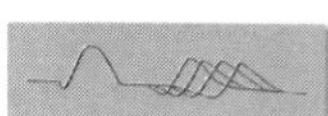

WEAKNESS OF SHOULDER GIRDLE MUSCLES AFTER ARTHROSCOPIC SURGERY IN THE SHOULDER

CASE PRESENTATION

A 46-year-old male weight lifter had arthroscopic surgery for a bony spur in the left shoulder joint 9 months previously. As soon as the swelling disappeared, he noticed difficulty raising his arm above shoulder level. Even with physical therapy and exercise, he noticed no improvement in strength but a gradual wasting of shoulder muscles. He also noticed a small area in the deltoid where sensation was lost. Abnormal neurological findings were marked atrophy, no trace movement, and decreased pin prick over a round 5-cm diameter area in the left deltoid muscle.

CASE ANALYSIS

This patient had motor and sensory deficits typical of axillary nerve palsy. The surgeon who performed the arthroscopic examination did not recognize the problem right away. Because there has not been any improvement for 9 months, it was important to make a decision regarding surgical exploration.

PLAN OF TESTING

1. NCS: Terminal latency study of the deltoid, triceps, and biceps muscles to document axillary nerve injury, evaluate the extent of injury, and rule out a brachial plexus injury (1).
2. Needle EMG: Three parts of the deltoid muscle to detect any sign of regeneration.

ELECTROPHYSIOLOGICAL TESTS AND FINDINGS (Fig. 7.6)

NCS Findings 1.75-mV CMAP with an initial positive deflection of 3.2-ms latency.

Needle EMG

1. Markedly decreased insertion activity, minimal fibrillation, and no MUP on maximal exertion in the left anterior and middle deltoid muscles.
2. Markedly decreased insertion activity, minimal fibrillation, and three MUPs generated in the left posterior deltoid muscle.

ELECTROPHYSIOLOGICAL INTERPRETATION

Severe left axillary nerve lesion with minimal evidence of regeneration in the left posterior deltoid muscle.

FINAL DIAGNOSIS

Left axillary neuropathy, postsurgical

TREATMENT AND FOLLOW-UP

Surgical exploration was done within a few days after the EMG study, and the damaged axillary nerve in the should joint was found to be razor thin. Frozen sections of the small excised nerve did not show any decent myelinated fibers. Thus, neurorrhaphy was performed with a resected sural nerve. Six months later, the first sign of small-amplitude polyphasic MUPs was observed in the needle EMG study before any trace movement was visible.

COMMENTS

The axillary nerve originates from the posterior cord of the brachial plexus formed from the C5 and C6 spinal roots. It innervates the teres minor and deltoid muscles and supplies the sensory fibers to the skin over the deltoid. The exposed position of the axillary nerve as it winds around the lateral aspect of the humerus makes this nerve especially liable to injury. Axillary neuropathy produces wasting and weakness of the deltoid muscle and sensory loss in a small area over the deltoid muscle. The most common cause of this neuropathy is trauma. The needle EMG shows denervation in the deltoid and teres minor muscles in this neuropathy.

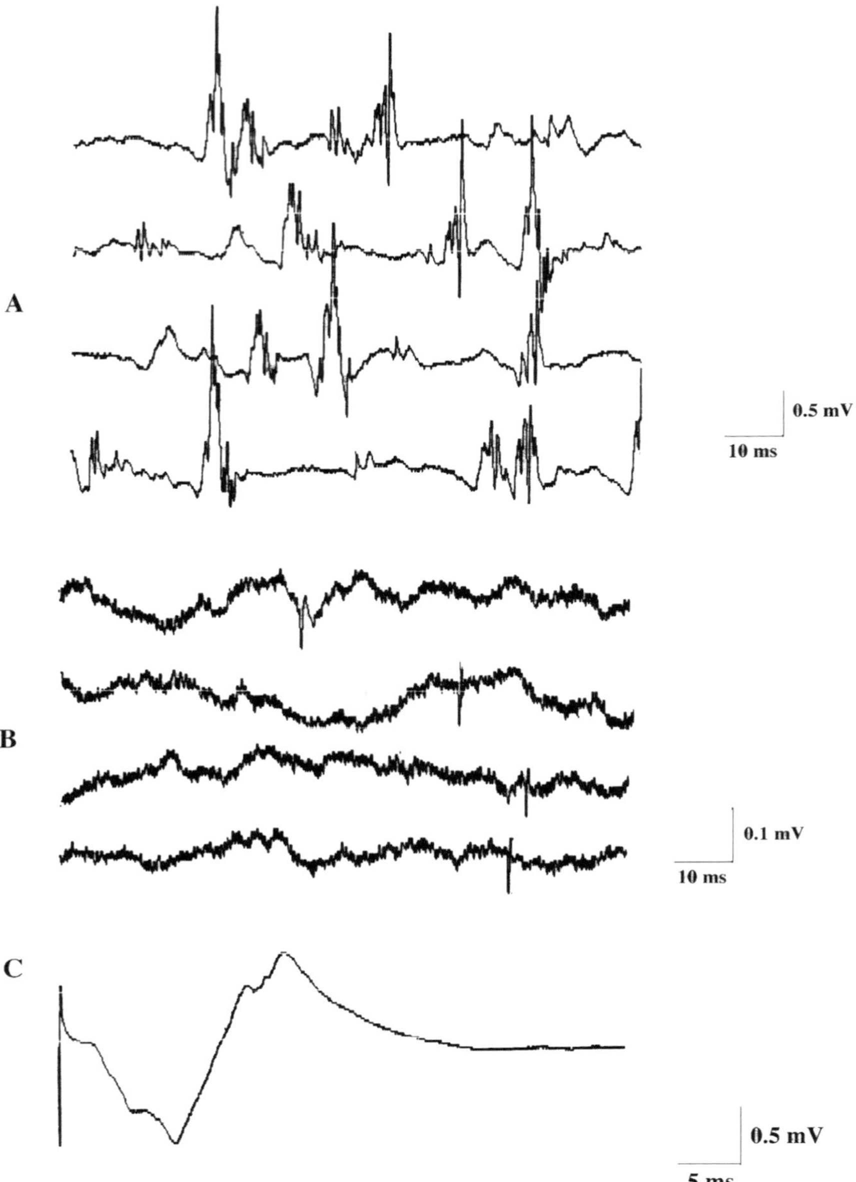

FIGURE 7.6. Three polyphasic MUPs **(A)** and fibrillations and PSWs **(B)** in the posterior deltoid muscle. **C.** CMAP response from the deltoid with Erb's point stimulation. Notice the initial positive deflection indicating a volume conduction response.

In axillary neuropathy, weakness of the teres minor muscle is not clinically testable because the infraspinatus muscle is the prime external rotator of the arm at the shoulder.

Serial EMG examinations are critically important in patients with severe nerve injury. Although there are divergent opinions regarding the best timing for surgical exploration and repair of a severe peripheral nerve injury, there seems to be common agreement on two points: the sooner the surgical repair is done, the greater is the chance of good recovery, and the rate of satisfactory improvement is poor when suturing is done more than 1 year after injury. On the basis of these principles, we recommend that surgical exploration should be carried out if there is no evidence of clinical and electrophysiological improvement 4 weeks after the first EMG study (ideally about 8 weeks after the injury) and preferably within the first 6 months after the injury. In this case, we did not wait another month because 9 months had already passed since the injury.

The needle EMG is more important than the NCS in follow-up studies after nerve repair. When reinnervation begins, there may be a reduction in the amount of fibrillation. However, the earliest positive evidence of reinnervation is the appearance of small-amplitude normal-duration polyphasic MUPs (often referred to as "reinnervation potentials"). Reinnervation potentials appear about 2 months before clinical evidence of improvement.

MAXIMS

1. The best results of surgical repair are obtained when the injured nerve is repaired within 6 months of injury.
2. Reinnervation potentials appear about 2 months before clinical evidence of improvement. Thus, the needle EMG is more helpful than the NCS in evaluation of regeneration after nerve injury or nerve repair.

REFERENCES

1. Oh SJ. Clinical electromyography. Nerve conduction studies. Baltimore, MD: Williams and Wilkins, 1993:174–175.
2. Oh SJ. Clinical electromyography. Nerve conduction studies. Baltimore, MD: Williams and Wilkins, 1993; Traumatic peripheral nerve injury, pp. 665–680.

CASE 6

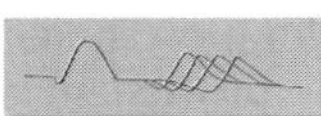

EXCRUCIATING PAIN FOLLOWED BY PARALYSIS OF THE ARM 5 DAYS AFTER NECK SURGERY

CASE PRESENTATION

Three months before the initial evaluation, a 59-year-old man experienced a sudden pain in his neck, radiating into his left hand, and followed by some atrophy of the biceps muscle. MRI showed cervical disc disease, and a cervical spinal fusion was done with marked improvement in pain and weakness. Five days after the surgery, however, the patient awoke with excruciating and unbearable pain in his right arm. This pain was followed a few days later by marked weakness of the entire right arm. The pain seemed to be subsiding over the last several weeks preceding our examination, but there was little movement in his right arm except for some slight flexion of fingers of his hand. Cervical myelogram showed spondylotic changes that could not explain his severe pain. Abnormal neurological findings in the left arm were 5 − MRC strength in the left infraspinatus and biceps muscles. Abnormal findings in the right arm were 0 strength in the infraspinatus, supraspinatus, deltoid, biceps, and triceps; 1 in wrist extension; 3 − in wrist flexion; 2 in hand grip; and 4 in flexion of the last two fingers; decreased pinprick involving the right C5–7 dermatomes; flaccid tone; atrophy of the shoulder girdle muscles; and absent reflexes in both upper extremities. Past history was significant for colon cancer. The patient had also been treated with one course of steroids during his hospitalization.

CASE ANALYSIS

This patient's examination and history were typical of acute brachial plexus neuropathy. Whether he had a left followed by a right APBN could not be resolved at this time. Clearly, surgery as an antecedent event for APBN has been reported, but what was unusual in this patient was the extensiveness of APBN.

PLAN OF TESTING

1. NCS: This should include the right median, ulnar, and radial nerves.
2. Needle EMG: This should include the right cervical paraspinal and one or two muscles innervated by each nerve from the right brachial plexus.
3. MRI of the right brachial plexus.

ELECTROPHYSIOLOGICAL TESTS AND FINDINGS

NCS Findings (Table 7.4)

1. No CMAP and sensory or mixed CNAPs in the right median nerves.
2. No sensory CNAP, low mixed CNAP amplitudes, and slow mixed NCV over the forearm segment; mildly prolonged terminal latency; and slow motor NCV in the right ulnar nerve.
3. Slow motor NCV, low CNAP amplitude, and slow sensory NCV in the right radial nerve.

Needle EMG (Table 7.5)

1. PSWs in the right C5 paraspinal muscle.
2. Fibrillations and PSWs and no MUP in the right infraspinatus, deltoid, biceps, triceps, and APB muscles.
3. Fibrillations, PSWs, normal MUPs, and RIP in the right FDI muscle.

OTHER TEST FINDINGS

MRI of the right brachial plexus showed no enhancing or mass lesion, ruling out a tumor-induced brachial plexopathy.

FINAL DIAGNOSIS

ABPN

TABLE 7.4. Nerve Conduction Data in Case 6

Right	Latent/NCV (ms/m/s)	Amplitude (mV/μV)		Latent/NCV (ms/m/s)	Amplitude (mV/μV)
	Median	**Motor N**		**Median**	**Sens/Mixed N**
TL	NP		F-W	NP	
E-W	NP		W-E	NP	
AX-E	NP		E-AX	NP	
F-wave	NP				
	Ulnar	**Motor N**		**Ulnar**	**Sens/Mixed N**
TL	3.0	6.0	F-W	NP	
BE-W	47.2	5.0	W-E	42.2	5
AE-BE	71.4	4.5	E-AX	71.4	4.5
AX-AE	60.7	4.3	AX-EB	60.7	4.3
EB-AX	62.4	4.0			
F-wave	31.2				
	Radial	**Motor N**		**Radial**	**Sens N**
TL	3.4	4.0	W-F	38.0	4.6
BE-AE	43.4	3.8			
AE-SG	56.7	3.6			

Height: 175 cm.

TREATMENT AND FOLLOW-UP

There was slow improvement over 1 year, at which time the patient still had substantial weakness in the right arm and hand.

COMMENTS

ABPN (neuralgic amyotrophy, Parsonage and Turner syndrome, paralytic brachial neuritis) is characterized by acute severe pain in the shoulder area followed by weakness of the muscles innervated by the brachial plexus. The proximal muscles of the arm and shoulder girdle are most frequently involved. In 65% of patients tested, the involvement was unilateral, and in 45% there had been an antecedent infection or other event. Clinical involvement is usually patchy and not strictly anatomic, in keeping with the scattered foci of inflammation, which is the pathological basis of this condition. In general, ABPN behaves like a restricted variety of GBS. It should also be noted that ABPN may present along with a distal mononeuropathy, such as anterior interosseous neuropathy, or in various combinations. The ultimate prognosis is good, with 80% of patients recovering within 2 years.

At present, the needle EMG is the best means of diagnosing ABPN and of delineating the anatomic extent and physiological severity of the disease. The needle EMG study shows fibrillation and PSWs and/or MUP changes indicative of denervation in the affected muscles. Paraspinal muscles are usually normal. In a small number of patients, the paraspinal EMG shows fibrillation and PSWs. About 50% of patients with unilateral clinical involvement have bilateral abnormalities on the needle EMG.

In general, routine motor and sensory nerve conduction studies are not particularly useful, unless the lower trunk is involved. The latency test to the shoulder girdle muscles and the sensory nerve conduction test from Erb's point through the brachial plexus are the most useful, but even they are of limited value in this disorder. The latency from Erb's point to the shoulder girdle muscle was abnormal in all cases in one study but in 50% of cases in another study. The sensory NCV through the brachial plexus was abnormal in two-thirds of cases in one study.

Tumor-induced brachial plexus neuropathy is characterized by subacute progressive painful plexopathy predominantly involving the lower trunk (C8–T1 roots) and often associated

TABLE 7.5. Needle EMG Data in Case 6

Muscle	Root	Nerve	Insertion Activity	Spontaneous Potentials				Motor Unit Potential				Interference	
				Fib	PSW	Fasc	CRD	Amplitude (mV)	Duration (ms)	Polyphasic Potential	HA MUP	Pattern	Mean Amplitude (mV)
Rt C5 PS			+	–	+	–	–						
C6-8 PS			N	–	–	–	–						
Infraspinatus	C5,6	Suprascapular	+	+ +	+ + +	–	–	No	MUP				
Deltoid	C5,6	Axillary	+	+ +	+ + +	–	–	No	MUP				
Biceps	C5,6	Musc cut	+	+ +	+ + +	–	–	No	MUP				
Triceps	C7,8	Radial	+	+ +	+ +	–	–	No	MUP				
APB	C8, T1	Median	+	+ +	+ + + +	–	–	No	MUP				
FDI	C8, T1	Ulnar	+	+	+ +	–	–	1–5	6–15	+	–	RIP	3

APB, abductor pollicis brevis.

with Horner's syndrome. The most common cause of this disorder is cancer of the lung and breast. Radiation-induced brachial plexopathy is characterized by painless neuropathy, more often involving the upper trunk (affecting the C5–7 roots), and is associated with progressive lymphedema and visible fasciculation or myokymia. The most typical EMG findings in this disorder are fasciculation and myokymia.

MAXIMS

1. The needle EMG is the best means of diagnosis of ABPN.
2. The most typical EMG findings in radiation-induced brachial plexopathy are fasciculation and myokymia.

REFERENCES

1. Flaggman P, Kelly JJ. Brachial plexus neuropathy: an electrophysiological evaluation. Arch Neurol 1980;37:160–164.
2. Lederman RJ, Wilbourn AJ. Brachial plexopathy: recurrent cancer or radiation? Neurology 1988;38: 546–550.

CASE 7

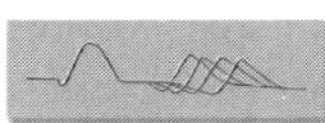

LOU GEHRIG'S DISEASE OR ANTERIOR INTEROSSEOUS NEUROPATHY?

CASE PRESENTATION

A 63-year-old woman sought a neurologist's opinion because of inability to flex the distal phalanx of the right thumb that began 3 weeks before her visit. This was followed by the same difficulty in the right index finger on the next day. After extensive evaluation with the needle EMG study, which documented denervation in the right C5-T1 innervated and left triceps muscles and right CTS, the possibility of motor neuron disease was raised. She was terrified and consulted her cousin, also a neurologist, who examined her and raised the possibility of AIO neuropathy. He referred the patient to us for a third opinion. Cervical spine MRI showed widespread degenerative changes with some foraminal narrowing but without any disc herniation. All other tests were unrevealing. Abnormal neurological findings in the right arm were "pinch sign" of the hand, MRC strength of 0 in the flexor pollicis longus, 4 in the right flexor digitorum superficialis II, and 4 in the opponens pollicis muscle. No sensory impairment, fasciculation, or reflex change was noted.

CASE ANALYSIS

Clearly, the diagnosis of AIO neuropathy was made by demonstration of the pinch sign. However, there was definite weakness in the APB and opponens pollicis muscles. Thus, this woman did not have a pure AIO, raising the possibility of a proximal median neuropathy. In view of the brief 5-week history and the possibility of a proximal median neuropathy, we asked the patient whether she had had any episode of pain before the onset of thumb weakness. She then stated that she had severe pain in the right scapular area, severe enough to seek medical attention, about a week before the thumb weakness. This pain was relieved by a local injection of steroid. The diagnosis of right acute brachial plexus neuropathy (Parsonage-Turner syndrome or neuralgic amyotrophy) was a definite possibility.

PLAN OF TESTING

1. NCS: This should include the median nerve and AIO nerve conduction (1).
2. Needle EMG: This should include a few muscles in the left arm and leg to rule out motor neuron disease.

ELECTROPHYSIOLOGICAL TESTS AND FINDINGS

NCS Findings (Table 7.6; Fig. 7.7)

1. Prolonged terminal latency, low CMAP, and slow sensory NCV over the finger-wrist segment in the right median nerve.
2. Prolonged latency to the flexor pollicis longus muscle and pronator quadratus.

Needle EMG (Table 7.7)

1. Normal needle EMG in the right pronator teres and FCR muscles.
2. Prominent fibrillations and PSWs and no MUPs in the right pronator quadratus, FPL, and FDP (median) muscles.
3. Moderate fibrillations and PSWs, normal MUPs, and RIP in the right APB muscle.
4. Normal needle EMG in the right deltoid, EIP, FDI, vastus lateralis, and anterior tibialis and the left triceps and FDI muscles.

ELECTROPHYSIOLOGICAL INTERPRETATION

AIO neuropathy and distal median neuropathy.

FINAL DIAGNOSIS

Right acute brachial plexus neuropathy involving predominantly the AIO nerve and the distal median nerve

TABLE 7.6. Nerve Conduction Data in Case 7

	Latent/NCV (ms/m/s)	Amplitude (mV/μV)		Latent/NCV (ms/m/s)	Amplitude (mV/μV)
Right	**Median**	**Motor N**		**Median**	**Sens/Mixed N**
TL	4.0	3.9	F-W	36.3	12.4
E-W	39.3	2.7	P-W	30.1	37
AX-E	50.0	2.5	W-E	51.5	14
F-wave	28.8		E-AX	55.8	13.2
	Ulnar	**Motor N**		**Ulnar**	**Sens/Mixed N**
TL	2.7	8.9	F-W	40.0	11.2
BE-W	51.2	8.2	W-E	50.3	18.8
AE-BE	52.4	7.4	E-AX	55.4	20.8
AX-AE	57.8	7.4			
F-wave	29.1				
	AIO	**Motor N**	**Left**	**AIO**	**Motor N**
TL (FPL)	9.8	0.7		3.8	6.3
TL (PQ)	6.4	0.9			

Height: 170.3 cm.
TL to flexor pollicis longus (FPL) and pronator quadratus (PQ) muscles.

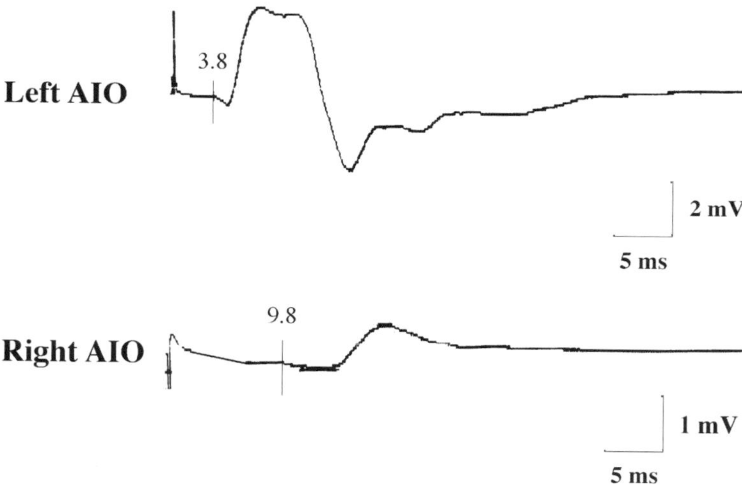

FIGURE 7.7. Anterior interosseous (AIO) nerve conduction with recording electrode in the flexor pollicis longus muscle.

TREATMENT AND FOLLOW-UP

With extensive physical therapy, the patient reported gradual but steady improvement during a 1-year follow-up period.

COMMENTS

The AIO nerve arises from the median nerve as it emerges between the two heads of the pronator teres muscle and courses deep in the forearm between the AIO membrane and the flexor digitorum profundus muscle. It is entirely motor and innervates the flexor pollicis longus, the II and III flexor digitorum profundus, and the pronator quadratus muscles. The characteristic clinical feature of AIO neuropathy is the inability to flex the terminal phalanges

TABLE 7.7. Needle EMG Data in Case 7

				Spontaneous Potentials				Motor Unit Potential				Interference	
Muscle	**Root**	**Nerve**	**Insertion Activity**	**Fib**	**PSW**	**Fasc**	**CRD**	**Amplitude (mV)**	**Duration (ms)**	**Polyphasic Potential**	**HA MUP**	**Pattern**	**Mean Amplitude (mV)**
Rt C5-8,T1			N	–	–	–	–						
Deltoid	C5,6	Axillary	N	–	–	–	–	1–2	6–10	N	–	FIP	1
EIP	C7,8	Radial	N	–	–	–	–	0.7–1.5	6–12	N	–	FIP	1
Pron teres	C6,7	Median	N	–	–	–	–	1–3	10–13	N	–	FIP	2
FPL	C7,8	AIO	+	+++	++	–	–	No	MUP				
FDP (med)	C7,8	AIO	+	++	–	–	–	No	MUP				
PQ	C7,8	AIO	+	+++	++	–	–	No	MUP				
APB	C8, T1	Median	+	++	+	–	–	1–4	9–14	N	–	RIP	2

Normal needle EMG findings in the right anterior tibialis, vastus lateralis, and left FDI and biceps muscles.

FPL, flexor pollicis longus; AIO, anterior interosseous.

of the thumb and index fingers. The patient typically forms a triangle with the thumb and index fingers (pinch sign) instead of forming a circle and has difficulty holding a cup tightly between the thumb and index fingers. Weakness of pronation with elbow flexion suggests weakness in the pronator quadratus. There is no sensory impairment in this neuropathy.

AIO neuropathy is induced by trauma or entrapment at the fibrous bands arising from the pronator teres or the flexor digitorum superficialis muscles. It can also be associated with acute brachial plexus neuropathy, as seen in this case. Routine median motor and sensory nerve conductions are normal in this neuropathy. The AIO NCS demonstrated an abnormal temporal dispersion in all of seven patients: a low CMAP amplitude in four and prolonged latency from the elbow to the pronator quadratus in five, confirming this neuropathy. We used a recently reported nerve conduction technique with the surface electrode on the flexor pollicis longus muscle. Needle EMG evidence of denervation occurs in the flexor pollicis longus, pronatur quadratus, and flexor digitorum profundus I and II but not in the flexor carpi radialis or flexor digitorum superficialis muscles.

MAXIMS

1. The pinch sign is indicative of AIO neuropathy.
2. The strength of the pronator quadratus muscle is tested with elbow flexion and of the pronator teres, with elbow extension.

REFERENCES

1. Felice KJ. Acute anterior interosseous neuropathy in a patient with hereditary neuropathy with liability to pressure palsies: a clinical and electromyographic study. Muscle Nerve 1995;18:1329–1331.
2. England JD, Summer AJ. Neuralgic amyotrophy: an increasingly diverse entity. Muscle Nerve 1967; 10:60–65.

CASE 8

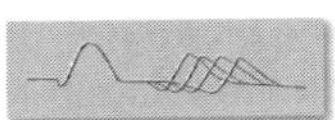

HAND NUMBNESS DUE TO CARPAL TUNNEL SYNDROME (CTS) OR PERIPHERAL NEUROPATHY?

CASE PRESENTATION

A 71-year-old woman with diabetes mellitus well controlled with Glucotrol had numbness and burning of the feet and hands for 4 years. For the past 1 year, there was worsening of pain in the hands, especially at night. Abnormal neurological findings were decreased pin-prick sensation over the distal half of the feet, absent vibration on the toes and decreased vibration on the ankles, areflexia, and positive Tinel's and Phalen's signs on both median nerves at the wrist.

CASE ANALYSIS

There was no doubt that this patient had diabetic sensory neuropathy. The question was whether the recent worsening of pain in her hands was caused by worsening of sensory neuropathy or to CTS. Certainly, Phalen's and Tinel's signs at the wrists were strongly suggestive of CTS. However, this impression had to be confirmed by the NCS before surgical decompression.

PLAN OF TESTING

1. NCS: Workup for peripheral neuropathy and CTS.
2. Needle EMG: Workup for peripheral neuropathy including the APB muscle.

ELECTROPHYSIOLOGICAL TESTS AND FINDINGS

`NCS Findings` (Table 7.8; Fig. 7.8)

1. Mildly prolonged terminal latency and mildly slow motor NCV in almost all tested nerves.
2. Mild slowing in the sensory and mixed NCV together with low CNAPs in all sensory and wrist-elbow segments of ulnar and median nerves.
3. Markedly prolonged terminal latency, low CMAP, and absent sensory CNAP over the finger-wrist segment in the right median nerve.
4. Mildly prolonged terminal latency and slow sensory NCV over the finger-wrist segment in the left median nerve.

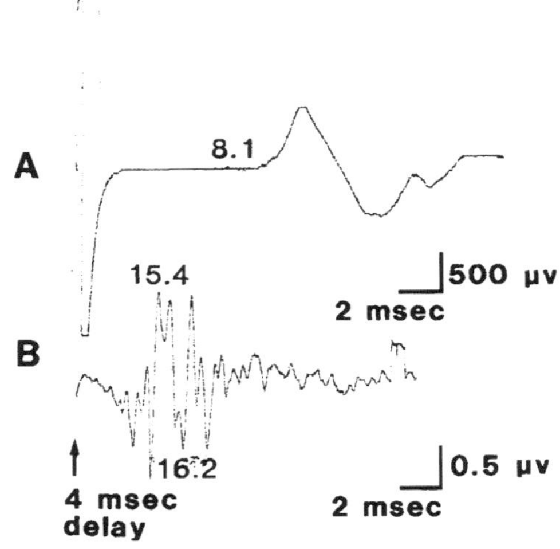

FIGURE 7.8. Motor and sensory nerve conduction in carpal tunnel syndrome. **A.** Prolonged terminal latency (8.1 ms) and low amplitude of the CMAP (1.5 mV). **B.** Sensory CNAP recorded with needle electrodes: the maximum NCV is 16.2 m/s; the negative peak NCV is 15.4 m/s; dispersion phenomenon is obvious. Surface electrodes were not able to record any sensory CNAP.

TABLE 7.8. Nerve Conduction Data in Case 8

	Latent/NCV (ms/m/s)	Amplitude (mV/μV)		Latent/NCV (ms/m/s)	Amplitude (mV/μV)	Shape
Right	**Median**	**Motor N**	**Right**	**Peroneal**	**Motor**	**Nerve**
TL	**8.1**	**1.25**	TL	**5.3**	**2.9**	
E-W	**45.2**	**1.0**	FH-A	**39.0**	**2.3**	
AX-E	68.1	**1.0**	PF-FH	64.3	**2.0**	
F-wave	**34.7**		F-wave	53.3		
	Ulnar	**Motor N**		**Post Tibial**	**Motor**	**Nerve**
TL	3.0	13.9	TL	**5.8**	9	
BE-W	**48.3**	13.0	PF-A	**38.2**	5.5	
AE-BE	59.4	12.5	F-wave	55.2		
AX-AE	56.3	12.0		**Sural**	**Sens**	**Nerve**
F-wave	30.0		MCA	33.2	4	
	Median	**Sens/Mixed N**		**Median***	**Sens***	
F-W	NP*		Max NCV	**16.2**	**2.5**	D
W-E	**46.2**	**8.0**	NP NCV	**15.4**		
E-AX	56.7	20				
	Ulnar	**Sens/Mixed N**	**Left**	**Median**	**Motor**	**Nerve**
F-W	**38.2**	**5.0**	TL	**4.5**	6.0	
W-E	**51.8**	10		**Median**	**Sens**	
E-AX	60.4	25.0	F-W	**36.0**	12	

Height: 170 cm.

* Near-nerve sensory nerve conduction in the finger-wrist segment.

FH, fibillar head; A, ankle; PF, popliteal fossa; MC, mid-calf; NP NCV, negative peak NCV; Max NCV, maximum NCV; D, dispersion.

Needle EMG in the Anterior Tibialis, Gastrocnemius, and APB Muscles

1. A few HA MUPs in the gastrocnemius muscles.
2. Fibrillations, PSWs, a few HA MUPs, and RIP in the right APB muscle.

ELECTROPHYSIOLOGICAL INTERPRETATION

Mild sensory-motor neuropathy with superimposed bilateral CTS, worse on the right.

FINAL DIAGNOSIS

Diabetic sensory neuropathy and superimposed bilateral CTS

TREATMENT AND FOLLOW-UP

Even though this patient had diabetic sensory neuropathy, clearly there was a well-documented superimposed CTS. Endoscopic decompression of the carpal tunnel was performed with complete relief of pain.

COMMENTS

The NCS is the most important diagnostic test for CTS, being positive in 91 to 98% of patients with clinically diagnosed CTS on the basis of their signs and symptoms. The NCS shows focal demyelination. The most sensitive diagnostic test is the sensory NCS, being positive in an average 87% of cases. The motor nerve conduction is less sensitive in the diagnosis of CTS, being positive in an average 67% of cases. The sensory NCS over the palm-wrist segment has further increased the diagnostic sensitivity in CTS, and in many laboratories it has become a standard test in the workup of CTS. To make the diagnosis of CTS, one or more of the following criteria has been used traditionally: abnormal sensory nerve conduction in the finger-wrist segment, abnormal sensory nerve conduction in palm-wrist segment, and prolonged terminal latency. Various comparison techniques have been tried to increase the diagnostic sensitivity in CTS, but this will never be 100% simply because a few rare CTS patients have pure C-fiber involvement alone.

The most challenging task for the electromyographer is to differentiate a superimposed CTS from diffuse peripheral neuropathy. This is because surgical decompression for CTS may be performed even in patients with diffuse polyneuropathy. Thus, it is important to identify an entrapment neuropathy even in the presence of axonal or demyelinating neuropathy. The most important criteria for this are based on a comparison between the segment of entrapment and other segments of the peripheral nerve. If the terminal latency and sensory nerve conduction in the finger-wrist segment are disproportionally more abnormal than those in the proximal segment or if the sensory NCV in the palm-wrist segment is disproportionally slower than the sensory NCV in the finger-wrist segment, then one can conclude that there is a superimposed CTS.

MAXIMS

1. The most sensitive electrophysiological test for CTS is the sensory NCS in the finger-wrist segment of the median nerve.
2. The diagnosis of superimposed CTS in peripheral neuropathy is based on a disproportionally more abnormal terminal latency and sensory NCS in the finger-wrist segment of the median nerve as compared with the proximal segments.

REFERENCES

1. Oh SJ. Clinical electromyography. Nerve conduction studies. Baltimore, MD: Williams and Wilkins, 1993; Carpal tunnel syndrome, pp. 517–526.
2. Morgenlander JC, Lynch JR, Sanders DB. Surgical treatment of carpal tunnel syndrome in patients with peripheral neuropathy. Neurology 1997;49:1159–1163.

CASE 9

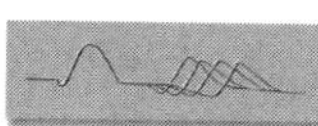

IS A MOTOR NCV OF 203 M/S IN THE FOREARM SEGMENT IN THE MEDIAN NERVE REAL?

CASE PRESENTATION

A 39-year-old woman was referred to the EMG Laboratory for evaluation of numbness in the left hand for 6 months. The numbness was worse while she was driving her car and awakened her at night. On examination, she had a Tinel's sign on the median nerve at the wrist and positive Phalen's sign in both hands, worse on the left. No atrophy or weakness of the hyperthenar muscle was observed. Sensory examination was also normal. Motor NCS in the left median nerve showed a terminal latency of 9.4 ms with a low CMAP amplitude, as expected. However, stimulation of the median nerve at the elbow (stimulus duration, 0.1 ms; stimulus intensity, 35 mA) showed an unexpected near-normal latency (10.5 ms) and CMAP with initial negative deflection. Repeated wrist stimulation confirmed that the stimulation was on the median nerve and that this was a genuine response. Motor NCV over the forearm segment was calculated to be 203 m/s.

CASE ANALYSIS

This patient had a typical history of CTS. NCS confirmed a severe CTS. The near-normal latency with elbow stimulation and NCV of 203 m/s over the forearm segment could not be explained by ordinary anatomical or physiological phenomena. A motor NCV of 203 m/s is extremely fast over this segment. Thus, technical problems must be ruled out, and the possibility of anomalous innervation must be suspected and studied.

PLAN OF TESTING

Martin-Grüber anastomosis is evaluated with the recording electrodes in the APB, ADQ, and FDI muscles and stimulation of the median and ulnar nerves at the wrist and elbow. A three-channel recording is essential. Sometimes the stimulus intensity has to be increased to stimulate anomalous nerve fibers.

ELECTROPHYSIOLOGICAL TESTS AND FINDINGS

NCS Findings (Table 7.9)

1. Routine study (Fig. 7.9)
   a. Markedly prolonged terminal latency, a low CMAP amplitude, absent F-wave, absent sensory CNAP over the finger-wrist and palm-wrist segments, and low mixed CNAP amplitude in the left median nerve.
   b. Mildly prolonged terminal latency and slow sensory NCV over the finger-wrist and palm-wrist segments in the right median nerve.

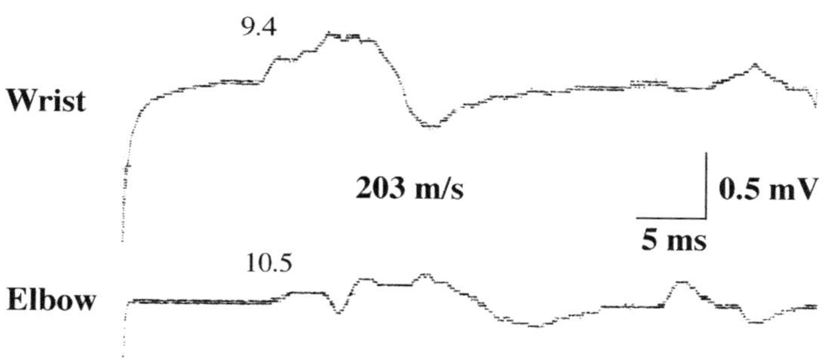

FIGURE 7.9. Median motor nerve conduction. Markedly prolonged terminal latency, erroneously calculated "extremely fast (203 m/s) NCV" and low CMAP amplitude. Notice that there is no initial positive deflection.

TABLE 7.9. Nerve Conduction Data in Case 9

	Latent/NCV (ms/m/s)	Amplitude (mV/μV)	Shape		Latent/NCV (ms/m/s)	Amplitude (mV/μV)
Right	**Median**	**Motor**	**Nerve**	**Left**	**Median**	**Motor N**
TL	9.4	0.75			3.7	12
E-W	203	0.4	IN*		61.6	10
AX-E						
F-wave	NP					
	Ulnar	**Motor**	**Nerve**		**Ulnar**	**Motor N**
TL	1.7	16				
BE-W	70.2	15				
AE-BE	60.5	14				
AX-AE	80.7	14				
EB-AX						
F-wave	24.4					
	Median	**Sens/Mixed**	**Nerve**		**Median**	**Sens/Mixed N**
F-W	NP				36.7	20
P-W	NP				29.5	90
W-E	50.0	3				
E-AX	52.2	20				
	Ulnar	**Sens/Mixed**	**Nerve**		**Ulnar**	**Sens/Mixed**
F-W	43.4	15				
W-E	59.5	30				
E-AX	62.0	20				

Height: 172 cm.
* Initial negative deflection.

2. Special study for Martin-Grüber anastomosis (Fig. 7.10)
   a. Median nerve stimulation at the elbow with stimulus duration of 0.2 ms and intensity of 35.0 mA (a much stronger stimulus than in the routine study) evoked 1.2-mV CMAP with initial positive deflection from the APB, 0.75-mV CMAP with initial negative deflection from the ADQ, and 0.65-mV CMAP with initial positive deflection from the FDI muscle.
   b. CMAPs from APB, ADQ, and FDI muscles were larger by at least 25% with median-elbow stimulation than with median-wrist stimulation.

ELECTROPHYSIOLOGICAL INTERPRETATION

1. Bilateral CTS, worse on the left.
2. Martin-Grüber type I (ADQ muscle) and II (FDI muscle) anastomosis.

FINAL DIAGNOSIS

CTS (bilateral) and Martin-Grüber anastomosis

COMMENTS

Martin-Grüber anastomosis (MGA; median-ulnar motor nerve anastomosis) is the most common form of anomalous innervation and has been found in 11 to 15% of cadavers. Various NCSs have revealed an anastomosis in 15 to 39% of normal controls and in 8 to 16% of patients with CTS. In normal individuals, it is difficult to recognize MGA without systematic analysis of the CMAP amplitude in the APB, ADQ, and FDI muscles with median and ulnar stimulation at the wrist and elbow. Thus, in practice, MGA is usually recognized in patients with CTS. It may produce additional electrophysiological changes that make interpretation

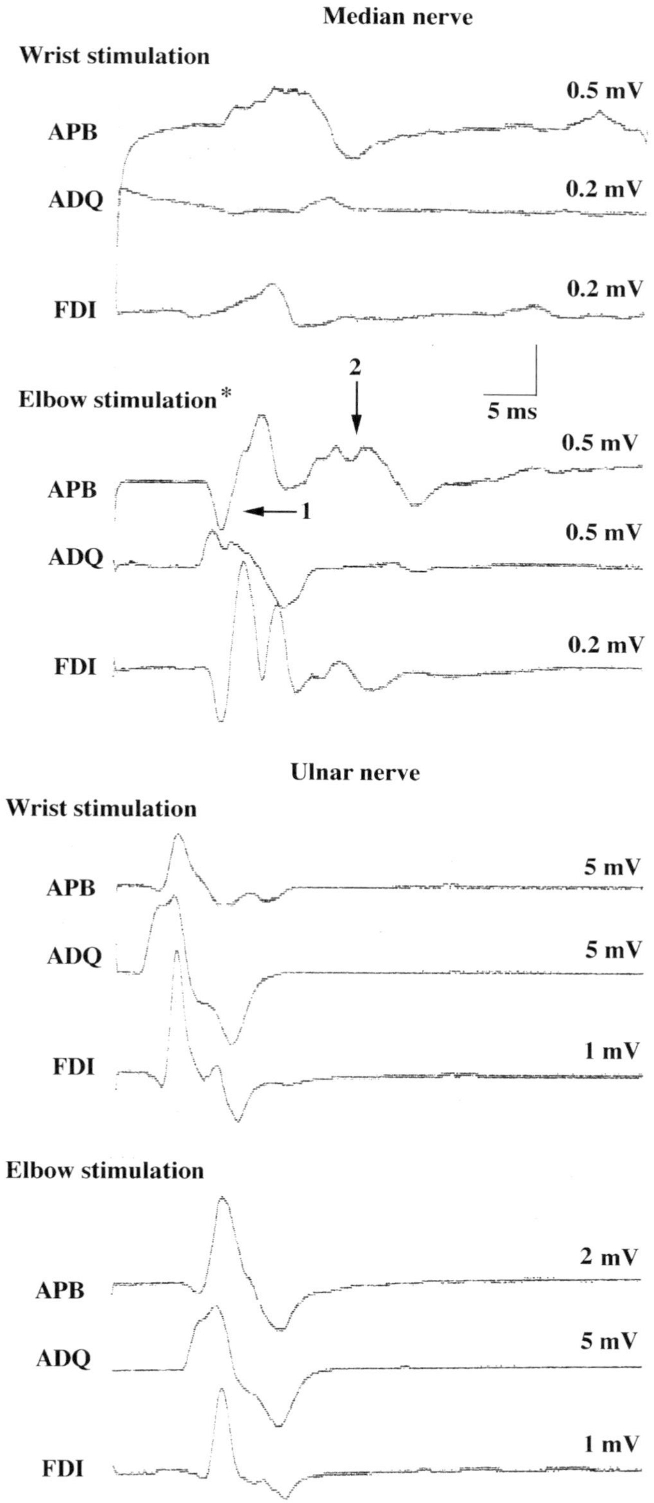

Median nerve

Wrist stimulation

APB 0.5 mV

ADQ 0.2 mV

FDI 0.2 mV

Elbow stimulation*

2

5 ms

APB 0.5 mV

1

ADQ 0.5 mV

FDI 0.2 mV

Ulnar nerve

Wrist stimulation

APB 5 mV

ADQ 5 mV

FDI 1 mV

Elbow stimulation

APB 2 mV

ADQ 5 mV

FDI 1 mV

FIGURE 7.10. Martin-Grüber anastomosis in a patient with carpal tunnel syndrome.* Stimulus stronger than that used for the response in Figure 7.8 is used here. Arrow 1 indicates an initial positive deflection (volume conduction response). Arrow 2 indicates the second component.

of the NCS difficult unless the electromyographer is aware of this anomaly. It is presented in three different conduction patterns in CTS:

1. Median nerve stimulation at the elbow evokes a thenar CMAP with an initial positive deflection not seen on stimulation at the wrist (Fig. 7.10, arrow 1). This is caused by a volume conduction response from the adductor pollicis muscle innervated by the ulnar nerve.
2. There is an erroneously normal proximal (elbow) motor latency in the median nerve with prolongation of the distal motor latency, producing an extremely fast NCV over the forearm segment. This is due to the rapid conduction of the stimulus along the noncompressed MGA.
3. A thenar CMAP with two components is seen upon median nerve stimulation at the elbow (Fig. 7.10, arrow 2). This is attributed to slower conduction in the median nerve at the wrist and faster conduction in those axons in MGA.

In our case, all three patterns were noted.

MAXIMS

1. The volume conduction response is recognized by an initial positive deflection of the CMAP.
2. MGA should be suspected in patients with CTS if the motor NCV over the forearm segment in the median nerve is extremely fast.

REFERENCES

1. Oh SJ. Clinical electromyography. Nerve conduction studies. Baltimore, MD: Williams & Wilkins, 1993:314–332. In: Anomalous Innervation of the Nerves.
2. Gutmann L. Important anomalous innervations of the extremities. AAEE Minimonograph #2, 1979.

CASE 10

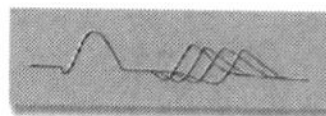

SEVERE ATROPHY OF THE LEFT HAND FOR 1.5 YEARS

CASE PRESENTATION

A 21-year-old patient noticed severe atrophy of the left hand muscles approximately 1.5 years previously while he was being evaluated for a minor injury to his wrist. He stated that the atrophy and weakness might have been present for 6 months before the wrist injury and also reported aching in his left forearm and wrist. He denied any preceding trauma or illness or any involvement of his right arm or leg. There did not seem to have been any obvious progression of weakness or atrophy or any sensory complaints for the preceding 1.5 years. Abnormal neurological findings were atrophy and 4 MRC strength in the FDI and intrinsic hand muscles, diminished pin-prick sensation over the ulnar aspect of the left hand and forearm, and a tender spot and Tinel's sign on the left supraclavicular area. Left APB muscle was of normal bulk.

CASE ANALYSIS

There was no question that this case represented an ulnar neuropathy by all accounts. A C8 radiculopathy was less likely because the APB muscle was not affected. The next question was localization of the lesion. Clearcut sensory deficits over the ulnar aspect of the forearm suggested a lesion in the proximal ulnar nerve because an entrapment neuropathy at the elbow produces sensory deficits over the ulnar nerve sensory territory on the dorsum and palmar aspects of the hand and the medial antebrachial cutaneous nerve that originates at the lower trunk of the plexus is responsible for sensory loss in the forearm. Clearly, the presence of Tinel's sign and tenderness over the Erb's point pinpointed the lesion at Erb's point.

PLAN OF TESTING

1. NCS: This should include the Erb's point-axilla segment of the ulnar nerve and medial antecubital sensory nerve conduction studies.
2. Needle EMG: This study should include cervical paraspinal and ulnar-innervated muscles and the APB muscle.
3. Special x-ray of the cervical spine to rule out cervical rib or MRI of the brachial plexus area.

ELECTROPHYSIOLOGICAL TESTS AND FINDINGS

NCS Findings (Table 7.10; Fig. 7.11)

1. A low sensory CNAP over the finger-wrist segment and mixed CNAP amplitude over the forearm segment, and slow mixed NCV over the elbow-axilla segment in the left ulnar nerve.
2. Relatively lower mixed CNAP amplitude over the elbow-axilla and axilla-Erb's point segments in the left ulnar nerve as compared with those in the right ulnar nerve.
3. A low sensory CNAP amplitude in the left medial antebrachial nerve.

Needle EMG

1. Increased insertion activity, fibrillation, and PSW; increased polyphasic MUPs; and RIP in the left FDI muscle.
2. Increased insertion activity, many giant MUPs, and RIP in the left ADQ muscle.

ELECTROPHYSIOLOGICAL INTERPRETATION

Proximal ulnar neuropathy with the lesion at the lower trunk, compatible with neurogenic thoracic outlet syndrome.

OTHER TEST FINDINGS

No cervical rib seen with special x-ray. Normal cervical MRI.

TABLE 7.10. Nerve Conduction Data in Case 10

	Latent/NCV (ms/m/s)	Amplitude (mV/μV)		Latent/NCV (ms/m/s)	Amplitude (mV/μV)
Left	**Median**	**Motor N**	**Right**	**Median**	**Motor N**
TL	3.0	18.7			
E-W	60	19			
AX-E	68.5	18			
F-wave	28.4				
	Ulnar	**Motor N**		**Ulnar**	**Motor N**
TL	3.0	6		2.2	12.5
BE-W	51.2	5.8		62.5	9.4
AE-BE	76.9	5.7		66.0	9.0
AX-AE	56.5	5.0		65.2	7.9
EB-AX	60.8	5.1			
F-wave	32.9			28.9	
	Median	**Sens/Mixed N**		**Median**	**Sens/Mixed N**
F-W	53.7	20			
W-E	59.0	52			
E-AX	65.4	33			
	Ulnar	**Sens/Mixed N**		**Ulnar**	**Sens/Mixed N**
F-W	43.4	4.8		44.0	14
W-E	57.0	6		56.8	38
E-AX	44.0	11		65.4	38
AX-EB	56.4	17		66.0	42
	Sup Radial	**Sensory N**			
W-F	52	11			
	Medial	**Antebrachial SN**		**Medial**	**Antebrachial SN**
Forearm	50	3.5		45.9	10

FINAL DIAGNOSIS

Left neurogenic thoracic outlet syndrome

TREATMENT AND FOLLOW-UP

Clearly, cervical rib is the most common cause for a proximal ulnar neuropathy at Erb's point. This was ruled out, however, by the normal x-ray. In view of the clinical and electrophysiological localization of the lesion, the Erb's point was surgically explored and a tight fibrous band from the first rib compressing the lower trunk was found and cut. Within 3 months, the patient's sensory deficits and motor weakness disappeared.

COMMENTS

In the 1970s, there was a period when the diagnosis of thoracic outlet syndrome was commonly made on the basis of "slow motor conduction" across the thoracic outlet between Erb's point and the axilla, and the first rib was resected. However, later studies were not able to confirm this nerve conduction abnormality. It now appears that these findings resulted from the inherent technical difficulty associated with motor NCS of the ulnar nerve in this segment. Neurogenic TOS is extremely rare and has distinct clinical features: pain and sensory loss in the C8-T1 dermatomes and selective weakness and wasting of the thenar muscles. In severe cases, weakness and wasting of all the intrinsic hand muscles were observed. In my experience, tenderness, "fullness," and the presence of Tinel's sign at Erb's point can localize the lesion

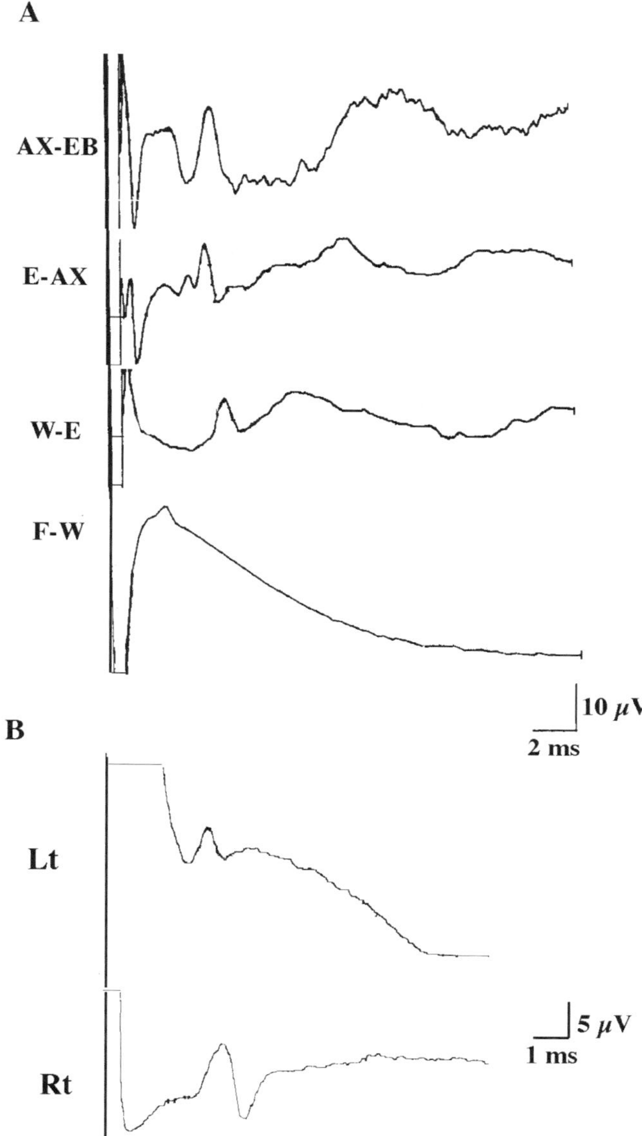

FIGURE 7.11. A. Sensory and mixed nerve conduction in the left ulnar nerve. Low CNAP amplitude in the sensory nerve conduction in the finger-wrist (*F-W*) segment and in the mixed nerve conduction in the wrist-elbow (*W-E*), elbow-axilla (*E-AX*), and axilla-Erb's point (*AX-EB*) segments. **B.** Lower CNAP amplitude in the left medial antebrachial cutaneous nerve compared with that on the right.

to the supraclavicular area. This patient had all the features of "neurogenic thoracic outlet syndrome" except for sensory deficits over the C8-T1 dermatomes. The most common causes of TOS are congenital abnormalities (cervical ribs, abnormal first rib with fibrous band, and scalenus muscle band). In most patients with neurogenic TOS, a distinct electrophysiological pattern exists: a low CNAP amplitude in the distal and thoracic outlet segments of the ulnar nerve, prolonged ulnar F-wave latency, and low CMAP, more often in the median nerve than in the ulnar nerve. Thus, this patient had all the typical electrophysiological findings. The low CMAP amplitude in the APB muscle was explained by the C8 motor nerve fiber traveling along the lower trunk and innervating the APB muscle through the median nerve. Our patient had neurogenic thoracic outlet syndrome due to compression of the lower trunk of the brachial plexus by a thick fibrous band from the first rib and thus did not have all the features described in this disorder. However, a proximal ulnar sensory neuropathy and medial antebrachial neuropathy due to Wallerian degeneration from a proximal lesion were clearly documented.

MAXIMS

1. The distinct clinical features of neurogenic TOS are pain and sensory loss in the C8-T1 dermatomes and selective weakness and westings of the thenar muscles. Local tenderness and fullness and Tinel's sign at the Erb's point are helpful in localizing the lesion to the supraclavicular area.
2. The most distinct electrophysiological pattern of neurogenic TOS includes a low CNAP amplitude in the distal and thoracic outlet segments of the ulnar nerve, a prolonged ulnar F-wave latency, and low CMAP more often in the median nerve than in the ulnar nerve.

REFERENCES

1. Oh SJ. Clinical electromyography. Nerve conduction studies. Baltimore, MD: Williams and Wilkins, 1993:536–540.
2. Wilbourn AJ, Hansen M, Hardy R. Neurogenic true thoracic outlet syndrome: electrodiagnostic features in 11 patients. Muscle Nerve 1982;5:558.

CASE 11

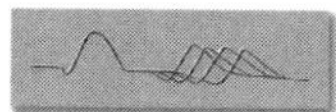

NUMBNESS IN THE HAND UPON WAKING AFTER SURGERY

CASE PRESENTATION

A 47-year-old woman, a professor at the local nursing school, developed a right rotator cuff tear in February 1995 as a result of a fall while carrying a very heavy bookbag. She developed severe pain in her shoulder, which was initially treated with conservative therapy, but had no weakness or numbness. Because of intractable pain, she underwent rotator cuff surgery under general anesthesia in November 1995. In the recovery room, she received a nerve block at Erb's point for pain relief. The patient awoke in her room several hours later, noting numbness in the entire right hand. Over the next 12 to 16 hours her sensation improved somewhat, but she was left with profound numbness in the ulnar distribution and prominent weakness in the right hand, especially in the thumb. Over the next 3 months, she did not improve at all despite physical therapy, and during the last several weeks before examination, she developed tremendous pain in the forearm, elbow, and upper arm areas. A subsequent right brachial plexus MRI was unremarkable. The patient thought that the nerve block was responsible for her problem. None of her local neurologists was willing to examine this patient and perform the EMG study because of possible medicolegal implications. An EMG study performed 500 miles from her home concluded the presence of a right ulnar neuropathy localized to between the elbow and medial cord of the brachial plexus.

Abnormal neurological findings were confined to the right upper extremity. There was 5 – weakness in the deltoid and triceps muscles, most likely due to shoulder pain. The biceps strength was full at 5. Wrist extensor and flexor, finger extensors, and thumb abduction were all 5 –. Hand interosseous muscle was 1 and hand grip was 4 in strength. Atrophy was noted in the intrinsic hand muscles and forearm flexors. Sensory function was normal except for hypoesthesia to pin prick in the ulnar distribution of the right hand, with some extension up to the medial forearm. Reflexes were normal.

CASE ANALYSIS

This patient's history and examination were consistent with a right brachial plexus lesion with predominant involvement of the ulnar nerve, possibly related to the previous "nerve block." Her findings were complicated by the sophistication of her medical knowledge and potential medicolegal implications. It was critical to localize the lesion accurately in this patient.

PLAN OF TESTING

1. NCS: This should include an ulnar nerve study to Erb's point and medial antebrachial cutaneous nerve and radial sensory nerve conduction.
2. Needle EMG: This should include the shoulder girdle, forearm, and hand muscles to identify the extent of the lesion.

ELECTROPHYSIOLOGICAL TESTS AND FINDINGS

NCS Findings (Table 7.11; Fig. 7.12)

1. Markedly slow motor NCV and conduction block across the elbow and absent mixed CNAP over the forearm segment in the right ulnar nerve.
2. Absent CNAP in the right dorsal cutaneous ulnar nerve.
3. Normal motor and mixed NCS over the axilla-Erb's point in the right ulnar nerve.
4. Normal NCS in the right medial antebrachial cutaneous nerve.
5. Inching study localized the lesion to between 0 and 2 cm distal to the medial epicondyle.

Needle EMG

1. Fibrillations, PSWs, and reduced interference pattern in the right FDI and FCU muscles.
2. HA MUPs in the right FCU muscle.
3. Normal EMG findings in the other tested muscles.

A

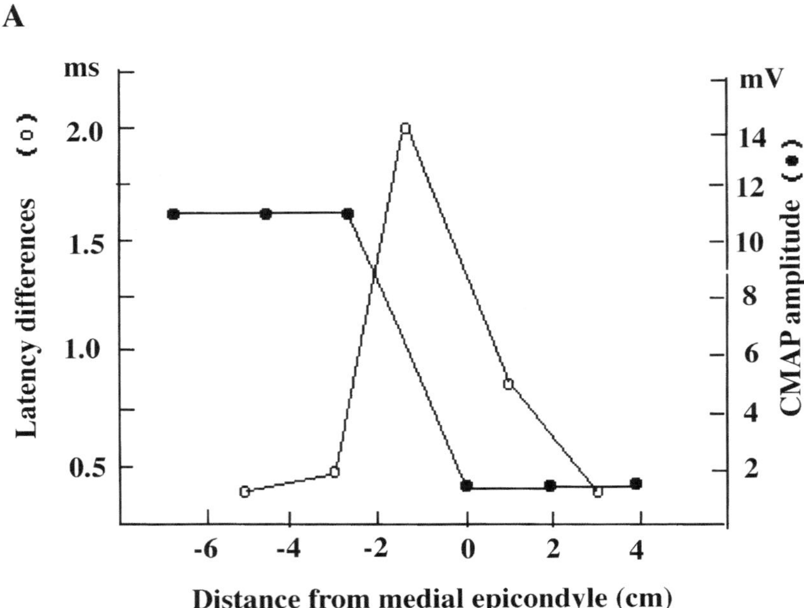

B

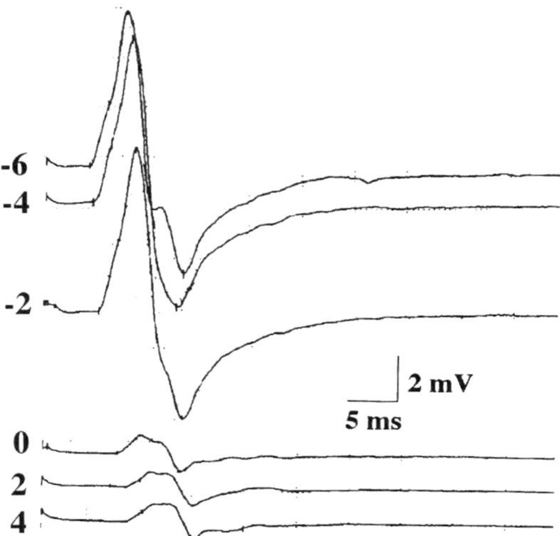

FIGURE 7.12. Graphic presentation of the CMAP and latency changes **(A)** and the actual tracing of the CMAPs **(B)** at six different sites along the elbow sulcus. Conduction block (89% decrease in the CMAP amplitude) and prolonged latency (2 ms) between 2 cm (−2) distal and 0 to the medial epicondyle.

TABLE 7.11. Nerve Conduction Data in Case 11

	Latent/NCV (ms/m/s)	Amplitude (mV/μV)	Others
Right	**Median**	**Motor**	**Nerve**
TL	3.2	10	
E-W	55.6	9.6	
AX-E	68.1	10.6	
F-wave	26.4		
	Ulnar	**Motor**	**Nerve**
TL	2.4	10.8	
BE-W	67.1	10.6	
AE-BE	24.4	1.42	CB
AX-AE	85.8	1.2	
EB-AX	64.7	0.9	
F-wave	NP		
	Median	**Sens/Mixed**	**Nerve**
F-W	44.7	20	
W-E	56.9	62	
E-AX	60.3	57	
	Ulnar	**Sens/Mixed**	**Nerve**
F-W	43.9	18	
W-E	NP		
E-AX	52.5	26.4	
AX-EB	59.1	11.6	
	Dorsal Cut	**Ulnar Sens**	**Nerve**
W-F	NP		
	Medial	**Antebrachial**	**Nerve**
Forearm	58.9	9.6	
	Superficial	**Radial**	**Nerve**
W-F	50.0	16	

Height: 180.3 cm.
CB, conduction block.

ELECTROPHYSIOLOGICAL INTERPRETATION

Right ulnar neuropathy at the elbow. No evidence of right brachial plexus neuropathy.

FINAL DIAGNOSIS

Perioperative right ulnar compression neuropathy at the elbow

TREATMENT AND FOLLOW-UP

MRI of the right brachial plexus was normal. The patient had a marked Tinel's sign at the elbow. She was assured that the nerve block was not responsible for her neurological deficits, some of which were attributable to her knowledge of brachial plexus lesions. This complicated the examination. Her ulnar neuropathy was due to acute perioperative ulnar compression neuropathy at the elbow. With physical therapy, she had slow but steady improvement.

COMMENTS

Ulnar nerve compression occurs most commonly at the elbow because of the superficial location of the ulnar nerve at the elbow sulcus. Acute compression of the ulnar nerve may occur after prolonged pressure on the nerve during surgery, which this patient had. This is a rare but well-known complication of operations under general anesthesia. Because this condition is due to acute decompression of the ulnar nerve, surgical treatment is not the best choice of treatment.

To differentiate a lower trunk brachial plexus lesion from an elbow lesion, it is essential to study the Erb's point-axilla segment of the ulnar nerve. The motor nerve conduction across the thoracic outlet is prone to technical errors caused by the changing distance between the electrode and the nerve trunk during stimulation. This difficulty is especially true in obese individuals. To document a conduction block in this segment, it is important to stimulate supramaximally, to obtain the same results on repeated studies, and to compare the findings with those on the other side. In our opinion, the mixed NCS across the thoracic outlet is a much more reliable measurement. It is also important to add the medial antebrachial cutaneous NCS because it is often involved in a lower trunk lesion.

MAXIMS

1. Sparing of the FCU and FDP (IV and V) muscles on the needle EMG does not necessarily localize the lesion to the wrist.
2. Surgical decompression or translocation of the ulnar nerve is not recommended for perioperative ulnar compression at the elbow.

REFERENCES

1. Oh SJ. Clinical electromyography. Nerve conduction studies. Baltimore, MD: Williams and Wilkins, 1993:194–197.
2. Miller RG, Camp PE. Postoperative ulnar neuropathy. JAMA 1979;242:1636–1639.

CASE 12

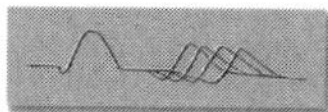

HAND WEAKNESS AFTER A 2000-MILE MOTORCYCLE RACE

CASE PRESENTATION

A 42-year-old man participated in a 2000-mile motorcycle race (300 miles a day) with his right hand on the throttle about 3 months previously. On the fifth to seventh days, the patient noted a sharp pain in his right wrist and palm that was relieved by rest at night. Minimal weakness of the right hand had been noted ever since. A month before his visit, the patient noticed wasting of the first web of the right hand. Neurological examination showed a positive Tinel's sign at the wrist on the right and left median nerves, abnormality in two-point discrimination in the right digit II, atrophy of the interosseous, and atrophy and weakness of the right first FDI and ADP muscles. Froment's sign was positive. No sensory abnormality was noted in the right ulnar nerve territory.

CASE ANALYSIS

Clinically, this patient had a bilateral CTS, worse on the right, and evidence of right ulnar neuropathy. The main question was location of the lesion in the right ulnar nerve. The absence of sensory loss in the ulnar nerve territory and normal hypothenar muscle ruled out the possibility of ulnar neuropathy at the elbow or thoracic outlet. Certainly, there was a possibility of C8-T1 radiculopathy, which was less likely in view of normal muscle strength in the right thenar muscle. Clinically, this patient had classic findings of neuropathy of the deep palmar branch of the right ulnar nerve.

PLAN OF TESTING

1. NCS: This should include a special study of the deep palmar branch of right ulnar nerve. This test is performed with the recording electrode on the FDI muscle (1).
2. Needle EMG: Needle EMG study in the right FDI, ADQ, and APB muscles after the NCS. Needle EMG in the ADQ was critical because it should be normal.

ELECTROPHYSIOLOGICAL TESTS AND FINDINGS

NCS Findings (Table 7.12; Fig. 7.13)

1. Prolonged terminal latency and slow sensory NCV over the finger-wrist segments in the right and left median nerves, worse on the left.
2. Low sensory CNAP amplitude in the finger-wrist segment in the right median nerve.
3. Prolonged terminal latency and low motor CMAP in the right FDI muscle.

Needle EMG

1. Normal needle EMG in the right ADQ and APB muscles.
2. Increased insertional activity, fibrillation and PSW, and DA in the right FDI muscle.

ELECTROPHYSIOLOGICAL INTERPRETATION

Bilateral CTS and neuropathy of the the deep palmar branch of the right ulnar nerve.

FINAL DIAGNOSIS

Symptomatic right CTS, asymptomatic left CTS, and neuropathy of the the deep palmar branch of the right ulnar nerve

TREATMENT AND FOLLOW-UP

The patient was told to avoid forceful and prolonged gripping of his motorcycle handlebars. Over next 2 years, he had gradual improvement of the atrophied muscles. His right CTS was relieved satisfactorily by endoscopic decompression.

TABLE 7.12. Nerve Conduction Data in Case 12

	Latent/NCV (ms/m/s)	Amplitude (mV/μV)		Latent/NCV (ms/m/s)	Amplitude (mV/μV)
Right	**Median**	**Motor N**	**Left**	**Median**	**Motor N**
TL	3.6	13.4		4.2	9.1
E-W	55	13.0			
AX-E	60	13.0			
	Ulnar	**Motor N**		**Ulnar**	**Motor N**
TL	2.5	13		2.5	18.6
BE-W	52	10		55.3	18.8
AE-BE	54	10			
AX-AE	63	10			
	Median	**Sens/Mixed N**		**Median**	**Sens/Mixed N**
F-W	37	9.5		24.3	13.2
W-E	54	12			
E-AX	58	14			
	Ulnar	**Sens/Mixed N**		**Ulnar**	**Sens/Mixed N**
F-W	46	12			
W-E	52	13			
E-AX	62	15			
	Ulnar	**Motor N**		**Ulnar**	**Motor N**
TL (FDI)	5.2	2		4.7	18.6

Height: 179.5 cm.

COMMENTS

The ulnar nerve can be compressed at various critical locations along its pathway at the wrist and hand. Proximally at the wrist, the entire ulnar nerve, containing both motor and sensory branches, passes through Guyon's canal. At the distal portion of the canal, the ulnar nerve divides into the superficial sensory and deep motor branches. The superficial sensory branch provides sensation to the ulnar 1.5 fingers on the palm of the hand. The deep motor branch, innervating the hypothenar muscles, takes an abrupt turn toward the thumb and follows along the deep palmar arch, innervating the small intrinsic muscles including the interosseous and adductor pollicis muscles. In neuropathy of the deep palmar branch, there is no sensory abnormality whatsoever; a pure motor deficit involving the intrinsic muscles is the cardinal finding. To confirm this disorder, extra recording electrodes in the FDI muscle are required.

This test is not done as part of a routine ulnar nerve study. Thus, neuropathy of the deep palmar branch of the ulnar nerve has to be suspected clinically before this test is performed. Marked prolongation of terminal latency to the FDI and dispersion phenomenon in the CMAP are cardinal findings in the presence of normal terminal latency to the ADQ muscle and normal sensory NCS.

MAXIMS

1. Atrophy of the intrinsic hand muscles alone without atrophy of the thenar and hypothenar muscles is diagnostic of a neuropathy of the deep palmar branch of the ulnar nerve until proven otherwise.
2. Ulnar nerve conduction with recording electrodes over the FDI is sine qua non for diagnosis of the deep palmar branch neuropathy of the ulnar nerve.

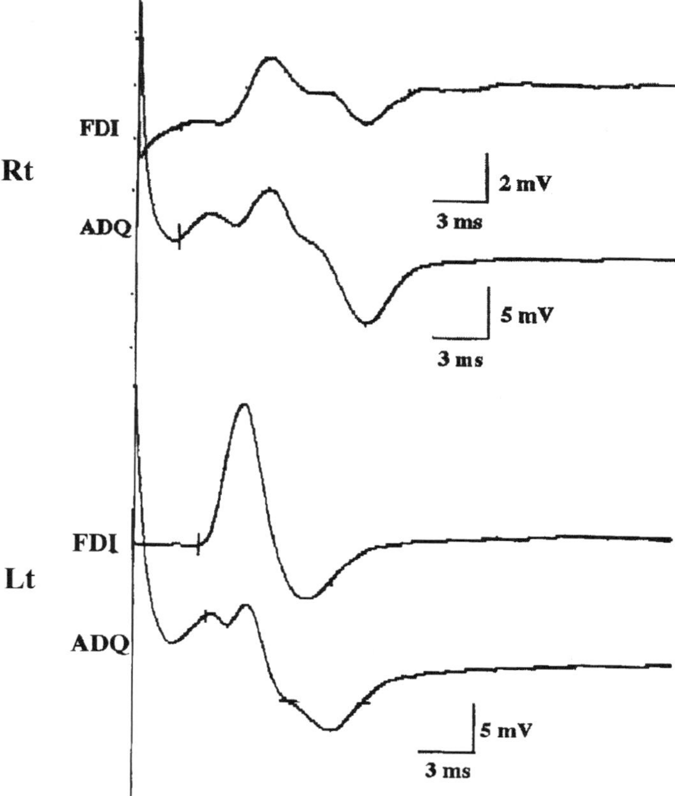

FIGURE 7.13. Mildly prolonged terminal latency and low CMAP amplitude in the right FDI muscle, indicative of a neuropathy of the deep palmar branch of the ulnar nerve.

REFERENCES

1. Oh SJ. Clinical electromyography. Nerve conduction studies. Baltimore, MD: Williams and Wilkins, 1993:197–199.
2. Shea JD, McAlain EJ. Ulnar nerve compression syndrome at and below the wrist. J Bone Joint Surg [Am] 1969;51:1095–1103.

CASE 13

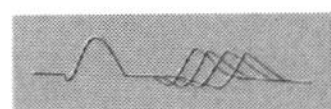

RADIAL NERVE PALSY OR POSTERIOR INTEROSSEOUS NEUROPATHY?

CASE PRESENTATION

A 35-year-old man first noted 3.5 months ago while playing pool that, he had trouble raising his finger to form a bridge. Since then, he noticed weakness in finger, thumb, and wrist extension. There was no sensory complaint or pain. When the referring neurologist evaluated him 1 month after onset of symptoms, he thought that the patient had a PIO because the brachioradialis was normal in strength and the needle EMG did not show any denervation. A review of the EMG report showed active denervation in the ECR muscle. On the basis of a "deposit of fat" in the arcade of Frohse in the MRI, decompression of the arcade of Frohse was done by anterior approach with incision in the antecubital area. After the surgery, the patient's condition became worse, with a new complaint of numbness over the lateral aspect of the forearm and weakness of thumb abduction. Another needle EMG now clearly documented active denervation in the brachioradialis. Because of "spreading of denervation process," he was sent to us for further evaluation. Abnormal findings were MRC strength of 0 in the left wrist extensor, EDC, brachioradialis, and finger extensors and 4 in the left APB muscle, with sensory loss over the lateral aspect of the left forearm corresponding to the territory of the lateral antebrachial cutaneous nerve. The left triceps muscle was normal.

CASE ANALYSIS

At the time of his evaluation at UAB, it was obvious that this patient had classic radial nerve palsy at the spiral groove. There was sufficient information to suggest that he had a radial nerve palsy from the beginning: wrist drop and active denervation in the ECR muscle, which do not occur in PIO neuropathy. In addition, there was weakness in the APB muscle and sensory loss over the lateral antebrachial cutaneous (musculocutaneous) nerve territory. The patient stated that these symptoms had occurred after the surgery in the antecubital area. Upon further questioning about any event near the time of onset of symptoms, he recalled that a few days before he had caught 80 fish and at one point he felt a "funny catch" between his scapula and axilla while trying to pull in a large fighting fish.

PLAN OF TESTING

1. NCS: This should include the radial motor and sensory and lateral antebrachial cutaneous nerve conduction studies (1).
2. Needle EMG: This should include the radial innervated muscles and APB muscles.

ELECTROPHYSIOLOGICAL TESTS AND FINDINGS

NCS Findings (Table 7.13)

1. Normal NCS in the left median, ulnar, and superficial radial nerves.
2. Low CMAP amplitude and normal NCV up to the spiral groove in the radial motor nerve.
3. Low CNAP amplitude in the left antebrachial cutaneous nerve.

Needle EMG (Table 7.14)

1. Moderate (+ + +) fibrillations and PSWs and no MUP in the left brachioradialis, ECR, EDC, and EIP muscles.
2. Normal needle EMG findings in the left triceps and deltoid muscles.
3. Normal needle EMG findings except for a few long-duration MUPs in the left APB muscle.

ELECTROPHYSIOLOGICAL INTERPRETATION

1. Left radial nerve palsy at the spiral groove.
2. Left lateral antebrachial cutaneous neuropathy.
3. Left partial median neuropathy involving the APB muscle.

TABLE 7.13. Nerve Conduction Data in Case 13

	Latent/NCV (ms/m/s)	Amplitude (mV/μV)		Latent/NCV (ms/m/s)	Amplitude (mV/μV)
	Median	**Motor N**		**Median**	**Sens/Mixed N**
TL	3.4	11	F-W	50.0	21
E-W	60.8	11	W-E	57.2	12
AX-E	63.3	12	E-AX	58.0	15
F-wave	30.4				
	Ulnar	**Motor N**		**Ulnar**	**Sens/Mixed N**
TL	2.4	15	F-W	45.8	15
BE-W	57.6	14	W-E	52.9	19
AE-BE	62.5	14	E-AX	58.3	15
AX-AE	66.6	14			
F-wave	29.2				
	Radial	**Motor N**		**Radial**	**Sens N**
TL	3.8	3.5	W-F	49.2	20
BE-AE	48.2	3.5			
AE-SG	75.0	2.0			

Height: 180 cm.
SG, spiral groove.

FINAL DIAGNOSIS

Radial nerve palsy at the spiral groove; postsurgical lateral antebrachial cutaneous and partial median neuropathy

TREATMENT AND FOLLOW-UP

Once the diagnosis of radial nerve palsy was made, intense physical therapy with daily "neuromuscular" stimulation was instituted. One month after the diagnosis, the patient reported no sign of improvement. However, the needle EMG in the brachioradialis muscle definitely showed a few small-amplitude polyphasic MUPs (reinnervation potentials) with distinct sounds. This convinced the patient that "regeneration" had begun. From that time, there has been gradual improvement of finger and wrist extensor function. Within 6 months, his brachioradialis improved in strength from 0 to 4.

COMMENTS

The radial nerve, a major continuation of the posterior cord of the brachial plexus, gives off branches to the triceps muscles before it reaches the spiral groove. At the distal portion of the spiral groove, the posterior antebrachial cutaneous nerve branches off from the main nerve. As the radial nerve emerges from the spiral groove, it sends out a first branch to the brachioradialis muscle and then to the extensor carpi radialis muscle. At the elbow, the radial nerve divides into the superficial branch—the superficial radial sensory nerve—and the deep branch—the PIO nerve.

The radial nerve is vulnerable to compression at the spiral groove in the upper arm. Radial nerve palsy is frequently seen in patients who have been in an alcoholic stupor after a weekend binge. Hence, this disorder is often called "Saturday night palsy." Clinically, the condition produces weakness or paralysis of the wrist and finger extensor muscles (wrist drop). The triceps muscle is spared, but the brachioradialis muscle is invariably involved. Sensory impairment is rare. There is no reliable motor nerve conduction technique to document a focal lesion in the spiral groove except the near-nerve needle technique. Thus, the routine nerve conduction study is rarely helpful in this disorder. Trojaborg's study with near-nerve needle stimulation and recording showed an acute compression block at the spiral groove. Diagnosis of this disorder is made by the needle EMG, which documents acute denervation in all radial-innervated muscles except the triceps and anconeus muscles.

TABLE 7.14. Needle EMG Data in Case 13

				Spontaneous Potentials				Motor Unit Potential				Interference	
Muscle	Root	Nerve	Insertion Activity	Fib	PSW	Fasc	CRD	Amplitude (mV)	Duration (ms)	Polyphasic Potential	HA MUP	Pattern	Mean Amplitude (K)
Lt deltoid	C5,6	Axillary	N	–	–	–	–	0.5–3	6–12	N	–	FIP	3
Triceps	C7,8	Radial	N	–	–	–	–	0.5–2	8–13	N	–	FIP	2
Brachiorad	C5,6	Radial	+	+++	+	–	–	No	MUP				
ECR	C7	Radial	+	++	+++	–	–	No	MUP				
EDC	C7	PIO	+	++	++	–	–	NO	MUP				
EIP	C7,8	PIO	+	+++	++	–	–	No	MUP				
APB	C8, T1	Median	+	+	++	–	–	1–5	6–13.3	+	–	FIP	2

ECR, extensor carpi radialis; EDC, extensor digitorum communis; EIP, extensor indices proprius; PID, posterior interosseous neuropathy.

***** END OF FILE *****

3893$$7t2a 02-26-98 18:11:42

The PIO nerve is the major terminal motor branch that passes through the supinator muscle (sometimes called the "radial tunnel" or "supinator channel"), entering the arcade of Frohse, and innervating the supinator, all the forearm and finger extensors except the extensor carpi radialis longus muscles. In contrast to the wrist drop seen in radial nerve palsy, this neuropathy produces "finger drop," an inability to extend the fingers at the metaphalangeal joint. The most common cause of PIO neuropathy is trauma. By performing a radial motor nerve conduction test with the needle in the extensor indices muscle and stimulation above the elbow, Carfi and Ma found normal responses in three of eight patients and prolonged latency or absent response in five. The superficial radial sensory nerve conduction is classically normal in PIO neuropathy. The needle EMG typically shows denervation in all the radial nerve-innervated forearm muscles except the extensor carpi radialis and brachioradialis.

MAXIMS

1. Wrist drop is the cardinal feature of radial nerve palsy and finger drop, the cardinal feature of PIO neuropathy.
2. Needle EMG study can detect small-amplitude polyphasic MUPs (reinnervation potentials) long before clinical improvement is noted.

REFERENCES

1. Oh SJ. Clinical electromyography. Nerve conduction studies. Baltimore, MD: Williams and Wilkins, 1993:202–211.
2. Trojaborg W. Rate of recovery in motor and sensory fibers of the radial nerve: clinical and electrophysiological aspects. J Neurol Neurosurg Psychiatry 1970;33:625–638.

CASE 14

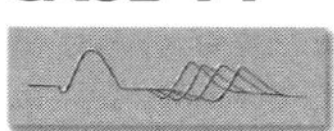

RADIAL SENSORY NEUROPATHY IN A PATIENT WITH NEUROFIBROMATOSIS

CASE PRESENTATION

A 10-year-old patient with generalized neurofibromatosis complained of tingling and numbness over the right thumb. A small, bean-sized neurofibroma was palpated over the upper portion of the forearm in the superficial radial sensory nerve. No motor weakness was observed. Minimally decreased sensation over the radial sensory dermatome on the web of the first and second digit was noted. Tinel's sign was present at the site of the neurofibroma.

CASE ANALYSIS

This patient had classic findings indicative of superficial radial sensory neuropathy. The question was the location of the lesion: at the wrist or forearm.

PLAN OF TESTING

1. NCS: This should include NCS of the superficial radial sensory nerve below the wrist and over the forearm (1).
2. Needle EMG: EDC muscle to rule out PIO neuropathy.

ELECTROPHYSIOLOGICAL TESTS AND FINDINGS

NCS Findings (Fig. 7.14)

1. Slow sensory NCV with normal CNAP amplitude in the distal radial sensory nerve.
2. Absent sensory CNAP in the forearm segment through the neuroma with both antidromic and orthodromic stimulation.
3. Normal sensory NCS in the lateral antebrachial cutaneous (sensory branch of the musculo-cutaneous nerve).

Needle EMG. Needle EMG in the EDC was normal.

ELECTROPHYSIOLOGICAL INTERPRETATION

Superficial radial sensory neuropathy.

FINAL DIAGNOSIS

Superficial radial sensory neuropathy due to neurofibroma in the forearm

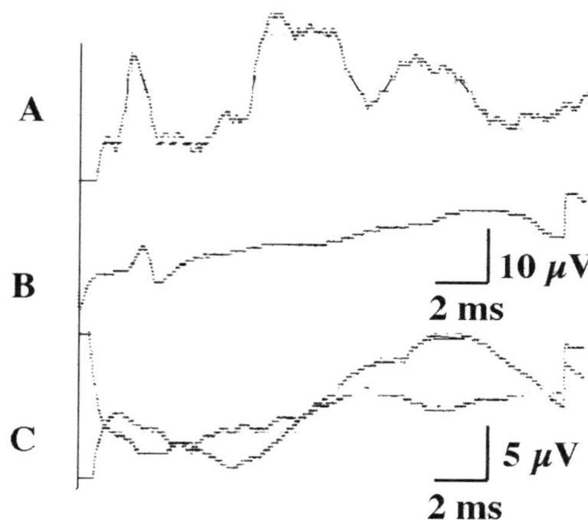

FIGURE 7.14. Sensory nerve conduction in the distal superficial radial **(A)**, lateral antebrachial cutaneous **(B)**, and the superficial radial **(C)** nerve of the forearm.

TREATMENT AND FOLLOW-UP

Because her superficial radial sensory neuropathy did not interfere with the patient's daily activity, the neurofibroma was left alone.

COMMENTS

The superficial radial sensory nerve is a long nerve, originating from the main radial nerve just above the elbow and dividing into terminal digital branches that supply the dorsolateral aspect of the hand and the first three digits. This neuropathy produces sensory impairment over the web of the first and second digits on the dorsum of the hand, which is usually compressed at the wrist where it lies close to the distal end of the radius. This produces cheiralgia paresthetica, or "handcuff neuropathy." In this neuropathy, the sensory CNAP is either absent or low in amplitude or the sensory NCV is slow in the superficial radial sensory NCS. Sometimes, handcuff neuropathy may involve the median or ulnar nerve in addition to the superficial radial sensory nerve. Entrapment of the superficial radial sensory nerve at the forearm, as seen in our case, has been reported. Clinically, distal and proximal radial sensory neuropathies cannot be distinguished from one another. In radial sensory neuropathy due to a lesion in the forearm, the radial sensory nerve conduction in the forearm is the critical test for confirmation of the lesion.

MAXIMS

1. Cheiralgia paresthetica or handcuff neuropathy refers to superficial radial sensory neuropathy.
2. Radial sensory neuropathy produces sensory impairment over the web of the first and second digits on the dorsum of the hand.

REFERENCES

1. Oh SJ. Clinical electromyography. Nerve conduction studies. Baltimore, MD: Williams and Wilkins, 1993:210–211.
2. Massey EW, Pleet AB. Handcuff and cheiralgia paresthetica. Neurology 1978;28:1312–1313.

CASE 15

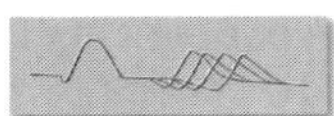

NUMBNESS AND PAIN IN THE RIGHT PUBIC AREA AFTER HERNIORRHAPHY

CASE PRESENTATION

A 43-year-old woman developed a right inguinal hernia after hysterectomy a few years ago. She reported numbness in the right lower abdomen and right half of the pubic area, together with pain along the inner side of the right thigh after herniorrhaphy 6 months before evaluation. Abnormal neurological findings were sensory loss over a small strip involving the right medial inguinal ligament and pubic areas lateral to the vagina and point tenderness at the surgical herniorrhaphy scar. There was no atrophy or weakness in the right thigh, and right iliopsoas and quadriceps were normal in strength. Right knee jerk was also normal.

CASE ANALYSIS

Consulting a sensory chart, we determined that the area of sensory loss in this patient matched best with the sensory territory of the ilioinguinal nerve.

PLAN OF TESTING

1. NCS: Right ilioinguinal motor nerve conduction study to confirm the clinical impression.
2. Needle EMG: In the right L1-2 paraspinal, internal oblique and transverse, iliopsoas and quadriceps muscles.

ELECTROPHYSIOLOGICAL TESTS AND FINDINGS

NCS Findings (Fig. 7.15)

1. Low CMAP amplitude in the right ilioinguinal nerve.
2. Normal femoral nerve conduction.

Needle EMG

1. Fibrillations and PSW in the right internal oblique and transverse muscles.
2. Normal needle EMG findings in the right iliopsoas and vastus lateralis muscles.
3. No fibrillations or PSW in the right L1 and L2 paraspinal muscles.

ELECTROPHYSIOLOGICAL INTERPRETATION

Right ilioinguinal neuropathy.

FINAL DIAGNOSIS

Postsurgical right ilioinguinal neuropathy

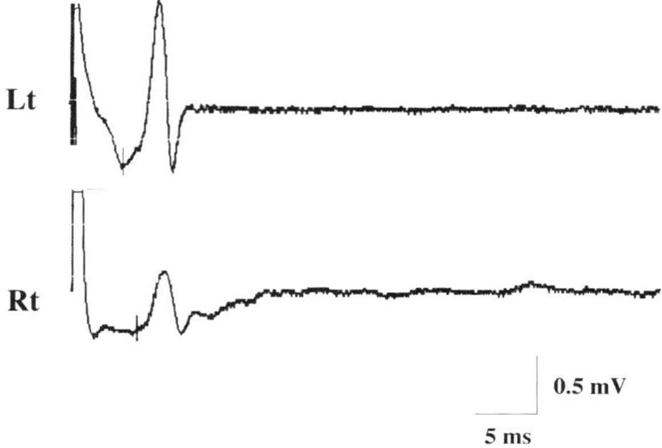

FIGURE 7.15. Low CMAP amplitude in the right ilioinguinal nerve conduction.

COMMENTS

Three nerves—the iliohypogastric, ilioinguinal, and genitofemoral nerves—innervate the small area around the inguinal ligament, the upper anterior and medial thigh, and part of the genital area. Like the thoracoabdominal nerves, the iliohypogastric and ilioinguinal nerves are derived from the first lumbar spinal nerve and follow a course that circles the trunk and innervates the skin and muscles of the abdominal wall. It is almost impossible to remember the exact map of the sensory territory of each nerve because of their complexity. Thus, it is always wise to consult a sensory chart for the final determination of the involved nerve.

Ilioinguinal neuropathy is usually due to surgical incision or postoperative adhesions in the lower abdomen and inguinal area, such as inadvertent damage to the nerve during herniorrhaphy and appendectomy. Considering the frequency of these surgeries, such neuropathy is extremely rare. Entrapment of the nerve as it passes through the muscles of the abdominal wall medial to the anterior superior iliac spine has also been reported. Injury to the ilioinguinal nerve is manifested by pain or numbness in the anatomical field of distribution of the nerve. This neuropathy is diagnosed by sensory loss or hyperesthesia in a small strip along the inguinal ligament and the pubic area. Although the internal oblique and transverse muscles are innervated by the ilioinguinal nerve, weakness or atrophy is usually asymptomatic. A technique of motor conduction of the ilioinguinal nerve has been reported. A difference of 50% or more in the CMAP amplitude between the normal and affected sides probably indicates abnormality in the affected side, as noted in this patient.

MAXIMS

1. Ilioinguinal neuropathy is usually due to a surgical incision or postoperative adhesion in the lower abdomen and inguinal area.
2. The internal oblique and transverse muscles are innervated by the ilioinguinal nerve.

REFERENCES

1. Oh SJ. Clinical electromyography. Nerve conduction studies. Baltimore, MD: Williams and Wilkins, 1993:215–216.
2. Stulz P, Pfeiffer KM. Peripheral nerve injuries from common surgical procedures in the lower portion of the abdomen. Arch Surg 1982;117:324–327.

CASE 16

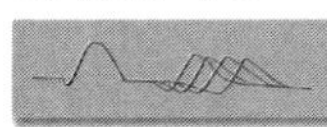

NUMBNESS OVER THE LATERAL ASPECT OF THE THIGH AFTER KIDNEY TRANSPLANTATION

CASE PRESENTATION

A 51-year-old man with uremia since 1965 and chronic hemodialysis since 1984 received a right kidney transplant 1 year ago. Since the surgery, he suffered from numbness over the lateral aspect of his right thigh. Examination showed decreased sensation to pin prick and touch over the lateral aspect of the right thigh corresponding to the lateral femoral cutaneous nerve territory, a surgical scar running medio-caudally from the right flank down to the midpubic area, normal muscle strength in the right iliopsoas and quadriceps muscles, and normal knee jerk.

CASE ANALYSIS

History and examination showed the classic features of meralgia paresthetica involving the lateral femoral cutaneous nerve.

PLAN OF TESTING

NCS: Sensory nerve conduction for the lateral femoral cutaneous nerve to confirm the clinical impression (1).

ELECTROPHYSIOLOGICAL TESTS AND FINDINGS

NCS Findings (Fig. 7.16)

1. Normal sensory NCS (56 m/s in NCV; 4 μ V in amplitude) in the left lateral femoral cutaneous nerve.
2. Absent sensory CNAP in the right lateral femoral cutaneous nerve.

ELECTROPHYSIOLOGICAL INTERPRETATION

Left lateral femoral cutaneous neuropathy typical of meralgia paresthetica.

FINAL DIAGNOSIS

Meralgia paresthetica due to previous surgery

TREATMENT AND FOLLOW-UP

Once the patient understood the cause of his problem, he was able to live with the numbness. There has not been any progression.

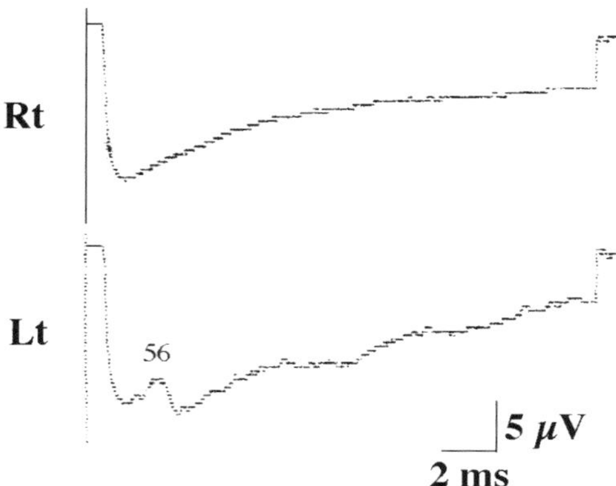

FIGURE 7.16. Lateral femoral cutaneous nerve conduction with near-nerve stimulation and recording. *Rt,* no CNAP is obtained; *Lt,* normal sensory NCV at 56.0 m/s.

COMMENTS

Meralgia paresthetica is a clinically benign entrapment neuropathy of the lateral femoral cutaneous nerve of the thigh. The site of entrapment is the point at which the nerve pierces the inguinal ligament or the fascia lata upon entering the thigh at or near the level of the anterior superior iliac spine. The diagnosis is usually based on the presence of dysesthesia over the territory of the lateral femoral cutaneous nerve. NCS of the lateral femoral cutaneous nerve can be used as an objective diagnostic aid in this disorder. The most prominent abnormality is an absence of sensory CNAP, as observed in 58% of the reported cases. The sensory NCV was slow in 17%.

One problem with the NCS in this nerve is the technical difficulty of obtaining reliable sensory CNAP. Unfortunately, many patients with this disorder are obese. In these patients, it is impossible to perform reliable sensory NCS in this nerve. In thin individuals, surface recording and stimulation electrodes are sometimes helpful. However, in many patients, a monopolar needle has to be used as the stimulating electrode or a near-nerve recording needle as the recording electrode. Because of this difficulty, it is always important to compare the test result in the involved side with that of the normal side. In this case, we obtained the sensory CNAP with the monopolar needle as a stimulating electrode 1 cm medial to the anterior superior iliac spine. Needle EMG is more helpful in ruling out L2 radiculopathy in this disorder.

MAXIMS

1. Meralgia paresthetica is a lateral femoral cutaneous neuropathy characterized by numbness and tingling sensation over the lateral aspect of the thigh.
2. The diagnosis of meralgia paresthetica can be made easily from history and findings without NCS in most cases. NCS of this nerve is technically difficult in obese individuals.

REFERENCES

1. Oh SJ. Clinical electromyography. Nerve conduction studies. Baltimore, MD: Williams and Wilkins, 1993:216–218.
2. Lagueny A, Deliac MM, Deliac P, Durandeau A. Diagnostic and prognostic value of electrophysiological tests in meralgia paresthetica. Muscle Nerve 1991;14:51–56.

CASE 17

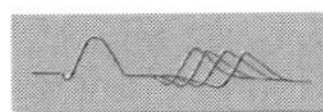

WEAKNESS OF THE LEG AFTER ARTERIOGRAM BY FEMORAL APPROACH

CASE PRESENTATION

Three months previously, a 45-year-old man had a cardiac arteriogram for chest pain performed by right femoral approach and immediately after this procedure developed a hematoma in the groin and numbness in the right leg. These symptoms were soon followed by weakness of the right leg, which progressed over the next 2 weeks and then stabilized. Sensation in the right leg improved somewhat. At the time of our initial evaluation, the patient's problems included difficulty walking and climbing a ladder or stairs, lack of sensation over the inner side of the right leg, and wasting of the right thigh. He denied any bowel or bladder dysfunction or back pain. Abnormal neurological findings were a limp with the right leg, gross atrophy of the right thigh, MRI strength of 4+ in the right iliopsoas and 3 in the right quadriceps, decreased pin-prick sensation on the anteromedial side of the right thigh and medial aspect of the right lower leg, and absent right knee reflex.

CASE ANALYSIS

Clinically, this patient's symptoms were consistent with a right femoral nerve injury in the groin. Historically, his symptoms began after a catheterization procedure to the right groin and became progressively worse before stabilizing. This pattern indicated that he suffered nerve damage, most likely at the time of the catheterization procedure, and that the progression had now stabilized.

TABLE 7.15. Nerve Conduction Data in Case 17

	Latent/NCV (ms/m/s)	Amplitude (mV/μV)		Latent/NCV (ms/m/s)	Amplitude (mV/μV)
Right	**Peroneal**	**Motor M N**	**Left**	**Peroneal**	**Motor N**
TL	3.6	9.5			
FH-A	50	9.1			
PF-FH	52	8.9			
F-wave	44.2				
	Posterior Tibial	**Motor N**		**Posterior Tibial**	**Motor N**
TL	4.0	19.5			
PF-A	51.0	13.5			
F-wave	48.7				
H-reflex	29.3			29.3	
	Femoral	**Motor N**		**Femoral**	**Motor N**
TL	5.3	3.0		4.3	23.9
	Sural	**Sensory N**		**Sural**	**Sensory N**
MC-A	42.0	23.8			
	Saphenous	**Sensory N**		**Saphenous**	**Sensory N**
MC-A	NP			41.0	4
	Medial Femoral Cutaneous	**Sensory N**		**Medial Femoral Cutaneous**	**Sensory N**
	NP			63.4	13.3

Height: 162.6 cm. Femoral nerve conduction: Stohr's method. Saphenous nerve conduction: Wainapel et al.'s method. Medial femoral cutaneous nerve conduction: Lee's method.

PLAN OF TESTING

1. NCS: This should include femoral (1), medial femoral cutaneous (2), and saphenous nerves (1).
2. Needle EMG: L3,4 paraspinal muscles, iliopsoas, rectus femoris, vastus lateralis and medialis, anterior tibialis, and peroneus longus muscles. These studies were done to rule out L3,4,5 radiculopathy and confirm femoral neuropathy at the inguinal ligament.

ELECTROPHYSIOLOGICAL TESTS AND FINDINGS

NCS Findings (Table 7.15; Fig. 7.17)

1. Low CMAP in the right femoral nerve.
2. Absent sensory CNAP in the right saphenous and medial femoral nerves.

Needle EMG (Table 7.16)

1. Fibrillations and PSW in the right vastus lateralis and medialis, rectus femoris, and iliopsoas muscles.

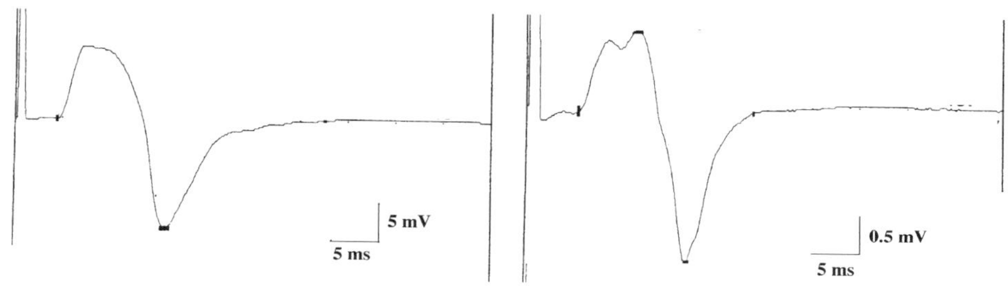

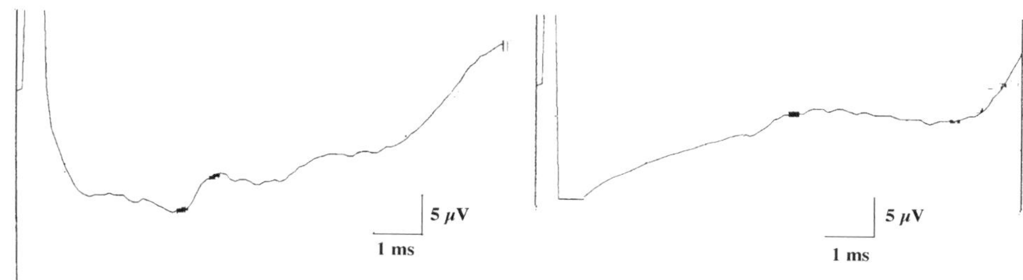

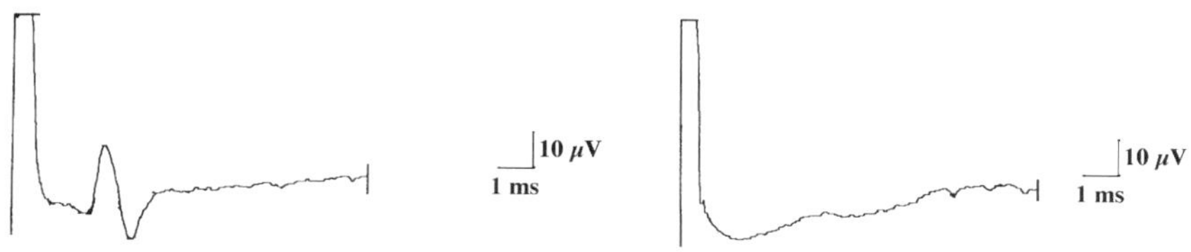

FIGURE 7.17. Low CMAP in the right femoral nerve and absent sensory CNAP in the right saphenous and medial femoral cutaneous nerves in a patient with right femoral neuropathy.

TABLE 7.16. Needle EMG Data in Case 17

				Spontaneous Potentials				Motor Unit Potential				Interference	
Muscle	**Root**	**Nerve**	**Insertion Activity**	**Fib**	**PSW**	**Fasc**	**Myotonia CRD**	**Amplitude (K)**	**Duration (ms)**	**Polyphasic Potential**	**HA MUP**	**Pattern**	**Mean Amplitude (K)**
Rt vast lat	L3,4	Femoral	+	+	+	–	–	1–3	6–18	+	–	DA	1
Vast med	L3,4	Femoral	+	+	+ +	–	–	NO MUP					
Rectus femoris	L3,4	Femoral	+	+ +	+ + +	–	–	1–5.5	6–16	+	+	DA	4
Ant tibial	L4,5	Peroneal	N	–	–	–	–	0.5–1.5	6–12	N	–	FIP	1.5
Gastroc	S1,2	Post tibial	N	–	–	–	–	0.5–1.5	6–12	N	–	FIP	1.5
Iliopsoas	L2-4	Femoral	+	+ +	+	–	–	0.5–3	6–12	+	–	RIP	2
L3,4 paraspinal	L3,4		N	–	–	–	–						

DA, discrete activity.

2. Marked loss of MUP recruitments in all muscles innervated by the right femoral nerve.
3. Increased polyphasic MUPs in the right vastus lateralis and rectus femoris muscles.
4. A few "HA MUPs" in the rectus femoris muscle.

ELECTROPHYSIOLOGICAL INTERPRETATION

Right femoral neuropathy at the inguinal area and superimposed local trauma to the distal portion of the right iliopsoas muscle.

FINAL DIAGNOSIS

Right femoral nerve injury due to hematoma associated with cardiac angiogram

TREATMENT AND FOLLOW-UP

No retroperitoneal hematoma was found by CT of the abdomen. The MRI of the lumbar spine showed several bulges. Intense physical therapy was instituted. Gradually over the next 6 months, there was improvement in motor and sensory functions of the right femoral nerve.

COMMENTS

The femoral nerve is formed from the posterior divisions of the L2,3,4 spinal nerves and emerges beneath the inguinal ligament lateral to the femoral artery and vein. In the thigh, it divides into a motor branch to the quadriceps muscle and a sensory branch to the anterior thigh. The saphenous nerve, the terminal branch of the femoral nerve, innervates the medial aspect of the lower leg and the arch of the foot. At present, the most common cause for femoral neuropathy is a local hematoma occurring during angiography performed through the femoral approach. In the past, the most common cause of femoral neuropathy was thought to be diabetes. Although the femoral nerve is predominantly involved in diabetic amyotrophy, there is a more widespread denervation process involving the lumbosacral roots and plexus in that disorder.

Femoral neuropathy is clinically characterized by the presence of one or more of the following three findings: weakness of the quadriceps, reduced or absent knee reflex, and sensory impairment over the anteromedial aspect of the thigh and the medial aspect of the lower leg. Weakness of the iliopsoas muscle indicates that either the proximal femoral nerve, the upper lumbar plexus, or the L2 or L3 roots are involved. Weakness of the hip adductors (innervated by the obturator nerve) means that the patient has either a lumbar plexopathy or an L2,3,4 radiculopathy.

The needle EMG study shows denervation process in the quadriceps muscles. It is always wise to examine the vastus lateralis, rectus femoris, and vastus medialis muscles separately in patients with femoral neuropathy because not all muscles are equally involved. The femoral, saphenous, and medial femoral cutaneous nerve conduction studies distinguish femoral neuropathy from lumbar radiculopathy. Even in patients with diabetic amyotrophy, a prolonged terminal latency in the femoral nerve was noted in 65% of cases. This finding is in addition to widespread evidence of polyradiculopathy and peripheral neuropathy. In patients with traumatic injury of the femoral nerve at the inguinal area, as in our case, prolonged latency of the femoral nerve and absence of the saphenous CNAP are consistent findings. A sensory nerve conduction technique for the medial femoral cutaneous nerve has recently been reported. According to our experience, this technique is easier to perform and more reliable than the saphenous nerve conduction study.

MAXIMS

1. The classic distribution of sensory loss in femoral neuropathy is over the anterior-medial aspect of the thigh (medial femoral and intermediate femoral nerve territory) and the medial aspect of the lower leg and foot (saphenous nerve territory).
2. Femoral neuropathy invariably produces weakness of the quadriceps muscles and impaired knee reflex.

REFERENCES

1. Oh SJ. Clinical electromyography. Nerve conduction studies. Baltimore, MD: Williams and Wilkins, 1993:218–225.
2. Lee HJ, Bach J, DeLisa JA. Medial femoral cutaneous nerve conduction. Am J Phys Rehabil 1995; 74:305–307.

CASE 18

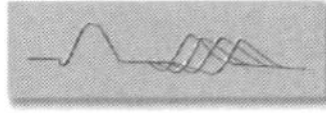

PAIN IN THE RIGHT HAMSTRING AREA FOR 3 MONTHS FOLLOWED BY URINARY RETENTION

CASE PRESENTATION

Three months before the initial evaluation, a 54-year-old man with a history of chronic hepatitis B developed aching pain in the right hamstring area. Occasionally, he also experienced "lightning pains" down to the calf. The pain had been intermittent, varied in its severity, was not aggravated by coughing, and was relieved by rest and ibuprofen. There was no complaint of back pain. One week before examination he noted the sudden onset of inability to urinate; 1400 mL of urine was drained by Foley catheter. The patient then noted a tingling pins-and-needles sensation from the posterior portion of the right leg down to the sole of his right foot but no obvious weakness. He also complained of constipation and some tingling/pain sensation around the right perineal area. Abnormal neurological findings were tenderness in the right sacroiliac joint; positive straight leg raise at 80 on the right; MRC strength of 4 in the right hamstring, anterior tibialis, and gastrocnemius and 5- in the right gluteus medius and maximus muscles; mild atrophy of the right gluteal and hamstring muscles; decreased sensation to pin prick over the right S3-5 area including the scrotum, penis, and medial aspect of the posterior thigh to the knee; and absent right ankle jerk. A CT a few years before revealed a suspicious lesion in the liver. The patient had a Foley catheter inserted.

CASE ANALYSIS

Urinary retention, weakness in the S1-2 innervated muscles, and sensory loss over the right S3-5 area localized the lesion to the sacral plexus or unilateral cauda equina. In view of his history of hepatitis B, abnormal CT, and subacute progression of disease, there was a definite possibility of a metastatic tumor. The question was whether this was in the sacral plexus or cauda equina.

PLAN OF TESTING

1. Needle EMG: To rule out the lumbosacral radiculopathy and determine the extent of denervation in the right leg, including the bulbocavernous (BC) muscle.
2. BC reflexes: To assess the degree of severity of neurogenic bladder.
3. NCS in the right posterior tibial, peroneal, superficial peroneal, posterior gluteal cutaneous, and sural nerves to assess the degree of involvement in these nerves.
4. MRI of the right pelvis and lumbosacral area to look for a mass in the cauda equina and sacral plexus.

ELECTROPHYSIOLOGICAL TESTS AND FINDINGS

NCS Findings (Table 7.17; Fig. 7.18)

1. Low CMAP amplitude and absent F-wave in the right peroneal and posterior tibial nerves.
2. Mild prolongation in the right H-reflex.
3. Absent posterior gluteal cutaneous sensory nerve CNAP.
4. Normal sural and superficial peroneal sensory nerve conduction.
5. Absent right BC reflex and normal latency on the left.

TABLE 7.17. Nerve Conduction Data in Case 18

	Latent/NCV (ms/m/s)	Amplitude (mV/μV)
Rt	**Peroneal**	**Motor N**
TL	5.6	0.7
FH-A	44.2	0.68
PF-FH	40.3	0.68
F-wave	NP	
	Post Tib	**Motor N**
TL	4.8	0.24
PF-A	42.5	0.29
F-wave	NP	
H-reflex	33.4	
	BC	**Reflex**
Rt	NP	
Lt	46	
	Sural	**Sensory**
MC-A	48.1	16.4
Rt	**Post Glut Cut**	**Sensory**
SG-PF	NP	
	Sup Peroneal	**Sensory**
MC-A	52.1	10.8

Height: 170.2 cm.

Needle EMG (Table 7.18)

1. Fibrillations and PSWs in the right medial gastrocnemius, BC, gluteus maximus, and medius muscles.
2. A few long-duration MUPs in the right gluteus maximus muscle.
3. No MUPs in the right gluteus medius and BC muscles.
4. Reduced recruitment in the MUPs in the S1- and 2-innervated muscles.

ELECTROPHYSIOLOGICAL INTERPRETATION

Right sacral plexus neuropathy.

OTHER TEST FINDINGS

MRI of the lumbosacral area showed a mass in the right sacral area. In view of the patient's history, the most likely diagnosis was metastatic hepatoma.

FINAL DIAGNOSIS

Right sacral plexus metastatic hepatoma

TREATMENT AND FOLLOW-UP

Radiation therapy was tried. During radiation therapy, the patient developed massive abdominal bleeding that could not be controlled and subsequently died.

COMMENTS

There are two trunks in the sacral plexus. The lateral trunk is derived from the dorsal branches of the S1 and S2 roots and becomes the peroneal nerve. The medial trunk is derived from

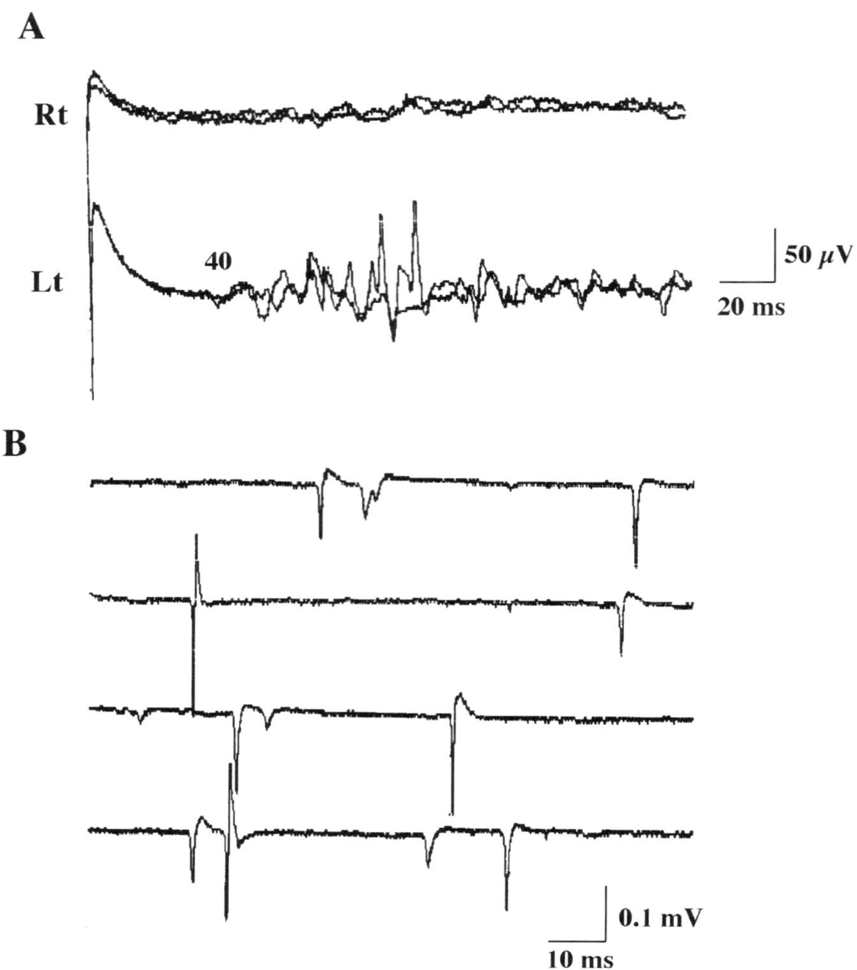

FIGURE 7.18. A. Bulbocavernous reflex: absent response on the right (*Rt*) and normal response on the left (*Lf*). **B.** Fibrillations and PSWs in the right bulbocavernous muscle.

the ventral branches of the S1, 2, 3, and 4 roots. Unlike the brachial plexus, there are only a handful of nerves arising from the sacral plexus: the superior and inferior gluteal, pudendal, and posterior gluteal cutaneous nerves and several smaller branches to muscles in the pelvic and hip regions. Because of this limited number of nerves arising from the sacral plexus, the needle EMG of these muscles becomes important in differentiating a plexus lesion from a sciatic nerve lesion. In differentiating sacral plexopathy from radiculopathy, the paraspinal needle EMG and posterior gluteal cutaneous sensory nerve conduction study were helpful in this case. The dorsal cutaneous nerve of the penis can also be tested, but unfortunately it can not be tested unilaterally. It should be noted that superficial peroneal and sural nerve conduction was normal in this case.

In the workup of sacral plexus and lower sacral radiculopathy, there are two pelvic muscles that can be easily tested with the EMG needle: the BC and external anal muscles. As seen in this case, a unilateral abnormality can be documented by testing both sides of BC muscles. Activation and relaxation of these muscles are not easy. MUP generation is easy in the anal sphincter because in the normal state this muscle is contracted. To relax this muscle, the

TABLE 7.18. Needle EMG Data in Case 18

				Spontaneous Potentials				Motor Unit Potential				Interference	
Muscle	**Root**	**Nerve**	**Insertion Activity**	**Fib**	**PSW**	**Fasc**	**Myotonia CRD**	**Amplitude (K)**	**Duration (ms)**	**Polyphasic Potential**	**HA MUP**	**Pattern**	**Mean Amplitude (K)**
Rt L4-S2	L4-S2		N	–	–	–	–						
Glut max	S1	Inf glut	+	++	++	–	–	0.5–3	8–22	N	0	DA	1
Glut med	L5	Sup glut	+	++	++	–	–	No	MUP				
Vast lat	L3,4	Femoral	+	–	–	–	–	0.5–2	8–12	N	0	FIP	1
Ant tibial	L4,5	Peroneal	N	–	–	–	–	0.5–2K	8–12	N	0	FIP	2
Peroneus	L5	Peroneal	N	–	–	–	–	0.5–2	8–12	+	0	RIP	2
Med gastroc	S1	Post tibial	+	+	++	–	–	0.5–1	10	+	0	DA	1
Lat gastroc	S2	Post tibial	+	–	–	–	–	0.5–3	8–12	+	0	RIP	3
BC	S1-3	Pudendal	+	++	++	–	–	No	MUP				1

BC, bulbocavernous.

patient is asked to push down as if attempting to expel feces during a bowel movement. It is not easy to achieve complete relaxation of the external anal sphincter. With the BC muscles, activation is not easy. We usually ask the patient to tighten up the pelvic muscles, and this is not easy to do. As far as the paraspinal muscles are concerned, one can test down to the S2 paraspinal muscle but not beyond that.

The BC reflex test is a useful tool for evaluation of neurogenic bladder, as seen in this patient. It is best to do this test by recording the response with a concentric needle from the BC muscle and stimulating the dorsal nerve of the penis in men or the clitoris in women. In patients with neurogenic bladder due to a cauda equina or conus medullaris lesion, the BC reflex is either absent or present with a prolonged latency. This technique is also helpful in distinguishing organic impotence from functional impotence and assessing neurogenic fecal incontinence.

MAXIMS

1. The needle EMG in the gluteal medius and maximus muscle is critical in differentiating sacral plexopathy from sciatic nerve lesions.
2. The BC reflex test is useful in evaluating neurogenic bladder, fecal incontinence, and organic impotence.

REFERENCES

1. Oh SJ. Clinical electromyography. Nerve conduction studies. Baltimore, MD: Williams and Wilkins, 1993; pp. 218–219 for posterior femoral cutaneous nerve conduction and pp. 393–400 for BC reflex.
2. Fower CJ. Pelvic floor neurophysiology. Methods in clinical neurophysiology. Skolunde, Denmark; Dantec, 1991:1–24.

CASE 19

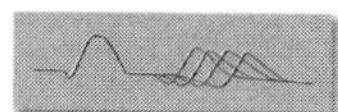

FOOT DROP AFTER A MOTORCYCLE ACCIDENT

CASE PRESENTATION

A 14-year-old boy was involved in a motorcycle accident with fracture of the right femur and tibia 7 months previously. After the cast was removed, he was found to have a right foot drop and was referred to the EMG laboratory for peroneal nerve palsy. Neurological examination showed 1 MRC strength in the right anterior tibialis and peroneus muscles and difficulty walking on his right heel. Right ankle and knee reflexes were well preserved. No obvious sensory loss or weakness in the right gastrocnemius was noted.

CASE ANALYSIS

Clinically, this patient had a right foot drop typical of peroneal nerve palsy. The referring orthopedic surgeon thought that this was due to common peroneal nerve palsy secondary to the cast compression at the fibular head. In view of the history of femur fracture, sciatic nerve injury had to be considered as a possibility, although clinically we did not have any finding suggestive of this.

PLAN OF TESTING

1. NCS: To identify or rule out a common peroneal nerve palsy.
2. Needle EMG: To sort out whether the sciatic nerve or the plexus was injured. To do this, the needle EMG in the gluteal muscles and the short and long heads of the biceps femoris muscle is crucial.

ELECTROPHYSIOLOGICAL TESTS AND FINDINGS

NCS Findings

1. Normal motor NCS in the right posterior tibial nerve.
2. Normal sensory NCS in the right sural and superficial peroneal nerves.
3. Absent CMAP from the EDB muscle in the right peroneal nerve.
4. With the recording electrode in the anterior tibialis muscle, low CMAP amplitude, but normal NCV across the fibular head.

Needle EMG (Table 7.19)

1. Prominent PSWs and fibrillations in the right anterior tibialis, peroneus longus, and EDB muscles.
2. Minimal fibrillations and PSWs in the right gastrocnemius and in the short and long heads of the biceps femoris muscle.
3. A few HA MUPs in the right anterior tibialis muscle and increased polyphasic MUPs in the right peroneus longus and biceps femoris muscles.
4. DA in the right EDB and RIP in the right anterior tibialis and peroneus longus muscles.

ELECTROPHYSIOLOGICAL INTERPRETATION

Right partial sciatic neuropathy.

FINAL DIAGNOSIS

Foot drop due to a right partial sciatic nerve injury

TREATMENT AND FOLLOW-UP

In view of the partial lesion, no surgical intervention was considered. There has been a slow but steady improvement in his foot drop.

COMMENTS

The sciatic nerve consists of two distinct nerve trunks, the medial trunk (posterior tibial nerve) and the lateral trunk (common peroneal nerve). The medial trunk arises from the posterior

TABLE 7.19. Needle EMG Data in Case 19

				Spontaneous Potentials				Motor Unit Potential				Interference	
Muscle	Root	Nerve	Insertion Activity	Fib	PSW	Fasc	CRD	Amplitude (mV)	Duration (ms)	Polyphasic Potential	HA MUP	Pattern	Mean Amplitude (mV)
Rt ant tibial	L4,5	Peroneal	+	++	+++	–	–	1–7	8–15	N	+	RIP	3.5
P longus	L5, S1	Peroneal	+	+	+	–	–	1–3	8–18	+	–	RIP	3
EDB	L5, S1	Peroneal	+	++	+++	–	–	0.5[a]	7	N	–	DA	0.5
Gastroc	S1,2	Post tibial	+	–	+	–	–	1–4	6–12	N	–	FIP	3
Biceps fem short		Sciatic	+	–	+	–	–	0.5–2	6–14	+	–	RIP	1
Biceps fem longus	S1,2	Sciatic	+	+	–	–	–	0.5–2	6–14	+	–	FIP	1
Glut max	S1,2	Inf glut	N	–	–	–	–	0.5–1.5	6–12	N	–	FIP	1.5

[a] One MUP.

EDB, extensor digitorum brevis.

divisions and the lateral trunk from the anterior divisions of the L4-S2 spinal nerves. The sciatic nerve innervates the hamstring muscles. The short head of the biceps femoris is the only muscle innervated by the lateral trunk, all other hamstring muscles being innervated by the medial trunk. No sensory branch arises from the sciatic nerve itself. Sciatic neuropathy should be differentiated clinically from common peroneal nerve palsy because the peroneal branch is always more involved in sciatic neuropathy. The greater vulnerability of the lateral trunk is most likely due to a combination of factors: it is more firmly fixed and angulated at the sciatic notch and it contains larger and fewer fascicles and less connective tissue than the medial trunk and so has less tensile strength. The most common cause of sciatic neuropathy is trauma because of the proximity of the sciatic nerve to the hip joint. Hip surgery and the insertion of prostheses can also cause sciatic nerve injuries. Sciatic neuropathy is the most common neurological complication from intramuscular gluteal injections, accounting for 96% of cases. Sciatic neuropathy usually develops immediately after the injection, mostly without pain, but a few patients develop neuropathy later, presumably due to scar formation. Compression of the proximal sciatic nerve occurs infrequently. In sciatic neuropathy, the lesion can be localized by the presence of denervation process in the sciatic nerve-innervated muscles, typically including the hamstrings, in the needle EMG study, and by a combined nerve conduction abnormality in the peroneal, posterior tibial, and sural nerves. In partial sciatic neuropathy, as in our patient, NCS in the posterior tibial and sural nerves can be normal. In this situation, the needle EMG in the short head of the biceps femoris muscle is the most crucial test, showing denervation process in patients with sciatic foot drop and normal findings in those with peroneal foot drop. A sciatic motor nerve conduction test is available, but we have rarely found it to be useful in cases of mild or partial sciatic neuropathy.

MAXIMS

1. The short head of the biceps femoris is the only muscle innervated by the lateral trunk, all other hamstring muscles being innervated by the medial trunk.
2. The needle EMG in the short head of the biceps femoris muscle is the most crucial test, revealing denervation process in cases of sciatic foot drop and normal findings in peroneal foot drop.

REFERENCES

1. Oh SJ. Clinical electromyography. Nerve conduction studies. Baltimore, MD: Williams and Wilkins, 1993:551–552.
2. Steward JD. Focal peripheral neuropathies. New York: Elsevier, 1987:270–289.

CASE 20

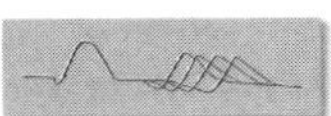

PERONEAL NEUROPATHY AND ABSENT REFLEX IN AN AVID JOGGER

CASE PRESENTATION

A 12-year-old avid jogger and high school long-distance champion noticed weakness and a tingling sensation over the lateral aspect of the left lower leg for 1 month. These symptoms were not progressive, and she could still jog without any difficulty. Abnormal neurological findings were MRC strength of 3 in the left anterior tibialis and 4 in the left peroneus muscle and absent left ankle jerk. No obvious sensory loss was observed. No Tinel's signs were noted in the peroneal nerve at the fibular head or in the posterior tibial nerve at the tarsal tunnel. Straight leg raise was negative. No mass was palpated along the sciatic nerve from the popliteal fossa to the sciatic notch.

CASE ANALYSIS

This patient's history and neurological findings were typical of crossed-leg palsy at the fibular head. Unlike classic crossed-leg palsy, this case did not occur acutely and we were not able to elicit any Tinel's sign at the fibular head. The absent ankle jerk clearly did not fit with peroneal nerve palsy, raising the possibility of a sciatic nerve lesion. L5 radiculopathy was also ruled out by the lack of any weakness in the foot inverter and negative straight leg raise.

PLAN OF TESTING

1. NCS: This should include the H-reflex, superficial peroneal, sural, and plantar nerves.
2. Needle EMG: This should include the anterior tibialis, peroneal, gastrocnemius, and short head of the biceps femoris muscles.

ELECTROPHYSIOLOGICAL TESTS AND FINDINGS

NCS Findings (Table 7.20; Fig. 7.19)

1. Slow sensory NCV in the left superficial peroneal nerve.
2. Borderline slowing in sensory NCV in the left medial plantar and sural nerves.

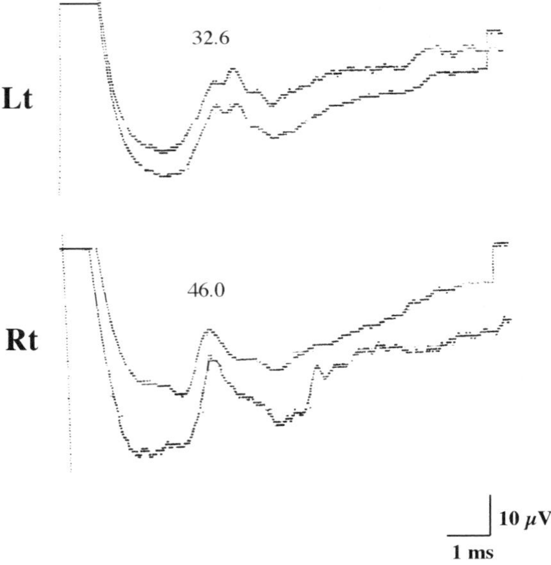

FIGURE 7.19. Slow (32.6 m/s) sensory NCV in the left superficial peroneal nerve compared with normal NCV (46.0 m/s) in the right.

TABLE 7.20. Nerve Conduction Data in Case 20

	Latent/NCV (ms/m/s)	Amplitude (mV/μV)		Latent/NCV (ms/m/s)	Amplitude (mV/μV)
Left	**Peroneal**	**Motor N**	**Right**	**Peroneal**	**Motor N**
TL	4.8	4.2		5.0	5.8
FH-A	41.4	4.0		48.3	5.8
PF-FH	50.0	3.8		50.0	5.0
F-wave	46.8			44.8	
	Posterior Tibial	**Motor N**		**Posterior Tibial**	**Motor N**
TL	4.2	15		3.0	20
PF-A	43.7	15		52.7	15
F-wave	42.0			42.8	
H-reflex	NP			27.2	
	Sural	**Sensory N**		**Sural**	**Sensory N**
MC-A	34.6	20		46.0	16
	Superficial Peron	**Sensory N**		**Superficial Peron**	**Sensory N**
MS-A	32.6	15		46.0	16
	Medial Plantar	**Sensory N**		**Medial Plantar**	**Sensory N**
Toe-A	30.4	3.8		39.4	6.8

Height: 157.5 cm.

3. Borderline CMAP amplitude but normal motor NCV in the left peroneal nerve.
4. Absent left H-reflex.

Needle EMG

1. Fibrillations and PSWs (+ +) and normal MUP (amp, 0.5 to 3.5 mV; 5 to 15 ms) with RIP (2 mV) in the left anterior tibialis muscle.
2. Normal needle EMG findings in the left gastrocnemius and short head of left biceps femoris muscles.

ELECTROPHYSIOLOGICAL INTERPRETATION

Left peroneal and posterior tibial neuropathy at the popliteal fossa.

FINAL DIAGNOSIS

Mild compression neuropathy of the left peroneal and posterior tibial nerves at the popliteal fossa probably caused by pressure against the side rail of a car seat

TREATMENT AND FOLLOW-UP

After discussing the difficulty of localizing the lesion to one nerve and the possible causes for her problem, we went over the details of the patient's daily activities just before the onset of her symptoms. Apparently, while reading a book, she had crossed her legs over the side rail of the back seat of a van for many hours during a family summer vacation. We believe that the compression occurred in the distal sciatic nerve at the popliteal fossa. Upon learning this, we followed the patient without any further workup. Gradually, her symptoms improved to normal in 6 months.

COMMENTS

Joggers are susceptible to two neuropathies: peroneal compression neuropathy and medial plantar neuropathy. In Leach et al.'s report, seven runners and one soccer player with peroneal compression neuropathies were identified. Running produced pain, numbness, and tingling on the lateral aspect of the lower leg, as in our case. Examination revealed muscle weakness and Tinel's sign. Nerve conduction studies were abnormal in five studied cases. Seven of eight had marked improvement after surgery. Three cases of reversible "jogger's foot" (medial plantar neuropathy) were also reported. Tenderness and Tinel's sign at the abductor tunnel behind the navicular tuberosity of the foot, where the medial plantar nerve is located, and sensory loss in the medial plantar nerve territory were found in these patients. All three improved with conservative treatment, which included local injection of lidocaine at the abductor tunnel, where the medial plantar nerve passes through. Running produces a pounding effect on the medial aspect of the foot, producing medial plantar neuropathy. In our case, we were not able to find "jogger's peroneal neuropathy" but instead found common peroneal and posterior tibial neuropathy at the popliteal fossa caused by prolonged compression of the distal sciatic nerve.

MAXIMS

1. Joggers are prone to develop peroneal neuropathy and medial plantar neuropathy.
2. The superficial peroneal nerve innervates sensory function over the lateral aspect of the lower leg.

REFERENCES

1. Dawson DM, Hallett M, Millender LH. Entrapment neuropathies, 2nd ed. Boston, MA: Little, Brown and Company, 1990:341–355.
3. Rask MR. Medial plantar neurapraxia (jogger's foot). Clin Orthop 1978;134:193–195.

CASE 21

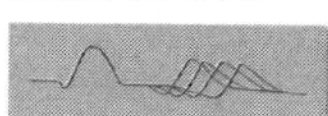

DEEP PERONEAL NEUROPATHY 4 WEEKS AFTER ARTHROSCOPIC SURGERY

CASE PRESENTATION

A 34-year-old man had three arthroscopic surgeries for a cartilage injury in the right knee joint. Four weeks after the surgery, he noted weakness in the right lower leg, which got worse over the next 2 months without any pain or numbness. Examination showed mild weakness in the right extensor hallucis longus and moderate atrophy of the right extensor digitorum brevis muscles. Normal strength was noted in the right anterior tibialis and peroneus longus muscles. No sensory impairment or Tinel's sign at the fibular head was observed. Right knee and ankle reflexes were normal.

CASE ANALYSIS

The constellation of findings indicated the possibility of a partial peroneal neuropathy. This patient was sent to the EMG laboratory to evaluate for a common peroneal neuropathy associated with the arthroscopic surgery. However, the history clearly suggested that his problem was not related to the surgery. Also, it appeared less likely that this was a peroneal compression neuropathy at the fibular head because of the slow progression over a period of 2 months.

PLAN OF TESTING

1. NCS: To confirm peroneal neuropathy and localize the site of the lesion.
2. Needle EMG: To document a partial lesion in the DPN. This should include the test in the anterior tibialis, extensor hallucis longus, extensor digitorum brevis, and peroneal longus muscles.

ELECTROPHYSIOLOGICAL TESTS AND FINDINGS

NCS Findings (Table 7.21; Fig. 7.20)

1. Low CMAP amplitude with conduction block and temporal dispersion in the ankle-fibular head segment of the right peroneal nerve.
2. Markedly slow motor NCV in the fibular head-ankle segment of the right peroneal nerve.
3. Normal sensory nerve conduction in the right superficial peroneal nerve.

TABLE 7.21. Nerve Conduction Data in Case 21

	Latent/NCV (ms/m/s)	Amplitude (mV/μV)	Shape		Latent/NCV (ms/m/s)	Amplitude (mV/μV)
Right	**Peroneal**	**Motor**	**Nerve**	**Left**	**Peroneal**	**Motor N**
TL	8.2	3.5			4.4	19
FH-A	23.2	0.5	D		46.7	17
PF-FH	?				50.0	16
F-wave	NP					
Right	**Posterior tibial**	**Motor**	**Nerve**	**Right**	**Peroneal**[a]	**Motor N**[a]
TL	4.0	25.6		TL	4.8	5
PF-A	46.9	19.0		PF-FH	50.0	5
F-wave	56.8					
H-reflex	31.6					
	Sural	**Sensory**	**Nerve**	**Right**	**Superficial peroneal**	**Sensory N**
MC-A	38.8	18.4		MS-A/P	36.6	20.8
				MS-A/O	50.0	20.8

Height: 183 cm. A/P, NCV with the negative peak latency; A/O, NCV with the onset latency.
[a] With the recording electrodes in anterior tibialis muscle.

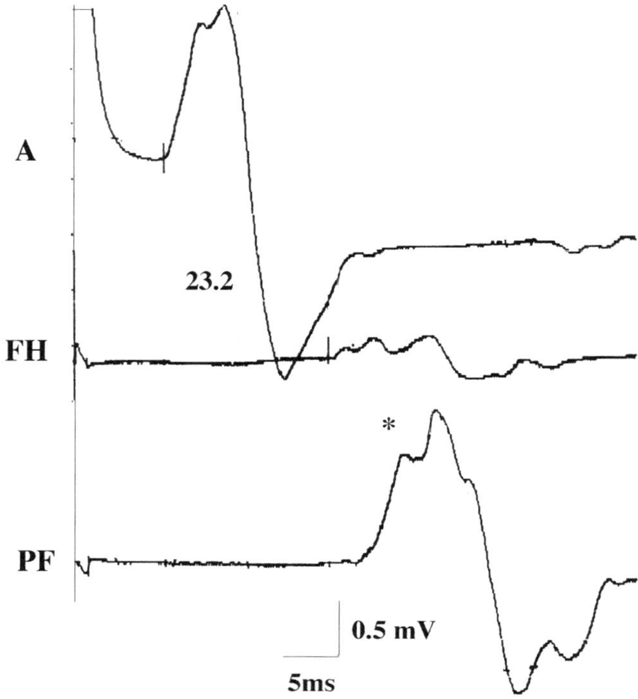

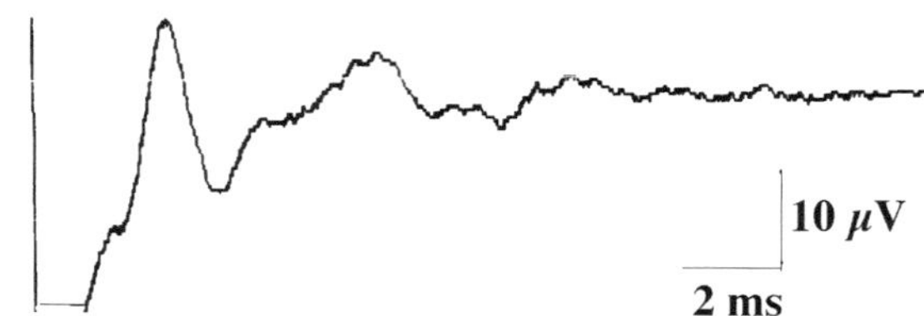

FIGURE 7.20. Nerve conduction in the right deep and superficial peroneal nerves. *A*, ankle; *FH*, fibular head; *PF*, popliteal fossa. Number between A and FH represents NCV.* Response through posterior tibial nerve.

Needle EMG

1. Fibrillations and PSWs in right extensor digitorum brevis muscle.
2. HA MUPs in right anterior tibialis and extensor digitorum brevis muscles.
3. Normal EMG findings in right peroneus longus muscle.

ELECTROPHYSIOLOGICAL INTERPRETATION

Right deep peroneal neuropathy between the fibular head and the ankle. There was no electrophysiological evidence of a right common peroneal neuropathy between the fibular head and popliteal fossa.

FINAL DIAGNOSIS

Right deep peroneal neuropathy

TREATMENT AND FOLLOW-UP

Because of the progressive nature of focal neuropathy below the fibular head, we decided to explore the DPN. There was a focal mass 5 cm distal to the fibular head that turned out to be a neurolemma.

COMMENTS

With the patient's history of arthroscopic surgery at the knee, common peroneal neuropathy between the fibular head and popliteal fossa was a definite possibility. However, electrophysiological studies did not show either such a lesion or a compression neuropathy across the fibular head. Instead, the study localized the lesion clearly to between the ankle and below the fibular head.

The common peroneal nerve is the continuation of the lateral trunk of the sciatic nerve, separating from the sciatic nerve in the upper popliteal fossa, descending downward and laterally through the popliteal fossa, and passing behind and around the fibular head. It divides into two major branches: the superficial and DPNs. Common peroneal neuropathy is clinically characterized by weakness of the anterior tibialis and peroneus muscles and sensory impairment in the territory of the superficial peroneal nerve (lower lateral aspect of the calf). Crossed-leg palsy is acute compression neuropathy caused by compression of the peroneal nerve across the fibular head after prolonged crossing of the legs, squatting, or incorrect positioning of the legs. Clinically, this palsy is characterized by acute onset of foot drop and weakness of eversion of the foot. Unlike in L5 radiculopathy, inversion of the foot (posterior tibial muscle) is unaffected in peroneal nerve palsy. This muscle is innervated by the posterior tibial nerve.

Crossed-leg palsy is commonly confirmed by the motor nerve conduction study in about 64% of cases. The most important point to remember in this process is to stimulate the peroneal nerve below and above the fibular head, thus assessing the segment of the fibular head, which is the most common site of compression. Selective slowing in NCV, conduction block, and abnormal temporal dispersion across the fibular head are the cardinal findings indicative of peroneal compression neuropathy at the fibular head. The test is severely limited by the frequent difficulty of obtaining the CMAP in the EDB muscle. An alternative method of nerve conduction is the recording of the CMAP in the anterior tibialis or peroneus longus muscle.

The DPN is the main branch of the common peroneal nerve that innervates the anterior tibialis, extensor hallucis and digitorum longus, and peroneus tertius muscles. Deep peroneal neuropathy is characterized by foot drop with sparing of the peroneus muscle and is a rare entity.

MAXIMS

1. The DPN innervates the anterior tibialis, extensor hallucis longus, and extensor digitorum brevis muscles.
2. The superficial peroneal nerve innervates the peroneus longus and brevis muscles.

REFERENCES

1. Oh SJ. Clinical electromyography. Nerve conduction studies. Baltimore, MD: Williams and Wilkins, 1993:227–228.
2. Sourkes M, Steward JD. Common peroneal neuropathy: a selective motor and sensory involvement. Neurology 1991;41:1029–1033.

CASE 22

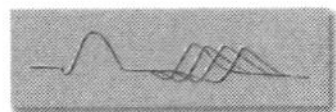

A HIGHER CMAP AMPLITUDE WITH PROXIMAL STIMULATION?

CASE PRESENTATION

A 33-year-old man was referred to the EMG Laboratory for evaluation of Charcot-Marie-Tooth disease because of bilateral pes cavus since childhood. Family history was unremarkable, and the remainder of his examination was normal. A nerve conduction study in the left peroneal nerve with stimulation at the fibular head showed CMAPs with a higher amplitude compared with those with stimulation at the ankle.

CASE ANALYSIS

In normal individuals, the CMAP amplitude with proximal stimulation of the nerve is the same as or smaller than that with distal stimulation. A higher CMAP amplitude with proximal than with distal stimulation is abnormal. Technical artifact has to be ruled out first, and then the possibility of an accessory DPN must be considered.

PLAN OF TESTING

NCS: To guarantee maximal stimulation, the peroneal nerve should be tested with maximal intensity and duration. Once this is done, the accessory DPN should be sought by adding stimulation at the lateral malleolus. If this nerve is found, then the accessory DPN should be located on the opposite side.

ELECTROPHYSIOLOGICAL TESTS AND FINDINGS

NCS Findings (Fig. 7.21)

1. Right peroneal nerve: prolonged terminal latency and low CMAP amplitude, abnormally higher amplitude with fibular-head stimulation than with ankle stimulation, and 2.9-mV CMAP response with stimulation of the accessory DPN behind the lateral malleolus.

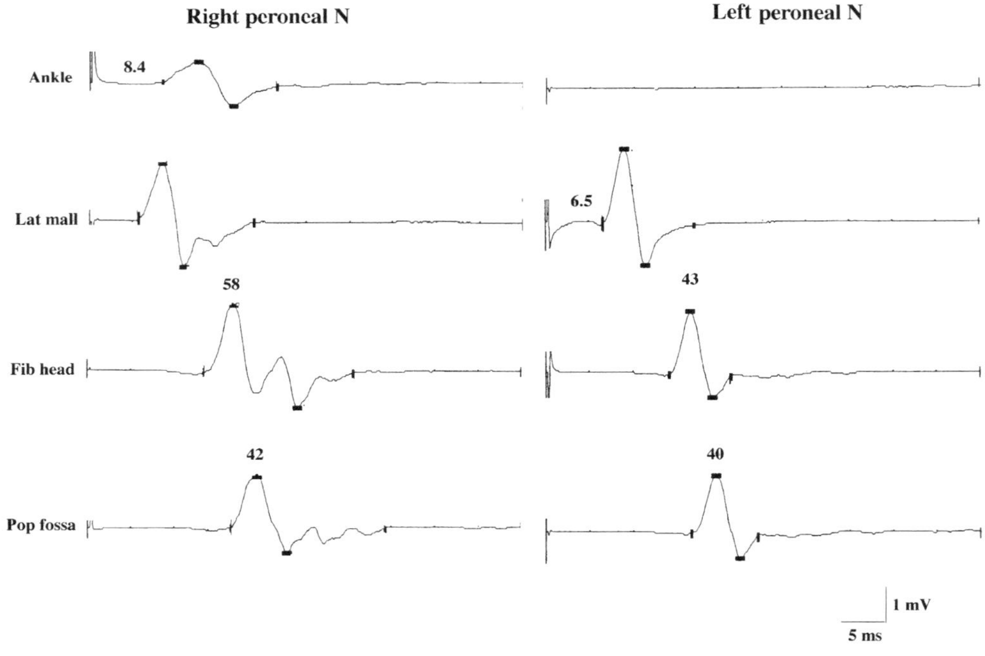

FIGURE 7.21. Partial accessory peroneal branch of the right peroneal nerve. Complete accessory peroneal branch of the left peroneal nerve. Numbers above the CMAPs represent either terminal latency in ms or NCVs in m/s. Notice in the left peroneal nerve there was no potential elicited with stimulation at the ankle.

2. Left peroneal nerve: no response with ankle stimulation and 2.4-mV CMAP response with stimulation of the accessory DPN behind the lateral malleolus.

ELECTROPHYSIOLOGICAL INTERPRETATION

Partial right accessory DPN and complete left accessory DPN.

FINAL DIAGNOSIS

Bilateral accessory DPN

TREATMENT AND FOLLOW-UP

Extensive NCS in this patient showed no other abnormality except for bilateral accessory DPN. This ruled out CMT disease type A (HMSN type 1: hypertrophic type).

COMMENTS

The accessory DPN is a common variant of the common peroneal nerve innervating the EDB. The EDB is usually innervated exclusively by the DPN, a main branch of the common peroneal nerve. However, in 19 to 22% of individuals, one or both of the EDBs are innervated partially by the accessory DPN, a branch of the superficial peroneal nerve, which passes deep and posterior to the peroneus brevis tendon and behind the lateral malleolus. This anatomical variation can be easily proved by stimulating the peroneal nerve at three locations: the DPN at the ankle, the common peroneal nerve at the fibular head, and the accessory DPN posterior at the lateral malleolus. The presence of this anomalous nerve is verified by the following typical findings: the amplitude of the EDB CMAP is 0.2 mV or greater upon stimulation of the accessory DPN behind the lateral malleolus, the EDB CMAP is abnormally smaller (less than 90%) after stimulation of the DPN on the dorsum of the ankle than it is after stimulation of the common peroneal nerve at the knee, and the amplitude of the EDB CMAP upon stimulation of the accessory DPN at the ankle is approximately equal to the difference between the CMAP of the DPN at the ankle and that of the common peroneal nerve at the knee.

An awareness of this variation in innervation of the EDB is important for the correct clinical and electromyographic evaluation of peroneal nerve lesions. The presence of the accessory DPN may cause confusion in the following clinical situations: a lesion in the accessory DPN might produce fibrillations and PSWs in the EDB muscle that can be misinterpreted as evidence of deep peroneal neuropathy, a complete lesion of the DPN can be misinterpreted as evidence of partial lesion in the DPN, and conduction block at the fibular head may be lost. Thus, the diagnosis of common peroneal nerve palsy can be missed.

MAXIMS

1. Accessory deep peroneal neuropathy should be suspected when the amplitude of the EDB CMAP is considerably smaller with distal stimulation of the DPN at the ankle compared with proximal stimulation of the common peroneal nerve at the knee.
2. Stimulation of the accessory DPN behind the lateral malleolus is an essential test for confirmation of accessory deep peroneal nerve.

REFERENCES

1. Oh SJ. Clinical electromyography. Nerve conduction studies. Baltimore, MD: Williams and Wilkins, 1993:327–330.
2. Gutmann L. Important anomalous innervations of the extremities. AAEM Minimonograph #2, 1979.

CASE 23

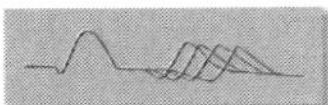

INTERMITTENT BURNING PAIN ON THE BOTTOM OF FOOT

CASE PRESENTATION

A 39-year-old woman was evaluated at the EMG Laboratory for intermittent burning pain and numbness on the bottom of her right foot, including the last two toes, for 6 months. These symptoms were relieved by rest and aggravated by a few hours' weight bearing on the left foot. She had a lumbar laminectomy for a right L5-S1 herniated disc 1 year before and still had recurrent episodes of aggravated lower back pain. The patient stated that the pain in her foot was different from that associated with lower back pain. On examination, she had mild tenderness in the right lumbar paraspinal area, negative straight leg sign, absent left ankle reflex, normal muscle strength, Tinel's sign in the posterior tibial nerve at the left ankle, minimal loss of pin-prick sensation in the medial and lateral aspects of the sole of her left foot, and marked loss of pin-prick sensation on the last two toes.

CASE ANALYSIS

The referring neurologist thought that this patient's problem was due to a lumbar radiculopathy associated with postlaminectomy subarachnoid adhesions. Except for the loss of ankle reflex, there was no definite objective finding suggestive of a right S1 radiculopathy. The key differential diagnosis from S1 radiculopathy is an objective sensory loss: S1 dermatome sensory loss is over the lateral aspect of the calf and foot and not on the medial aspect of the bottom of foot. In fact, this patient had the classic history and findings of TTS, but her past history of a lumbar laminectomy complicated the clinical analysis.

PLAN OF TESTING

1. NCS: Right peroneal, sural, and posterior tibial NCS to rule out a distal sensory neuropathy.
2. Near-nerve needle sensory nerve conduction of the plantar nerve to confirm TTS (1).
3. Needle EMG: To sort out the role of lumbosacral radiculopathy.

ELECTROPHYSIOLOGICAL TESTS AND FINDINGS

NCS Findings (Table 7.22; Fig. 7.22)

1. Normal motor NCS in the left peroneal and posterior tibial nerves and normal sensory NCS in the left sural nerve, including the terminal latency of the lateral plantar nerve.
2. Normal terminal latencies in the left abductor hallucis and abductor digiti quinti muscles.

TABLE 7.22. Nerve Conduction Data in Case 23

	Latent/NCV (ms/m/s)	Amplitude (mV/μV)	Shape
	Medial Plantar	**Motor**	**Nerve**
TL	4.7	10	
	Lateral Plantar	**Motor**	**Nerve**
TL	5.4	8	
	Interdigital	**Sensory**	**Nerve**
I	23.2	1.4	
I-II	22.4	0.6	D
II-III	22.0	0.8	D
III-IV	21.3	0.7	
IV-V	21.0	0.5	
V	NP		

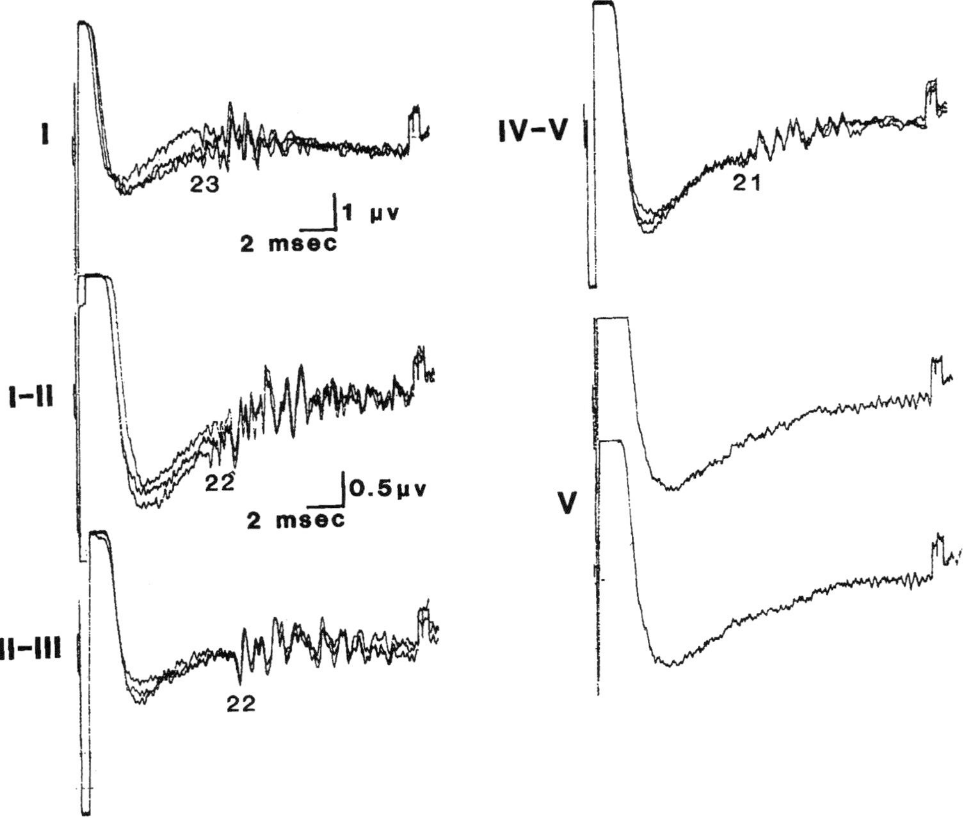

FIGURE 7.22. Sensory nerve conduction abnormalities in tarsal tunnel syndrome. The CNAPs are obtained with the near-nerve technique. Roman numerals indicate the stimulating digit; arabic numbers under each CNAP denote the maximum sensory NCV in m/s. No CNAP is obtained with digit stimulation.

3. Slow maximum NCVs and low CNAPs in I digital, I-II, II-III, III-IV, and IV-V interdigital nerves.
4. Prolonged duration of the CNAPs (dispersion phenomenon) in the I-II and II-III interdigital nerves.
5. Absent response in V digital nerve.

`Needle EMG`. Normal needle EMG in the left lumbosacral radiculopathy workup (see Chapter 9). In the left abductor hallucis muscle, a few 8-mV HA MUPs were present.

ELECTROPHYSIOLOGICAL INTERPRETATION

Left medial and lateral plantar neuropathy typical of TTS.

FINAL DIAGNOSIS

Left TTS

TREATMENT AND FOLLOW-UP

Decompression surgery of the left flexor retinaculum down to the abductor tunnel was performed. Focal compression of the medial plantar nerve by the thickened flexor retinaculum was found in the tarsal tunnel. The patient's symptoms were relieved.

COMMENTS

The routine NCS ruled out a diffuse sensory distal neuropathy in this case. Findings in the near-nerve needle sensory NCS in the plantar nerves were indicative of medial and lateral plantar neuropathy with marked slowing in NCV, which is typical of a focal entrapment neuropathy. The needle EMG study ruled out any role of lumbosacral radiculopathy for her neurological deficit. The few HA MUPs in the left abductor hallucis muscle were compatible with left TTS.

TTS is a compression neuropathy of the posterior tibial nerve and its branches within the fibro-osseous tunnel that lies beneath the flexor retinaculum on the medial side of the ankle. Typical symptoms of TTS include burning pain and paresthesia on the toes and along the sole of the foot. Classically, the symptoms are increased by activity, are diminished by rest, and often become worse at night. The most helpful diagnostic criteria are a positive Tinel's sign (radiating pain from the spot of tapping, not local tenderness) at the ankle and objective sensory loss in the territory of the plantar nerve. This does not include sensory loss over the dorsum of the foot, which is a key finding in distal sensory neuropathy. Weakness of flexion and atrophy of the medial intrinsic foot muscles are rare.

The NCS is the test of choice for confirming the diagnosis of TTS. The overall diagnostic sensitivity of the terminal latency is 47%. In contrast, the sensory NCS with the near-nerve needle technique improves the diagnostic sensitivity to 96%. We use the near-nerve needle technique because the sensory CNAP in the plantar nerve is not easily obtained, even in normal older individuals. The medial plantar nerve is more commonly involved in TTS. Slow NCV and dispersion phenomenon are the common nerve conduction abnormalities, suggesting a focal demyelination in this disorder.

Sensory NCS of the plantar nerve can be done with the surface recording electrode in younger patients. A technique for recording mixed nerve conduction in the medial and lateral plantar nerves is also available. The needle EMG in the abductor hallucis and abductor digiti quinti muscles may show denervation process, but it is painful and does not add any more information. In our case, we did the needle EMG to assess the role of lumbar radiculopathy in this patient's problem.

With this technique, one can confirm the diagnosis of medial and plantar neuropathy and interdigital neuropathy. The medial plantar nerve can be compressed in isolation along its pathway distal to the tarsal tunnel, thereby producing medial plantar neuropathy (MPN). The common site of compression in the medial plantar nerve is at the abductor tunnel (the fibromuscular tunnel behind the navicular tuberosity). Clinically, these patients have burning pain/tingling numbness over the medial two-thirds of the sole of the foot and Tinel's sign and tenderness over the medial plantar nerve at the entrance of the abductor tunnel. The sensory nerve conduction study of the plantar nerves can confirm the diagnosis of MPN, being selectively abnormal in the medial plantar nerve and normal in the lateral plantar nerve.

With lateral plantar neuropathy (LPN), sensory loss is confined to the lateral one-third of the sole of the foot. The sensory nerve conduction of the plantar nerve can confirm the diagnosis of LPN. Morton's neuroma refers to an interdigital neuropathy of the third and fourth digits. Typically, the patient complains of pain on the plantar aspect, precisely localized between the third and fourth metatarsal heads, often with radiation to the toes. Nearly all patients have tenderness on the interdigital nerve between the metatarsal heads. Sensory impairment is often detectable in the affected clefts and toes. With this technique, one can document a selective decrease in the amplitude of the CNAP in the involved interdigital nerve ("abnormal dip phenomenon"), a relative normal NCV, and normal duration of CNAP.

MAXIMS

1. Sensory deficits over the dorsum of the foot are incompatible with TTS and rule out that diagnosis.
2. Tinel's sign and sensory deficits over the plantar nerve territory are typical of TTS.

REFERENCES

1. Oh SJ. Clinical electromyography. Nerve conduction studies. Baltimore, MD: Williams and Wilkins, 1993:247–248.
2. Oh SJ, Kim HS, Ahmad B. The near-nerve sensory nerve conduction in TTS. J Neurol Neurosurg Psychiatry 1985:45:999–1003.

CASE 24

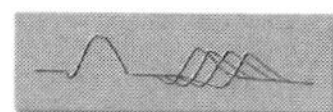

BURNING PAIN ON THE DORSUM OF THE FOOT RADIATING TOWARD THE SECOND AND THIRD TOES

CASE PRESENTATION

A 53-year-old woman complained of "burning pain" on the dorsum of the right foot radiating toward the second and third toes for 3 weeks. Loosening her shoe laces reduced the pain somewhat. She denied any back pain. Abnormal findings were tenderness and Tinel's sign at the midpoint of the ankle, hypoalgesia over the midportion of the dorsum of the right foot including the first four toes, and absent ankle reflexes. Straight leg raise was absent. Differential diagnoses by the referring physician includes lumbar radiculopathy, interdigital neuropathy, and superficial peroneal neuropathy.

CASE ANALYSIS

Interdigital neuropathy of the foot was easily ruled out by the patient's history because its classic complaint is pain on the plantar surface of foot. Although the L5 dermatome involves the dorsum of foot, it usually extends above the ankle. The absence of a straight leg raise, and low back pain suggested the less likely possibility of lumbar radiculopathy. The area of sensory impairment corresponded to the sensory territory of the medial branch of the superficial peroneal nerve. The presence of Tinel's sign and tenderness at the mid-portion of the ankle pinpointed the compression site.

PLAN OF TESTING

1. NCS: Special study should include the NCS in the peroneal superficial nerve below ankle (1).
2. Needle EMG: To rule out lumbosacral radiculopathy.

ELECTROPHYSIOLOGICAL TESTS AND FINDINGS

NCS Findings (Fig. 7.23)

1. Normal motor NCS in the right peroneal and posterior tibial nerves.
2. Normal sensory NCS in the right sural and superficial peroneal nerves.
3. Slow sensory NCV and low sensory CNAP amplitude of the medial dorsal cutaneous branch of the right superficial peroneal nerve in the low dorsum of foot-ankle segment.

Needle EMG. Increased insertion activity and fibrillation and PSW in the right peroneus longus and L5 and S1 paraspinal muscles.

ELECTROPHYSIOLOGICAL INTERPRETATION

Medial dorsal cutaneous neuropathy of the right superficial peroneal nerve below the ankle and asymptomatic right L5 and S1 radiculopathy.

FINAL DIAGNOSIS

Compression neuropathy of the medial dorsal cutaneous branch of the right superficial peroneal nerve at the ankle

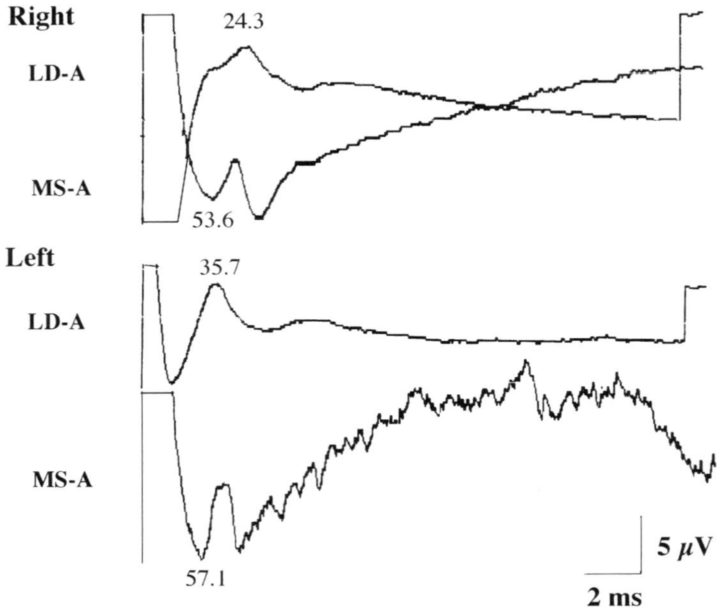

FIGURE 7.23. Sensory CNAPs in the medial dorsal cutaneous branch of the superficial peroneal nerve. *MS-A*, midshin to ankle (antidromic test); *LD-A*, low dorsum of foot to ankle (orthodromic test): 10 cm distance.

TREATMENT AND FOLLOW-UP

On her birthday, the patient's husband had given her fancy new shoes with tight shoelaces. We asked her to wear loose old shoes. Her symptoms disappeared in a month.

COMMENTS

Because there was no description of a technique or normal data for the medial dorsal cutaneous nerve conduction below the ankle, we placed the recording electrodes at the ankle following Izzo's method (1) and stimulated this nerve 10 cm distal to the recording electrodes on the dorsum of the foot. We compared the results of this test with those on the asymptomatic side.

The superficial peroneal nerve is a branch of the common peroneal nerve innervating the peroneus longus and brevis muscles and then becoming a pure sensory nerve with two terminal branches (the medial dorsal and intermediate dorsal nerves). Thus, it supplies sensory function to the lateral portion of the lower leg and almost all the dorsum of the foot except for the adjoining web of the first and second toes, which is supplied by the DPN. Superficial peroneal neuropathy can occur in rare peroneal compartment syndrome and is characterized by motor weakness of the peroneus muscle (eversion of the foot) and sensory impairment over the sensory territory. Pure superficial peroneal neuropathy can also occur due to compression at the site where it passes through the deep fascia and becomes a superficial sensory branch. Patients with this neuropathy complain of paresthesia, pain, and sensory impairment in its entire sensory territory. The sensory NCS of this nerve over the midshin to ankle segment can confirm this neuropathy. The terminal branches of this nerve can be compressed or injured at the ankle, as seen in this patient, usually as a result of local trauma or tight shoes such as roller skates or ski boots. This terminal lesion should be confirmed by testing this nerve over the dorsum of the foot, as in this case.

MAXIMS

1. The sensory branch of the DPN innervates the sensory fibers to the dorsal web space of the first and second toes.
2. The superficial peroneal nerve innervates two muscles: the peroneus longus and peroneus brevis muscles.

REFERENCES

1. Oh SJ. Clinical electromyography. Nerve conduction studies. Baltimore, MD: Williams and Wilkins, 1993:230–233.
2. Gersini L, Jandolo B, Piertrangeli A. The anterior tarsal tunnel syndrome. J Bone Joint Surg [Am] 1984:66:786.

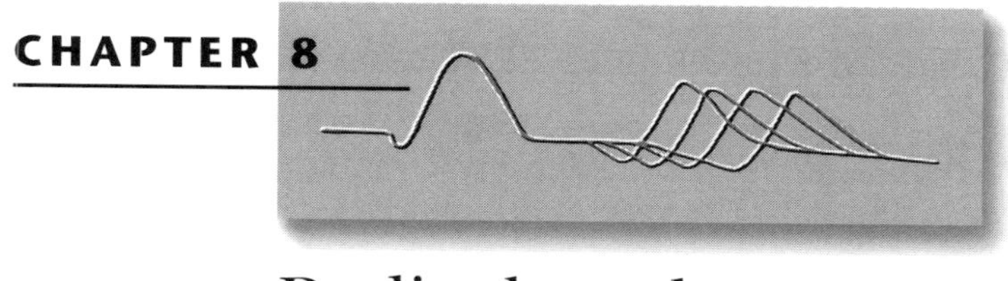

CHAPTER 8

Radiculopathy

CLINICAL FEATURES OF RADICULOPATHY

Radiculopathy is one of the most common causes of patient referrals to the electromyography (EMG) laboratory and can be divided into cervical, thoracic, and lumbosacral radiculopathies depending on the site of involvement. Cervical and lumbosacral radiculopathies are most frequently attributed to root compression, resulting from disc herniation or protrusion, and/or osseoligamentous hypertrophy associated with disc degeneration, whereas thoracic radiculopathy is most commonly due to diabetic radiculopathy. In general, lumbosacral radiculopathy is more often due to disc herniation or protrusion, and cervical radiculopathy is caused by osseoligamentous hypertrophy. Thus, acute radiculopathy is more common in lumbosacral radiculopathy than in cervical radiculopathy. In the cervical region, the C7, C8, C6, and C5 roots are compressed, and in lumbosacral lesions, the L5, S1, and L4 roots are compressed in the order of decreasing frequency. The clinical features of cervical and lumbosacral radiculopathies due to herniated discs are shown in Table 8.1.

Radicular pain has three characteristics that are helpful in distinguishing it from other pains: radiation from the involved spinal region along the involved individual sensory dermatome, aggravation of pain by any maneuver that increases the intraspinal pressure, and aggravation of pain by a maneuver that stretches the involved root. Classically, radicular pain is aggravated by coughing or straining that increases the intra-abdominal pressure and subsequently the intraspinal pressure. The straight-leg raising maneuver stretches the L5 and S1 roots and is thus positive in L5 and S1 radiculopathies, and the femoral stretch maneuver stretches the L4 root, being positive in L4 radiculopathy. Unfortunately, there is not a good maneuver that stretches the cervical roots.

Radiculopathy is suspected when a patient presents with the classic description of radicular pain and confirmed clinically by objective demonstration of sensory loss over the individual dermatomes and the presence of motor weakness confined to the muscles innervated by the involved roots (Table 8.1). Although these diagnostic features are generally held to be true, one has to remember that because of contiguous dermatome overlap and multiple root innervations in many muscles, the classic pattern may not be present in a given patient.

ROLE OF THE EMG STUDY IN THE ERA OF MRI

With the widespread availability of the MRI, the role of the EMG study has dramatically changed. In the days before the MRI, the needle EMG study was used as the screening test for the conventional or CT myelogram. Because it is painless, the MRI has become the first test of choice in the workup of radiculopathy. In fact, most patients with neck or lower back pain in the United States demand a cervical or lumbar MRI, usually before having an EMG study. On many occasions, a definite diagnosis of cervical or lumbar radiculopathy can be confirmed by unequivocal abnormalities in the MRI, and surgical decompression of roots or cord is performed on the basis of the clinical and MRI findings without requiring a needle EMG study. This is rightly so in some cases. Unfortunately, unnecessary surgery has been performed in many patients on the basis of a "minor" abnormality on the MRI (e.g., disc bulge or facet narrowing), which is usually due to "over-reading" without regard for the clinical findings. The chief reason for this is the frequency of abnormalities on the MRI of

TABLE 8.1. Clinical Findings in Cervical and Lumbosacral Radiculopathy

Root	Involved Disc Space	Pain Distribution	Sensory Deficit	Main Motor Weakness	Reflex Others
Cervical radiculopathy					
C5[a]	C4–5	Neck pain radiating down to anterior arm (above elbow)	C5 dermatome over anterior upper arm	Rhomboids infra- and supraspinatus, deltoids	Biceps
C6	C5–6	Neck pain radiating along arm and dorsum of forearm to thumb	C6 dermatome over radial forearm and thumb	Biceps, and brachioradialis	Biceps
C7	C6–7	Neck pain radiating along lateral arm and dorsum of forearm to middle finger	C7 dermatome over midportion of forearm and middle finger	Triceps, and pronator teres	Triceps
C8	C7–8	Neck pain radiating along ulnar side of arm and forearm to ring and little finger	C8 dermatome over ulnar portion of forearm and little finger	Intrinsic hand muscles Extensor indicis proprius	Triceps
Lumbosacral radiculopathy					
L4[b]	L3–4	Low back pain (LBP) radiating over the anterior-medial thigh and lower leg (above ankle)	L4 dermatome	Quadriceps Iliopsoas	Knee reflex Femoral stretch test: positive
L5	L4–5	LBP radiating along the posterior thigh to the big toe	L5 dermatome involving medial aspect of foot and big toe	Peroneus Posterior tibial Extensor hallucis longus	Straight leg raising test: positive
S1	L5–S1	LBP radiating along the posterior thigh to the little toe	S1 dermatome involving lateral aspect of foot and little toe	Gastrocnemius	Ankle reflex Straight leg raising test: positive

[a] Corresponding root is placed above the vertebral body except C8 root that is coming out below C7. There is an extra C8 root.

[b] Corresponding root is exited below the vertebral body.

the lumbar area in asymptomatic individuals. Recent studies have shown that substantial abnormalities were observed in 33 to 52% of asymptomatic adult individuals, indicating oversensitivity of the MRI test. Another problem is that the MRI cannot confirm radiculopathy in all cases of radiculopathy, especially in diabetic, inflammatory, or paraneoplastic radiculopathies. Because of these limitations of the MRI, there is a definite role for the needle EMG in the workup of radiculopathy. The EMG study has a distinct advantage over the MRI in that it identifies physiological abnormalities in contrast to the structural abnormalities observed on the MRI. Thus, these two tests can be complimentary and certainly are not mutually exclusive. Thus, the judicious use of the needle EMG is warranted even in the era of the MRI.

The needle EMG is indicated clearly under the following conditions:

1. When a radiculopathy is clinically suspected but the MRI is unrevealing. This includes metabolic or inflammatory radiculopathies. The best example of a metabolic radiculopathy is diabetic radiculopathy, and radiculopathies due to herpes zoster are good examples of inflammatory radiculopathy. In these cases, the needle EMG is definitely indicated because it is the only means of confirming the diagnosis.
2. When there is a discrepancy between the MRI and clinical findings and an additional test is needed to confirm the clinical impression of radiculopathy. As discussed above, the

MRI is sometimes too sensitive. Because of this, there is a definite potential for unnecessary surgical treatment because of mistaken diagnosis. Clearly, the EMG study is indicated in such cases.

3. When radiculopathy cannot be differentiated clinically from plexopathy or mononeuropathy, the needle EMG and nerve conduction test is indicated because it can identify plexopathies, mononeuropathies, and polyneuropathies.

When neuroimaging is not available, as in many developing countries, the EMG is indicated as the first objective test for radiculopathy.

ELECTROPHYSIOLOGICAL FINDINGS IN RADICULOPATHY

Needle EMG

The needle EMG study is the most important test in the workup of radiculopathy, because it is the only diagnostic tool capable of assessing the physiological status or integrity of nerve roots with a reasonably high sensitivity, being positive in 85% of clinically diagnosed radiculopathy patients. The needle EMG in radiculopathy should include both paraspinal and limb muscles. Among the various EMG abnormalities, fibrillations and positive sharp waves (PSWs) are the most reliable EMG parameters for diagnosis of radiculopathy. Another reliable EMG parameter is evidence of chronic denervation, or HALD MUPs. Increased polyphasic MUPs or fasciculation alone should not be taken as EMG evidence of radiculopathy. In this regard, the rules for time factors for fibrillations and PSWs become important: fibrillations and PSWs may be absent in the first 2 weeks after the injury, these abnormal spontaneous potentials develop earlier in the muscles proximal to the lesion, and PSWs develop earlier than fibrillations by 1 week. Thus, it is important to do a needle EMG study in the third or fourth week after onset of an acute herniated disc, when the EMG features of acute denervation are expected to be full-blown.

Nerve Conduction Study

Sensory nerve conduction should be unequivocally normal in radiculopathy because the dorsal root ganglia are located distal to the roots and are not affected by the radiculopathy. If the dorsal root ganglia are involved, then the peripheral nerves are definitely affected by the disease process, indicating peripheral neuropathy. This is used as the cardinal rule for differentiating plexopathy from radiculopathy. Thus, when the sensory nerve conduction is abnormal in patients with radiculopathy, both processes of radiculopathy and neuropathy coexist in the same individual and the more appropriate term, radiculoneuropathy, is applicable. On the other hand, the motor nerve conduction study may show a motor neuronopathy pattern in severe cases of radiculopathy. This is because a proximal root lesion can induce Wallerian degeneration in the distal motor axon, producing a low CMAP amplitude and minimal slowing in the motor NCV. In practice, this occurs rarely in radiculopathy and is seen in only about 29% of cases of lumbar radiculopathy. An important point to remember is that this finding does not have any diagnostic value with regard to radiculopathy.

Late Responses

Because the F-wave travels through the proximal segment of the motor nerve including the root, theoretically it is expected to be abnormal in radiculopathy. However, because of the input of many roots in producing peripheral nerves, the F-wave is rarely abnormal, being abnormal in about 13% of cases of lumbar radiculopathy. Earlier studies reported higher values that subsequent studies were not able to confirm. The F-wave is either absent or mildly prolonged in latency in severe cases of radiculopathy. Again, the F-wave has no diagnostic value with regard to radiculopathy. The H-reflex represents a monosynaptic reflex, involving sensory and motor fibers. Thus, the H-reflex should show a higher sensitivity of abnormality than the F-wave. Among the various H-reflexes that test other roots, the only H-reflex that is reliable and simple in practice is the H-reflex from the gastrocnemius-soleus muscle, which tests the S1 root. Side-to-side latency difference greater than 1.5 ms or latencies that exceed those predicted by height have been used to diagnose S1 radiculopathy. H-reflex was abnormal in 32% of cases of lumbar radiculopathy. For reasons similar to that described above, the H-reflex alone cannot be used as a diagnostic tool for S1 radiculopathy.

PARASPINAL MUSCLE NEEDLE EMG

The EMG of the paraspinal muscles is a "must test" in evaluation of radiculopathy. The paraspinal muscles are innervated by the posterior primary rami in contrast to all the limb muscles that are innervated by the anterior primary rami. Thus, fibrillations and PSWs found in paraspinal muscles indicate that the responsible lesion is located proximally along the motor nerve fibers and, in combination with a normal sensory nerve conduction, are absolute evidence of a lesion lying proximal to the dorsal root ganglia, namely in the nerve root or anterior horn cells. Another advantage of paraspinal muscle testing is that fibrillations and PSWs develop 1 week earlier in the paraspinal than in distal muscles, and thus that abnormal EMG findings may be found in isolation in paraspinal muscles alone. According to our study, fibrillations and PSWs were observed in paraspinal muscles in 82% of patients with clinically diagnosed lumbosacral radiculopathy and only in paraspinal muscles in 20% of these cases.

The nerve supply of the superficial layer of paraspinal muscles has considerable segmental overlap and therefore cannot be used as a means of identifying a specific spinal root level. On the other hand, in the lumbar area, segmental representation of the deep paraspinal muscles, especially the multifidus spinae, is specific enough to be used as a marker for identifying a specific root level. Thus, it is important to insert the EMG needle into the multifidus as accurately as possible. To do this, the needle has to be inserted more than 2.5 cm deep and medially (from 2 to 3 cm from the midline) close to the spinous process following the anatomical guideline (Figs. 8.1 and 8.2).

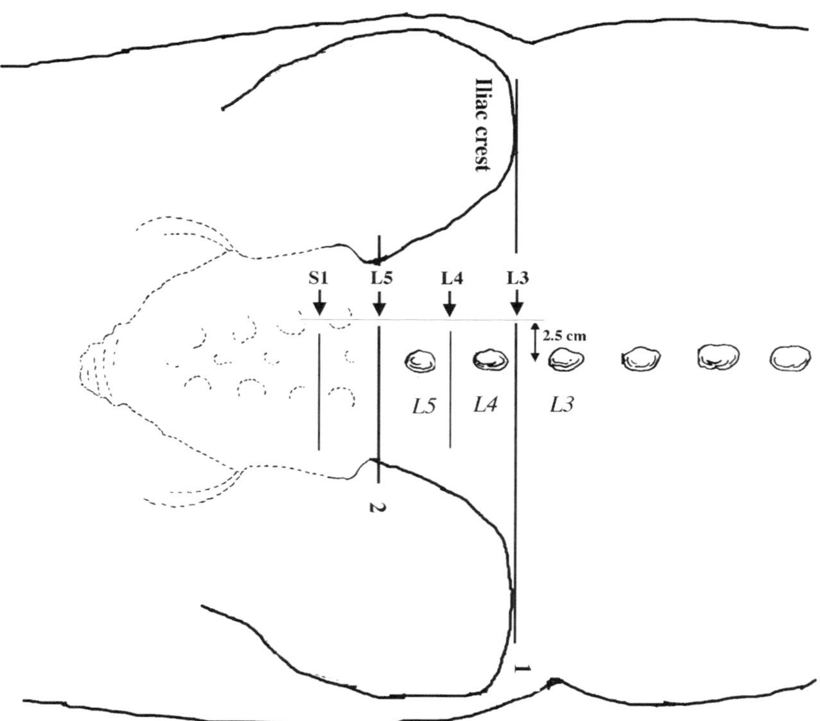

FIGURE 8.1. Location of EMG needle insertion in the lumbar paraspinal muscles. **1.** Line connecting the iliac crests, crossing the L3-4 intervertebral space. **2.** The last palpable intervertebral space, representing the L5-S1 intervertebral space. *L3, 4,* and *5*, Corresponding spinous processes. **L3**, **4**, **5** and **S1** indicate the location of EMG needle insertion in the corresponding segments.

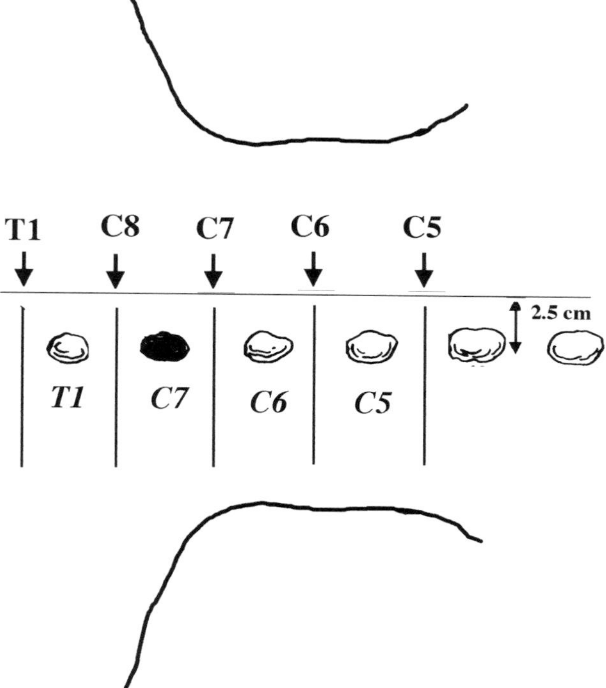

FIGURE 8.2. Location of EMG needle insertion in the cervical paraspinal muscles. C7 spinous process is the best lowest palpable spinous process. *C5, 6, 7, T1* indicate the corresponding spinous processes. **C5, 6, 7, 8, T1** indicate the location of EMG needle insertion in the corresponding segments.

Because fibrillations and PSWs are important in detection of radiculopathy, it is important to relax the paraspinal muscles fully and look for these potentials. By nature, human paraspinal muscles are not made to be relaxed and thus it is not easy to achieve relaxation. For this purpose, Johnson recommended placing the patient in a prone position with pillows under the abdomen and ankles for the lumbar paraspinal EMG study. In our laboratory, we have the patient lie on one side with the side to be examined upward and with the lower leg extended and the upper leg flexed for the unilateral lumbar needle EMG. For the bilateral needle EMG, the prone position is used with the hip on the examined side somewhat raised. We do not recommend looking for other evidence of denervation of MUPs in paraspinal muscles. For the thoracic paraspinal needle EMG, we have the patient lie down with the side to be examined downward and both legs fully flexed to the abdomen. This method works wonders for the thoracic paraspinal muscles. For the cervical paraspinal EMG, we prefer to have the patient lie on one side, with the side to be tested uppermost, and gently bend the head forward against the examiner's fist placed under the patient's chin. Because the relaxation of paraspinal muscles is the most important part of the needle EMG study in radiculopathy, we do not usually examine MUPs in these muscles.

To interpret abnormal spontaneous potentials, one has to consider several issues. The presence of CRDs alone in paraspinal muscles is not abnormal. The paraspinal muscles are one of three muscles in the body in which CRDs are normally observed, the other two being the iliopsoas and sphincter muscles. Thus, CRDs are clinically significant only when observed together with fibrillations or PSWS. Another issue is that these abnormal potentials were seen in a substantial number of asymptomatic individuals over 40 years of age in a recent study. In asymptomatic individuals under 30 years of age, fibrillations and PSWs are rarely seen in paraspinal muscles and thus are clinically significant as an indication of radiculopathy. However, in individuals over 40 years of age, fibrillations and PSWs in paraspinal muscles must always be correlated with the clinical findings because they have been detected in approximately 32% of clinically asymptomatic individuals. A third issue is localization of the involved roots. Considering the anatomical and technical factors in performance of the needle EMG, a one-level difference in fibrillations and PSWs in the paraspinal muscles is within the technical limit, and thus we interpret this as a normal variation.

"ROOT SEARCH" IN THE LIMB MUSCLES

There are very few limb muscles that are innervated by a single root, one exception being the rhomboid muscle, which is innervated by C5. All other muscles are innervated by several neighboring roots. Because of this, the EMG localization of root abnormalities depends primarily on the detection of abnormalities in a group of muscles that share innervation from a single root, or myotome. The most important principle of the "root search" in the limb muscles is examination of two or three muscles with the same root but with different peripheral nerve innervation. By this strategy, one can avoid the pitfall of difficulty in distinguishing radiculopathy from peripheral neuropathy. The best example is performing an L5 root search by examining the posterior tibial (L5; posterior tibial nerve) and peroneus longus (L5; peroneal nerve) muscles in a patient with foot drop. If the foot drop is due to L5 radiculopathy, EMG abnormalities will be observed in the posterior tibial and the peroneus longus muscles. On the other hand, if the foot drop is caused by peroneal neuropathy, needle EMG examination of the posterior tibial muscle should be normal. This rule is also applicable in the clinical setting: the posterior tibial muscle is the foot inverter and the peroneus longus muscle, the foot everter.

Unfortunately, no single standardized clinical and EMG myotome chart exists. To cause further confusion, each textbook has a chart showing different groupings of muscles in a myotome. In our laboratory, Haymaker's myotome is used as the standard reference and we follow the guidelines in Table 8.2 in doing a root search in the limb muscles. These guidelines have proved to be practical and valuable in localizing root detection according to our experience. There is no set rule for the root search, which depends heavily on the clinical history and findings. If clinical findings are strongly indicative of radiculopathy, the needle EMG may have to be performed in more than two muscles in a myotome. On the other hand, if radiculopathy is not suspected clinically but a workup is requested, then a basic workup for radiculopathy is sufficient. For cervical radiculopathy, a basic workup consists of examination of the C5-8 paraspinal, deltoid, biceps, triceps, and FDI muscles. We prefer the FDI muscle

TABLE 8.2. Choice of Muscles for the Radiculopathy Workups

Root	First Choice	Second Choice	Third Choice
Cervical roots			
C5	Rhomboids (C5) (dorsal scapular)	Supraspinatus (C5 and 6) (suprascapular)	Deltoids (C5 and 6) (axillary)
C6	Biceps (C5 and 6) (musculocutaneous)	Brachioradialis (C5 and 6) (radial)	Pronator teres (C6 and 7) (median)
C7	Triceps (C6 and 7) (radial)	Pronator teres (C6 and 7) (median)	Flexor carpi ulnaris (C7 and 8) (ulnar)
C8	FDI (C8 and T1) (ulnar)	Extensor indicis proprius (C8) (radial)	APB (C8 and T1) (median)
Lumbosacral roots			
L4	Vastus lateralis (L3 and 4) (femoral)	Adductor brevis (L3 and 4) (obturator)	Anterior tibialis (L4 and 5) (peroneal)
L5	Peroneus longus (L5 and S1) (peroneal)	Gluteus medius (L5 and S1) (superior gluteal)	Posterior tibial (L5 and S1) (posterior tibial)
S1	Gastrocnemius med (S1 and 2) (posterior tibial)	Gluteus maximus (L5 and S1) (inferior gluteal)	Soleus (S1 and 2)[a] (posterior tibial)

[a] Third peripheral nerve is not available.

to the C8 muscle because of the better tolerance of EMG needle by the patient. For lumbar radiculopathy, the basic study includes the L3-5 and S1 paraspinal, gluteus medialis and maximus, vastus lateralis, anterior tibialis, peroneus longus, and medial gastrocnemius muscles. If this basic work is normal, then no further testing is performed. On the other hand, depending on the finding of abnormalities in the tested muscles, we choose a second or third muscle in the same myotome.

POSTLAMINECTOMY EMG EXAMINATION

In the practice of EMG, it is not unusual to have a request for an EMG study on patients with previous laminectomy. There are several special problems associated with the postlaminectomy EMG examination, especially in the interpretation of findings. These patients fall into two major groups: those in whom the laminectomy was a failure and those in whom symptoms have recurred after a symptom-free period. For the first group, clinicians are interested in knowing whether persistence of symptoms is due to persistence of previous disc disease or to epidural or subarachnoid adhesion of roots. The EMG study is often requested a few months after the laminectomy. For the second group of patients, clinicians want to know whether the recurrence of symptoms is due to recurrence of previous disc disease, new disc disease, or epidural or subarachnoid adhesion. The EMG study is usually requested a few years after the laminectomy.

There are a few general rules to follow in the postlaminectomy EMG. The first is that a preoperative EMG is crucial in interpretation of the findings. This is the only way that the issues involved in the first group of patients can be resolved. Unfortunately, however, a first EMG was often not done or is not available. A second problem is that the benefit of the paraspinal muscle EMG is severely compromised in postlaminectomy patients. The presence of fibrillations and PSWs in the paraspinal muscles can be an expression of denervation due to terminal axonal injury during the surgical procedure. As a rule, fibrillations or PSWs due to muscle trauma involve many roots and are superficially located. Thus, a more extensive EMG study is required in the limb muscles. Several authors have recommended a modified technique in assessing paraspinal muscles in postlaminectomy patients, but there is no effective way to avoid this dilemma.

For the first group, especially if potential medicolegal issues are involved, it is imperative to do the needle EMG within the first 10 days after surgery. If the needle EMG detects fibrillations or PSWs in the first 10 days, they cannot be explained as the result of intraoperative trauma to the root. The lesion thus antedates the surgery because it takes 7 to 10 days for fibrillations or PSWs to develop after injury to the nerve. The needle EMG study soon after the surgery cannot answer whether the root compression was adequately relieved by the surgery. This is because it takes a few weeks or months before one observes a change in the needle EMG abnormality. Among the various EMG parameters, an improvement of fibrillations or PSWs is the best index of improvement.

For the second group of postlaminectomy patients, the general rule is that radiculopathy at other levels can be identifiable, but whether this radiculopathy is caused by new disc disease or by epidural or subarachnoid adhesions is not answerable. In the same root, in general, the longer the time interval, the more likely it is that any abnormalities seen have been caused by a "new" lesion. Thus, there are substantial limitations in the needle EMG study in postlaminectomy patients. For this reason, the MRI has a definite advantage in addressing these issues in postlaminectomy patients.

CASE 1

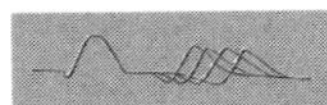

INTERMITTENT PARESTHESIA OF THE LEFT ARM WITH TILTING OF THE HEAD FOR 3 YEARS

CASE PRESENTATION

A 50-year-old man had intermittent paresthesia in the left arm for 3 years. This intermittent paresthesia radiated downward from the neck to the middle two fingers of the left hand along the dorsum of the forearm. In the previous 1 year, the patient also noticed some weakness in the left arm. Abnormal neurological findings were 4+ MRC strength in the left triceps muscle, absent left triceps reflexes, and reproducible paresthesia as described above on extreme tilting of the head to the left.

CASE ANALYSIS

This patient had classic sensory symptom suggestive of a C7 radiculopathy: paresthesia radiating downward to the middle finger (C6 dermatome). Neurological examination clearly documented C7 radiculopathy: triceps weakness and absent triceps reflexes.

PLAN OF TESTING

1. NCS: To rule out any concomitant CTS.
2. Needle EMG: Needle EMG workup for the cervical radiculopathy
3. Other tests: MRI of the cervical spine

ELECTROPHYSIOLOGICAL TESTS AND FINDINGS

`NCS Findings.` Normal motor and sensory nerve conductions in the left median and ulnar nerves.

`Needle EMG` (Table 8.3; Fig. 8.3)

1. Increased insertion activity, rare PSWs, and increased polyphasic MUPs in the left biceps muscle.
2. Increased insertion activity and PSWs, increased polyphasic MUPs, and a few HA MUPs in the left triceps muscle.
3. Increased insertion activity, prominent PSW, and rare HA MUPs in the left FCU muscle.
4. Prominent fibrillations, PSWs, and CRD in the left C7 paraspinal muscle.

ELECTROPHYSIOLOGICAL INTERPRETATION

Left C7 radiculopathy.

OTHER TEST FINDINGS

MRI of the cervical spine showed a herniated disc at the C6-7 intervertebral space with obliteration of the neuroforamina and central disc bulging at C3-4 and minimal flattening of the cervical cord.

FINAL DIAGNOSIS

Left C7 radiculopathy due to herniated disc at C6-7 intervertebral space

TREATMENT AND FOLLOW-UP

The patient had surgical removal of the herniated disc with complete disappearance of paresthesia and minimal improvement in strength in the left triceps muscle.

COMMENTS

In the needle EMG workup of radiculopathy, one has to remember two cardinal principles: the needle test in the paraspinal muscles and needle test in at least two muscles that are innervated by the same root but by a different peripheral nerve must be performed. The paraspinal muscle needle EMG is important because, if abnormal, it pinpoints the lesion to a site proximal to the paraspinal muscle: the root or anterior horn cells. Thus, the paraspinal needle test is critical for differentiation between radiculopathy and plexopathy. In plexopathy,

TABLE 8.3. Needle EMG Data in Case 1

				Spontaneous Potentials				Motor Unit Potential				Interference	
Muscle	**Root**	**Nerve**	**Insertion Activity**	**Fib**	**PSW**	**Fasc**	**Myotonia CRD**	**Amplitude (K)**	**Duration (ms)**	**Polyphasic Potential**	**HA MUP**	**Pattern**	**Mean Amplitude (K)**
Lt C5, 6 paraspinal	C5,6		N	–	–	–	–						
C7 paraspinal	C7		+	–	+ +	–	–						
C8 paraspinal	C8, T1		–	–	–	–	–						
Deltoid	C5	Axillary	–	–	–	–	–	0.5–3	6–15	–	–	FIP	1.8
Biceps	C5,6	Musc cut	+	–	±	–	–	0.5–3	6–12	+	–	FIP	2
Brachioradialis	C6	Radial	–	–	–	–	–	0.5–3	6–15	–	–	FIP	1.5
Triceps	C7,8	Radial	+	–	+	–	–	0.5–6	8–15	+	+	RIP	6
Pron teres	C6,7	Median	+	+ +	+	–	–	0.5–5.5	6–12	N	+	FIP	3
FDI	C8, T1	Ulnaris	–	–	–	–	–	0.5–3	6–14	N	–	FIP	3

Fib, fibrillations; PSW, positive sharp wave; Fasc, fasciculations; CRD, complex repetitive discharge; HA, high amplitude; N, normal; –, absent; +, present or increased; FIP, full interference pattern; RIP, reduced interference pattern.

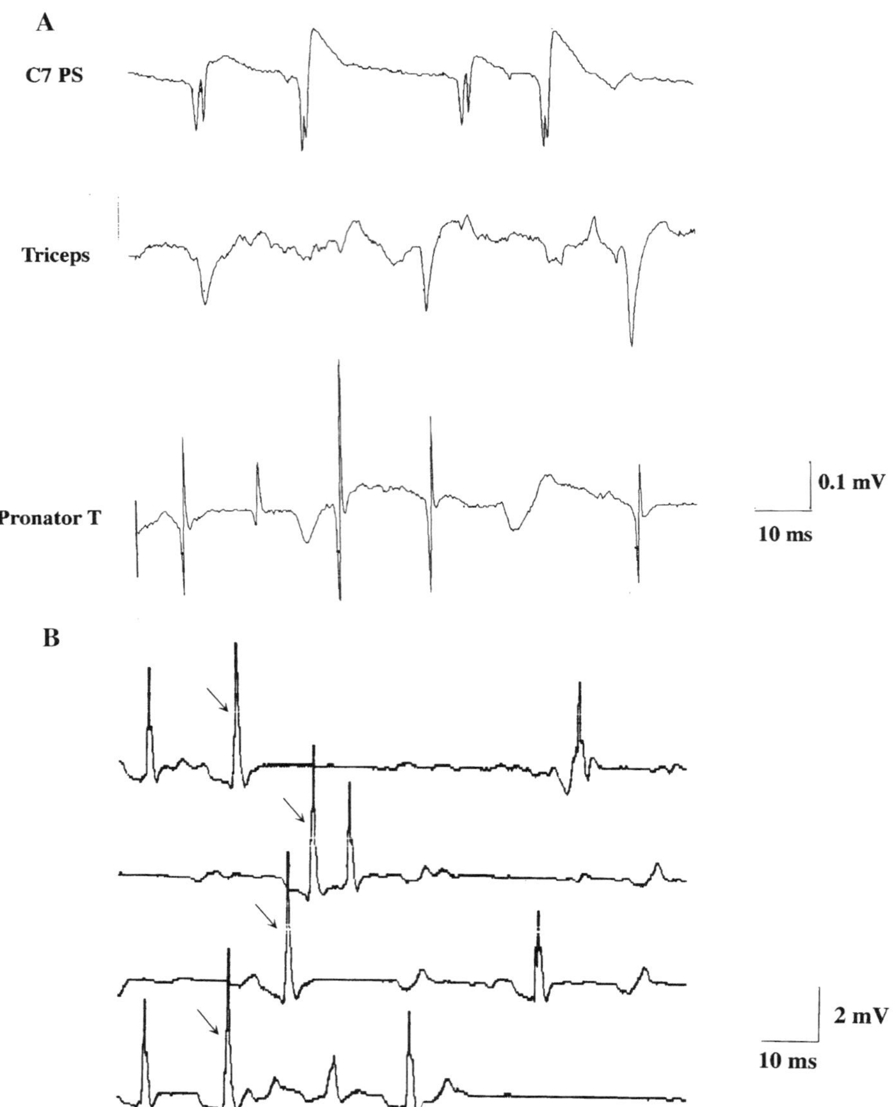

FIGURE 8.3. **A.** Fibrillations and PSWs in the C7 paraspinal (*PS*), triceps, and pronator teres (*T*) muscles. **B.** HA MUPs in the triceps muscle.

the needle EMG in the paraspinal muscles should be normal. Paraspinal muscles are involved in 82% of patients with clinically proven radiculopathy and 95% of patients with EMG abnormalities. In the limb muscles, if two muscles that are innervated by the same root but by different peripheral nerves show denervation process, then one can assume that the radiculopathy is more responsible than a peripheral nerve lesion. In about 4% of cases, the limb muscles alone are involved.

C7 radiculopathy is the most common cervical radiculopathy, accounting for 70% of cases. The frequency of other cervical radiculopathies is as follows: C6, 20%; C8, 8%; and C5, 2%. Because of extensive overlapping of root innervation of the muscles in the upper extremities, it is often difficult to identify a single root by the clinical evaluation alone. There are a few clinical caveats that are helpful in identifying the involved level. First, when the rhomboid muscle is weak, it is always related to C5 radiculopathy. Unfortunately, the demonstration of rhomboid weakness is not easy clinically. Second, when C5-6 radiculopathy is suspected clinically, the diagnosis of C6 radiculopathy is safe by statistics, because C5 radiculopathy is extremely rare. Third, subjective description of radiation of sensory symptoms to specific fingers and objective sensory loss in specific fingers (C6 to thumb, C7 to middle finger, and C8 to little finger) are reliable indicators of root involvement. Fourth, the biceps muscle and biceps reflexes are always involved in C6 radiculopathy. Fifth, the triceps muscle and triceps reflexes are always involved in C7 radiculopathy. Finally, the intrinsic hand muscles are always involved in C8 radiculopathy. In the EMG workup for cervical radiculopathy, there are several helpful guidelines to follow. First, a single radiculopathy can mimic brachial plexopathy, for example, C6 radiculopathy mimicking an upper trunk brachial plexopathy and C8 radiculopathy mimicking a lower trunk plexopathy. In this regard, two procedures are helpful: the needle EMG study in paraspinal muscles, where the presence of fibrillations and PSWs indicates radiculopathy, and evaluation of appropriate sensory nerve conduction studies, where low-amplitude or absent response indicates a plexopathy. Lateral antebrachial cutaneous (musculocutaneous) and superficial radial sensory NCS for C6 radiculopathy and medial and ulnar NCS for C8 radiculopathy. Second, C6 or C7 radiculopathy can mimic CTS. This can easily be ruled out by the routine nerve conduction study. Routine NCS should be done in all suspected cases of cervical radiculopathy. In fact, CTS is more commonly diagnosed in patients suspected of having cervical radiculopathy. Finally, when multiple level radiculopathy is diagnosed, the needle EMG study should be performed in the contralateral limb because cervical stenosis (cervical spondylotic myelopathy) is the most likely diagnosis and also in the lower extremity muscle to rule out motor neuron disease.

MAXIMS

1. The paraspinal needle EMG study is critical in the workup of radiculopathy.
2. For the workup of radiculopathy, the needle EMG should be done in two limb muscles innervated by the same root but by the different peripheral nerve.

REFERENCES

1. Wilbourn AJ, Aminoff MJ. AAEE Minimonograph #32. The electrophysiological examination in patients with radiculopathies. Muscle Nerve 1988;11:1099–1114.

CASE 2

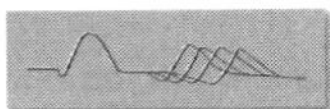

INCREASING "MUSCLE CRAMPS" AND WEAKNESS IN THE LOWER EXTREMITIES FOR 3 MONTHS

CASE PRESENTATION

A 42-year-old man had a 3-month history of worsening "muscle cramps" and weakness in the lower extremities. He was able to walk only with a cane in the previous few days and also noticed involuntary jerking movements in the lower extremities. He denied any weakness of the arms, sensory deficits, or bladder or bowel dysfunction. Abnormal neurological findings were MRC strength of 4 with fasciculation and mild atrophy in the right deltoid, biceps, and triceps muscles; 3 in the proximal and 4 in the distal muscles of both legs with spasticity; brisk reflexes all over with clonus in ankle and knee reflexes; Babinski signs; and scissors gait. No fasciculations were noted in any leg muscles. No obvious sensory abnormality was found except for loss of vibratory sense on the ankles and toes, and no cranial nerve abnormality, including jaw jerk, was observed.

CASE ANALYSIS

Neurological examination clearly showed a combination of lower and upper motor neuron signs without any definite sensory deficits. Vibratory abnormalities could have been attributable to the aging process. The possibility of amyotrophic lateral sclerosis was raised. In view of the poor prognostic implications, all treatable diseases must first be ruled out, the first being cervical spondylotic myelopathy. The needle EMG study was critical in this regard.

PLAN OF TESTING

1. NCS: To rule out any entrapment neuropathy in the right arm.
2. Needle EMG: To document cervical radiculopathy and to rule out widespread denervation process.
3. Other tests: Median somatosensory evoked potentials. CT metrazimide myelogram.

ELECTROPHYSIOLOGICAL TESTS AND FINDINGS

NCS Findings. Normal NCS in the right median and ulnar nerves.

Needle EMG (Table 8.4; Fig. 8.4)

1. Occasional fasciculations in the right deltoid, biceps, and FDI and left deltoid and FDI muscles.
2. HA MUPs and reduced recruitment in all tested muscles.

Median SEPs (Fig. 8.5)

1. Prolonged interpeak EP (Erb's point potential)–N13 (cervical potential) latencies (6.3 ms for the left and 6.5 ms for the right versus normal, 4.3 ms).

ELECTROPHYSIOLOGICAL INTERPRETATION

Chronic denervation process in the right and left C6-8 innervated muscles compatible with bilateral cervical polyradiculopathy.

OTHER TEST FINDINGS

Cervical CT metrizamide myelogram showed an incomplete block at the C7-T1 level in addition to bar defects at C6-7, and narrowing of the cervical canal secondary to degenerative disc degeneration and enlarged ligamentum flavum at the C5-6 levels.

FINAL DIAGNOSIS

CSM

TREATMENT AND FOLLOW-UP

The patient refused surgery and was conservatively treated with a cervical collar and intensive physical therapy at a rehabilitation facility with minimal improvement.

TABLE 8.4. Needle EMG Data in Case 2

Muscle	Root	Nerve	Insertion Activity	Spontaneous Potentials				Motor Unit Potential				Interference	
				Fib	PSW	Fasc	Myotonia CRD	Amplitude (K)	Duration (ms)	Polyphasic Potential	HA MUP	Pattern	Mean Amplitude (K)
Rt C6-8 paraspinal	C6-8		N	–	–	–	–						
Deltoids	C5,6	Axillary	+	–	–	+	–	2–11	10–15	N	++	RIP	3
Biceps	C6	Musc cut	+	–	–	+	–	2–8	10–15	N	++	FIP	3
Triceps	C7	Radial	+	–	–	–	–	1–9	8–16	N	++	RIP	3
FDI	C8, T1	Ulnar	+	–	–	++	–	2–5	9–16	N	+	RIP	3
Lt deltoids	C5,6	Axillary	+	–	–	+	–	1–6	7–15	N	+	RIP	
Triceps	C7	Radial	+	–	–	–	–	1–8	8–16	N	+	RIP	4
FDI	C8, T1	Ulnar	+	–	–	+	–	1–7	7–15	N	+	DA	4

Normal needle EMG findings in the left vastus lateralis, anterior tibialis, and gastrocnemius muscles.
DA, discrete activity.

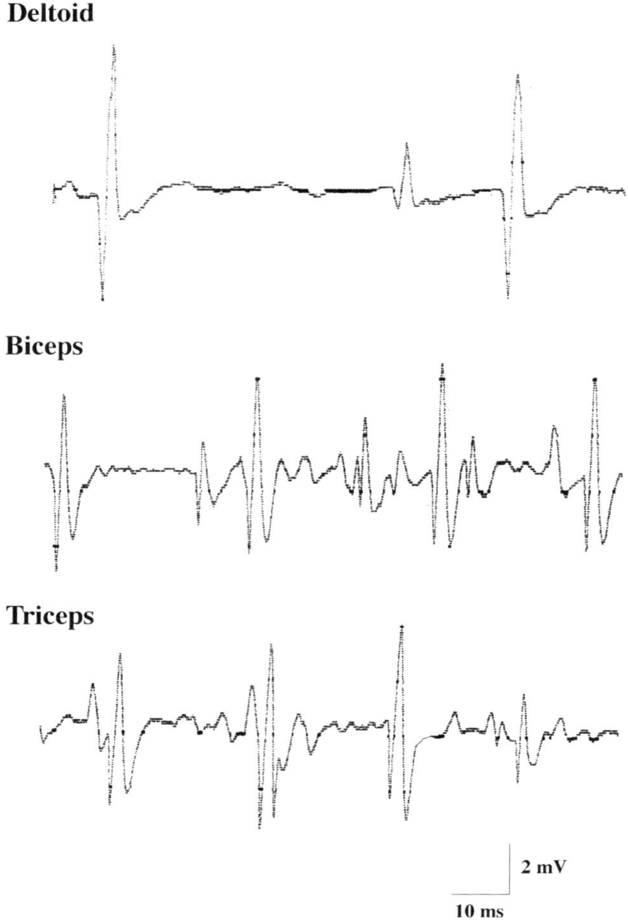

FIGURE 8.4. HA MUPs in the right deltoid, biceps, and triceps muscles.

COMMENTS

Cervical spondylosis is caused by extensive degeneration of the intervertebral discs in the cervical area and produces two neurological syndromes: cervical spondylotic radiculopathy caused by nerve root compression in the neural foramina and CSM resulting from cord compression by thickened ligaments, degenerated disc materials, and osteophytes. Cervical spondylotic radiculopathy affects more than one cervical root, thus producing bilateral and more diffuse symptoms than those associated with a single unilateral herniated disc. The C6 and C7 roots are the most commonly affected, producing various combinations of motor, sensory, and reflex impairments depending on the roots involved. A definitive diagnosis of CSM is made either by MRI of the cervical cord or CT myelogram. The advantage of the CT myelogram is assessment of the degree of cord compression between extension and flexion of the neck.

In cervical spondylotic radiculopathy, the most typical needle EMG findings are chronic polyradiculopathy involving multiple levels and often both sides. Thus, whenever multisegmental abnormalities are found in the upper extremities, EMG testing in the contralateral limb is mandatory because similar changes may be seen in that limb, frequently in multiple root distribution. A more important role for the EMG study in cervical spondylotic radiculopa-

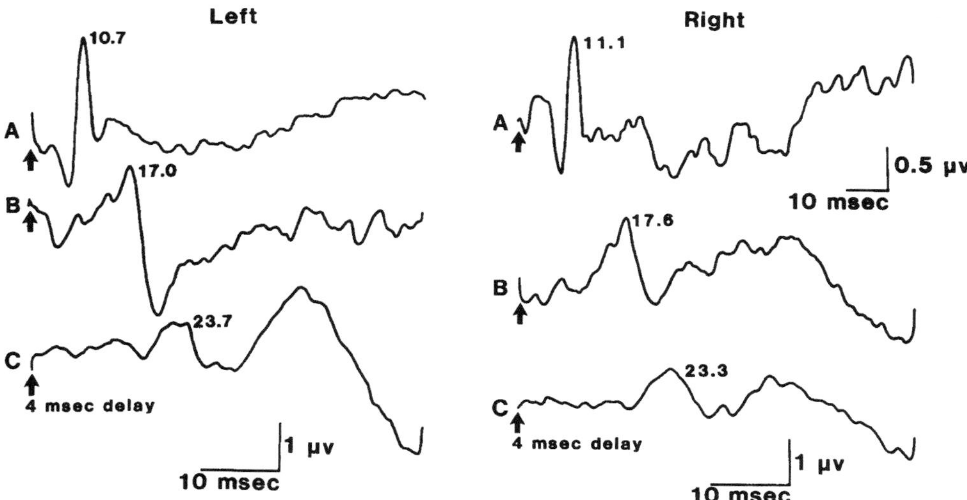

FIGURE 8.5. The median nerve evoked SEP abnormalities in cervical spondylotic myelopathy. **A.** EP (N9). **B.** Cervical SEP (N13). **C.** Cortical SEP (N20). Left indicates the left median nerve evoked SEPs and right, the right median nerve evoked SEPs. Latencies to EP are normal. EP-N13 interpeak latencies are prolonged bilaterally (normal, 4.3 ms), whereas N13-N20 interpeak latencies are normal (normal, 7.1 ms). Number at the peak of potentials refers to latency in ms.

thy is to rule out a common entrapment neuropathy and brachial plexus neuropathy in the upper extremities. In cervical spondylotic myelopathy, patients usually have the cervical radiculopathy features with cord compression signs in the legs. Depending on which tract and level of the cord are involved, various spinal cord syndromes may be observed, ranging from central cord syndrome to Brown-Séquard syndrome. CSM can often mimic amyotrophic lateral sclerosis, presenting as a pure motor syndrome with combined lower and upper motor neuron signs. This group of patients are referred to the EMG laboratory first for evaluation of ALS. Certainly, this is a subset of patients where the EMG study can make a crucial difference. Because ALS involves the lower cranial motor and lumbosacral motor neurons, the needle EMG study in the cranial muscles (tongue and masseter muscles in that order) and in several muscles of the legs should be performed. In CSM, there should be no active denervation process in either cranial or leg muscles. If active denervation is found (the tongue muscle is most commonly checked), the diagnosis of ALS is favored. We have observed three patients with "tandem" cervical and lumbar stenosis mimicking ALS who violated this rule. In these cases, we were not able to distinguish ALS from tandem cervical and lumbar stenoses by EMG testing.

The SEP test is also helpful in differentiation between CSM and ALS. In CSM, cervical SEPs are abnormal in most patients, with a prolonged EP-N13 interwave latency and low amplitude of N13; the posterior tibial SEP is also markedly abnormal in most patients. In ALS, the SEP is normal. We found these tests extremely helpful in differentiating between CSM and ALS.

MAXIMS

1. The presence of fibrillations, PSWs, and fasciculations in the tongue and lower extremity muscle rules out CSM.
2. The SEP study is abnormal in CSM and normal in ALS.

REFERENCES

1. McCormack BM, Weinstein PR. Cervical spondylosis, an update. WJM 1996;165:43–51.
2. Yu YL, Jones SJ. Somatosensory evoked potentials in cervical spondylosis. Correlation of median, ulnar and posterior tibial nerve responses with clinical and radiological findings. Brain 1985;108: 273–300.

CASE 3

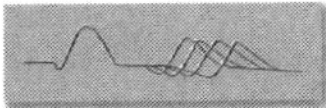

"FLAIL ARM" AFTER A MOTORCYCLE ACCIDENT

CASE PRESENTATION

A 16-year-old boy was involved in a serious motorcycle accident 7 weeks previously. After recovery from a head injury accompanied by loss of consciousness for 2 hours, the patient was noted to have paralysis of the right arm, which was initially thought to be due to cerebral contusion. However, CT of the head did not show cerebral hematoma or contusion. Apparently, there were extensive muscle contusions in various parts of the body, but the patient did not notice any improvement whatsoever in his right arm deficits. Abnormal neurological findings were a flaccid total paralysis of the right arm including the hand, absent right biceps and triceps reflexes, total loss of sensation below the elbow, and decreased sensation in the triceps area. Sensation was normal in the deltoid area. No obvious Horner's syndrome was noted, and neurological findings were normal in the other extremities.

CASE ANALYSIS

Although initially the right arm paralysis was thought to be due to cerebral contusion, there were no neurological findings suggestive of an upper motor neuron lesion. All the motor findings were indicative of a lower motor neuron lesion involving the C5-T1 innervated muscles. On the other hand, sensory examination showed severe sensory loss over the C6-8 and T1 area and partial loss over the C5 dermatome. Because Horner's syndrome, which is indicative of T1 radiculopathy, was absent, there were no clearcut neurological abnormalities indicative of radiculopathy. Clinically, "flail arm" with marked sensory loss in this setup is strongly suggestive of cervical avulsion. However, electrophysiological tests are critical in differentiating between cervical avulsion and a brachial plexus lesion.

PLAN OF TESTING

1. NCS: To see whether the brachial plexus was injured.
2. Needle EMG: To see the extent of cervical radiculopathy.
3. Other tests: SEP study. Cervical myelogram.

ELECTROPHYSIOLOGICAL TESTS AND FINDINGS

NCS Findings

1. Absence of any CMAP in the right median and ulnar nerves.
2. Normal sensory NCS in the right median and ulnar nerves.

Needle EMG (Table 8.5; Fig. 8.6)

1. Prominent fibrillations and PSWs, and no MUP generated with maximal attempt in any tested muscles.
2. Prominent fibrillations and PSWs in the right C5–8 and T1 paraspinal muscles.

SEP Findings on the Right Median Nerve SEP (Fig. 8.7)

1. Normal Eerb's point potential for his height and no reproducible cervical or cortical potentials.

ELECTROPHYSIOLOGICAL INTERPRETATION

Right C5–8 and T1 radiculopathy typical of cervical avulsion.

OTHER TEST FINDINGS

Cervical myelogram confirmed cervical avulsion in the C6, 7, and 8 roots.

FINAL DIAGNOSIS

Traumatic cervical avulsion involving the right C6, 7, and 8 roots

TABLE 8.5. Needle EMG Data in Case 3

				Spontaneous Potentials				Motor Unit Potential				Interference	
Muscle	**Root**	**Nerve**	**Insertion Activity**	**Fib**	**PSW**	**Fasc**	**Myotonia CRD**	**Amplitude (K)**	**Duration (ms)**	**Polyphasic Potential**	**HA MUP**	**Pattern**	**Mean Amplitude (K)**
Rt C5-8, T1			+	+ + +	+ + +	–	–						
Infraspinatus	C5	Suprascapular	+	+ + +	+ + +	–	–	No	MUP	on	maximal	attempt	
Supraspinatus	C5	Suprascapular	+	+ + +	+ + +	–	–	No	MUP				
Deltoid	C5,6	Axillary	+	+ + +	+ + +	–	–	No	MUP				
Biceps	C5,6	Musc cut	+	+ + +	+ + +	–	–	No	MUP				
Triceps	C7	Radial	+	+ + +	+ + +	–	–	No	MUP				
Extensor digitorum communis	C7	Radial	+	+ + +	+ + +	–	–	No	MUP				
Flexor carpi radialis	C7	Median	+	+ + +	+ + +	–	–	No	MUP				
Flexor carpi ulnaris	C8, T1	Ulnar	+	+ + +	+ + +	–	–	No	MUP				
Pron teres	C6,7	Median	+	+ + +	+ + +	–	–	No	MUP				

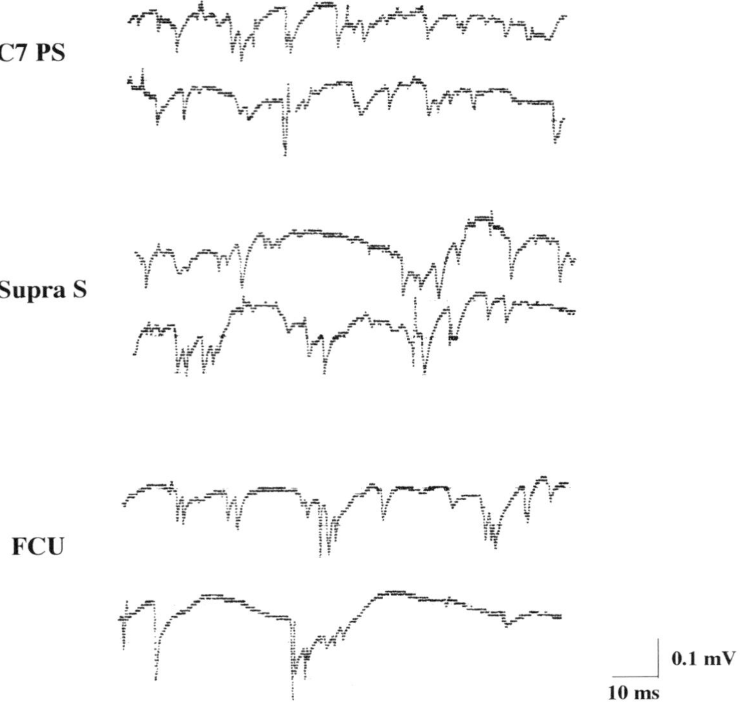

FIGURE 8.6. Prominent PSWs and a few fibrillations in the C7, supraspinatus (*Supra S*), and flexor carpi ulnaris (*FCU*) muscles.

TREATMENT AND FOLLOW-UP

Because a needle EMG performed 3 months later did not show any improvement, the cervical roots were explored. Complete avulsion was found in the C6, 7, and 8 roots with partial avulsion in the C5 and T1 roots. Intraoperative SEP with stimulation at the C5 stump recorded a small but definite cortical response. Thus, the upper trunk plexus was attached to the C5 stump. Three years later, the supraspinatus muscle showed a minimal but definite recovery of function.

COMMENTS

Because of the poor prognosis of cervical avulsion, differentiation between cervical avulsion and brachial plexopathy is critical in the management of patients. In this sense, the NCS, needle EMG, and SEP tests are extremely helpful.

The most dramatic dissociation between the EMG and clinical findings is observed in root avulsion: totally normal sensory NCS in the presence of total anesthesia in involved dermatomes. This occurs because the dorsal root ganglia are intact while the roots are avulsed, producing objective sensory loss. If the sensory nerve conduction is abnormal in root avulsion, this has to be interpreted as evidence of an additional brachial plexus lesion. The motor nerve conduction shows a pattern typical of axonal neuropathy: low CMAP amplitude or mild slowing in NCV or absent responses. The critical needle EMG findings are fibrillations and PSWs in the paraspinal muscles. All other involved muscles show severe denervation. Thus, our patient had all the typical findings of cervical avulsion.

The SEP test is essential in the diagnosis of a root avulsion. Characteristic findings are normal sensory CNAPs at Erb's point in the presence of clinical sensory impairment and

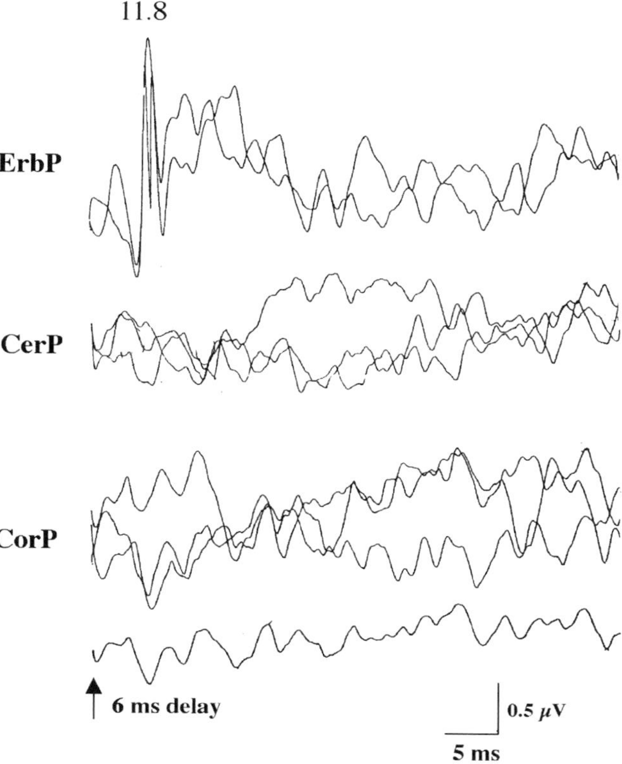

FIGURE 8.7. The median nerve evoked SEP abnormalities typical of cervical root avulsion. Normal Erb's point SEP (*ErbP*) with 11.8-ms latency and no reproducible cervical SEP (*CerP*) or cortical SEP (*CorP*).

markedly abnormal cervical and cortical SEPs. Early in the 1970s, two articles reported normal sensory CNAPs and an absence of cortical SEPs in the presence of total anesthesia in the involved dermatomes in patients with root avulsion. A later study in 1979 reported normal sensory CNAPs and abnormal cervical SEPs. Subsequent studies in patients with brachial plexus injuries have confirmed that the preservation of antidromic sensory CNAP with absent cervical and cortical SEPs is a reliable indicator of a root lesion proximal to the dorsal root ganglia. As expected, if the Erb's point potential latency is delayed, then it is indicative of an additional brachial plexus lesion.

MAXIMS

1. The sensory NCS is completely normal in patients with root avulsion in the presence of total anesthesia in the involved dermatome.
2. A normal SEP at the Erb's point in the presence of clinical sensory impairment and markedly abnormal cervical and cortical SEP is pathognomonic of cervical root avulsion.

REFERENCES

1. Jones SJ. Investigation of brachial plexus traction lesions by peripheral and spinal somatosensory evoked potentials. J Neurol Neurosurg Psychiatry 1979;49:107–116.
2. Trojaborg W. Clinical, electrophysiological, and myelographic studies of 9 patients with cervical spinal root avulsions: discrepancies between EMG and X-ray findings. Muscle Nerve 1994;17:913–922.

CASE 4

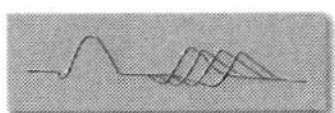

SUDDEN ONSET OF LOW BACK PAIN RADIATING DOWN TO THE FEET

CASE PRESENTATION

A 38-year-old man was in his usual state of good health until 1 month before examination when he developed a sudden onset of low back pain while lifting furniture at home. Soon thereafter, he began experiencing episodic shooting pains into the left buttock region. These pains gradually worsened to the point of persistent pain down the back of the left leg, associated with persistent numbness over the lateral aspect of the left foot. The pain was aggravated by coughing or sitting and failed to respond to a trial of treatment with Medrol dose pack. A poor-quality MRI of the lumbar spine did not show any herniated or bulging disc. Abnormal neurological findings included an absent left ankle reflex and a positive straight leg raise test at 30 on the left.

CASE ANALYSIS

This patient had a rather typical history of acute lumbar herniated disc with radicular pain. The constellation of history and findings, including radiating pain into the left buttock and leg, numbness along the lateral aspect of the left foot, and an absent left ankle jerk, suggested the possibility of a left S1 radiculopathy. However, no obvious motor or sensory deficit indicative of an S1 radiculopathy was found.

PLAN OF TESTING

1. Motor (peroneal, posterior tibial) and sensory (sural) nerve conduction studies.
2. F-wave studies of tested motor nerves.
3. H-reflex on gastrocnemius-soleus muscle in both legs.
4. Needle EMG of lumbar paraspinal, gluteus, vastus lateralis, anterior tibialis, peroneus longus, and gastrocnemius muscles.

ELECTROPHYSIOLOGICAL TESTS AND FINDINGS

NCS Finding (Fig. 8.8)

1. Prolonged F-wave latencies in left peroneal (55.7 ms) and posterior tibial (60.0 ms) nerves.
2. Prolonged H-reflex (36.5 ms) from the left gastrocnemius-soleus muscle in contrast to normal H-reflex (32.9 ms) from the right gastrocnemius-soleus muscle.
3. Mildly prolonged terminal latency (4.9 ms) in the left peroneal nerve.
4. Normal NCS findings in the left posterior tibial and sural nerves.

Needle EMG (Table 8.6; Fig. 8.9)

1. Increased insertion activity and fibrillations and PSWs in the left L5 and S1 paraspinal muscles.
2. Increased insertion activity with fibrillations and PSWs in the left gluteus maximus muscle.
3. Increased insertion activity with PSWs in left medial gastrocnemius.
4. Normal EMG findings in the remainder of tested muscles in the left anterior tibialis and vastus lateralis muscles.

ELECTROPHYSIOLOGICAL INTERPRETATION

Left S1 radiculopathy.

OTHER TEST FINDINGS

For better quality, a repeat MRI of the lumbar spine was requested but denied by the patient's insurance company. Surgery showed a laterally situated herniated disc compressing the root on the left at the L5-S1 intervertebral space without distortion of any dural sac.

FINAL DIAGNOSIS

Left S1 radiculopathy

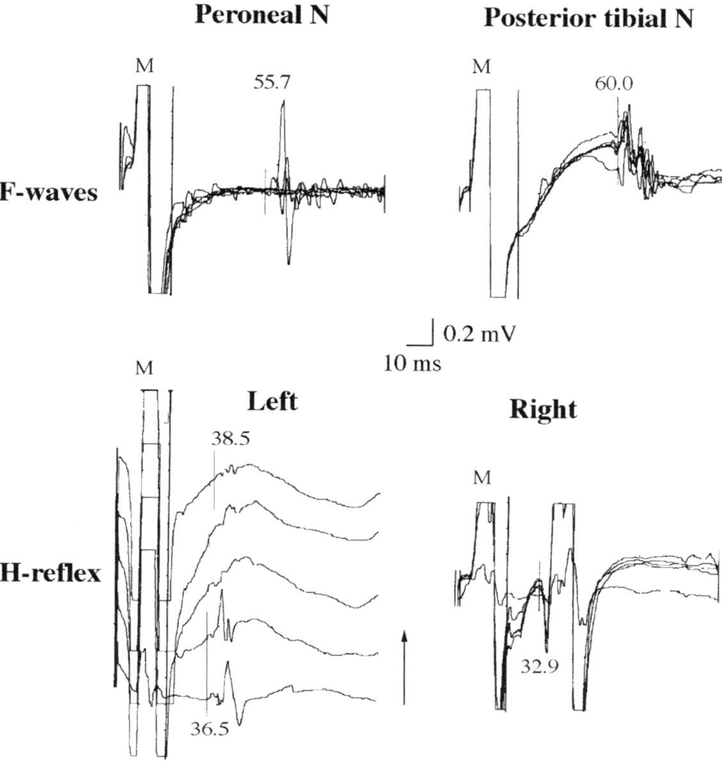

FIGURE 8.8. Prolonged F-wave and H-reflex latencies in the left posterior tibial nerve in the split screen. Numbers above the potentials represent F-wave latencies. Numbers below the potentials represent H-reflex latencies. *M* represents the CMAPs. *Arrow* indicates an increasing stimulus intensity.

TREATMENT AND FOLLOW-UP

Conservative treatment did not relieve the pain, and the patient underwent a lumbar laminectomy with complete relief of pain.

COMMENTS

This case clearly shows the value of the electrodiagnostic workup in lumbar radiculopathy, even in the "MRI era." The EMG study showed a rather classic pattern of S1 radiculopathy: fibrillations and PSWs in paraspinal and S1 innervated muscles (medial gastrocnemius and gluteal maximus), and prolonged F-wave and H-reflex latencies. Fibrillation and PSWs in the L5 paraspinal muscle are acceptable because there is a one-level error limit in the paraspinal EMG for localization of the root level. What is important is to document fibrillations and PSWs in the paraspinal muscles that definitely indicate a radiculopathy. Prolonged F-wave latency in the posterior tibial nerve and H-reflex latency, although rarely observed, are indicative of S1 radiculopathy. A simple and practical way of judging H-reflex abnormality is to compare the values on the affected and unaffected sides. A difference of more than 1.5 ms in the H-reflex latency between normal and abnormal side has been considered objective evidence of S1 radiculopathy.

Lumbosacral radiculopathy is most commonly involved with herniated disc disease. Its major difference from cervical radiculopathy is that a single-level herniated disc may compress

TABLE 8.6. Needle EMG Data in Case 4

				Spontaneous Potentials				Motor Unit Potential				Interference	
Muscle	**Root**	**Nerve**	**Insertion Activity**	**Fib**	**PSW**	**Fasc**	**Myotonia CRD**	**Amplitude (K)**	**Duration (ms)**	**Polyphasic Potential**	**HA MUP**	**Pattern**	**Mean Amplitude (K)**
Lt L3, 4			N	–	–	–	–						
L5, S1			+	+	++	–	–						
Glut med	L5	Sup glut	+	–	±	–	–						
Glut max	S1	Inf glut	+	+	++	–	–	0.5–4	6–12	N	0	RIP[a]	2
Vast lat	L3,4	Femoral	N	–	–	–	–	0.5–4	6–12	N	0	FIP	3
Ant tibial	L4,5	Peroneal	N	–	–	–	–	0.5–3	6–12	N	0	FIP	4
Peroneus	L5	Peroneal	N	–	–	–	–	0.5–3	6–13	N	0	FIP	3
Gastroc med	S1	Post tibial	+	+	++	–	–	0.5–3	6–12	N	0	RIP*	2

[a] Rapid firing.

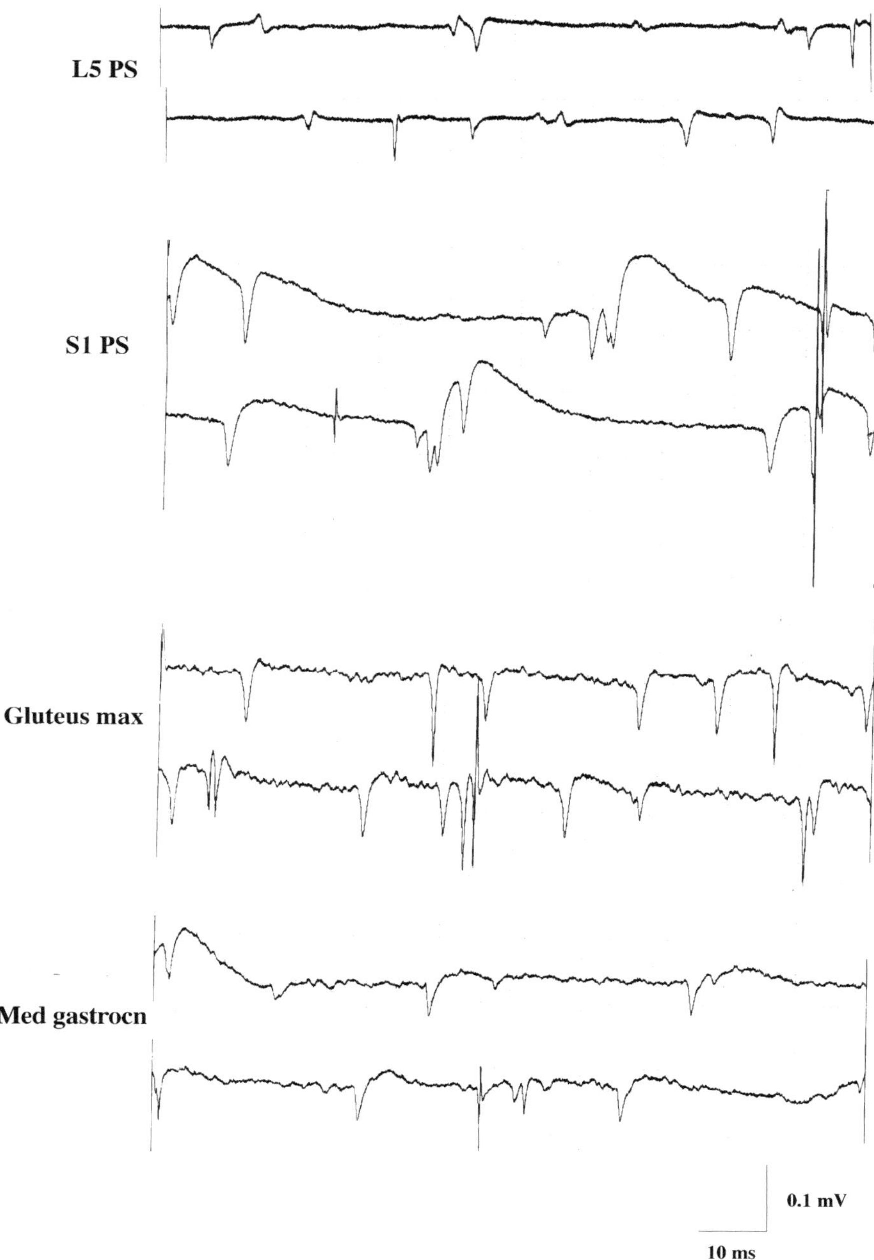

FIGURE 8.9. Fibrillations and PSWs in the left L5 and S1 paraspinal (*PS*), gluteus maximus (*max*), and medial gastrocnemius (*med gastrocn*) muscles indicative of left S1 radiculopathy.

multiple roots depending on the location of the herniated disc. In classic L5 radiculopathy, the L5 root is compressed due to lateral herniation of the disc at the L4–5 intervertebral disc space. If this disc is herniated closer to the midline, then the S1 root can also be compressed. This difference is anatomical; in cauda equina lesion, many root filaments are closely situated together in small space until they exit through their own foramen. This anatomical difference explains why in lumbosacral radiculopathy often more than one root is involved with one level herniated disc.

Isolated L4 radiculopathy due to a herniated disc is extremely rare. The clinical hallmarks of L4 radiculopathy are weakness in the iliopsoas and quadriceps muscles and decreased or absent patellar reflexes. Because similar findings are observed in lumbar plexopathy and femoral neuropathy, it is not easy to differentiate these disorders on clinical grounds alone. Theoretically, weakness in adduction of the thigh (L3,4; obturator nerve) is supposed to differentiate L4 radiculopathy from femoral neuropathy, but it is not easily demonstrable because the adductor magnus, the most powerful adductor, is jointly co-innervated through the sciatic nerve. Femoral neuropathy or diabetic amyotrophy is observed more commonly than L4 radiculopathy. The femoral nerve conduction and paraspinal needle EMG study are two crucial tests in this respect: the paraspinal EMG is abnormal in L4 radiculopathy and the latency is prolonged in femoral neuropathy. The saphenous nerve conduction is not very helpful because it is technically difficult to obtain even in normal individuals. The newly described medial femoral cutaneous nerve conduction test is potentially useful, showing abnormality in lumbar plexopathy and femoral neuropathy. Lumbosacral polyradiculopathy together with femoral neuropathy is a classic EMG feature of diabetic amyotrophy. Thus, the femoral nerve conduction study has been a crucial test in documenting femoral neuropathy in patients with diabetic amyotrophy.

The clinical hallmark of L5 radiculopathy is foot drop, which is also seen in peroneal neuropathy and sciatic neuropathy. Although the L4 root innervates the anterior tibialis muscle, foot drop due to weakness of the anterior tibialis is indicative of L5 radiculopathy. L5 radiculopathy classically produces weakness in foot eversion (peroneus muscle) and inversion (posterior tibial muscle), but no weakness is observed in foot inversion in peroneal neuropathy. In the workup for L5 radiculopathy, it is important to test L5 innervated muscles, the gluteus medius (innervated by the superior gluteal nerve), flexor digitorum longus and posterior tibial muscles (posterior tibial nerve). If these muscles show abnormality, L5 radiculopathy, not peroneal neuropathy, is definitely indicated. In peroneal palsy, the peroneal motor NCS shows focal slowing or conduction block across the fibular head, and the superficial peroneal sensory nerve conduction is abnormal. On the other hand, the superficial peroneal sensory nerve conduction is normal in L5 radiculopathy. Abnormality in the short head of the biceps femoris is indicative of sciatic neuropathy in patients with foot drop because this muscle is normal in peroneal palsy. In differentiation of sciatic neuropathy from L5 radiculopathy, the sural nerve conduction is also crucial, being normal in L5 radiculopathy and abnormal in sciatic neuropathy.

The clinical hallmarks of S1 radiculopathy are weakness of the gastrocnemius muscle and decreased or absent ankle reflexes. Differentiation from posterior tibial neuropathy is almost impossible clinically. In this regard, the needle EMG in the gluteal muscles is extremely helpful. In posterior tibial neuropathy, the needle EMG in the gluteal maximus is normal, but sural and plantar nerve conductions are abnormal. A problem with these NCS is that sometimes no response can be elicited in normal individuals over 60 years of age. In S radiculopathy, when it is observed in connection with lumbar stenosis, the soleus and lateral gastrocnemius muscles must be assessed along with the external anal sphincters and S2 paraspinal muscles because the S2 root innervates these muscles. Thus, such studies are needed in all patients with bowel or bladder disturbance of lower motor neuron origin.

MAXIMS

1. The H-reflex of the gastrocnemius-soleus muscle may be absent or prolonged in latency on the involved side in S1 radiculopathy. A more than 1.5-ms difference in the H-reflexes between the normal and involved sides is indicative of S1 radiculopathy.

2. In classic radiculopathy, the sensory nerve conduction is always normal, and the motor nerve conduction is either normal or shows a motor neuronopathy pattern (low CMAP amplitude; prolonged F-wave latency) if the radiculopathy is severe or multiple roots are involved.

REFERENCES

1. Braddom RI, Johnson EW. Standardization of H reflex and diagnostic use in S1 radiculopathy. Arch Phys Med Rehabil 1974;55:161–166.
2. Kuruoglu R, Oh SJ, Thompson B. Clinical and electromyographic correlations of lumbosacral radiculopathy [letter]. Muscle Nerve 1994;17:250–251.

CASE 5

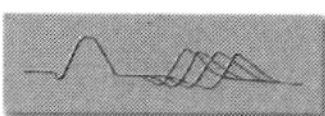

RECURRENCE OF LUMBAR RADICULOPATHY IN A POSTLAMINECTOMY PATIENT?

CASE PRESENTATION

A 56-year-old man was evaluated in 1985 for low back pain radiating down to both feet, followed by progressive weakness of the left leg for 3 months. Additionally, he had urinary urgency. Abnormal neurological findings were MRC strength of 1 in the left posterior tibialis, anterior tibialis, and peroneus muscles; 4 in the left quadriceps and glutei, and in the right peroneus longus and gastrocnemius muscles; absent ankle jerks; decreased knee jerks; and positive straight leg raise in both legs. Sensory examination was normal. EMG study showed bilateral L4,5, S1 polyradiculopathy (Table 8.7). A CT myelogram revealed severe three-level lumbar stenosis for which the patient had lumbar decompression surgery. After the surgery, he recovered quite well with an improvement in strength. In 1990, he was sent for another EMG evaluation because of a 2-month recurrence of low back pain radiating along the posterior part of the left leg to the lateral aspect of the feet. Abnormal findings were MRC strength of 4 in the left quadriceps, anterior tibialis, and gastrocnemius muscles; decreased knee reflexes; and absent ankle reflexes.

CASE ANALYSIS

This patient with a history of previous laminectomy developed subacute progression of motor weakness involving predominantly the left L4,5 and S1 innervated muscles. Considering his diminished knee jerk, clearly the L4 root was also involved. Although there had been definite improvement as compared with the previous evaluation, the patient insisted on knowing exactly whether there had been any recurrence of his lumbar stenosis, considering his previous "bad" experience. The most likely possibility, in view of his surgical history, was epidural or subarachnoid adhesion (scarring) of multiple lumbosacral roots.

PLAN OF TESTING

1. NCS: To compare with previous findings.
2. Needle EMG: To compare with previous findings.

ELECTROPHYSIOLOGICAL TESTS AND FINDINGS

NCS Findings (Table 8.8)

1. Normal NCS in the left peroneal, posterior tibial, and sural nerves.
2. Absent left H-reflex.

Needle EMG (Table 8.9; Fig. 8.10)

1. Prominent fibrillations and PSWs in the left L3-5 paraspinal muscles.
2. Fibrillations and PSWs in the left anterior tibialis, peroneus longus, and gastrocnemius muscles.
3. HALD and HA MUPs and RIP in all tested muscles of the left leg.

TABLE 8.7. Needle EMG Data, 9/25/85, in Case 5

				Spontaneous Potentials				Motor Unit Potential				Interference	
Muscle	Root	Nerve	Insertion Activity	Fib	PSW	Fasc	Myotonia CRD	Amplitude (K)	Duration (ms)	Polyphasic Potential	HA MUP	Pattern	Mean Amplitude (K)
Lt and rt L4-5, S1	L3,4 5, S1		+	+	++	–	+						
Lt L3 paraspinal	L3		+	+	–	–	–						
Lt gluteus med and max	L5, S1	Sup and inf glut	N	–	–	–	–	0.5–2	7–14	N	–	RIP	1.5
Rt gluteus med and max	L5, S1	Sup and inf glut	+	++	+	–	–	0.5–1.5	8–15	N	–	RIP	1
Lt vast lat	L3,4	Femoral	+	–	++	–	–	1–2	10–16	N	–	RIP	2
Rt vast lat	L3,4	Femoral	+	++	++	–	–	1–6	12–15	N	+	RIP	3
Lt ant tibial	L4,5	Peroneal	+	++	++	–	–	No MUP					
Rt ant tibial	L4,5	Peroneal	+	++	++	–	–	1–14	16–22	N	HALD	DA	6
Lt peroneus longus	L5, S1	Peroneal	+	++	++	–	–	No MUP					
Lt med gastroc	S1,2	Post tibial	+	++	++	–	–	1–4	10–15	N	–	RIP	3
Rt med gastroc	S1,2	Post tibial	+	+	+	–	–	1–7	10–16	N	HA	RIP	3
Lt posterior tibial	L5	Post tibial	+	+++	+++	–	–	1–4	10–20	N	–	DA	4

[a] Rt L3 paraspinal muscle: no fibrillations or PSWs.
HALD, high-amplitude long-duration.

TABLE 8.8. Nerve Conduction Data in Case 5

	9/25/85				2/13/90	
	Latent/NCV (ms/m/s)	**Amplitude (mV/μV)**	**Latent/NCV (ms/m/s)**	**Amplitude (mV/μV)**	**Latent/NCV (ms/m/s)**	**Amplitude (mV/μV)**
	Rt Peroneal	**Motor N**	**Lt Peroneal**	**Motor N**	**Lt Peroneal**	**Motor N**
TL	4.3	8.0	6.1	3.5	4.8	5.0
FH-A	49.2	8.0	36.0	3.0	43.9	4.0
PF-FH			59.2			
F-wave	53.9		61.6		50.8	
	Rt Posterior Tibial	**Motor N**	**Lt Posterior Tibial**	**Motor N**	**Lt Posterior Tibial**	**Motor N**
TL	44	6.2	4.8	10.5	4.6	12.0
PF-A	45.1	6.0	39.0	10.5	42.2	12.0
F-wave	53.6		63.0		52.8	
H-reflex	NP		NP		NP	
	Rt Sural	**Sensory N**	**Lt Sural**	**Sensory N**	**Sural**	**Sensory N**
MC-A	38.8	10	40.0	10	48.0	30

Height: 173 cm.

TL, terminal latency; FH, fibular head; A, ankle; PF, popliteal fossa; MC, mid-calf; NP, no potential.

TABLE 8.9. Needle EMG Data, 2/13/90, in Case 5

				Spontaneous Potentials				Motor Unit Potential				Interference	
Muscle	**Root**	**Nerve**	**Insertion Activity**	**Fib**	**PSW**	**Fasc**	**Myotonia CRD**	**Amplitude (K)**	**Duration (ms)**	**Polyphasic Potential**	**HA MUP**	**Pattern**	**Mean Amplitude (K)**
Lt L3-5 PS	L3-5		+	+++	+++	–	+						
S1 PS	S1		N	–	–	–	–						
Glut med	L5	Sup glut	N	–	–	–	–	1–10	7–14	N	+	RIP	2
Glut max	S1	Inf glut	N	–	–	–	–	1–8	8–15	N	+	RIP	2
Vast lat	L3,4	Femoral	N	–	–	–	–	1–12	7–15	N	+	RIP	4
Ant tibial	L4,5	Peroneal	+	–	+	–	–	2–20	6–20	+	HALD	DA	5
Peroneus longus	L5, S1	Peroneal	+	+	+	–	–	2–10	8–24	+	HALD	DA	6
Med gastroc	S1,2	Post tibial	+	+	++	–	–	2–16	8–16	N	++	DA	4

PS, paraspinal muscles.

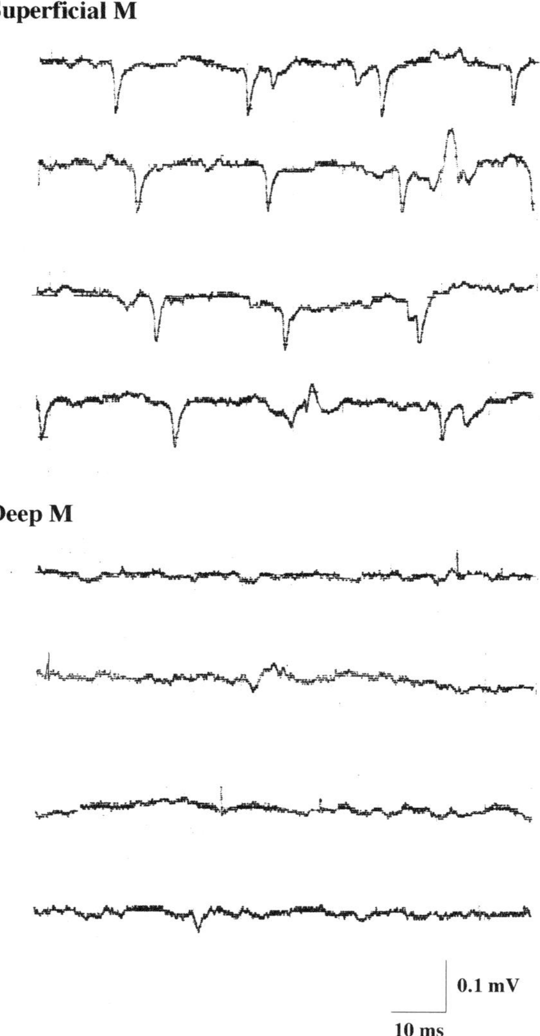

FIGURE 8.10. Fibrillations and PSWs in the superficial and deep paraspinal muscles due to the trauma of muscle. Usually, fibrillations and PSWs due to the trauma of muscle are more prominent in the superficial muscle. However, this alone does not distinguish fibrillations and PSWs due to the radiculopathy from those due to the trauma of muscle.

ELECTROPHYSIOLOGICAL INTERPRETATION

Left L5 and S1 radiculopathy. Compared with the previous test on 9/25/85, there had been definite improvement.

FINAL DIAGNOSIS

Improved state from the previous lumbar stenosis. No evidence of recurrence of lumbar stenosis.

TREATMENT AND FOLLOW-UP

With definite improvement on the recent EMG, the physician was able to convince the patient that there had not been any recurrence of lumbar stenosis. His low back pain was well relieved with nonsteroidal antiinflammatory medication alone.

COMMENTS

In the EMG evaluation of postlaminectomy patients, comparison with a previous EMG report is the most important part of the workup, as seen in this case. Without the previous study, it is almost impossible to determine whether there has been any improvement, recurrence, persistence, or worsening of radiculopathy. Unfortunately, an EMG study is requested in many postlaminectomy patients who did not have a previous EMG study. To accommodate this problem, we used the following guidelines in interpreting the needle EMG findings in patients in whom radiculopathy is suspected.

1. In individuals who have not had a previous laminectomy:
   a. When fibrillations and PSWs are seen in paraspinal muscles, findings are indicative of radiculopathy.
   b. When fibrillations and PSWs together with denervation pattern are found in limb muscles alone, findings are compatible with radiculopathy.
2. In individuals with previous laminectomy:
   a. When fibrillations and PSWs are found in paraspinal muscles with concomitant EMG abnormalities in the limb muscles, findings are indicative of radiculopathy. However, we cannot differentiate among recurrence of radiculopathy, persistence of radiculopathy, or subarachnoid adhesions. Clinical correlation is needed.
   b. When fibrillations and PSWs are found in paraspinal muscles without any EMG abnormalities in the limb muscles, findings are most likely due to trauma on muscles. We cannot completely rule out radiculopathy. Clinical correlation is needed.
   c. When fibrillations or PSWs and/or HA and HALD MUPs are found in the limb muscles without any EMG abnormalities in the paraspinal muscles, findings are compatible with radiculopathy. However, we cannot differentiate among recurrence of radiculopathy, persistence of radiculopathy, or subarachnoid adhesion. Clinical correlation is needed.

MAXIMS

1. The importance of needle EMG abnormalities in the paraspinal muscles in postlaminectomy patients is extremely limited because fibrillations and PSWs in these muscles are most likely due to trauma on muscle.
2. Without the presurgery EMG report in postlaminectomy patients, it is impossible to differentiate among recurrence of radiculopathy, persistence of radiculopathy, or subarachnoid adhesion by means of the postlaminectomy EMG study.

REFERENCES

1. Wilbourn AJ. The value and limitations of electromyographic examination in the diagnosis of lumbosacral radiculopathy. In: Hardy RW, ed. Lumbar disc diseases. New York: Raven Press, 1982:65–109.

CASE 6

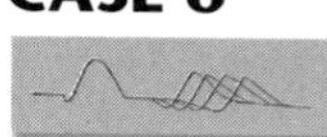

NERVE BIOPSY FOR PERIPHERAL NEUROPATHY OF UNKNOWN ETIOLOGY

CASE PRESENTATION

A 76-year-old woman was referred for evaluation of peripheral neuropathy and possible nerve biopsy. She had numbness in the toes of her right foot about 2 years before, and this gradually spread toward the knees. She complained of weakness and numbness in the right lower leg, which had grown worse in the previous 6 months. For the past 3 to 4 months, she had begun to notice the same numb feelings on the toes of her left foot, and for the past 2 weeks, on the first three fingers of her left hand as well. About 4 years before, she had "pulled a muscle" in her right arm with symptoms persisting for 7 to 8 weeks. She also complained of difficulty with urination and experienced incontinence if she could not get to the bathroom right away.

Abnormal neurological findings were MRC strength of 4 in the right deltoid (due to previous brachial plexopathy), 4 in the right and left anterior tibialis muscles, absent vibratory sensation on toes and ankles, decreased pinprick below the ankles in stocking distribution, absent ankle reflexes, decreased knee reflexes, mild pes cavus, and difficulty walking on her heels. Tinel and Phalen's signs were positive on the median nerve at the wrist.

CASE ANALYSIS

This patient had all the symptomatic triad of polyneuropathy: symmetrical distal motor weakness, stocking-distribution of sensory loss, and areflexia. These were followed by a recent diagnosis of right carpal tunnel syndrome. Certainly, with this constellation of findings, it was reasonable to think of peripheral neuropathy as the first diagnostic impression. Sphincter disturbance would be extremely unusual unless we were dealing with diabetic or amyloid neuropathy.

PLAN OF TESTING

1. NCS: To document peripheral neuropathy.
2. Needle EMG: To document denervation process in the limb and paraspinal muscles.
3. Other tests: MRI. Fasting blood sugar and HbAic.

ELECTROPHYSIOLOGICAL TESTS AND FINDINGS

NCS Findings

1. Markedly prolonged (10.9 ms) terminal latency and absent sensory CNAP in the finger-wrist segment in the left median nerve.
2. No CMAP response from the extensor digitorum brevis muscle and low CMAP from the anterior tibialis muscle in the right peroneal nerve.
3. Low CMAP and slow motor NCV in the bilateral posterior tibial and left peroneal nerves.
4. Normal NCS in the bilateral sural nerves.

Needle EMG (Table 8.10; Fig. 8.11)

1. Fibrillations and PSWs in the bilateral anterior tibialis, gastrocnemius, and lumbosacral paraspinal muscles.
2. CRD in the left vastus lateralis and right gastrocnemius muscles.
3. HALD MUPs and DA in all tested muscles.

ELECTROPHYSIOLOGICAL INTERPRETATION

1. Bilateral lumbosacral polyradiculopathy (cauda equina syndrome).
2. No evidence of peripheral neuropathy.

OTHER TEST FINDINGS

MRI of the lumbosacral area that showed a severe stenosis at T12-L1 and L3-4 levels. Normal fasting blood sugar and hemoglobulin Aic.

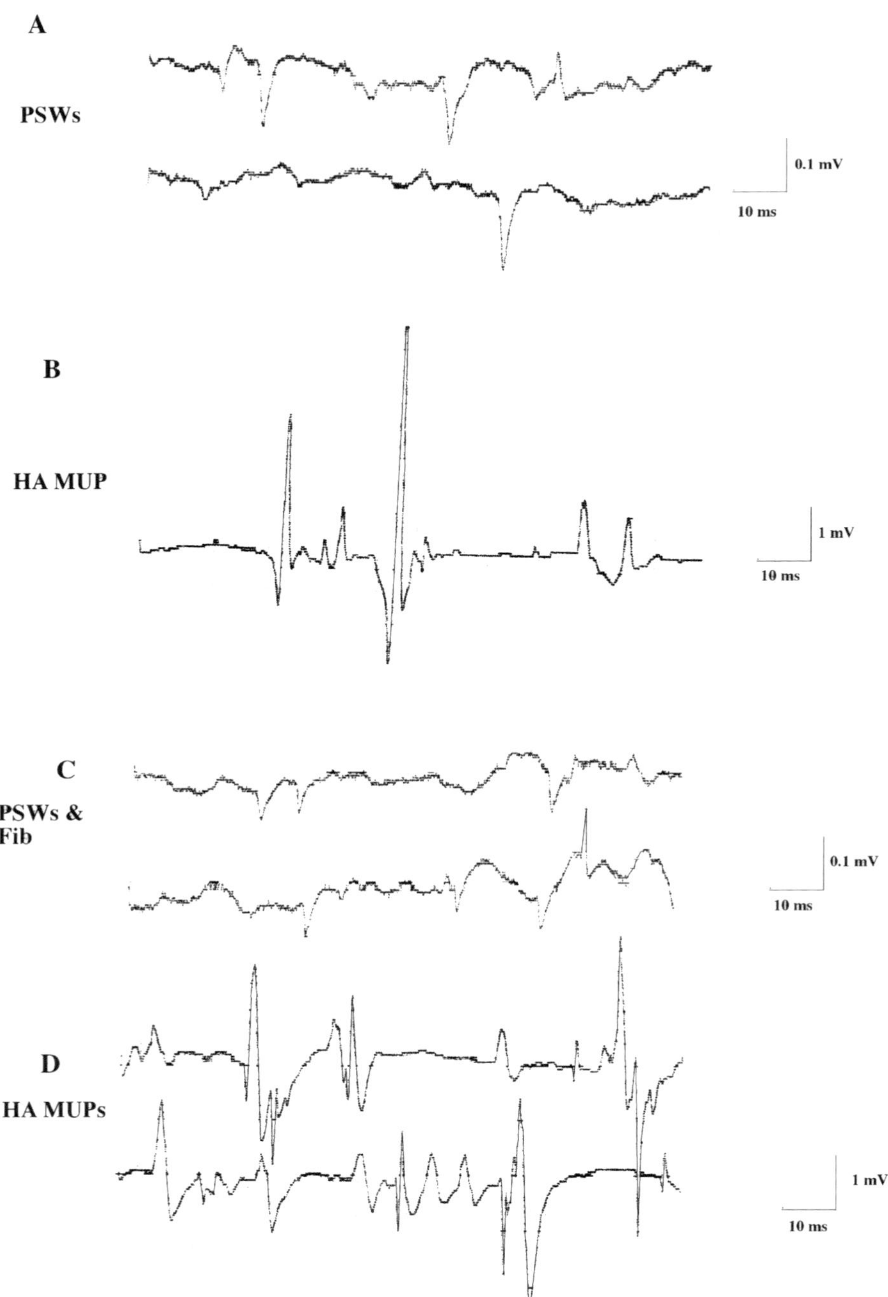

FIGURE 8.11. **A.** PSWs in the left L4 paraspinal muscles. **B.** HA MUPs in the left anterior tibialis. **C.** PSWs and fibrillations in the right S1 paraspinal muscles. **D.** HA MUPs in the right gastrocnemius muscle.

TABLE 8.10. Needle EMG Data in Case 6

				Spontaneous Potentials				Motor Unit Potential				Interference	
Muscle	**Root**	**Nerve**	**Insertion Activity**	**Fib**	**PSW**	**Fasc**	**Myotonia CRD**	**Amplitude (K)**	**Duration (ms)**	**Polyphasic Potential**	**HALD MUP**	**Pattern**	**Mean Amplitude (K)**
Lt ant tibial	L4,5	Peroneal	+	+++	+++	−	−	1–9	6–18	N	+	DA	5
Gastroc	S1,2	Post tibial	+	+++	+++	−	−	1–14	6–20	N	+	DA	4
Vast lateral	L3,4	Femoral	N	−	−	−	+	0.5–6	6–18	N	+	DA	3
Glut med	L5	Sup glut	+	++	++	−	−	1–12	6–18	N	+	DA	5
Rt ant tibial	L4,5	Peroneal	+	++	+	−	−	1–6	6–20	N	+	DA	4
Gastroc	S1,2	Post tibial	+	+	++	−	+	1–7	8–18	N	+	DA	5
Lt,5,S1 PS	L5, S1	Post rami	+	+	+	−	−						
L3 PS	L3		−	−	−	−	−						
Rt L5,S1,PS	L5, S1	Post rami	+	+	+	−	−						

FINAL DIAGNOSIS

1. Severe bilateral lumbar stenosis
2. Left carpal tunnel syndrome

TREATMENT AND FOLLOW-UP

In view of the electrodiagnostic findings, a nerve biopsy was not performed. MRI of the lumbar area was ordered. With the diagnosis of lumbar stenosis, the patient was referred to neurosurgery for lumbar decompression and decompression of the carpal tunnel. She experienced good recovery from pain, walking difficulty, and sphincter disturbance.

COMMENTS

There were two striking findings in this patient's EMG study that are unusual for peripheral neuropathy: normal sural nerve conduction and lumbosacral polyradiculopathy in the presence of clinically suspected peripheral neuropathy. It is extremely unusual to have completely normal sural nerve conduction in peripheral neuropathy. Thus, until proven otherwise, this pattern was indicative of a polyradiculomyelopathy. In patients of this age group, lumbar stenosis is the most common cause for lumbar polyradiculopathy. The complaint of sphincter difficulty in this patient was certainly suggestive of cauda equina lesion. Thus, an MRI was ordered and identified severe lumbar stenosis.

Lumbar stenosis refers to the cauda equina syndrome associated with nerve root compression by soft tissues and osseous lesions in the lumbar area. It is common in elderly patients and can produce one or both of two clinical syndromes: neurogenic claudication and chronic painful cauda equina syndrome producing motor-sensory impairment, areflexia in the legs, and sphincter problems in severe cases. This disorder can mimic peripheral neuropathy, motor neuron diseases, or distal myopathy. The clinical hallmark of lumbar stenosis is neurogenic claudication. This refers to pain, paresthesia, and rarely weakness in the legs, which are exacerbated by lumbar extension (as in walking and prolonged standing) and relieved by rest and lumbar flexion. This postural relationship is the most important differential point from vascular claudication. In lumbar stenosis, lumbar extension increases nerve root compression, producing an acute neural ischemic syndrome that is manifested as neurogenic claudication.

Lumbar stenosis can be diagnosed by the MRI or CT myelogram, which shows the classic multilevel hour-glass compression of nerve roots in the cauda equina. The electrodiagnostic study is important in confirming bilateral lumbosacral radiculopathy and ruling out other causes of neurological dysfunction, such as polyneuropathy, motor neuron disease, or myopathy. Because the definitive diagnosis of lumbar stenosis is made by the MRI or CT myelogram, electrodiagnostic tests are not necessary in classic cases of neurogenic claudication. We believe that EMG studies are necessary, however, in the subset of patients with cauda equina syndrome but without neurogenic claudication.

The classic EMG abnormalities in lumbar stenosis are a combination of lumbosacral polyradiculopathy and a normal or motor neuronopathy pattern in the NCS. Lumbosacral polyradiculopathy is commonly bilateral and usually involves the lower lumbosacral roots. NCS show the classic features of the motor neuropathy pattern; sural and superficial peroneal nerve conductions are characteristically normal and the peroneal and posterior tibial motor nerve conductions show a low or unelicitable CMAP amplitude. Motor NCV and distal latencies are either normal or mildly slow due to wallerian degeneration of the fastest conducting motor fibers. H-reflexes are usually absent bilaterally because the S1 roots are usually involved. The needle EMG shows fibrillations and PSWs, a chronic denervation pattern of MUPs (HALD or HA MUPs), or some combination of both in multiple root distributions in paraspinal muscles and both lower extremities. According to Wilbourn, multiple bilateral lumbosacral radiculopathies (cauda equina syndrome) are observed in 50% of cases of lumbar stenosis, a single radiculopathy in 20% of cases, non specific EMG changes in 20%, and normal findings in the remaining 10% of cases. Thus, the EMG findings with lumbar canal stenosis are quite variable, depending on the severity of the compression. The degree of dural sac stenosis correlated with the severity of EMG abnormalities in Johnson's study in 1987: EMG abnormality in all cases of complete block and neurogenic claudication, in 94% of patients with neurogenic claudication and partial block, and in 54% with neurogenic claudication but with no block. Thus, a normal EMG study does not rule out lumbar stenosis, especially in patients with radiologically mild cases.

MAXIMS

1. Neurogenic claudication is the clinical hallmark of lumbar stenosis and refers to pain in the legs that is aggravated by lumbar extension, including walking, and relieved by lumbar flexion and rest.
2. The typical EMG findings in lumbar stenosis are bilateral polyradiculopathy and a normal or motor neuronopathy pattern of nerve conduction abnormality.

REFERENCES

1. Katz JN, Dalgas M, Stucki G, Lipson SJ. Diagnosis of lumbar spinal stenosis. Rheum Dis Clin North Am 1994;20:471–483.
2. Johnson KE, Rosen I, Uden A. Neurophysiologic investigation of patients with spinal stenosis. Spine 1987;12:483–487.

CASE 7

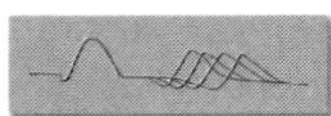

RIGHT LOWER ABDOMINAL PAIN WITH NEGATIVE FINDINGS AFTER EXHAUSTIVE STUDIES

CASE PRESENTATION

A 24-year-old woman was admitted to the GI service at UAB hospital for workup of a 3-month history of right lower abdominal quadrant pain. This pain was described as a "constant tightness" with episodic sharp pain radiating to the back. The patient had been admitted to a local hospital three times. All workups for lower abdominal pain, including CT and ultrasound scan of the abdomen, a barium study, pelvic examination, and endoscopic study of the upper and lower abdomen, had been negative. GTT was also normal. Exploratory laparascopy showed diffuse adenopathy, a biopsy of which showed a "reactive lymph node." The patient looked chronically ill without any obvious abnormality on general or neurological examinations. To complete the diagnostic workup, a GI attending ordered a needle EMG study with a specific request to rule out thoracic radiculopathy.

CASE ANALYSIS

Despite exhaustive studies, the cause for this patient's right lower abdominal quadrant pain had not been found. As a final diagnostic test, the EMG study was ordered for thoracic radiculopathy. This practice is not uncommon at the UAB EMG laboratory. Although no obvious neurological abnormality may be found on examination to suggest a thoracic radiculopathy, the needle EMG can still detect radiculopathy if present. Our experience is that the needle EMG is positive in roughly 1 of 10 referred patients of this type.

PLAN OF TESTING

1. NCS: To detect any asymptomatic neuropathy. Usually in diabetic radiculopathy, NCS is abnormal.
2. Needle EMG: To document clinically nondetected radiculopathy, the needle EMG in paraspinal muscles corresponding to the dermatome of "pain." If paraspinal muscles are normal, the rectus abdominalis muscles should be tested.

ELECTROPHYSIOLOGICAL TESTS AND FINDINGS

NCS Findings. Normal motor NCS in the left median, ulnar, posterior tibial, peroneal and sural nerves.

Needle EMG (Fig. 8.12)

1. Fibrillations and PSWs in the right T10-12 and L1-4 paraspinal muscles.
2. Minimal PSWs but normal MUPs in the right anterior tibialis muscle.
3. Normal needle EMG findings in the right vastus lateralis and gastrocnemius muscles.

ELECTROPHYSIOLOGICAL INTERPRETATION

Right thoracic 10-12 and lumbar 1-4 radiculopathies.

OTHER TEST FINDINGS

Persistent low white blood cell count (3,700) and platelets (83,000).

FINAL DIAGNOSIS

Neoplastic right thoraco-lumbar radiculopathy

TREATMENT AND FOLLOW-UP

After the diagnosis of right thoracolumbar radiculopathy was made and a malignancy was suggested as a diagnostic possibility, an astute resident ordered a bone marrow biopsy on the basis of agranulocytosis. This confirmed the diagnosis of acute lymphoblastic leukemia. Subsequently, the patient was treated with chemotherapy with remission of leukemia for 5 years.

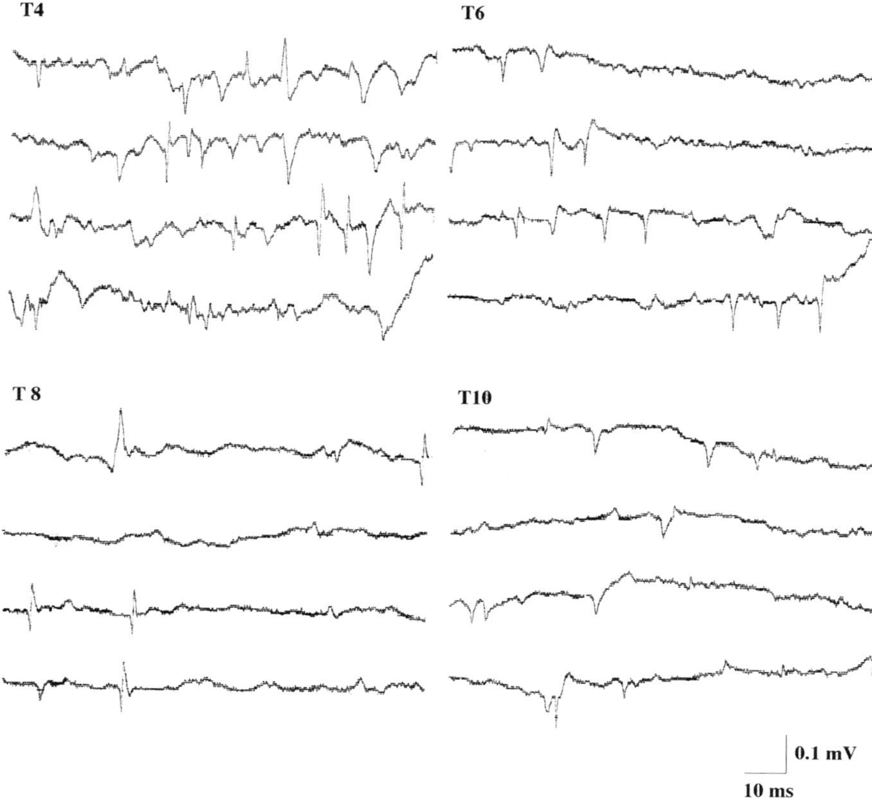

FIGURE 8.12. Fibrillations and PSWs in the right T4, 6, 8, and 10 paraspinal muscles.

COMMENTS

It is extremely gratifying to find an organic cause for pain of unknown origin, as seen in this patient. On many occasions, these patients are labeled as "functional." The only means of finding thoracolumbar radiculopathy is the needle EMG study. It is not easy to relax the thoracic muscles for this study. Among the various methods we have tried, the best relaxation is achieved by having the patient lie on the table on the side to be examined. This is the opposite of what we do for the cervical or lumbar radiculopathy workup. Even in this position, it is not easy to achieve 100% relaxation of the thoracic paraspinal muscles.

LaBan and Grant reported a special pattern of needle EMG abnormalities in occult spinal metastases in 38 patients with back pain and a history of malignant neoplasm: profound denervation in the paraspinal muscles innervated by the posterior rami and relatively little involvement of the anterior ramus. In all these cases, the predominant symptom was back pain, and metastasis was suspected on clinical grounds but was not confirmed by routine neurological, radiological, or radioisotope procedures. Needle EMG showed polyradiculopathy only in the paraspinal muscles. In three autopsies, gross evidence of posterior ramus involvement was found. In the last three cases, these authors were able to suggest the presence of metastatic disease before the discovery of the primary cancer. This was the case in our patient. Watson and Waylonis analyzed 91 cases with this pattern of needle EMG abnormality and found herniated discs in 28%, occult metastatic carcinoma in 24%, degenerative disc disease in 16%, diabetes in 9%, and miscellaneous disorders in 8%, indicating that "metastatic carcinoma" is the second most common cause for this pattern of needle EMG abnormality.

The etiologies for polyradiculopathy limited to the paraspinal muscles are not always apparent. Certainly, diabetic radiculopathy and multiple disc disease, such as cervical or lumbar stenosis, are the two most common causes for polyradiculopathy. These have to be ruled out by the MRI and appropriate blood tests for diabetes. Once they have been excluded, a malignancy must be considered. We suggested this possibility in the report in this patient. An astute intern carefully went over the patient's laboratory workup and found unexplainable "agranulocytosis" in this patient. A bone-marrow study was performed, and the patient was found to have leukemia. Rare causes for polyradiculopathy include myelopathy, anterior horn cell diseases, postepidural block, Paget's disease, and active myopathy.

MAXIMS

1. To achieve the best relaxation of the thoracic muscles, the patient should lie with the side to be tested against the examining table. This is opposite of what is recommended for cervical or lumbar radiculopathy workups.
2. Once diabetes and multiple disc disease are ruled out, the possibility of malignancy must be considered as the etiology of polyradiculopathy confined to the paraspinal muscles.

REFERENCES

1. LaBan MM, Grant AE. Occult spinal metastases—early electromyographic manifestations. Arch Phys Med Rehabil 1971;52:223–226.
2. Watson R, Waylonis G. Paraspinal electromyographic abnormalities predictor of occult metastatic carcinoma. Arch Phys Med Rehabil 1975;56:216–218.

CASE 8

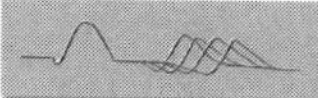

DIABETIC AMYOTROPHY OR INCLUSION BODY MYOSITIS

CASE PRESENTATION

A 74-year-old man with diabetes mellitus being treated with insulin had developed lower back pain, which radiated down along the backs of both legs, and weakness in both lower extremities 4 years before. The weakness progressed slowly to the point that he had difficulty walking, climbing stairs, and eventually had to use a cane to ambulate. The patient denied any sensory symptoms in the lower extremities, bowel or bladder problems, or claudication. Previous tests revealed an increased CPK (four times normal) and an EMG was requested to rule out polymyositis. The EMG diagnosis was polyradiculopathy with signs of reinnervation and peripheral neuropathy as seen in diabetes (Table 8.11; Fig. 8.13). However, there was a disclaimer: coexisting myopathy could not be ruled out. Abnormal neurological findings were MRC

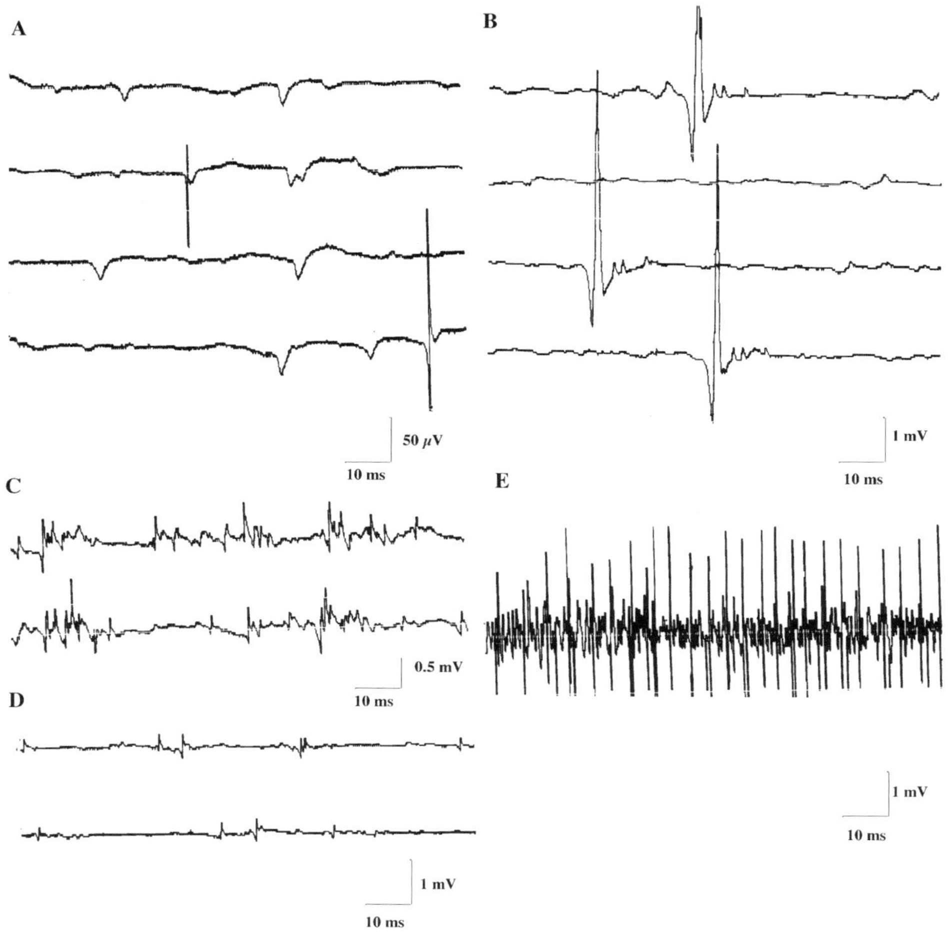

FIGURE 8.13. Mixed myopathic and denervation pattern in the first EMG study. **A.** PSWs and fibrillations in the left L5 paraspinal muscle. **B.** HA MUP in the left vastus lateralis muscle. **C.** Some SASD MUPs in the left anterior tibialis muscle. Some polyphasic MUPs have normal duration and thus were misinterpreted as "regeneration MUPs." **D.** Obvious SASD MUPs in the anterior tibialis muscle on the minimal contraction in some area. **E.** RIP with mean amplitude of 4 mV in the vastus lateralis muscle.

TABLE 8.11. Needle EMG Data in Case 8

				Spontaneous Potentials				Motor Unit Potential				Interference	
Muscle	Root	Nerve	Insertion Activity	Fib	PSW	Fasc	CRD	Amplitude (mV)	Duration (ms)	Polyphasic Potential	HA MUP	Pattern	Mean Amplitude (mV)
8/21/97													
Lt vast lat	L3,4	Femoral	+	++	++	−	−	1.5–7	7–19	+++	+	RIP	2
Gastroc	S1,2	Post tibial	+	+++	++	−	−	0.4–2	4–12	+++	−	RIP	1
Ant tibial	L4,5	Peroneal	+	++	++	−	+	0.3–2.5	2–10	+++	−	RIP	1.5
L3–5, S1			+	++	+	−	−	1–3	5–12	+	−		
Rt 3–5, S1			+	+	+								
10/3/97													
Lt iliopsoas	L3,4	Femoral	+	+	+	−	−	0.3–1	2–10	++	−	FIP[a]	0.7
Rectus fem	L3,4	Femoral	+	++	++	−	−	0.3–1.5	2–10	++	−	FIP[a]	0.8

[a] Early recruitment.

strength of 2 in the iliopsoas, 4 − in the anterior tibialis, 5 − in the gastrocnemius muscles, atrophy of the thighs, and absent patellar and ankle reflexes. The patient walked slightly slowly with foot drop and could not walk on tiptoes or heels. Sensory evaluation was completely normal. No fasciculation was observed.

CASE ANALYSIS

This patient's problems began with low back pain radiating down to the legs and eventually showing a pure proximal muscle weakness with areflexia and thigh atrophy. Diagnostic possibilities included diabetic amyotrophy, lumbar stenosis, spinal muscular atrophy, and polymyositis. EMG findings were compatible with the first three possibilities. Diabetic amyotrophy is usually asymmetrical and extremely painful at onset but does not last 4 years. Lumbar stenosis was a definite possibility but usually involves the L5 and S1 roots more severely. Neurogenic claudication and sphincter dysfunction were absent. Spinal muscular atrophy as an expression of ALS could explain all the findings: elevated CPK, proximal muscle weakness, thigh atrophy, areflexia, and polyradiculopathy. In polymyositis, thigh atrophy and areflexia are extremely unusual. One attending predicted a diagnosis of inclusion body myositis before muscle biopsy.

PLAN OF TESTING

1. Needle EMG: The previous needle EMG was reviewed. Additional needle EMG studies were performed in a limited number of muscles to analyze the MUPs.
2. NCS: Previous NCS was reviewed for any peripheral neuropathy as seen in diabetes mellitus.
3. Other tests: Muscle biopsy.

ELECTROPHYSIOLOGICAL TESTS AND FINDINGS

NCS Findings on 8/21/97 **(Table 8.12).** Generalized axonal neuropathy with carpal tunnel syndrome.

Needle EMG (Table 8.11; Fig. 8.14)

1. Minimal fibrillations and PSWs in the left rectus femoris and iliopsoas muscles.
2. Many simple and polyphasic SASD MUPs with early recruitment.

ELECTROPHYSIOLOGICAL INTERPRETATION

Active myopathy typical of inclusion body myopathy, considering the previous EMG findings.

OTHER TEST FINDINGS

Muscle biopsy confirmed inclusion body myositis.

FINAL DIAGNOSIS

Inclusion body myositis and asymptomatic diabetic neuropathy

TREATMENT AND FOLLOW-UP

Because of his diabetes mellitus, the patient was treated with azathioprine.

COMMENTS

As predicted by one of the attendings, this patient had all the typical findings of IBM: proximal weakness, thigh atrophy, areflexia, an increased CPK, and a combination of HALD and SASD MUPs (see case 6 in Chapter 11). Quadriceps atrophy and areflexia were tips for a diagnosis of IBM. Because of peripheral neuropathy and polyradiculopathy, polyphasic SASD MUPs were interpreted as a sign of regeneration. Because a combination of polyradiculopathy and peripheral neuropathy is typical of diabetic amyotrophy, it was concluded that this patient had diabetic amyotrophy. We concluded that his peripheral neuropathy was due to diabetes. However, one-third of IBM patients have peripheral neuropathy by NCS. This patient exemplifies a case of myopathy that can be misinterpreted as lumbosacral polyradiculopathy.

TABLE 8.12. Nerve Conduction Data in Case 8

	Latent/NCV (ms/m/s)	Amplitude (mV/μV)		Latent/NCV (ms/m/s)	Amplitu (mV/μV)
	Median	**Motor Nerve**		**Peroneal**	**Motor N**
TL	5.8	4.3	TL	4.6	0.20
E-W	48.2	4.2	FH-A	38.3	0.18
AX-E	50.0	4.2	PF-FH	50.0	0.18
F-wave	36.8			F-wave	NP
	Ulnar	**Motor Nerve**		**Post Tibial**	**Motor N**
TL	3.0	7.8	TL	4.6	0.66
BE-W	50.0	7.8	PF-A	36.0	0.56
AE-BE	39.2	7.8			
AX-AE	75.0	7.8			
F-wave	32.8		F-wave	63.6	
	Median	**Sens/Mixed Nerve**		**Sural**	**Sens Ner**
F-W	NP		MC-A	32.4	3.8
W-E	44.4	14.0			
E-AX	50.0	58.8			
	Ulnar	**Sens/Mixed Nerve**		**Superficial Peroneal**	**Sens Ner**
F-W	37.5	5.6	MC-A	NP	
W-E	46.5	8.8			
E-AX	39.4	7.2			

Height: 182.9 cm.
E, elbow; W, wrist; AX, Axilla; F, finger.

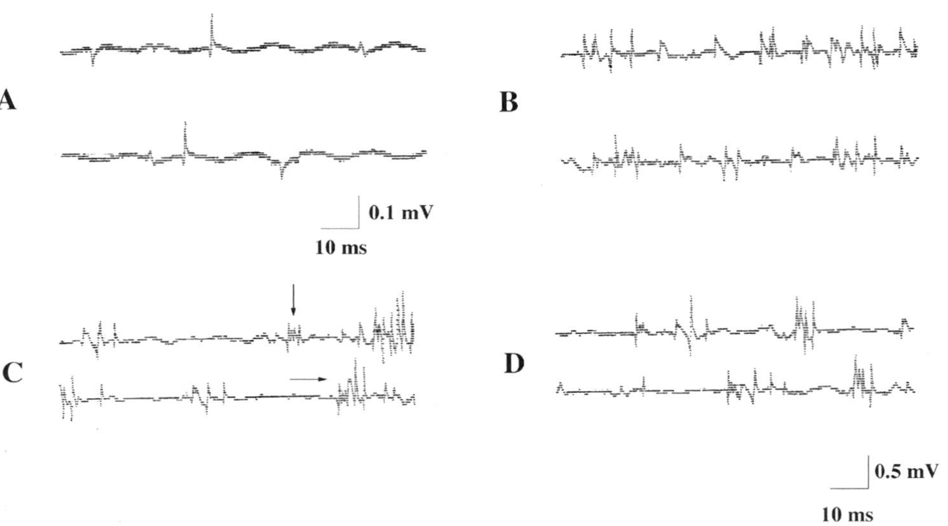

FIGURE 8.14. Typical myopathic EMG pattern in the second EMG study in the rectus femoris muscle. **A.** Fibrillations and PSWs. **B.** Many simple and polyphasic SASD MUPs with early recruitment. **C.** A *downward arrow* indicates one polyphasic SASD MUP and a *sideward arrow*, polyphasic MUP with normal duration. **D.** Combination of many SASD MUPs and polyphasic MUPs with normal duration.

Multiple lumbosacral radiculopathies in the EMG can be observed classically in lumbar stenosis, as discussed in case 6. However, such findings can also represent a diabetic radiculopathy including diabetic amyotrophy, demyelinating peripheral neuropathy, metastatic disease, motor neuron disease, the neuronal type of Charcot-Marie-Tooth disease, and active myopathy. In classic "dying-back axonal neuropathy," the sural nerve conduction is abnormal and paraspinal EMG is normal. In demyelinating neuropathies such as CIDP, the paraspinal EMG is often involved, showing fibrillations and PSWs, but the sural nerve conduction is abnormal. Diabetes mellitus is notorious in involving roots producing polyradiculopathy. Polyradiculopathy in relation to metastatic disease has already been discussed in case 7.

Another entity that can be mistaken for multiple bilateral lumbosacral radiculopathy is motor neuron disease. Although ALS classically starts with weakness and wasting of the upper extremities, there is a small number of patients whose symptoms begin in the lower extremities. This disorder is purely motor and is often accompanied by hyperreflexia. In ALS, much more florid EMG evidence of active denervation and fasciculation is seen. Spinal muscular atrophy, a form of motor neuron disease, and the neuronal type of Charcot-Marie-Tooth disease are other entities that can produce a lumbosacral polyradiculopathy EMG pattern. As noted in our case, active myopathy including IBM should be considered as another possibility that can be mistaken for polyradiculopathy. In these cases, SASD MUPs are critical in differentiating between polyradiculopathy and myopathy. In IBM, this differentiation is more difficult because of the mixed pattern of MUPs seen in one-third of cases including the present one.

MAXIMS

1. A polyradiculopathy EMG pattern, a classic EMG pattern of multiple level disc diseases, can be seen in metastatic disease, peripheral neuropathy, motor neuron disease, and active myopathy.
2. Quadriceps and forearm flexor atrophy is common in inclusion body myopathy.

REFERENCES

1. Joy JL, Oh SJ, Baysal AL. Electrophysiological spectrum of inclusion body myositis. Muscle Nerve 1990;13:949–951.
2. Wilbourn AJ, Aminoff MJ. AAEE Minimonograph #32. The electrophysiological examination in patients with radiculopathies. Muscle Nerve 1988;11:1099–1114.

CASE 9

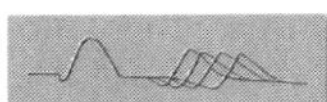

NORMAL PARASPINAL EMG IN A PATIENT WITH SUSPECTED DIABETIC RADICULOPATHY

CASE PRESENTATION

A 55-year-old woman with a history of noninsulin-dependent diabetes mellitus for 16 years had experienced epigastric pain beginning at the midline and radiating laterally beneath the left breast toward the flank and midback. This pain was described as a constant, dull ache with intermittent episodes of sharper discomfort. It was not associated with any other GI symptoms. All GI workups including endoscopy were negative. MRI of the thoracolumbar cord was also normal. Needle EMG study in the left thoracic paraspinal muscles performed by the local neurologist was normal. The patient was referred to us for further study. Neurological evaluation was completely normal, including pinprick and touch examination over the left T6-10 dermatome areas. No tenderness was noted in the rectus abdominalis muscles.

CASE ANALYSIS

Because thoracic radiculopathy is not uncommon in long-term diabetics, this should be suspected. The lack of any obvious demonstrable sensory loss even in the involved area in this case was not unexpected in diabetic thoracic radiculopathy. The local neurologist was not able to confirm thoracic radiculopathy, possibly due to the inherent technical difficulty of performing the needle EMG in thoracic paraspinal muscles. Thus, we had to repeat the needle EMG study in the left thoracic paraspinal muscles.

PLAN OF TESTING

1. NCS: To document diabetic neuropathy.
2. Needle EMG: To document thoracic radiculopathy.

ELECTROPHYSIOLOGICAL TESTS AND FINDINGS

NCS Findings. Normal motor, sensory, and mixed NCS in all tested nerves.

Needle EMG (Table 8.13; Fig. 8.15)

1. No fibrillations or PSW in the left T5-T12 paraspinal muscles.
2. Prominent fibrillations and/or PSW in the left rectus abdominalis and T6-L1 paraspinal muscles.

ELECTROPHYSIOLOGICAL INTERPRETATION

Compatible with left T6-L1 intercostal neuropathy or T6-L1 radiculopathy.

FINAL DIAGNOSIS

Diabetic left thoracic radiculopathy

TREATMENT AND FOLLOW-UP

The patient's pain was partially relieved with Elavil and Neurontin.

COMMENTS

In this patient, we were not able to find any fibrillations or PSW in thoracic paraspinal muscles even in the relaxed state. Thus, the rectus abdominalis was examined and confirmed the denervation in the rectus abdominalis muscles. In view of the absence of fibrillation and PSW in paraspinal muscles, these findings were not indicative of thoracic radiculopathy. These findings were certainly compatible with thoracic intercostal neuropathy. Because we do not have a practically applicable intercostal nerve conduction method, we could not resolve this issue.

The needle EMG study in thoracic paraspinal muscles is most difficult because of the inherent difficulty of relaxation of these muscles. The best position for testing of the thoracic paraspinal muscles is with the patient lying on the table on the side to be tested downward, in contrast to the recommended position for testing of the cervical and lumbar paraspinal

TABLE 8.13. Needle EMG Data in Case 9

				Spontaneous Potentials				Motor Unit Potential				Interference	
Muscle	Root	Nerve	Insertion Activity	Fib	PSW	Fasc	Myotonia BHFD	Amplitude (K)	Duration (ms)	Polyphasic Potential	Giant MUP	Pattern	Mean Amplitude (K)
Lt T5-12 paraspinal	T5-12		N	–	–	–	–						
Rectus abd T6	T6	IC T6	+	–	+	–	–	0.5–2	6–12	+	–		
Rectus abd T7	T7	IC T7	+	+	+++	–	–	0.5–1.5	6–10	+	–		
Rectus abd T8-12	T8-12	IC T8-12	+	–	+++	–	–	0.5–2.0	6–14	+	–		
Rectus abd L1	L1	IC L1	+	–	++	–	–	0.5–1.0	8–15	N	–		

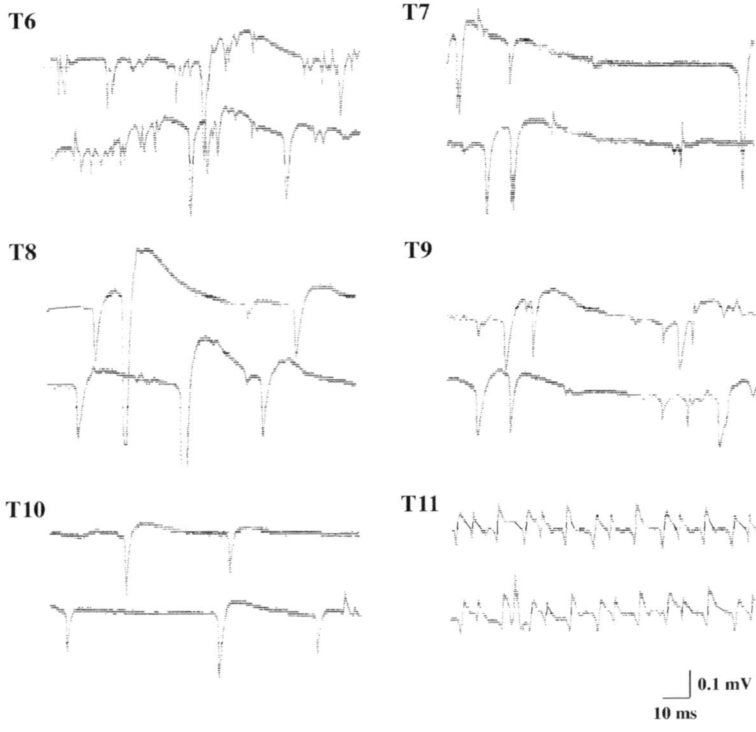

FIGURE 8.15. Fibrillations and PSWs in the rectus abdominalis muscle innervated by T6-11.

muscle where the patient lies with the side to be tested uppermost.

The needle EMG test is essentially the sole means of identifying diabetic thoracic radiculopathy. Fibrillation and PSWs are typically found in the involved thoracic paraspinal muscles but usually in multiple contiguous segments beyond the clinically involved segment. Sometimes they are observed in paraspinal muscles corresponding almost exactly to the area of maximal pain. Fibrillations are observed on both sides of the spine in most patients. Thus, the characteristics of diabetic thoracic radiculopathy is "polyradiculopathy" beyond the clinically suspected area, as seen in this patient. This is an example of EMG overload syndrome.

Because of the inherent difficulty of relaxation of the thoracic paraspinal muscles, Streib et al. recommended the needle EMG in the abdominal muscles in patients suspected of having diabetic thoracic radiculopathy; in three cases in which the thoracic needle EMG was impossible because of poor relaxation, the needle EMG in the abdominal muscles showed abnormalities, identifying diabetic thoracic radiculopathy. Concomitant polyneuropathy has been reported in 33 to 75% of patients with diabetic thoracic radiculopathy.

MAXIMS

1. The needle EMG test is essentially the sole means of identifying diabetic thoracic radiculopathy. Polyradiculopathy is the characteristic finding in diabetic radiculopathy.
2. The rectus abdominals muscle should be examined in patients suspected of having diabetic thoracic radiculopathy if the paraspinal muscles are normal.

REFERENCES

1. Sun SF, Streib EW. Diabetic thoraco-abdominal neuropathy: clinical and electrodiagnostic features. Ann Neurol 1981;9:75–79.
2. Streib EF, Sun SF, Paustian FF et al. Diabetic thoracic radiculopathy: electrodiagnostic study. Muscle Nerve 1986;9:548–553.

CASE 10

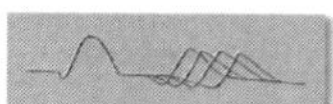

BELL'S PALSY FOLLOWED BY THORACIC RADICULOPATHY

CASE PRESENTATION

A 58-year-old woman began to notice pain in the left midthoracic area of the back radiating around to the abdomen about 4 months ago, followed shortly thereafter by right midthoracic pain that radiated to the abdomen. The pain was described as sharp and constant without any apparent alleviating or aggravating factors. Three months ago, she also developed a left Bell's palsy that improved spontaneously over the course of 4 weeks. One month ago, she developed a right Bell's palsy for which 40 mg of prednisone was given, with dramatic improvement of pain over the back area for 5 days. The pain returned with cessation of prednisone. The needle EMG study performed by a referring neurologist documented multiple thoracic radiculopathy. There was no history of weight loss or shingles. Past history was noncontributory except for gastric bleeding due to ulcers. Abnormal neurological findings were peripheral right facial paresis, hyperesthesia on the right and left T9-T12 dermatomes, and decreased ankle reflexes.

CASE ANALYSIS

This patient had bilateral thoracoradiculopathy associated with alternating left and right Bell's palsy. This history is thought to be typical of Lyme disease, which should be the diagnosis until proven otherwise. However, there was no history of travel to a Lyme disease endemic area or of chronic erythema migrans. Other possibilities included diabetes mellitus, sarcoidosis, lymphoma, and a motor sensory demyelinating mononeuropathy multiplex (multifocal demyelinating motor and sensory neuropathy).

PLAN OF TESTING

1. Needle EMG: To confirm the extent of radiculopathy.
2. NCS: To see whether this represented a radiculoneuropathy.
3. Other tests: Cerebrospinal fluid including cytospin. Myelogram.

ELECTROPHYSIOLOGICAL TESTS AND FINDINGS

NCS Findings (Table 8.14)

1. Mild slowing in motor and sensory NCV in the distal segments of almost all tested nerves.
2. Mildly prolonged terminal latency and F-wave latencies in the peroneal and posterior tibial nerves.
3. Moderately slow NCV in the sural nerve.

Needle EMG (Table 8.15; Fig. 8.16)

1. Prominent fibrillations and PSWs in the right and left T7-T12 and right L3-5 S1 paraspinal muscles.
2. Minimal fibrillations and PSWs in the gluteus medius and maximus muscles.

ELECTROPHYSIOLOGICAL INTERPRETATION

Thoracolumbar polyradiculopathy and mild peripheral neuropathy with some suggestion of demyelination.

OTHER TEST FINDINGS

CSF protein of 61 mg/dL with 3 WBC/mm^3 and normal glucose. No malignant cells were found. Normal Lyme titer, angiotensin-converting enzyme, GTT, myelogram, and muscle biopsy. Nerve biopsy showed minimal demyelinating neuropathy.

FINAL DIAGNOSIS

MSDMM

TABLE 8.14. Nerve Conduction Data in Case 10

	Latent/NCV (ms/m/s)	Amplitude (mV/μV)		Latent/NCV (ms/m/s)	Amplitude (mV/μV)
	Median	**Motor Nerve**		**Peroneal**	**Motor Nerve**
TL	3.6	8.2	TL	7.8	4.2
E-W	48.6	8.0	FH-A	34.2	4.1
AX-E	55.5	8.0	PF-FH	44.1	4.0
F-wave	30.0		F-wave	66.4	
	Ulnar	**Motor Nerve**		**Post Tibial**	**Motor Nerve**
TL	2.8	10.2	TL	7.5	3.8
BE-W	30.4	9.5	PF-A	31.1	3.0
AE-BE	52.3	9.4			
AX-AE	62.5	9.0			
F-wave	30.4		F-wave	69.6	
	Median	**Sens/Mixed Nerve**		**Sural**	**Sens Nerve**
F-W	35.8	22	MC-A	23.7	3.2
W-E	48.6	32			
E-AX	62.3	40			
	Ulnar	**Sens/Mixed Nerve**		**Plantar**	**Sens Nerve**
F-W	38.1	21	Medial		
W-E	48.0	35	Lateral		
E-AX	60.2	38			

Height: 167.2 cm.

TREATMENT AND FOLLOW-UP

The patient was treated with prednisone for 1.6 years with one relapse, and her radiculopathy was completely cured. Six years later, she again came to the clinic with complaints of back pain. Studies did not show any sign of recurrence of radiculopathy but just lumbar strain.

COMMENTS

Even though the history and findings are so classical for Lyme disease, this was ruled out by negative serological titer. Diabetes mellitus and sarcoidosis were also ruled out by the appropriate tests. In view of her polyradiculopathy, mildly high CSF protein, and neuropathy by NCS, the diagnosis of chronic polyradiculoneuropathy was justified. This is the term originally used by Dyck in describing CIDP. There were three pieces of NCS data that suggested the possibility of demyelination: sural NCV of 23.7 m/s and terminal latencies of 7.5 ms in the peroneal and posterior tibial nerves. Sural nerve biopsy confirmed a mild demyelinating neuropathy in this patient. It is extremely unusual for CIDP to have facial paresis as an initial symptom and thoracic radiculopathy as the predominant symptom. This patient had all the typical findings of MSDMM: motor and sensory mononeuropathy multiplex, demyelinating nerve conduction data, high CSF protein, and demyelination in the sural nerve biopsy, which was recently reported by us. The patient was treated successfully with steroids (see case 3 in Chapter 9).

Lyme disease is a systemic illness caused by the tick-borne spirochete *Borrelia burgdoferi*. Neuropathy occurs in 36 to 40% of patients with symptomatic late Lyme disease. In Europe, the name Garin-Boujadoux or Barnwarth syndrome is used to describe the presence of a neurological triad of lymphocytic meningitis, cranial neuritis, and radiculoneuritis that follows days to weeks after erythema chronicum migrans spreading from the bitten area, the pathognomonic marker of this disease. Sural nerve biopsy in this disorder is characterized by perivascular collections of inflammatory cells and axonal degeneration in a majority of cases. Neurop-

TABLE 8.15. Needle EMG Data in Case 10

				Spontaneous Potentials				Motor Unit Potential				Interference	
Muscle	**Root**	**Nerve**	**Insertion Activity**	**Fib**	**PSW**	**Fasc**	**Myotonia CRD**	**Amplitude (K)**	**Duration (ms)**	**Polyphasic Potential**	**HA MUP**	**Pattern**	**Mean Amplitude (K)**
Rt T7-12	T7-12		+	+	+	–	–						
Lt T7-12	T7-12		+	+++	++++	–	–						
Rt L3-4	L3-4		+	+++	+++	–	–						
Rt L5, S1	L5, S1		+	++	++	–	–						
Glut med	L5, S1	Sup glut	+	+	–	–	–	1–4	10–15	+	–	RIP	1.5
Glut max	S1,2	Inf glut	N	–	–	–	–	1–2	10–15	+	–	RIP	1.5
Vast lat	L3,4	Femoral	N	–	–	–	–	1–2	10–15	+	–	FIP	1.5
Ant tibial	L4,5	Peroneal	N	–	–	–	–	0.8–2	8–15	N	–	FIP	1.5
Gastroc	S1,2	Post tibial	N	–	–	–	–	0.7–2	8–15	N	–	FIP	1.5

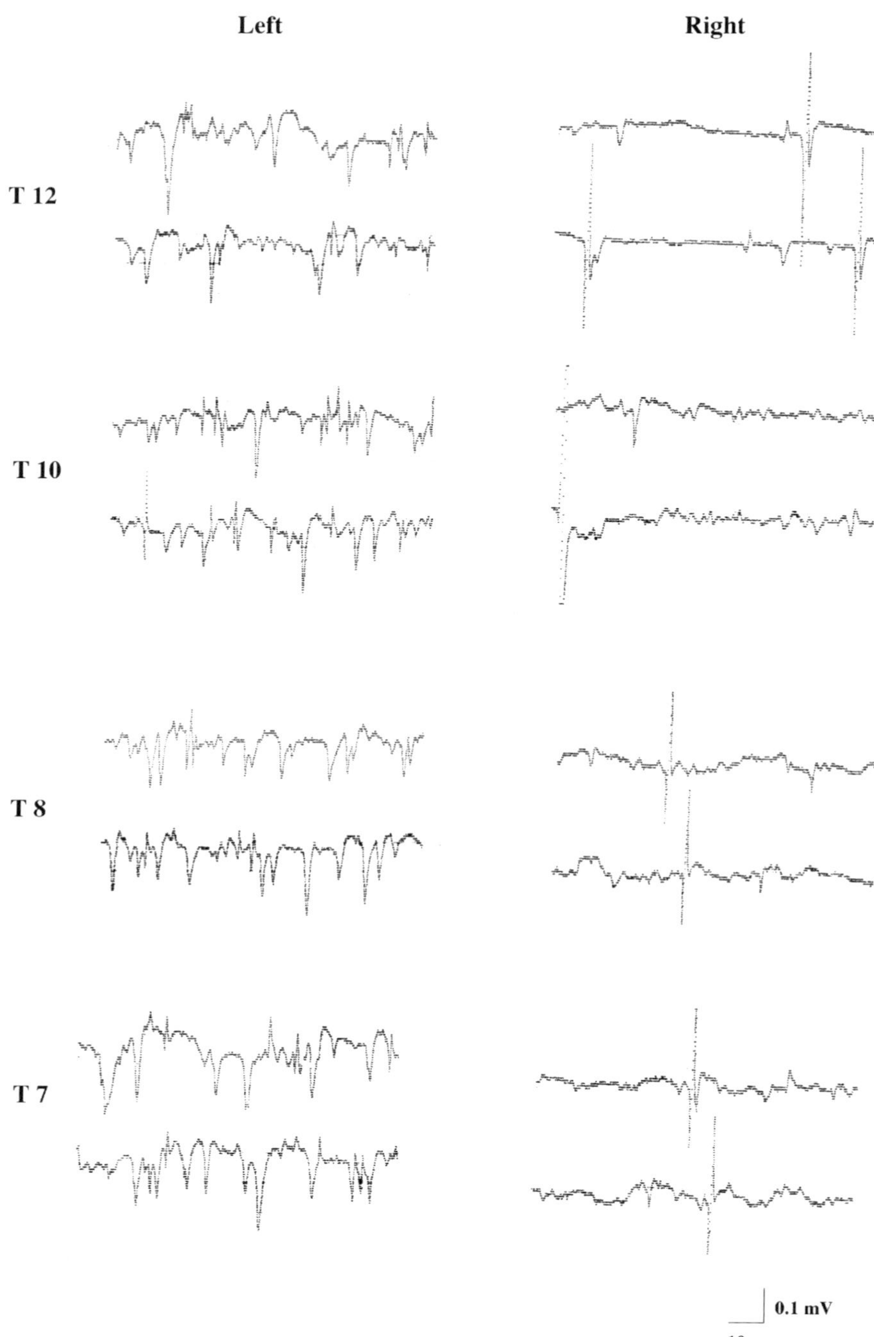

FIGURE 8.16. Fibrillations and PSWs in the right and left *T7*, *8*, *10*, and *12* paraspinal muscles.

athy in Lyme disease can be loosely divided into acute and chronic Lyme neuropathy. Lyme neuropathy can present in three distinct patterns: cranial neuropathy, painful radiculopathy, and peripheral neuropathy. Cranial neuropathy occurs early in the disease and can affect any cranial nerve. However, facial palsy is most common and often occurs bilaterally. Radiculopathy is usually painful and can involve the thoracic and the cervical and lumbar areas. Peripheral neuropathy is usually characterized by nonpainful intermittent paresthesia and asymmetrical distribution. If some of these features are combined, then the clinical presentation is typical of mononeuropathy multiplex. Motor weakness or hyporeflexia is rare. According to Halperin et al., sensory neuropathy is the most common form of Lyme neuropathy, followed by painful radiculopathy and Bell's palsy. In Barnwarth syndrome, lymphocytic pleocytosis, often with elevated protein, is a uniform finding in the spinal fluid. In chronic Lyme neuropathy, a high protein is the most common abnormality in the spinal fluid. Electrophysiological findings in Lyme neuropathy are as follows: in Barnwarth syndrome, facial nerve latency is abnormal in most cases: in three of four tested cases, the facial nerve latency was abnormal; in polyradiculopathy, the needle EMG showed denervation in paraspinal and limb muscles; and in sensory neuropathy, sensory conduction abnormalities are the characteristic finding: NCV is slow and CNAP amplitude is reduced. In motor nerve conduction, terminal latencies and late responses were the values most likely to be affected. Nerve conduction abnormalities were usually minimal and not seen in all nerves but rather were scattered. Despite the broad clinical spectrum of presenting manifestations, the nerve conduction and needle EMG abnormalities were surprisingly uniform in frequency and distribution, being found in both paraspinal and limb muscles.

MAXIMS

1. NCV below 60% of normal means and terminal latencies above 150% of normal means are indicative of demyelination.
2. The clinical triad of Lyme disease is cranial neuropathy, polyradiculopathy, and aseptic meningitis.

REFERENCES

1. Oh SJ, Claussen GC, Kim DS. Motor and sensory demyelinating mononeuropathy multiplex (multifocal motor and sensory demyelinating neuropathy): a separate entity or a variant of chronic inflammatory demyelinating polyneuropathy? JPNS 1997;2:362–369.
2. Logigian EL, Steere AC. Clinical and electrophysiological findings in chronic neuropathy of Lyme disease. Neurology 1992;42:303–311.

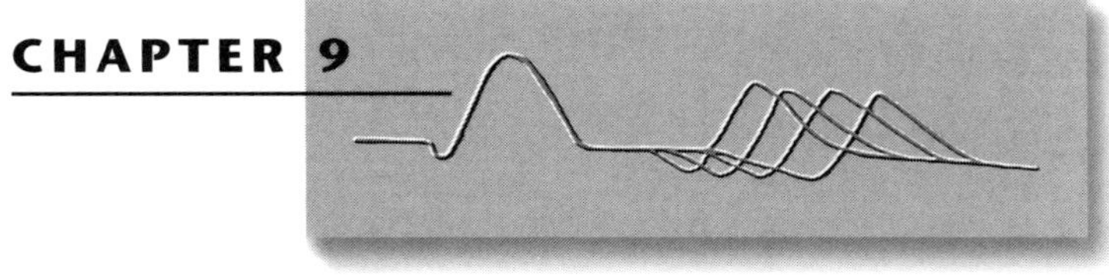

CHAPTER 9

Polyneuropathy

Peripheral neuropathy is produced by a disease process of the peripheral nerves with clinical manifestation of flaccid weakness, impairment of sensation, loss of muscle stretch reflexes, and atrophy.

CLASSIFICATION OF PERIPHERAL NEUROPATHY

There are two major anatomical components in peripheral nerve: axon and myelin. Of the two major components, myelin is the most effective in conduction of action potential. This is due to saltatory conduction of myelinated fibers.

Depending on which component of peripheral nerve is predominantly involved, the pathological process of neuropathy can be classified into two main categories: axonal degeneration and segmental demyelination. There are also clear pathophysiological differences between axonal degeneration and segmental demyelination, as noted in Table 3.5.

Thus, it is logical to classify peripheral neuropathy into two major types: axonal neuropathy with predominant axonal degeneration and demyelinating neuropathy with predominant segmental demyelination (see Table 3.5).

ETIOLOGIES OF PERIPHERAL NEUROPATHY

The most common known cause of peripheral neuropathy in the United States is diabetes mellitus, followed by chronic alcoholism, whereas in the world as a whole it is leprosy. For neurology patients, the most common cause of peripheral neuropathy is the Guillain-Barré syndrome (GBS). Despite extensive and costly evaluations, the causes of peripheral neuropathy remain unknown in a substantial number of cases. In two recent studies in the 1980s, the causes were undetermined in only 13 to 24% of cases. These figures were reported from centers where the sural nerve biopsy is extensively used in identifying the cause of peripheral neuropathy. Compared with 70 to 52% in 1960s, the frequency of unknown causes has decreased over the years. This decrease is mainly due to four factors: greater sophistication of the electrophysiological study in differentiation between axonal neuropathy and demyelinating neuropathy, classification of inflammatory neuropathies such as GBS as a "known" cause, monoclonal gammopathy and paraneoplastic neuropathy as now known causes of some neuropathies, and increasing use of the nerve biopsy in the workup for peripheral neuropathy.

DIAGNOSIS OF PERIPHERAL NEUROPATHY

The first step in the diagnosis of peripheral neuropathy is to rule out other lower motor neuron diseases following the guidelines in Table 11.1. The major manifestations of neuropathy are muscle weakness, sensory loss in all modalities, weak or absent reflexes, and trophic changes. Among these, sensory impairment is the most important clue for peripheral neuropathy.

The second step is to decide what kind of neuropathy the patient has: polyneuropathy, mononeuropathy multiplex, or mononeuropathy. This distinction is important because it suggests the etiology.

Polyneuropathy is a symmetrical, distal, usually ascending neuropathy due to involvement of distal branches of the nerves. Stocking-glove dysesthesia is the classic term describing the distribution of sensory impairments. "Foot drop" is common. Mixed sensorimotor polyneu-

TABLE 9.1. Helpful Tips in Etiological Diagnosis of Peripheral Neuropathy

1. Family history, pes cavus, "stork-leg"	Charcot-Marie-Tooth disease
2. Relapse	Chronic inflammatory demyelinating neuropathy HNPP
3. Acute	GBS, acute intermittent porphyria, diphtheric neuropathy
4. Alopecia, sensory neuropathy	Thallium neuropathy
5. Painful opthalmoplegia with sparing of pupil	Diabetes mellitus
6. Gum lead line, wrist drop	Lead neuropathy
7. Anesthetic depigmented skin	Leprosy
8. Angiokeratoma, sensory neuropathy	Fabry's disease
9. Mee's line, sensory neuropathy, hyperkeratosis of skin	Arsenic neuropathy
10. Femoral neuropathy	Diabetes mellitus
11. Palpable thick nerves	Leprosy, Charcot-Marie-Tooth disease Dejerinne-Sottas disease
12. Charcot-Joint	Diabetes mellitus, leprosy
13. Trophic ulcer, insensitivity to pain	Diabetes mellitus, amyloidosis, leprosy, hereditary sensory neuropathy
14. Dysautonomia	Diabetes mellitus, amyloidosis
15. Kaposi sarcoma, lymphadenopathy	AIDS neuropathy
16. Erythema chronicum migrans, facial palsy	Lyme disease

ropathy suggests nutritional neuropathy (alcoholism, beriberi, vitamin B deficiency, pernicious anemia) and metabolic neuropathy (diabetes mellitus or uremia). Sensory polyneuropathy suggests arsenic or carcinomatous polyneuropathy. Motor polyneuropathy suggests GBS, chronic inflammatory demyelinating neuropathy (CIDP), or multifocal motor neuropathy (MMN).

Mononeuropathy multiplex occurs in two or more nerves in more than one involved extremity (e.g., left ulnar neuropathy and right peroneal neuropathy). This is typically seen in vasculitic neuropathy. Two other causes of mononeuropathy multiplex are leprosy and diabetes mellitus. Rare causes of this disorder include MMN and motor sensory demyelinating mononeuropathy multiplex (multifocal motor sensory demyelinating neuropathy).

In mononeuropathy, the most common cause is entrapment neuropathy due to compression of a nerve in an anatomically narrow area. The best example is carpal tunnel syndrome. Certain mononeuropathy is common to certain diseases: femoral neuropathy and ophthalmoplegic neuropathy with pupil sparing in diabetes mellitus, recurrent or bilateral facial nerve palsy in sarcoidosis and Lyme disease, and radial nerve palsy in lead neuropathy.

The third step is to search for the cause of peripheral neuropathy. A complete history, including any history of drugs or exposure to toxins, and thorough general and neurological examinations are most important in detection of the cause. A partial guide in this regard is given in Table 9.1. These will suggest the need for any special laboratory workup.

NERVE CONDUCTION STUDIES AND NEEDLE ELECTROMYOGRAPHY

The most important test in polyneuropathy is the nerve conduction study (NCS), which is an objective means of confirming peripheral neuropathy, identifying mononeuropathy, and determining the entrapment site in compression neuropathy. Nerve conduction is abnormal in peripheral neuropathy but is normal in myopathy and anterior horn cell disease. It is also helpful in differentiating between axonal neuropathy and demyelinating neuropathy. The hallmark of nerve conduction abnormalities in axonal degeneration is the diminution of the amplitude of the CMAP and CNAP in the presence of normal or near-normal maximal NCVs. On the other hand, the hallmarks of nerve conduction abnormalities in demyelinating neuropathy are conduction block, abnormal temporal dispersion (dispersion phenomenon), and marked slowing in the NCV. NCS can provide a certain pattern of abnormalities specific enough to be of value in localizing the lesions to specific parts of the nerve and in suggesting the nature of a neuropathy, as discussed in Chapter 3. The best example is the pure sensory neuronopathy pattern; the sensory nerve conduction is markedly abnormal, but the motor nerve conduction is completely normal. This pattern is pathognomonic of a sensory neuronopathy involving the dorsal root sensory ganglia.

The needle electromyography (EMG) test is invaluable in ruling out myopathy and in confirming denervation process. In myopathy, MUPs are short in duration and small in amplitude. In denervation process, MUPs are either normal or high in amplitude and long in duration (HALD MUPs). The needle EMG is also helpful in identifying "activity" of neuropathy. In active (ongoing) denervation, fibrillations and positive sharp waves (PSWs) are prominent with increased polyphasic MUPs and reduced MUP recruitment. On the other hand, in inactive (usually chronic) denervation, fibrillations and PSWs are minimal together with HALD MUPs. The needle EMG is also helpful in distinguishing axonal neuropathy from demyelinating neuropathy. Fibrillations and PSWs, electrophysiological hallmarks of axonal degeneration, are prominent in axonal neuropathy but are absent or scarce in demyelinating neuropathy. Fasciculation or myokymia is a more prominent finding in demyelinating neuropathy.

LABORATORY STUDIES

Laboratory tests are most important in finding the etiology of peripheral neuropathy (Table 9.2). The first-line tests should be performed in all patients suspected of peripheral neuropathies. The second-line tests are selected depending on the clinician's suspicion, which is based

TABLE 9.2. Basic Laboratory Tests for Peripheral Neuropathy

Test	Diagnostic Possibilities
First-line tests	
CBC, sedimentation rate	Collagen disease, leukemia, vasculitis
Renal and liver functions	Uremic and hepatic neuropathy
Rheumatoid profiles	Collagen disease, vasculitis
Blood sugar, HbA1C, GTT	Diabetes
Serum B12 and folate level, Schilling test	Neuropathy with macrocytosis
Thyroid functions	Hypothyroid neuropathy
Immunoelectrophoresis of serum protein by immunofixation test	Dysproteinemias, monoclonal gammopathy lymphoma, amyloidosis
Second-line tests	
Porphobilinogen in urine	Acute porphyria
Heavy metals in urine	Lead, arsenic, thallium, mercury
Arsenic in hair and nails	Arsenic neuropathy
Hepatitis B antigen	Polyarteritis nodosa
Antineutrophile cytoplasmic antibody	Wegener's granulomatosis
CT scan of chest, cancer survey	Carcinomatous neuropathy
High CSF protein	GBS, CIDP
Increase cell in CSF	Lyme disease; AIDS, paraneoplastic neuropathy
Serum HIV antibody	AIDS neuropathy
Serum Borellia Burgdoferri antibody	Lyme disease
Metastatic bone survey	Sclerotic multiple myeloma
Anti-Hu antibody	Paraneoplastic neuropathy
GM_1 and MAG antibody	Autoimmune neuropathy
CMT1A DNA duplication test	CMT 1A disease
HNPP DNA deletion test	HNPP

on clinical, electrophysiological, and laboratory data. For example, if monoclonal gammopathy is found in the serum of patient, then a metastatic bone survey and 24-hour urine immunoelectrophoresis by immunofixation are ordered to differentiate benign monoclonal gammopathy from malignant gammopathy.

NERVE BIOPSY

The most common nerve for biopsy is the sural nerve. When the sural nerve conduction is normal, the superficial peroneal or radial nerve is biopsied in rare cases. Etiological diagnosis can be made by sural nerve biopsy in vasculitis, amyloidosis, leprosy, sarcoidosis, hypertrophic, inflammatory, and tomaculous neuropathies. The nerve biopsy is clearly indicated in two groups of patients: those suspected of vasculitis and those with clinically significant peripheral neuropathy without known cause. The sural nerve biopsy is best indicated in patients suspected of having vasculitis, with or without the clinical features of neuropathy. This is because the nerve is more commonly involved than other readily available biopsied tissues, such as skin and muscle, and the diagnostic yield of the sural nerve biopsy is high in vasculitis. Peripheral neuropathy was reported in 52 to 60% of patients with vasculitis. The nerve conduction test was crucial in these patients because it detected neuropathy in asymptomatic patients and because vasculitis was invariably found in the sural nerve when the nerve conduction was abnormal. The reason for indication of the sural nerve biopsy in neuropathy without known cause is obvious, because a definite diagnosis and other clinically helpful information can be obtained in some patients. Based on data obtained in 385 sural nerve biopsies, we found clinically helpful or relevant information in 45% of the cases. Specific diagnoses were obtained in 24% of cases; diagnosis of subacute or chronic inflammatory neuropathy was confirmed in 12%, and hereditary neuropathy was diagnosed in 9% of cases. Among the specific diagnoses, vasculitic neuropathy was the most common form of neuropathy, accounting for 12% of 385 nerve biopsies. Once a specific diagnosis is made, it dictates the clinical management of the disorder. This is best exemplified in vasculitic neuropathy where steroid and cytotoxic agents are very helpful in inducing remission. In subacute or chronic inflammatory neuropathy, long-term steroid treatment, often for many years, is required. Thus, it is essential to confirm such diagnoses by the nerve biopsy before steroid is administered. Confirmation of hereditary neuropathy is helpful in predicting the progression of disease and in genetic counseling of patients. This outlook is changed now because of the easy availability of CMT1A and HNNP DNA testing. The nerve biopsy was not clinically helpful in 55% of cases.

Again, it is important to recognize that in only 24% of cases were specific diagnoses made. In 55% of cases, the diagnosis of demyelinating or axonal neuropathy was made without further elucidation of any specific cause. In these cases, the nerve biopsy findings have to be correlated with the clinical information to reach a final diagnosis. This underlines the importance of exhaustive and detailed clinical examinations in the workup of neuropathy.

CASE 1

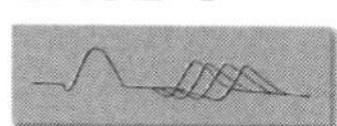

ACUTE WEAKNESS IN THE LEGS FOR 5 DAYS IN A TWO-AND-A-HALF-YEAR-OLD BOY

CASE PRESENTATION

A two-and-a-half-year-old boy was in good health until 5 days before admission, when he refused to walk and had a temperature of 100 F. He was evaluated by his pediatrician, who placed him on amoxicillin for otitis media. On the day of admission, he became very irritable, complained of "hurting all over," and could not stand by himself. Vital signs were normal. Examination showed an alert boy who could not sit or stand without support with a slight left facial droop, neck stiffness, decreased tone, absent reflexes, poor head control, and a hoarse voice. Pin-prick response was normal. Cerebrospinal fluid on the day of admission showed 26 WBC (predominantly lymphocytes)/mm^3, 436 mg/dL protein, and normal glucose.

CASE ANALYSIS

In the days of polio, this patient's first diagnosis would have been poliomyelitis: acute weakness with a fever, pleocytosis, and elevated protein in CSF. At present, however, poliomyelitis is almost nonexistent in the United States. Other diagnostic possibilities had to be considered: myasthenia gravis, GBS, and botulism. Absent reflexes were clearly suggestive of the latter two possibilities. The lack of oculobulbar signs was a strong point against botulism. GBS was a definite possibility, but CSF findings were atypical in view of the mild pleocytosis. GBS had to be confirmed by NCS and a repeat study of CSF.

PLAN OF TESTING

1. NCS: This is a critical test to rule out or confirm GBS.
2. Other tests: Another CSF evaluation.

ELECTROPHYSIOLOGICAL TESTS AND FINDINGS

NCS on Hospital Day 7 (Table 9.3; Fig. 9.1)

1. Markedly prolonged terminal latency and markedly slow NCV in all nerve tested.
2. Conduction block and marked temporal dispersion.

TABLE 9.3. Nerve Conduction Data in Case 1

	Latent/NCV (ms/m/s)	Amplitude (mV/μV)	Shape		Latent/NCV (ms/m/s)	Amplitude (mV/μV)	Shape
	Median	**Motor**	**Nerve**		**Peroneal**	**Motor**	**Nerve**
TL	17.2	0.6	D	TL	8.1	0.4	N
E-W	2.8	0.4	D	FH-A	21.2	0.09	CB
AX-E	10.0	0.1	D	PF-FH			
F-wave	NP			F-wave	NP		
	Ulnar	**Motor**	**Nerve**		**Post Tibial**	**Motor**	**Nerve**
TL	6.0	0.15	D	TL	12.2	0.3	D
BE-W	14.2	0.3	D	PF-A	20.4	0.12	CB
AE-BE	6.0	0.3	D				
F-wave	NP			F-wave	NP		
	Median	**Sens/Mixed**	**Nerve**		**Sural**	**Sens**	**Nerve**
F-W	NP			MC-A	NP		
	Ulnar	**Sens/Mixed**	**Nerve**		**Facial**	**Motor**	**Nerve**
F-W	NP			TL	16.3	0.8	

TL, terminal latency; E, elbow; W, wrist; AX, axilla; BE, below elbow; AE, above elbow; F, finger; FH, fibula head; A, ankle; ML, mid-calf; NP, no potential; Sens, sensory; N, normal; D, dispersion; CB, conduction block.

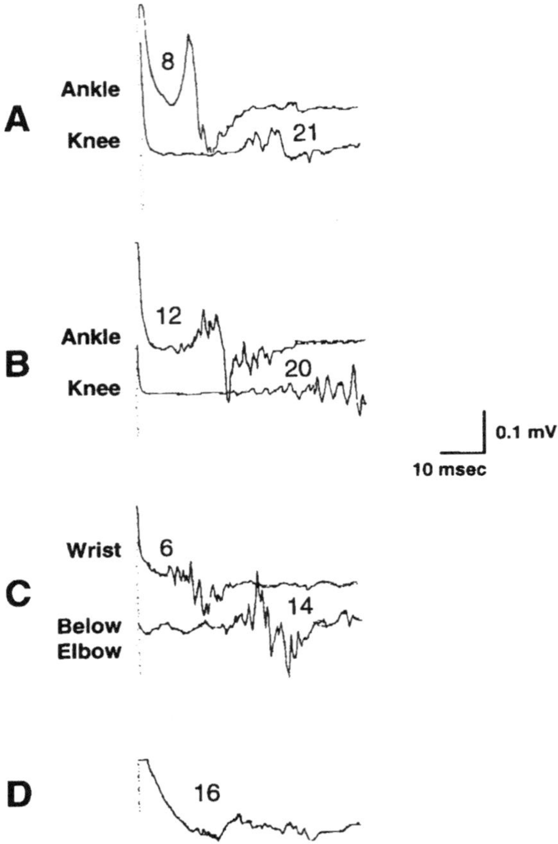

FIGURE 9.1. Conduction block. **A** and **B.** Abnormal temporal dispersion and slow NCVs typical of acquired demyelinating neuropathy in the GBS. Low CMAP amplitudes are also obvious. **A.** Peroneal nerve. **B.** Posterior tibial nerve. **C.** Ulnar nerve. **D.** Facial nerve. Numbers on the left represent the terminal latencies in ms. Numbers on the right represent the NCVs by m/s.

3. Markedly prolonged terminal latency in the facial nerve.
4. Absent sensory CNAP in median, ulnar, and sural nerves.

ELECTROPHYSIOLOGICAL INTERPRETATION

Demyelinating neuropathy typical of GBS.

OTHER TEST FINDINGS

CSF on day 5 of admission showed 6 WBC/mm^3 and 400 mg/dL protein.

FINAL DIAGNOSIS

GBS

TREATMENT AND FOLLOW-UP

The child's weakness did not progress and he experienced no respiratory failure. Treatment was supportive. The patient was discharged on hospital day 17 with a stronger voice, improved head control, and some movement in the lower extremities. Over the next 6 months, he gradually regained his lost muscle strength.

COMMENTS

GBS is an acutely evolving areflexic and usually symmetrical neuropathy that is commonly associated with antecedent infection and a high CSF protein and that reaches its maximum severity within 4 weeks. The mandatory diagnostic criteria of GBS include a progressive motor weakness of more than one limb, areflexia, and maximum severity within 4 weeks. Supportive diagnostic criteria include elevated spinal fluid protein with 10 or fewer cells/mm^3 and nerve conduction evidence of demyelination. An antecedent event is evident within 1 month in 70% of cases, most commonly a respiratory tract infection or gastroenteritis. GBS has been associated with AIDS, Lyme disease, Hodgkin's disease, and non-Hodgkin's lymphoma. The pathological changes in the peripheral nerves in GBS are those of primary demyelination and endoneurial inflammatory cells. In recent years, the concept of GBS has expanded to include acute motor axonal neuropathy and acute motor-sensory axonal neuropathy, and GBS has been classified under two subgroups: demyelinating and axonal forms. Because the classic and most common form of GBS is the demyelinating type, we regard GBS as representing a classic demyelinating neuropathy. In this regard, it is essential to have evidence of demyelination in the NCS as a supportive diagnostic criterion. Recent studies have shown nerve conduction abnormalities in almost all cases and evidence of demyelination in 80% of GBS patients. In a few patients, the NCS in the first week could be normal, and thus it is important to repeat these studies during the following weeks to document demyelination. Demyelination in GBS can be either expressed as marked NCV slowing, temporal dispersion, or conduction block.

The diagnosis of the axonal form of GBS is made typically on the basis of inexcitability of motor nerve fibers and widespread fibrillations within 2 to 5 weeks of onset and very poor recovery in an otherwise classic case of GBS. The pathological studies of one patient who died revealed an acute axonal neuropathy. One has to remember that inexcitability of motor nerve fibers can be due to an extreme distal conduction block. A few recent studies on patients with inexcitability of motor nerve fibers within the first 2 weeks of GBS reported that serial testing is critical in assessing prognosis and that patients who showed an improvement in the second test had a good recovery. Thus, authors concluded that distal conduction block is not uncommon in GBS and that "axonal changes" in such patients are due to distal conduction block. On this basis, they challenged the notion that inexcitability of motor nerves and low CMAP amplitude are indicative of axonal degeneration and stated that such observations early in the course of disease are not necessarily definite evidence of axonal degeneration. Serum IgG GM1 antibody was reported to be present in 18 to 42% of cases of GBS in recent studies. GBS with serum IgG GM1 antibody was characterized by a predominantly motor neuropathy, axonal neuropathy in the NCS, poor prognosis, and a high association of *Camphobactor jejuni* infection. AMAN is also known to be associated with a high frequency of GM1 antibody and *C. jejuni*.

MAXIMS

1. The classic nerve conduction abnormalities in GBS are marked NCV slowing, temporal dispersion, and/or conduction block typical of a demyelinating neuropathy.
2. Inexcitability of motor nerve fibers is due either to axonal neuropathy or to an extreme distal conduction block.

REFERENCES

1. Albers JW, Kelly JJ. Acquired inflammatory demyelinating polyneuropathies: clinical and electrodiagnostic features. Muscle Nerve 1989;12:435–451.
2. Dyck PJ. Is there an axonal variety of GBS? Neurology 1993;43:1277–1280.

CASE 2

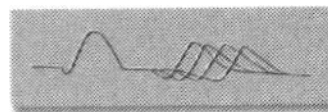

SYMMETRICAL WEAKNESS OF THE ARMS AND LEGS FOR 4 MONTHS

CASE PRESENTATION

In 1973, 4 months before the first evaluation, a 24-year-old woman first noticed weakness of both arms, which had spread to her legs. The patient reported a viral infection 3 weeks before the onset of this weakness. At the time of the first evaluation, she was unable to get up from her chair, climb stairs, button her clothes, or comb her hair but could still walk slowly. With a high spinal fluid protein (173 mg/dL) and NCS abnormalities, she was told that she had chronic GBS. She was treated with high-dose steroids for 2 months with improvement to almost her normal state. With tapering of steroid, however, her weakness recurred in 2 months. This relapse was again treated with high-dose steroids for 3 months with clinical improvement, which lasted about 4 months before she had another relapse of weakness. At that point, the patient was referred to us for further evaluation. Abnormal neurological findings were MRC strength of 2 in hand grip, wrist extensors and flexors, and biceps muscles; 3 in triceps, deltoids, iliopsoas, and gastrocnemius muscles; 4 in quadriceps and hamstring muscles; 0 in anterior tibialis muscles. Reflexes were absent, and the patient walked with footdrop. Occasional fasciculations were visible in the vastus lateralis and deltoid muscles. Sensory evaluation was completely normal.

CASE ANALYSIS

This patient had a rather typical history of CIDP by the present criteria: subacute progression (4 months) of symmetrical motor neuropathy, a high spinal fluid protein, and "demyelinating neuropathy." However, in 1973, the concept of CIDP was not fully understood. With Austin's classic paper on steroid effectiveness in "relapsing neuropathy," continued steroid therapy was thought to be indicated only for relapsing neuropathy. In this case, steroid was used for chronic GBS. The diagnosis of GBS was made in view of a motor neuropathy 3 weeks after an antecedent viral infection and high spinal fluid protein. It was considered to be "chronic" because of 4 months progression of neuropathy. In this case, steroid was effective twice in treating "relapsing neuropathy," for which continued steroid treatment was indicated at that time.

PLAN OF TESTING

1. NCS: To document demyelinating neuropathy.
2. Needle EMG: To see whether secondary axonal changes had occurred.
3. Spinal fluid evaluation and nerve biopsy.

ELECTROPHYSIOLOGICAL TESTS AND FINDINGS

`NCS Findings` (Table 9.4; Fig. 9.2)

1. Prolonged terminal and F-wave latencies and slow motor NCV to the degree of demyelination criteria in many motor nerves.
2. Conduction block and dispersion phenomenon in three of four tested motor nerves.
3. Mild slowing in sensory and mixed NCV and low CNAP amplitude in sensory NCS in median and ulnar nerves.

`Needle EMG` **(Table 9.5; Fig. 9.3).** Rare fibrillations and PSWs, fasciculations, many HALD MUPs (10 to 28 ms; 1 to 12 mV) and discrete activity in most tested muscles.

ELECTROPHYSIOLOGICAL INTERPRETATION

Demyelinating neuropathy typical of CIDP.

OTHER TEST FINDINGS

CSF protein, 240 mg/dL. Nerve biopsy showed demyelinating neuropathy with a few endoneurial inflammatory cells.

FINAL DIAGNOSIS

CIDP

TABLE 9.4. Nerve Conduction Data in Case 2

	Latent/NCV (ms/m/s)	Amplitude (mV/μV)	Shape		Latent/NCV (ms/m/s)	Amplitude (mV/μV)	Shape
	Median	**Motor**	**Nerve**		**Peroneal**	**Motor**	**Nerve**
TL	5.0	7.2		TL	11.5	2.8	
E-W	34.6	2.8	CB	FH-A	18.3	2.0	
AX-E	50.0	2.1	D	PF-FH	19.7	1.4	
F-wave	45.0			F-wave	7.0		
	Ulnar	**Motor**	**Nerve**		**Post Tibial**	**Motor**	**Nerve**
TL	5.5	5.0		TL	7.0	2.0	D
BE-W	24.7	1.4	CB	PF-A	24.6	0.6	CB/D
AE-BE	22.2	1.0	D				
AX-AE	38.7	1.2	D				
F-wave	45.6			F-wave	75		
	Median	**Sens/Mixed**	**Nerve**		**Sural**	**Sens**	**Nerve**
F-W	33.6	15		MC-A	37.4	10	
W-E	42.8	25					
E-AX	48.3	2.5					
	Ulnar	**Sens/Mixed**	**Nerve**		**Plantar**	**Sens**	**Nerve**
F-W	30.3	7.5		Medial			
W-E	35.3	10		Lateral			
E-AX	48.0	5					

Height: 167.6 cm.

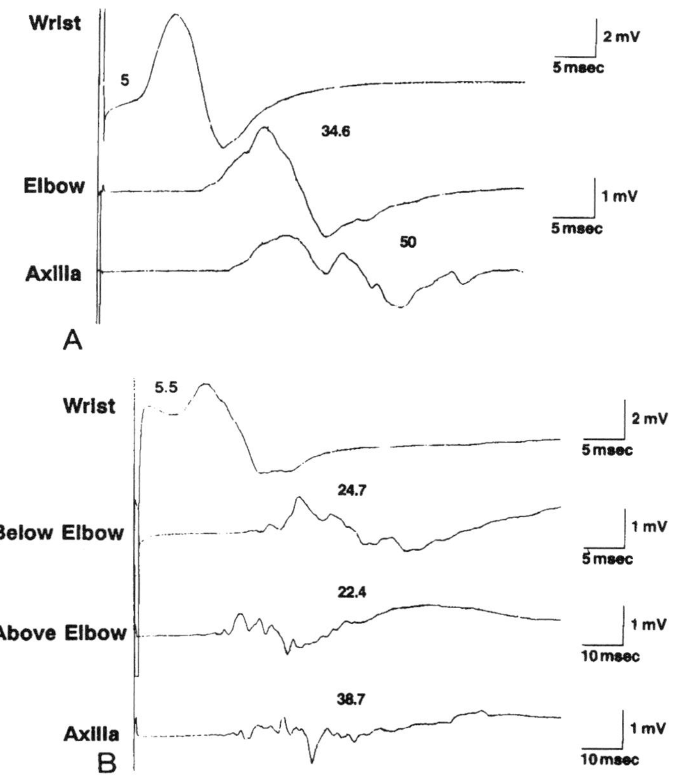

FIGURE 9.2. Conduction block, abnormal temporal dispersion, and nonuniform slowing of NCVs, typical of acquired demyelinating neuropathy, in CIDP. **A.** Median nerve. **B.** Ulnar nerve.

TABLE 9.5. Needle EMG Data in Case 2

				Spontaneous Potentials				Motor Unit Potential				Interference	
Muscle	**Root**	**Nerve**	**Insertion Activity**	**Fib**	**PSW**	**Fasc**	**CRD**	**Amplitude (mV)**	**Duration (ms)**	**Polyphasic Potential**	**HALD MUP**	**Pattern**	**Mean Amplitude (mV)**
Rt biceps	C6,7	Musc cut	+	−	+	+	−	1–6	10–18	N	+	RIP	4
FDI	C8, T1	Ulnar	+	±	−	+	−	1–7	10–21	N	+	DA	5
Vast lat	L3, 4	Femoral	+	−	−	+ +	−	1–10	8–28	N	+ +	DA	7
Ant tibial	L4, 5	Peroneal	+	+	+	+	−	1–8	8–24	N	+ +	DA	6
Gastroc	S1, 2	Post tibial	+	±	+	+	−	1–12	8–20	N	+ +	DA	7

Fib, fibrillations; PSW, positive sharp wave; Fasc, fasciculations; CRD, complex repetitive discharge; HALD, high-amplitude long-duration; RIP, reduced interference pattern; DA, discrete activity; −, absent; +, present or increased; N, normal.

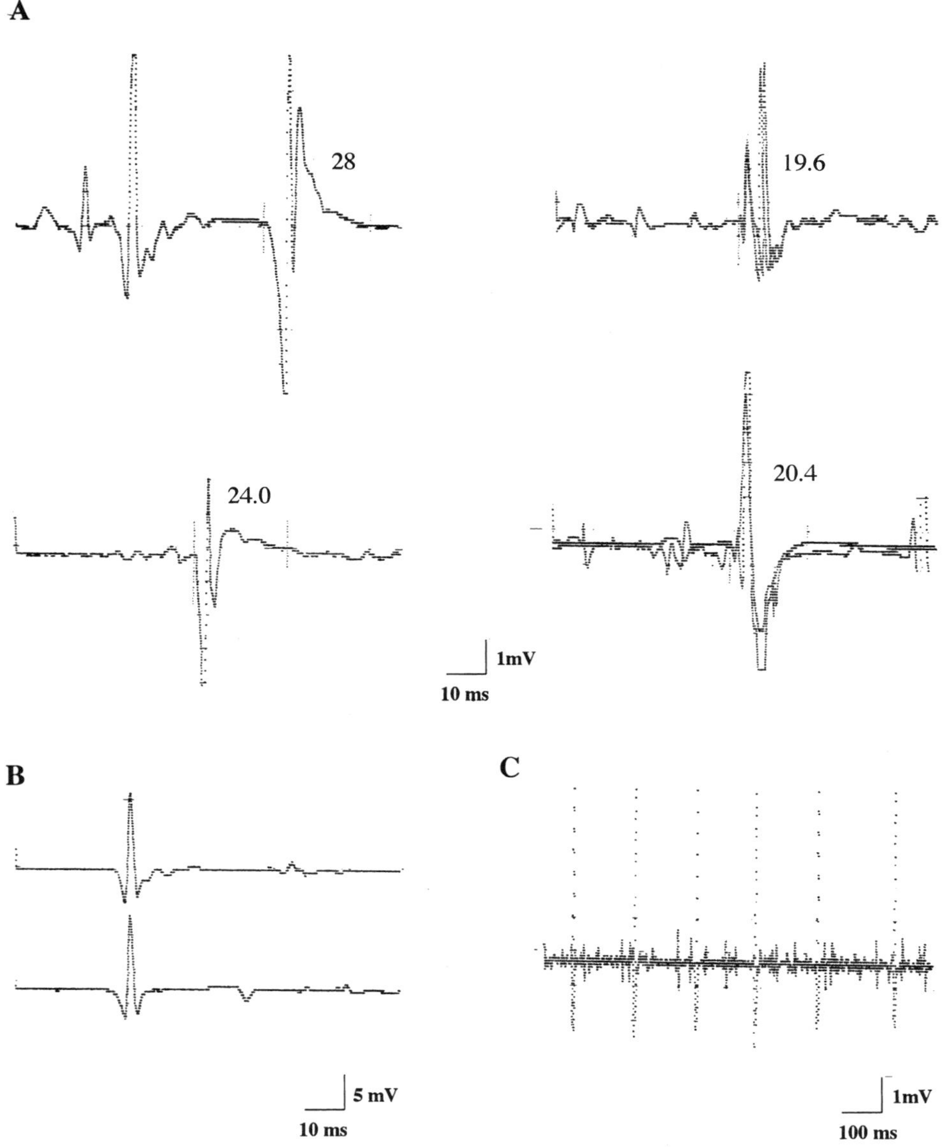

FIGURE 9.3. MUPs from the various muscles. **A.** HALD MUPs. **B.** HA MUP. **C.** Discrete activity. The number above MUPs indicates the duration of MUP by msec.

TREATMENT AND FOLLOW-UP

This patient was followed with continued steroid treatment for more than 20 years. When steroid withdrawal was attempted on several occasions, the patient experienced relapses, with her longest period of remission being 1 year. Plasma exchanges were used twice and IVIg once to reverse her relapses. At the present time, she has been off any medications for 2 years without any relapse. Hopefully, her CIDP is cured. She has not experienced any major side reactions from the long-term steroid treatment.

TABLE 9.6. Differences Between GBS and CIDP

Features	GBS	CIDP
Onset	Acute: maximum deficit < 4 weeks	Subacute; maximum debit in 1–12 mo
Antecedent infection	Present in 70%	Absent
Cranial nerve deficit	Facial palsy common	Rare
Respiratory muscle	Commonly involved	Rare
Nerve conduction study	Markedly slow in 50% of cases Mildly slow in 42% of cases	Markedly slow
Relapse	Rare	Common
Response to steroids	None	Yes
Plasma exchange, IVIg	Effective	Effective

COMMENTS

CIDP is a chronic progressive or relapsing neuropathy that resembles AIDP (GBS). Pathologically it is characterized by demyelinating neuropathy and, in some cases, endoneurial inflammatory cells as noted in GBS. However, CIDP is different from GBS in its subacute progression of polyneuropathy, high rate of relapse, and response to steroid treatment (Table 9.6). The diagnosis of CIDP is based on the typical clinical features of subacute progression of diffuse polyneuropathy, high spinal fluid protein, and marked nerve conduction abnormalities indicative of acquired demyelinating neuropathy. CIDP is known to occur in association with other diseases: AIDS, dysproteinemia, systemic lupus erythematosus, and lymphoma.

The most helpful objective diagnostic finding is the typical pattern of nonuniform demyelinating neuropathy. Without this pattern, it is impossible to make the diagnosis of CIDP. The nerve conduction test in this disorder shows findings typical of extensive segmental demyelination: marked slowing in NCV, conduction block, and dispersion phenomenon. The nerve conduction abnormalities are diffuse, involving the distal and proximal segments of the nerves. All nerves are affected in this disorder, although the degree of abnormality varies from nerve to nerve. Motor nerve conduction is universally abnormal in CIDP, showing evidence of demyelination. Sensory nerve conduction also shows marked abnormalities. Sensory CNAPs are either absent or low in amplitude, and the F-wave and H-reflex are either absent or markedly prolonged in latencies. Compared with GBS, CIDP is characterized by more typical evidence of demyelination. In this case, unlike the classic cases of CIDP, sensory nerve conduction was relatively less affected. In small numbers of GBS and CIDP patients, motor fibers may be affected predominantly. Needle EMG findings in this case is typical of chronic demyelinating neuropathy: scarce or absent fibrillation and PSWs, fasciculations, and HALD MUPs.

CIDP is the second most common type of neuropathy after distal sensory axonal neuropathy in AIDS. Peripheral neuropathy is one of the most common neurological manifestations of AIDS. It may occur in as many as 20% of these patients and in all stages of AIDS infections. Four distinct types of peripheral neuropathy are observed: predominantly sensory neuropathy, the most common; acute or chronic inflammatory demyelinating neuropathy; mononeuritis multiplex due to vasculitis; and lumbosacral polyradiculopathy due to cytomegalic virus. Distal painful sensory neuropathy is an axonal neuropathy that usually occurs in the later stage of AIDS. Unlike the classic GBS and CIDP, CSF pleocytosis is the rule in AIDS inflammatory neuropathy. AIDS inflammatory neuropathy is usually observed early in AIDS and responds well to immunotherapies, as does the classic inflammatory neuropathy.

MAXIMS

1. The major difference between GBS and CIDP is the duration of disease up to maximum disability; the duration of CIDP is greater than 4 weeks and that of GBS, less than 4 weeks. CIDP in AIDS is different from the classic CIDP in that there is spinal fluid pleocytosis.
2. Nerve conduction findings in CIDP are classic for acquired demyelinating neuropathy: markedly slow NCV, abnormal temporal dispersion, and conduction block.

REFERENCES

1. Oh SJ. Subacute demyelinating polyneuropathy responding to corticosteroid treatment. Arch Neurol 1978;35:509–516.
2. Dalakas MC, Pezeschkpour G. Neuromuscular diseases associated with human immunodeficiency virus infection. Ann Neurol 1988;23(suppl):S38–S48.

CASE 3

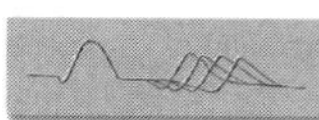

A 3-MONTH HISTORY OF PROGRESSIVE WEAKNESS OF THE RIGHT HAND

CASE PRESENTATION

A 56-year-old man presented with a 3-month history of progressive weakness, loss of grip strength, and atrophy, primarily of the first web space and hypothenar eminence in the right hand. He specifically denied any pain or sensory changes associated with this weakness or any weakness in the left hand. Cervical MRI showed diffuse degenerative arthritic changes in the cervical spine with no significant cord compression. Routine peripheral nerve laboratory workup was negative. Abnormal neurological findings included mild atrophy of the intrinsic, thenar, hypothenar, wrist flexor, and extensor muscles; MRC strength of 5− in the wrist extensors, 4+ in the wrist flexors, 4 in the thenar and hypothenar muscles, and 3 in the hand intrinsic muscles of the right arm. Reflexes were brisk throughout, and plantar responses were flexor. Sensory examination was perfectly normal in all modalities. Fasciculation was not present. Past history was not significant.

CASE ANALYSIS

This patient had a subacute motor weakness and atrophy without any sensory or reflex involvement. The presence of brisk reflexes together with motor weakness and atrophy raised the possibilities of early amyotrophic lateral sclerosis and cervical spondylotic myelopathy. MRI of the cervical spine ruled out cervical spondylotic myelopathy. Other differential diagnoses included benign focal amyotrophy and MMN.

PLAN OF TESTING

1. Needle EMG in the right and left cervical paraspinal, proximal, and distal muscles. If the needle EMG in the left arm EMG was abnormal, the needle EMG study in one lower extremity would be needed. The study was to document either a focal or widespread denervation process.
2. NCS: To document peripheral neuropathy, especially demyelinating neuropathy, and conduction block in the right median, ulnar, and radial nerves.
3. GM1 antibody test: To confirm MMN.

ELECTROPHYSIOLOGICAL TESTS AND FINDINGS

`NCS Findings` (Table 9.7; Fig. 9.4)

1. Prolonged terminal latency, low CMAP amplitude, conduction block in the forearm segment, slow NCV over the forearm and upper arm segments, and prolonged F-wave latency in the right median nerve.
2. Initial positive deflection of the CMAP with stimulation at the elbow in the right median nerve.
3. Prolonged terminal latency, low CMAP amplitude, slow NCV over the forearm segment, and prolonged F-wave latency in the right ulnar nerve.
4. Slow sensory and mixed NCV with normal CNAP amplitude in the right median nerve.
5. Slow sensory NCV with low CNAP amplitude and slow mixed NCV over the forearm segment in the right ulnar nerve.
6. Normal motor and sensory NCS in the right radial nerve.

TABLE 9.7. Nerve Conduction Data in Case 3

	Latent/NCV (ms/m/s)	Amplitude (mV/μV)	Shape
Rt	**Median**	**Motor**	**Nerve**
TL	4.7	0.53	
E-W	37.9	0.25	CB/Pos
AX-E	42.6	0.25	
F-wave	34.3		
Rt	**Ulnar**	**Motor**	**Nerve**
TL	3.3	4.4	
BE-W	48.6	4.4	
AE-BE	50.0	4.2	
AX-AE	52.0	4.2	
EB-AX	55.7	3.2	
F-wave	35.6		
Rt	**Radial**	**Motor**	**Nerve**
TL	2.8	4.3	
AE-BE	53.5	3.8	
Rt	**Median**	**Sens/mixed**	**Nerve**
F-W	45.1	15	
W-E	46.5	23	
E-AX	59.6	18	
Rt	**Ulnar**	**Sens/mixed**	**Nerve**
F-W	41.1	5.7	
W-E	46.1	14.6	
E-AX	54.4	17	
AX-EB	54.0	26	
Rt	**Superf. Radial**	**Sensory**	**Nerve**
W-F	48.1	21.5	

CB/Pos, conduction block/initial positive deflection. Normal NCS in the lt median, ulnar, peroneal, posterior tibial, and sural nerves.

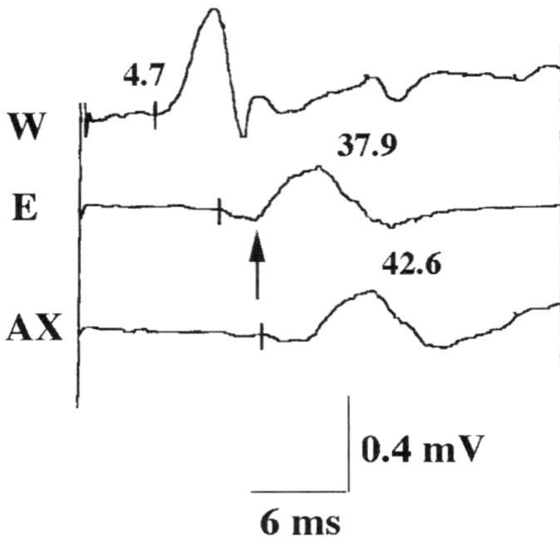

FIGURE 9.4. Motor nerve conduction in the median nerve. Conduction block in the forearm segment with slower motor NCV. Notice initial positive deflection indicating Martin-Grüber anastomosis. *W*, wrist stimulation; *E*, elbow stimulation; *AX*, axilla stimulation. Numbers between the responses represent motor NCV.

7. Normal motor and sensory NCS in the left median and ulnar nerves except for prolonged F-wave latencies in both nerves.
8. Normal NCS in the right peroneal, posterior tibial, and sural nerves.

Needle EMG

1. PSWs, many high-amplitude MUPs, and RIP in the right FDI muscle.
2. Normal MUPs but RIP in many tested muscles in the right arm.
3. Normal needle EMG in all tested muscles in the left arm.

ELECTROPHYSIOLOGICAL INTERPRETATION

Demyelinating neuropathy in the right median and ulnar nerves typical of MMN. In addition, a Martin-Grüber anastomosis was identified on the basis of initial positive deflection of the CMAP from the APB muscle with median nerve stimulation at the elbow.

OTHER TEST FINDINGS

IgM GM1 and asialo-GM1 antibody tests were normal. However, IgG GM1 antibody titer was positive at 1400 (normal, <800) and asialo-GM_1 antibody titer at 1200 (normal, <1000).

FINAL DIAGNOSIS

MMN

TREATMENT AND FOLLOW-UP

The patient was treated with a high dose of prednisone (60 mg/day) and one course of IVIg (0.4 g/1 kg BW for 5 days). This treatment was followed by gradual reduction of prednisone and a 2-day IVIg treatment each month. After 3 months of treatment, there was improvement in the trophic state and muscle strength of the right forearm and hand.

COMMENTS

Our patient had a subacute MMN with conduction block in the median nerve and positive anti-GM1 antibody. The diagnosis of MMN was confirmed. In benign focal amyotrophy, the needle EMG shows chronic denervation without any evidence of peripheral neuropathy, usually in one limb, more commonly in the upper extremity. Hemiatrophy of the cervical cord has been documented in a few cases of benign focal amyotrophy. The absence of a widespread denervation process and evidence of peripheral neuropathy rules out amyotrophic lateral sclerosis. Brisk reflexes are not an uncommon finding in MMN. In recent years, MMN has emerged as a distinct entity. This neuropathy is characterized clinically by pure motor mononeuropathy multiplex, electrophysiologically by multifocal motor conduction block with sparing of sensory nerve conduction, therapeutically by a lack of steroid response but a fair response to cyclophosphamide and IVIg, and immunologically by a strong association with the anti-GM_1 antibody. Anti-GM_1 antibody was positive in 90% of MMN cases. However, it is not specific because a low anti-GM_1 antibody has been reported in some cases of amyotrophic lateral sclerosis and often in the axonal form of the GBS. Our case was atypical of MMN because of the sensory nerve conduction abnormality and good response to steroid and IVIg treatments.

Motor-sensory demyelinating mononeuropathy multiplex (MSDMM; multifocal motor-sensory demyelinating neuropathy [MMSDN]) has been recently reported. MSDMM resembles MMN because it is a multifocal neuropathy, involves the arms predominantly, and shows demyelination in the NCS. However, it is different from MMN because of the presence of sensory deficits, sensory nerve conduction abnormalities, good response to immunotherapies, and absence of GM_1 antibody. This is a clinically recognizable entity and is characterized by subacute or chronic motor-sensory mononeuropathy multiplex, electrophysiological evidence of demyelination, high CSF protein in 60% of patients, demyelination in the nerve biopsy, and good response to the immunotherapies. There are also some similarities between MSDMM and CIDP: subacute or chronic progression of neuropathy, electrophysiological evidence of demyelination, demyelination in the sural nerve biopsy, and good response to corticosteroid therapy. The main differences between MSDMM and CIDP are the clinical pattern of neuropathy and spinal fluid protein: an asymmetrical mononeuropathy multiplex, starting usually from the arms in MSDMM, compared with a symmetrical polyneuropathy, starting usually in the legs, in CIDP; and high spinal fluid protein, less frequent in MSDMM and more frequent in CIDP. Most likely, MSDMM is a link between MMN and CIDP.

MAXIMS

1. MMN is characterized by multifocal motor conduction block, positive anti-GM1 antibody, and nonresponsiveness to steroid.
2. MMSDN is different from MMN in its sensory deficis, sensory nerve conduction abnormalities, good response to immunotherapies, and lack of GM_1 antibody.

REFERENCES

1. Parry G, Sumner A. Multifocal motor neuropathy. Neurol Clin 1992;10:671–683.
2. Oh SJ, Claussen GC, Kim DS. Motor and sensory demyelinating mononeuropathy multiplex (multifocal motor and sensory demyelinating neuropathy): a separate entity or a variant of chronic inflammatory demyelinating neuropathy? JPNS 1997;2:362–369.

CASE 4

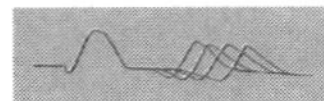

NUMBNESS AND TINGLING SENSATION IN THE HANDS FOR 12 YEARS

CASE PRESENTATION

A 61-year-old man began to have numbness and tingling in the left hand 12 to 13 years ago, followed by similar symptoms in the right hand. He underwent a left carpal tunnel release and a left cubital tunnel release approximately 10 years ago without any benefit although the symptoms progressively worsened in his hands, there was no pain or weakness. In the past 5 years, he had numbness and tingling sensations in his right foot, followed by similar complaints in the left foot, spreading further to involve the lower third of his leg. He reported that his toes had curled and caused him discomfort with walking. He denied any burning pain, but reported occasional sharp, needle-like sensations extending into his feet. He had no history of diabetes but did have a history of moderate ethanol abuse and was told that his neuropathy was due to alcoholism. His neuropathy was treated with Dilantin, Tegretol, Imipramine, and TENS unit. Normal laboratory studies included ANA, rheumatoid factor, sedimentation rate, folic acid and B12 and a negative urine screen for heavy metal. He had three previous NCS and EMG studies.

Examination showed normal muscle strength, mild pes cavus with hammer toes, pin-prick loss below the wrists and midcalves, loss of position sense on the toes, absent vibratory sensation below the ankles, absent ankle reflexes, but otherwise normal reflexes.

CASE ANALYSIS

This patient had a pure sensory neuropathy for 12 years that was thought to be due to alcoholism. He told us at the beginning that if there were nothing to be done for his neuropathy, he would not have another electrodiagnostic study. We were able to convince him that not all NCS were the same and that we wanted to do a fourth NCS to identify the pathology of his sensory neuropathy. This is the first step in determining the cause of neuropathy. It is dangerous to assume that sensory neuropathy is due to chronic alcoholism simply because of a patient's history. In older patients, it is always important to check for monoclonal gammopathy as a cause of neuropathy, because it is one of the major neuropathies in this age group.

PLAN OF TESTING

1. NCS: To identify the nature of sensory neuropathy.
2. Needle EMG: To identify the nature of sensory neuropathy.
3. Serum protein immunoelectrophoresis, anti-GM1 and MAG serum autoantibodies, spinal fluid study, and nerve biopsy.

TABLE 9.8. Nerve Conduction Data in Case 4

	Latent/NCV (ms/m/s)	Amplitude (mV/μV)	Shape		Latent/NCV (ms/m/s)	Amplitude (mV/μV)	Shape
	Median	**Motor**	**Nerve**		**Peroneal**	**Motor**	**Nerve**
TL	10.0	0.7		TL	15.6	2.0	
E-W	34.7	0.7		FH-A	16.8	1.8	
AX-E	40.0	0.8		PF-FH	28.1	1.7	
F-wave	48.0			F-wave	NP		
	Ulnar	**Motor**	**Nerve**		**Post Tibial**	**Motor**	**Nerve**
TL	5.0	6		TL	9.2	0.24	
BE-W	43.7	6		PF-A	25.5	0.16	D
AE-BE	33.3	6					
AX-AE	63.6	5.5					
F-wave	41.6			F-wave	NP		
	Median	**Sens/Mixed**	**Nerve**		**Sural**	**Sens**	**Nerve**
F-W	NP			MC-A	NP		
W-E	NP						
E-AX	45.8	4					
	Ulnar	**Sens/Mixed**	**Nerve**		**Plantar**	**Sens**	**Nerve**
F-W	NP			Medial			
W-E	NP			Lateral			
E-AX	NP						

Height: 176 cm.

ELECTROPHYSIOLOGICAL TESTS AND FINDINGS

NCS Findings (Table 9.8; Fig. 9.5)

1. Markedly prolonged terminal latencies, markedly slow motor NCV, low CMAP amplitude, and absent F-waves in the peroneal and posterior tibial nerves.
2. Markedly prolonged terminal and F-wave latencies and slow motor NCV in the median and ulnar nerves.
3. Absent CNAP in median and ulnar sensory and mixed nerve conduction.
4. Low CMAP amplitude in the median nerve.
5. Conduction block in the peroneal nerve.

Needle EMG Findings in the Gastrocnemius, Anterior Tibialis, Vastus Lateralis, FDI, Deltoids, and L3-5, S1 Paraspinal Muscles

1. A few HA MUPs and DA in the gastrocnemius and anterior tibialis muscles.
2. Otherwise, normal needle EMG findings.

ELECTROPHYSIOLOGICAL INTERPRETATION

Demyelinating neuropathy with disproportionate distal slowing.

OTHER TEST FINDINGS

1. SGPG autoantibody TLC: positive.
2. SGPG-Elisa: 51200.
3. MAG autoantibody-ELISA: <800.
4. MAG-autoantibody-Western: positive.
5. GD1B, GD1B: all negative.
6. CSF protein, 86 mg/dL.
7. One kappa oligoclonal band in serum and in CSF.

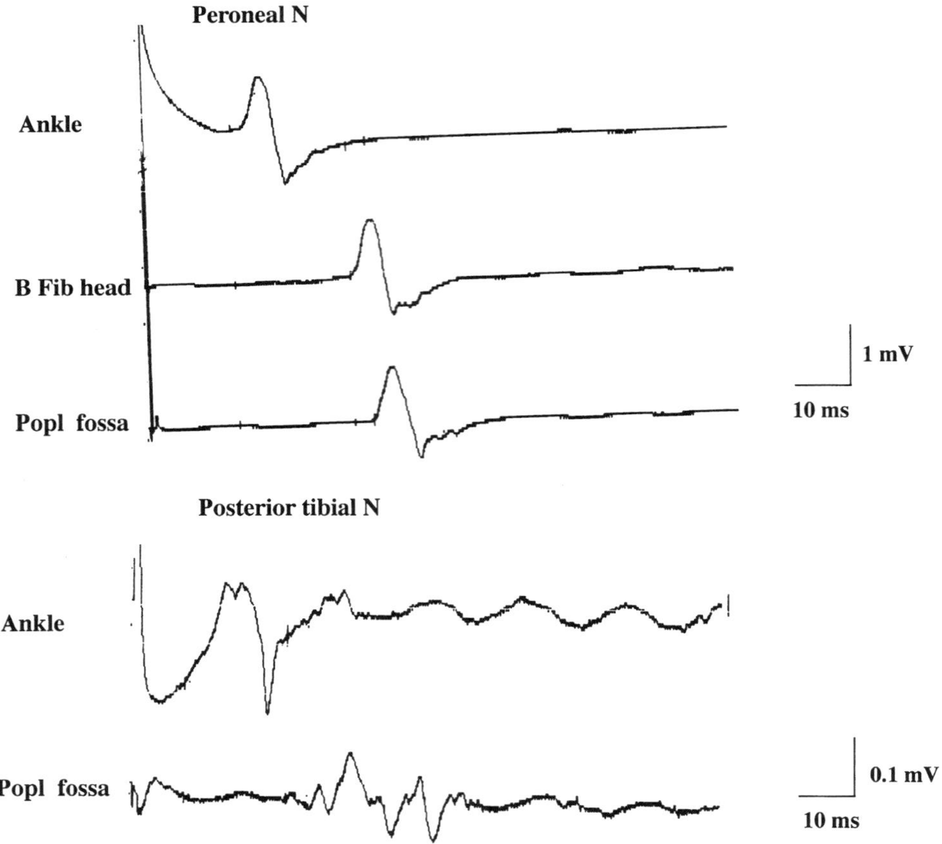

FIGURE 9.5. Motor nerve conduction in the peroneal and posterior tibial nerves. In the posterior tibial nerve, conduction block is obvious; 60 Hz artifact is present in the CMAP response with ankle stimulation. *B fib head,* below fibular head; *popl fossa,* popliteal fossa.

FINAL DIAGNOSIS

MAG-positive chronic sensory demyelinating neuropathy

TREATMENT AND FOLLOW-UP

With azathioprine and intermittent IVIg treatment, this patient's neuropathy has gradually improved. This was not expected in view of the long 12-year history.

COMMENTS

CSDN is an entity recently described by us and is characterized by subacute or chronic progression over months or years, pure sensory neuropathy (no motor weakness), high spinal fluid protein in most cases, electrophysiological evidence of demyelination affecting motor and sensory nerve fibers, demyelination on sural nerve biopsy, and good response to immunotherapy in the progressive phase of disease. In our experience, CSDN is the most common treatable form of neuropathy among the sensory neuropathies. We believe that this entity represents a CIDP presenting as a pure sensory neuropathy.

The most important diagnostic test in CSDN is the motor nerve conduction study, which is usually the first objective clue suggestive of demyelinating neuropathy, as noted in our case. In some patients, the near-nerve needle sensory nerve conduction study is needed to make a definite diagnosis. Neuropathy is monophasic in most cases. In many patients, the neuropathy seemed to have stabilized after a certain period of progression, either spontaneously or with immunotherapy. Immunotherapies (steroid, IVIg, immunosuppressive, plasmapheresis) are effective in the progressive phase of disease in most cases.

MAG-positive neuropathy is also a recently described autoimmune neuropathy and has distinct features: predominantly sensory neuropathy, IgM paraprotein, high CSF protein, and unsatisfactory response to immunotherapies. Unlike our patient, previously described cases had some motor involvement. In 27 patients with neuropathy and IgM monoclonal gammopathy, antibodies to MAG were found in 59% in one series. The sural nerve biopsy showed demyelinating neuropathy. Nerve conduction study showed findings typical of demyelinating neuropathy in all cases; the motor NCV was markedly slow, terminal latencies were markedly prolonged, sensory CNAPs were either absent or reduced in amplitude, but when present the sensory NCV was markedly slow. The most conspicuous finding in MAG-positive neuropathy is a disproportionate distal slowing of motor conduction expressed by markedly prolonged terminal latency in comparison with other demyelinating neuropathies. Thus, the motor nerve conduction abnormalities in the median and ulnar nerves in this case are typical of MAG-positive demyelinating neuropathy.

MAXIMS

1. In CSDN, the most important diagnostic test is the motor nerve conduction study, which shows a typical demyelinating neuropathy.
2. In MAG-positive neuropathy, NCS shows a typical demyelinating neuropathy with a disproportionately prolonged terminal latency compared with the NCV slowing in proximal segments.

REFERENCES

1. Oh SJ, Joy JL, Kuruoglu R. "Chronic sensory demyelinating neuropathy": chronic inflammatory demyelinating polyneuropathy as a pure sensory neuropathy. J Neurol Neurosurg Psychiatry 1992; 55:677–680.
2. Kaku DA, England JD, Sumner AJ. Distal accentuation of conduction slowing in polyneuropathy associated with antibodies to myelin-associated glycoprotein and sulphated glucuronyl paragloboside. Brain 1994;117:941–947.

CASE 5

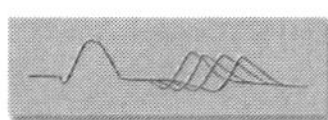

A 2-MONTH HISTORY OF NUMBNESS OF HANDS AND FEET IN A 68-YEAR-OLD MAN

CASE PRESENTATION

Two months previously, a 68-year-old man noticed some tingling in his fingers after prolonged use of a chain saw and later experienced some numbness of both feet, which gradually progressed over the course of 1.5 months. He became mildly unsteady on his feet and the numbness extended up to his ankles. He continued to have occasional numbness and tingling in the fingertips of both hands but no particular pain.

Abnormal neurological findings level 5− MRC strength in the gastrocnemius and anterior tibialis muscles, areflexia, decreased vibration, proprioception, and pin-prick to just above the ankles bilaterally. The patient had mild unsteadiness of gait and was unable to heel, toe, or tandem walk. Romberg was borderline positive.

Serum vitamin B12 and folic acid level, thyroid and rheumatology profiles, serum glycogenated hemoglobin and sedimentation rate, which were ordered by his primary physician, were normal. He was a social drinker. There was no family history of pes cavus or neurological deficit.

CASE ANALYSIS

This patient had a 2-month history of mostly symmetrical sensory neuropathy with minimal motor deficits. The basic neurology workup was normal, ruling out the more common neuropathies. Even though a vitamin B12 deficiency could have produced similar symptoms, such rapid progression would have been unusual. The first neuropathy to rule out was CIDP, because this is a treatable disease, despite his predominantly sensory complaints. At this age, we always have to consider also the possibility of a paraneoplastic sensory neuronopathy. The first step was to do a thorough NCS to define the nature of his neuropathy and help decide on the direction of further evaluation.

PLAN OF TESTING

NCS, needle EMG, nerve biopsy, spinal fluid study, immunoelectrophoresis of serum protein by immunofixation method.

ELECTROPHYSIOLOGICAL TESTS AND FINDINGS

NCS Findings (Table 9.9; Fig. 9.6)

1. Marked prolongation in terminal latency and slowing in NCV in the median nerve.
2. Mild to moderate slowing in NCV in other tested nerves.
3. Marked prolongation in F-wave latencies in the median and ulnar nerves and moderate prolongation of F-wave latencies in the peroneal and posterior tibial nerves.
4. Absent sensory and mixed CNAPs in the median, ulnar, and sural nerves.
5. Conduction block in the ulnar, peroneal, and posterior tibial nerves.
6. Low CMAP amplitude in the median nerve.

Needle EMG

1. Some LDMUPs and increased polyphasic MUPs in the right anterior tibialis muscle.
2. HA MUPs (giant MUPs) in the left anterior tibialis, abductor hallucis, and FDI muscles.
3. Increased polyphasic MUPs in many tested muscles.

ELECTROPHYSIOLOGICAL INTERPRETATION

Demyelinating neuropathy typical of CIDP.

OTHER TEST FINDINGS

CSF protein, 142 mg/dL; cell, 2; IgG monoclonal gammopathy (kappa spike); IFE urine, faint IGG-related paraprotein; light chain-unidentified. Normal GM1 and MAG autoantibodies. Metastatic bone survey did not show any abnormalities. Thus, a bone marrow study was done, which confirmed multiple myeloma by showing 12% of plasma cells.

TABLE 9.9. Nerve Conduction Data in Case 5

	Latent/NCV (ms/m/s)	Amplitude (mV/μV)	Shape		Latent/NCV (ms/m/s)	Amplitude (mV/μV)	Shape
	Median	**Motor**	**Nerve**		**Peroneal**	**Motor**	**Nerve**
TL	4.2	2.7		TL	4.6	1.7	
E-W	28.8	2.2		FH-A	34.6	0.7	CB
AX-E	25.7	2.3		PF-FH	35.4	0.7	
F-wave	42.0			F-wave	66.4		
	Ulnar	**Motor**	**Nerve**		**Post Tibial**	**Motor**	**Nerve**
TL	3.0	6.6		TL	6.0	5.2	
BE-W	37.5	2.7	CB	PF-A	30.3	1	CB
AE-BE	45.4	2.3					
AX-AE	38.3	1.9					
F-wave	38.4			F-wave	66.4		
	Median	**Sens/Mixed**	**Nerve**		**Sural**	**Sens**	**Nerve**
F-W	NP			MC-A	NP		
W-E	NP						
E-AX	NP						
	Ulnar	**Sens/Mixed**	**Nerve**		**Superficial Peroneal**	**Sens**	**Nerve**
F-W	NP			MC-A	NP		
W-E	NP						
E-AX	NP						

Height: 182 cm.

FINAL DIAGNOSIS

CIDP associated with IgG kappa myeloma

TREATMENT AND FOLLOW-UP

The diagnosis of CIDP was well established on this patient. Because an immunofixation serum protein immunoelectrophoresis showed monoclonal gammopathy, we ordered a 24-hour IFE urine test and metastatic bone survey. Initially, this patient was treated with IVIg, prednisone, and azathioprine with moderate improvement. Once multiple myeloma was found, azathioprine was switched to melphalan. Over a 2-year period, he had two relapses that were controlled with IVIg. Now his CIDP is in remission without any medication.

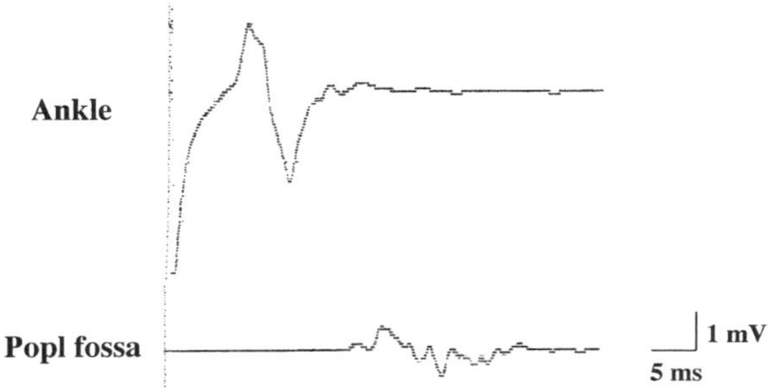

FIGURE 9.6. Motor nerve conduction in the posterior tibial nerve showing a conduction block. *Popl fossa*, popliteal fossa.

COMMENTS

NCS clearly indicated that this patient had demyelinating neuropathy. High spinal fluid protein and demyelinating neuropathy in the sural nerve biopsy were indicative of CIDP. Further studies confirmed that monoclonal gammopathy was due to IgG kappa myeloma. CIDP in myeloma is usually seen in osteosclerotic myeloma, which was not observed in this case.

Peripheral neuropathy associated with myeloma is a heterogenous disorder: demyelinating or axonal neuropathy. CIDP is the classic peripheral neuropathy associated with osteosclerotic myeloma, showing a predominantly motor disability, high CSF protein, and marked NCS abnormalities. Some patients develop a dramatic POEMS syndrome (polyneuropathy, organomegaly, endocrinopathy, M-protein, and skin changes). A skeletal survey reveals osteosclerotic lesions in the spine, pelvic bones, and ribs. Open biopsy of suspicious bony lesions is mandatory for confirmation of diagnosis. The treatment of solitary lesions with tumoricidal irradiation usually improves the neuropathy. On the other hand, peripheral neuropathy associated with multiple myeloma can be divided into two categories: myeloma neuropathy with or without amyloidosis. Myeloma neuropathy without amyloidosis bears a close resemblance to carcinomatous neuropathy. The basic pathological process in peripheral nerves is axonal degeneration. Myeloma neuropathy with amyloidosis is not clinically different from nonhereditary systemic amyloidosis. Of patients with multiple myeloma and polyneuropathy, about two thirds have amyloid neuropathy. A predominantly sensory neuropathy, carpal tunnel syndrome, and autonomic neuropathy are common findings.

CIDP can be associated with monoclonal gammopathy of unknown significance (MGUS). This gammopathy is originally called "benign" because many patients follow a benign course, but extended follow-up revealed an 11% conversion to a malignant plasma dyscrasia. Monoclonal gammopathy is usually absent in the urine, and metastatic bone marrow survey is negative. NCS shows a classic demyelination pattern with markedly slow NCVs. No significant difference is found in the various nerve conduction parameters between CIDP and CIDP associated with MGUS. Usually, the latter group responds less well to immunotherapy than do patients who have CIDP without MGUS. Thus, our patient was exceptional in that his CIDP responded quite well to immunotherapies.

MAXIMS

1. CIDP is the classic peripheral neuropathy associated with osteosclerotic myeloma. Treatment of solitary lesions with tumoricidal irradiation usually improves the neuropathy as well.
2. POEMS stands for polyneuropathy, organomegaly, endocrinopathy (gynecomastia), M-protein, and skin changes.

REFERENCES

1. Kelly J, Kyle RA, Miles JM, O'Brien PC, Dyck PJ. The spectrum of peripheral neuropathy in myeloma. Neurology 1981;31:24–31.
2. Bardwick PA, Zvaifler NJU, Gill GN, et al. Plasma cell dyscrasia with polyneuropathy, organomegaly, endocrinopathy, M-protein and skin changes: the POEMS syndrome. Medicine 1980;59:311–322.

CASE 6

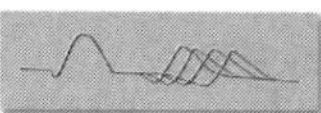

LEFT FOOT DROP IN A CHRONIC ALCOHOLIC

CASE PRESENTATION

A 43-year-old man noticed numbness in his left foot 4 weeks previously and then observed that he was dragging his left foot. He also complained of some numbness in the right foot and of low back pain radiating down to the left foot. He drank heavily, up to 8 to 12 cans of beer a day. Over the ensuing weeks, no major change was noticed. Abnormal neurological examination showed MRC strength of 2 in the left peroneus and anterior tibialis muscles, Tinel's sign at the left fibular head, symmetrical stocking-glove distribution of pin-prick loss over the lower quarter of the calf, and moderate decrease in vibratory sensation on the toes of both feet, absent ankle reflexes, and decreased patellar reflexes. The patient walked with a left foot drop. Straight leg raise was negative. There was no weakness in foot inversion.

CASE ANALYSIS

The history and findings were typical of a left peroneal nerve palsy. However, examination showed a symmetrical sensory neuropathy in addition to the left peroneal mononeuropathy. In view of the patient's history of chronic alcoholic abuse, alcoholism was thought to be most likely responsible for his sensory neuropathy and left peroneal palsy. Because he also complained of low back pain radiating down to the left foot, it was important to rule out L5 radiculopathy by the needle EMG, although this was less likely in view of his normal strength in left foot inversion.

PLAN OF TESTING

1. NCS: To document diffuse peripheral neuropathy and compression neuropathy of the left peroneal nerve at the fibular head.
2. Needle EMG: To document left peroneal neuropathy and rule out L5 radiculopathy.
3. Other tests: Peripheral neuropathy workup.

ELECTROPHYSIOLOGICAL TESTS AND FINDINGS

NCS Findings (Table 9.10; Fig. 9.7)

1. Mild prolongation of terminal latencies in all tested motor nerves.
2. Minimal slowing in motor NCV and mildly prolonged F-wave latencies in the peroneal and posterior tibial nerves.
3. Mild slowing in the sural NCV.

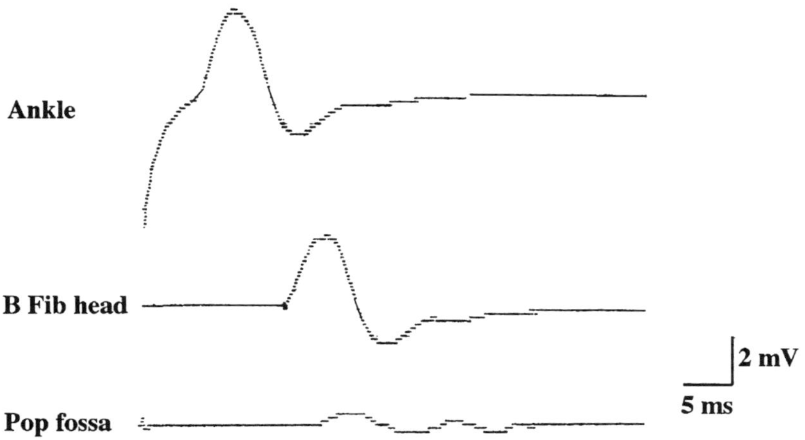

FIGURE 9.7. Motor nerve conduction in the peroneal nerve showing a conduction block across the fibular head, typical of the compression neuropathy at the fibular head. *B fib head*, below fibular head; *pop fossa*, popliteal fossa.

TABLE 9.10. Nerve Conduction Data in Case 6

	Latent/NCV (ms/m/s)	Amplitude (mV/μV)	Shape		Latent/NCV (ms/m/s)	Amplitude (mV/μV)	Shape
	Median	**Motor**	**Nerve**		**Peroneal**	**Motor**	**Nerve**
TL	3.6	15.4		TL	8.6	6	
E-W	59.8	15.6		FH-A	41.2	5	
AX-E	56.9	15.0		PF-FH	31.2	1	CB
F-wave	29.6			F-wave	63.9		
	Ulnar	**Motor**	**Nerve**		**Post Tibial**	**Motor**	**Nerve**
TL	3.0	13.6		TL	7.2	6.5	
BE-W	64.5	12.6		PF-A	30.4	4.0	
AE-BE	47.5	12.4					
AX-AE	60.0	12.2					
F-wave	30.4			F-wave	69.2		
	Median	**Sens/Mixed**	**Nerve**		**Sural**	**Sens**	**Nerve**
F-W	48.4	24		MC-A	32.0	18	
W-E	54.1	29					
E-AX	59.1	30					
	Ulnar	**Sens/Mixed**	**Nerve**		**Plantar**	**Sens**	**Nerve**
F-W	46.2	11.6		Medial			
W-E	51.9	27.2		Lateral			
E-AX	56.9	12.6					

Height: 173 cm.

Needle EMG

1. Fibrillations, PSWs, and two or three normal MUPs with rapid firing on maximal contraction in the left peroneus longus and anterior tibialis muscles.
2. Normal needle EMG findings in the left posterior tibialis and gastrocnemius, right anterior tibialis and gastrocnemius, and left L3-5 and S1 paraspinal muscles.

OTHER TEST FINDINGS

All other diagnostic workups were normal.

FINAL DIAGNOSIS

Alcoholic neuropathy with left peroneal nerve palsy

TREATMENT AND FOLLOW-UP

The patient was advised to quit drinking and take high doses of vitamin B complex. With physical therapy and abstention from alcohol, his foot drop gradually improved to normal in 3 months, but his sensory neuropathy remained unchanged.

COMMENTS

This patient developed a left peroneal compression neuropathy at the fibular head. Patients with diffuse peripheral neuropathy have a higher tendency to develop a compression focal neuropathy, as noted in this case. In fact, his left foot drop led us to make a diagnosis of alcoholic neuropathy in this patient. The diagnosis of alcoholism is elusive, because we do not have any single diagnostic test for chronic alcoholism. Liver dysfunction is at best an indirect evidence of chronic alcoholism.

Alcoholic neuropathy is one of the most common forms of peripheral neuropathy. It is a mixed sensory and motor disorder, involving predominantly the distal nerve segments and legs. Sensory neuropathy is typical in mild cases, with complaints of burning feet or painful paresthesia. In advanced cases, motor weakness is present along with sensory impairment. The neuropathy develops slowly, and recovery is slow. The predominant pathological process in this disorder is axonal degeneration of the heavily myelinated fibers. Thus, the nerve conduction abnormalities are typical of axonal degeneration; the amplitude of the CMAP and sensory CNAP is markedly reduced, whereas the motor and sensory NCVs are only mildly slow and the H-reflex and F-wave latencies are mildly prolonged. Because this is a "dying-back neuropathy," the nerve conduction abnormalities are more frequent and more severe distally and in the legs. Needle EMG shows fibrillations and other denervation changes in the distal leg muscles.

Foot drop is the chief complaint in peroneal nerve palsy and L5 radiculopathy. Thus, it is important to differentiate between these two disorders clinically as well as in the EMG laboratory. In peroneal neuropathy, the peroneus longus muscle is involved, thus causing weakness of foot eversion. In L5 radiculopathy, foot inversion is also weak because of involvement of the posterior tibialis muscle, which is innervated by the posterior tibial nerve.

MAXIMS

1. Foot drop in peroneal nerve palsy is different from that seen in L5 radiculopathy in that the foot inverter (posterior tibial muscle function) is normal.
2. Alcoholic neuropathy is one of the classic examples of axonal neuropathy.

REFERENCES

1. Behse F, Buchthal F. Alcoholic neuropathy: clinical, electrophysiological and biopsy findings. Ann Neurol 1977;2:95–110.

CASE 7

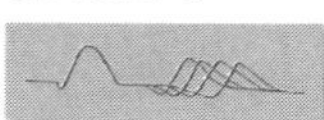

SUBACUTE NEUROPATHY IN A 19-YEAR-OLD GIRL WITH POSSIBLE ANOREXIA NERVOSA

CASE PRESENTATION

A 19-year-old girl was admitted to the UAB hospital at night through the emergency room with the diagnosis of GBS. For the preceding 5 months, she had been admitted to local hospitals twice for two short episodes of nausea and vomiting that were initially thought to be due to gastroenteritis. She did well again in the hospital; however, she was losing weight because of anorexia. The patient was transferred to the psychiatric unit at another hospital for treatment of anorexia nervosa with several psychotropic medications. One week after admission, she began to have trouble with lower-extremity weakness and fell several times on the ward. A bone marrow study was performed for an unknown reason during hospitalization. Because her stepmother was not allowed to stay in the hospital room, she signed the girl out against medical advice and brought her to the UAB emergency room in the middle of the night. Abnormal neurological findings were as follows: MRC strength of 4 in the hand grip, proximal leg, and gluteus muscles; 3 in hamstrings, anterior tibialis, and peroneus muscles; stocking-glove dysesthesias of the feet and hands with loss of position and vibration sensation on the toes and moderate sensory impairment on the fingers and ankles; mild atrophy of the anterior tibialis muscles; and absent DTRs. She walked with foot drop.

CASE ANALYSIS

The neurology resident on call admitted her under the diagnosis of GBS in view of the progression of neuropathy over a 3-week period after an episode of gastrointestinal illness. Spinal tap on the night of admission showed normal findings, with 32 mg/dL protein, which was unusual for GBS. Gastrointestinal upset seen as an antecedent event in GBS is usually noted within 4 weeks before onset of illness, whereas in this case the two gastrointestinal episodes had occurred in the preceding 5 months. The performance of a bone marrow study was unusual for GBS unless lymphoma was suspected. In essence, other causes for neuropathy had to be sought.

PLAN OF TESTING

1. NCS: To document neuropathy and identify the nature of the abnormality.
2. Needle EMG: To document denervation process.
3. Other tests: Detailed medical examination and complete workup for neuropathy.

ELECTROPHYSIOLOGICAL TESTS AND FINDINGS

NCS Findings (Table 9.11; Fig. 9.8)

1. Low CMAP amplitude in the peroneal and posterior tibial nerves.
2. Absent sensory CNAP in all sensory nerves.
3. Low CNAP amplitude or absent CNAP in the mixed nerve conduction in the median and ulnar nerves below the elbow.
4. Mild slowing in NCV and mildly prolonged terminal latency in most tested motor nerves.
5. Mildly prolonged F-wave latencies in the median and ulnar nerves and absent F-waves in the peroneal and posterior tibial nerves.

Needle EMG

1. Prominent fibrillations and PSWs, increased polyphasic MUPs, normal MUPs, and reduced interference pattern in the right and left anterior tibialis and gastrocnemius muscles.

ELECTROPHYSIOLOGICAL INTERPRETATION

Acute axonal neuropathy with predominant sensory nerve conduction involvement.

OTHER TEST FINDINGS

Twenty-four-hour urine test showed an arsenic level 1.5 times normal. Fingernail and pubic hair testing showed a high level of arsenic.

TABLE 9.11. Nerve Conduction Data in Case 7

	Latent/NCV (ms/m/s)	Amplitude (mV/μV)		Latent/NCV (ms/m/s)	Amplitude (mV/μV)
	Median	**Motor N**		**Peroneal**	**Motor N**
TL	3.9	5.0	TL	6.2	0.8
E-W	43.1	5.2	FH-A	36.2	0.8
AX-E	40.4	5.5	PF-FH	38.5	
F-wave	33.5		F-wave	NP	
	Ulnar	**Motor N**		**Post Tibial**	**Motor N**
TL	2.7	10.2	TL	3.2	0.5
BE-W	47.3	10.5	PF-A	32.0	0.5
AX-AE	52.4	10.6			
F-wave	34.2		F-wave	NP	
	Median	**Sens/Mixed N**		**Sural**	**Sens N**
F-W	NP		MC-A	NP	
W-E	NP				
E-AX	46.0	20			
	Ulnar	**Sens/Mixed N**		**Plantar**	**Sens N**
F-W	NP		Medial	NP	
W-E	38.6	5	Lateral		
E-AX	44.7	20			
	Super Radial	**Sens N**			
W-F	NP				

Height: 155 cm.

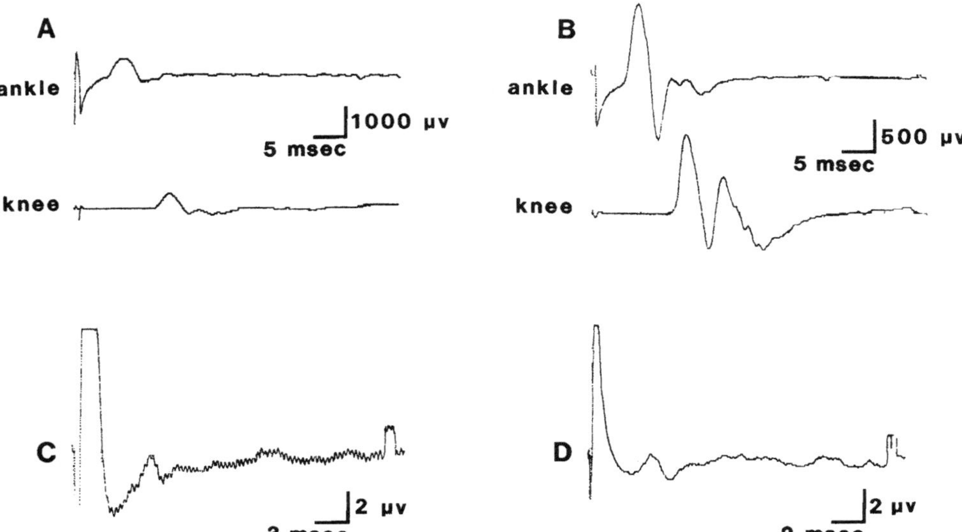

FIGURE 9.8. Motor and sensory nerve conduction in arsenic neuropathy. **A.** The amplitude of CMAP in the peroneal nerve is markedly reduced. Terminal latency and motor NCV are minimally abnormal. **B.** Improved CMAP in the peroneal nerve 2 years later. **C.** Markedly reduced amplitude and mild slowing of the sensory NCV (34.3 m/s) over the finger-wrist segment of the median nerve. **D.** Reduced amplitude and mild slowing in the sensory NCV (33.3 m/s) over the finger-wrist segment of the ulnar nerve. **C.** and **D.** The CNAPs represent an improvement from no CNAP 2 years earlier.

FINAL DIAGNOSIS

Arsenic polyneuropathy

TREATMENT AND FOLLOW-UP

The Neurology Attending examined the patient's fingernails and found a Mee's line during the morning rounds. Arsenic neuropathy was suspected. The diagnosis of arsenic neuropathy was confirmed by the 24-hour urine and fingernail and hair testing. Gradually, the patient improved over a 2-year period. In the meantime, an investigation by law enforcement authorities implicated the girl's stepmother as the culprit, who had poisoned her and the stepmother's two former husbands. In fact, in the other hospital, our patient had been given two injections of "drugs" by her stepmother. This patient's father, who had died a year before, and the stepmother's first husband were found to have been poisoned with arsenic. She was convicted of homicide.

COMMENTS

Our patient had the classic features of arsenic neuropathy: subacute mixed sensory-motor polyneuropathy. Other systemic features of arsenic intoxication included a history of severe gastrointestinal upsets, multiple organ failure, dermatological lesions, and Mee's line. The most helpful diagnostic finding of arsenic polyneuropathy is the presence of Mee's line in the fingernails and toenails and is observed in 80% of cases. Mee's line may not be seen in the early stage of neuropathy because it takes 4 to 6 weeks to develop. Arsenic neuropathy in the United States is most commonly due to homicidal intent, as noted in our case. The diagnosis of arsenic intoxication is confirmed by 24-hour urinalysis in the acute stage and by fingernail, toenail, and hair analysis in the chronic stage.

The most prominent electrophysiological finding is marked abnormalities in the sensory and mixed nerve conduction in the presence of moderate abnormalities in motor conduction. In almost all cases, the CNAPs are not obtainable. This prominent finding is seen in the early stage and in the recovery stage of neuropathy. In one of our cases, the sensory nerve conduction was abnormal even 9 years after exposure. We believe that this is a distinct finding in arsenic neuropathy due to the more severe involvement of sensory fibers. In contrast to the marked sensory nerve conduction abnormalities, motor conduction abnormalities are moderate. The most prominent abnormalities in motor nerve conduction parameters are abnormal CMAP and mild slowing in NCV, which are typical of axonal neuropathy. Needle EMG findings are also typical of axonal neuropathy. These electrophysiological findings are well supported by the histological observation of axonal degeneration as the predominant process in the sural nerve biopsy. Needle EMG study shows active denervation process in all cases. Prominent fibrillations and PSWs in the presence of normal or long-duration MUPs are indicative of axonal degeneration.

Other heavy metal neuropathies include lead, thallium, gold, and platinum neuropathies. Lead neuropathy is predominantly a motor polyneuropathy accompanied by wrist drop and occasional foot drop and occurs rarely in those who work with lead. It can thus mimic motor neuron disease. Anemia and basophilic stippling are noted in the peripheral blood. Nephropathy (common in adults) and encephalopathy (common in children) may be present. Although lead neuropathy in animals is referred to as a classic example of segmental demyelination, axonal degeneration is a leading process in human lead neuropathy. Thallium neuropathy is a predominantly sensory neuropathy. It may mimic arsenic neuropathy in that they both produce hyperkeratosis and Mee's lines. The hallmark of thallitoxicosis is alopecia, which rarely occurs, however, until 2 to 4 weeks after the patient is poisoned with thallium. Thallium neuropathy is a clearcut polyneuropathy of axonal degeneration. Gold salts are sometimes used in the treatment of rheumatoid arthritis. Gold neuropathy is an infrequent complication of gold therapy and is predominantly sensory. Axonal degeneration is the predominantly pathological finding. Generalized myokymia syndrome has also been reported with gold therapy. In this syndrome, motor and sensory conductions are normal. The needle EMG shows typical myokymic discharges. Platinum in the form of cisplatin is used in the chemotherapeutic treatment of cancer. Sensory neuropathy is a common complication of cisplatin therapy. The neuropathy is dose dependent. Nerve conduction studies show a distinct neuronopathy pattern.

MAXIMS

1. Mee's line is typical of arsenic neuropathy although it is also seen in thallium neuropathy. In thallium neuropathy, alopecia is the other hallmark to look for.
2. The most distinct electrophysiological finding in arsenic neuropathy is marked abnormality in the sensory and mixed nerve conduction in the presence of moderate abnormality in motor conduction.

REFERENCES

1. Oh SJ. Electrophysiological profile in arsenic neuropathy. J Neurol Neurosurg Psychiatry 1991;54: 1103–1105.
2. Jenkins R. Inorganic arsenic and the nervous system. Brain 1966;89:479–498.

CASE 8

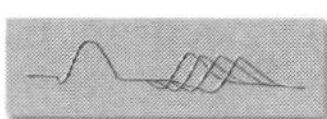

MALABSORPTION, IMPOTENCE, AND BURNING PAIN IN THE FINGERS

CASE PRESENTATION

A 56-year-old man developed severe diarrhea and dramatic weight loss 3 years before the initial evaluation. Within a month, he lost 40 pounds of body weight. Extensive studies, including a small bowel biopsy, showed bowel malabsorption and pancreatic dysfunction of undetermined etiology. Soon the patient developed burning pain in his fingertips that spread up to the wrists and numbness over the medial aspect of the calves. In the meantime, he also experienced profound fatigue, slight weakness in the hands and proximal portions of the legs, and impotence. CSF protein was 68 mg/dL. All workups for peripheral neuropathy were negative except for low serum B12 and 68 mg/dL CSF protein. Subsequently, the patient received monthly IM vitamin B12 injections without much benefit. Abnormal neurological findings included mild weakness of hand grip and interosseous muscles, mild right thenar atrophy, decreased pin prick in a stocking-glove distribution up to the wrists, and medial aspect of both legs. Position sense was normal; vibration was decreased on the toes and fingers. Reflexes were 1+ in the arms and absent in the legs. Plantar responses were flexor. Mild difficulty in tandem gait was also noted.

CASE ANALYSIS

This patient had a predominantly subacute sensory neuropathy that was thought to be due to vitamin B12 deficiency and nutritional neuropathy. Impotence and small bowel malabsorption raised the possibility of autonomic neuropathy. Two diseases can classically present with sensory neuropathy and autonomic neuropathy: diabetes mellitus and amyloid neuropathy. Because diabetes was well ruled out by the appropriate studies, a definite possibility of amyloid neuropathy remained.

PLAN OF TESTING

1. NCS and needle EMG: To rule out CIDP in view of the high CSF protein and to confirm axonal neuropathy with predominant sensory involvement.
2. Nerve biopsy: To confirm the diagnosis of amyloid neuropathy.
3. Immunofixation immunoelectrophoresis of serum and 24-hour urine: To confirm monoclonal gammopathy often associated with amyloidosis.

ELECTROPHYSIOLOGICAL TESTS AND FINDINGS

NCS Findings (Table 9.12)

1. Low CNAP amplitude over the finger-wrist-elbow segments in the median and ulnar nerves.
2. Low CNAP amplitude in the left sural nerve.
3. Slow sensory NCV over the finger-wrist segment in the left ulnar and median nerves.
4. Low CMAP amplitude in the peroneal, median, and ulnar nerves.
5. Prolonged terminal latencies in the median, ulnar, and left peroneal nerves.
6. Slow motor NCV in the right peroneal nerve.

Needle EMG

1. Many high amplitude, long duration MUPs, increased polyphasic MUPs, RIP, or DA in all tested muscles.
2. Fibrillation and PSW in the left gastrocnemius, vastus lateralis, and deltoid muscles.
3. Occasional fasciculations in the left gastrocnemius muscle.

ELECTROPHYSIOLOGICAL INTERPRETATION

Chronic sensory motor axonal neuropathy.

OTHER TEST FINDINGS

Although immunoelectrophoresis of serum protein did not show any monoclonal gammopathy, we continued with a 24-hour urine test for monoclonal gammopathy. It showed mono-

TABLE 9.12. Nerve Conduction Data in Case 8

	Latent/NCV (ms/m/s)	Amplitude (mV/μV)		Latent/NCV (ms/m/s)	Amplitude (mV/μV)
	Median	**Motor N**		**Peroneal**	**Motor N**
TL	4.0	3.6	TL	5.2	2.1
E-W	38.9	3.6	FH-A	36.3	1.5
AX-E	60.0	3.4	PF-FH	46.1	1.5
F-wave	29.6		F-wave	60.4	
	Ulnar	**Motor N**		**Post Tibial**	**Motor N**
TL	3.0	4	TL	4.4	5.4
BE-W	55.2	4	PF-A	41.5	4
AE-BE	54.5	4			
AX-AE	61.2	4			
F-wave	32.8		F-wave	58.8	
	Median	**Sens/Mixed N**		**Sural**	**Sens N**
F-W	39.2	2.0	MC-A	40.6	3
W-E	49.1	9.0			
E-AX	58.9	17			
	Ulnar	**Sens/Mixed N**		**Plantar**	**Sens N**
F-W	34.7	1.0	Medial		
W-E	45.5	4	Lateral		
E-AX	58.9	17			

Height: 170 cm.

clonal immunoglobulin of free lambda chain specificity in the urine. Sural nerve biopsy confirmed that this patient had amyloid neuropathy.

FINAL DIAGNOSIS

Amyloid neuropathy

TREATMENT AND FOLLOW-UP

Pain was improved with Zostrix cream. There has been a slow but gradual progression with more weakness in the arms and legs. The patient died 1 year after the diagnosis of amyloidosis.

COMMENTS

Nonhereditary amyloid neuropathy can be divided into two groups: primary and secondary, associated with malignant dysproteinemia. The neuropathy is sensory dominant with prominent early loss of small-fiber function followed by progressive weakness and large-fiber involvement. Dysautonomia is often severe and disabling, as is the pain associated with small-fiber damage. Systemic manifestations include common renal insufficiency with proteinuria, abnormal monoclonal gammopathy in the serum in about half the patients and in the urine in 90%, and increased plasma cells on bone marrow examination in about two-thirds of patients. Diagnosis depends on the histological demonstration of amyloid either in the rectal or nerve biopsy. Clinically, electrophysiologically, and morphologically, the primary type resembles dominantly inherited amyloidosis of the lower limbs (type 1 or Andrade type) with axonal degeneration of small myelinated and unmyelinated fibers. The nerve conduction findings are typical of axonal degeneration in sensory and motor nerve conduction.

Peripheral neuropathy is a prominent feature in all four types of inherited amyloidosis. All show an autosomal-dominant inheritance pattern. Amyloid deposits in the nerve fibers and vessels are pathognomonic of amyloid neuropathy. Axonal degeneration is the predominant feature, and thus the nerve conduction findings are typical of axonal degeneration. In type 2 (Indiana; Rukavian type), carpal tunnel syndrome is the common manifestation. In type 3 (Iowa; Van Allen type), painful distal sensorimotor polyneuropathy is most typical. In type 4 (Finnish; Meretoja type), cranial neuropathy associated with corneal lattice dystrophy and cutaneous laxity are the cardinal features.

MAXIMS

1. Amyloid neuropathy is characterized by dysautonomic and sensory neuropathy.
2. Two diseases associated with sensory and dysautonomic neuropathy are diabetes mellitus and amyloidosis.

REFERENCES

1. Kelly JJ Jr, Kyle RA, O'Brien PC, Dyck PJ. The natural history of peripheral neuropathy in primary systemic amyloidosis. Ann Neurol 1979;6:1–7.
2. Trotter JL, Engel WK, Ignaszak TF. Amyloidosis with plasma cell dyscrasia: an overlooked cause of adult onset sensorimotor neuropathy. Arch Neurol 1977;34:209–214.

CASE 9

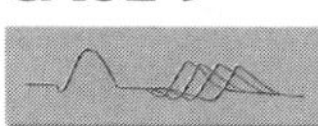

NUMBNESS OF HANDS AND FEET FOR 2 YEARS AND UNSUCCESSFUL CARPAL TUNNEL SURGERY

CASE PRESENTATION

This 76-year-old man had numbness of the hands followed by numbness of the feet for the preceding 2 years. Apparently, NCSs 2 years ago showed diffuse neuropathy, and another test repeated this year showed no essential change. Two years ago, he had carpal tunnel syndrome surgery without much relief except for "relaxation of hand muscles." Spinal fluid protein was 57 mg/dL without any cells. The following workups were normal: sulfatide, GM1, and MAG antibodies; urine heavy metals; and thyroid and rheumatology profiles. The patient was sent for a nerve biopsy.

Abnormal neurological findings included absent vibration on the toes and moderately decreased vibratory sensation on the ankles, impaired position on the left toes, and a decreased pin prick below the midcalf in the left leg. Reflexes and gait were all normal. Plantar responses were flexor.

CASE ANALYSIS

This patient developed a sensory neuropathy with numbness in the hands at the onset. This presentation is unusual for the chronic small fiber neuropathy that is commonly seen in older patients and that usually starts with burning feet. When sensory neuropathy begins with numbness in the hands, demyelinating neuropathy and vitamin B12 deficiency have to be considered among the differential diagnoses. Because of the easy availability of the serum vitamin B12 and folic acid assays today, deficiencies of these nutrients as a cause of neuropathy are usually identified long before the patient is referred to a tertiary care center. We were convinced that these tests had not been performed by simple omission in this case. Thus, the nerve biopsy was deferred and these tests were ordered.

PLAN OF TESTING

1. NCS: To confirm peripheral neuropathy and determine the nature of the neuropathy.
2. Needle EMG: To see whether there was any active denervation process in the muscles.
3. Other tests: Immunoelectrophoresis of serum protein by immunofixation test. Serum vitamin B12 and folic acid. Schilling test.

ELECTROPHYSIOLOGICAL TESTS AND FINDINGS

NCS Findings (Table 9.13)

1. Mild slowing in sensory NCV in the median, ulnar, and sural nerves.
2. Mild slowing in mixed NCV in the wrist-elbow segments in the median and ulnar nerves.
3. Mild slowing in motor NCV in all tested nerves.
4. Low CMAP amplitude in the peroneal and posterior tibial nerves.
5. Mild prolongation in the F-wave latency in the peroneal nerves.

Needle EMG

1. HA MUPs in all three tested muscles: FDI, APB, and anterior tibialis muscles.
2. Otherwise, normal needle EMG findings.

ELECTROPHYSIOLOGICAL INTERPRETATION

Axonal peripheral neuropathy.

OTHER TEST FINDINGS

Serum vitamin B12 level was 45 (normal, >200). Schilling test was 0.6% excretion (normal, >6%) in the first stage test and 4.5% excretion in the second stage test. Serum parietal cell antibodies were negative.

FINAL DIAGNOSIS

Vitamin B12 deficiency neuropathy

TABLE 9.13. Nerve Conduction Data in Case 9

	Latent/NCV (ms/m/s)	Amplitude (mV/μV)		Latent/NCV (ms/m/s)	Amplitude (mV/μV)
	Median	**Motor N**		**Peroneal**	**Motor N**
TL	3.4	9.5	TL	4.8	3.3
E-W	48.2	9.6	FH-A	36.1	2.0
AX-E	53.8	9.0	PF-FH	42.9	2
F-wave	30.9		F-wave	64.4	
	Ulnar	**Motor N**		**Post Tibial**	**Motor N**
TL	2.5	9.6	TL	4.1	3.2
BE-W	48.9	9.3	PF-A	32.6	2.8
AE-BE	43.5	9			
AX-AE	63.2	8.6			
F-wave	31.7		F-wave	54.2	
	Median	**Sens/Mixed N**		**Sural**	**Sens N**
F-W	39.2	15	MC-A	28.6	8
W-E	43.6	13			
E-AX	54.1	82			
	Ulnar	**Sens/Mixed N**		**Superficial Peroneal**	**Sens N**
F-W	35.6	14	MC-A		
W-E	47.7	12			
E-AX	59.3	15			

Height: 178 cm.

TREATMENT AND FOLLOW-UP

Schilling test confirmed that vitamin B12 deficiency in this patient was due to intrinsic-factor deficiency. With the continued vitamin B12 injections, his sensory deficits improved gradually.

COMMENTS

Vitamin B12 deficiency usually occurs in individuals with pernicious anemia but may also be seen rarely in those with blind loop syndrome, ileal resection, or fish tapeworm and in strict vegetarians. Peripheral neuropathy, posterior column signs, and pyramidal tract signs are the classic triad of this disorder (subacute combined degeneration). Megaloblastic anemia and dementia are usually present. In the 1990s, when the serum B12 test is easily available, full-blown subacute combined degeneration syndrome is rare. Vitamin B12 deficiency neuropathy is classically a sensory neuropathy that invariably begins in the hands. Motor weakness is a late manifestation and is usually due to myelopathy. Although the central nervous system pathology is known to be caused by demyelination in the white matter, peripheral neuropathy is typically of axonal degeneration. Thus, the nerve conduction abnormalities are typical of axonal neuropathy, as seen in this case. With treatment, neuropathy and nerve conduction abnormalities usually improve.

Vitamin B12 deficiency neuropathy is a rare cause of peripheral neuropathy. However, because this is one of the treatable causes of neuropathy, it is important to check the serum vitamin B12 routinely in any patient with peripheral neuropathy. Other vitamin deficiencies that can produce peripheral neuropathies are folic acid, thiamine, niacin, pyridoxin, and vitamin E. Vitamin B1 deficiency produces beriberi, which is characterized by edema, cardiomegaly, and predominantly sensory neuropathy. Beriberi neuropathy is typical of axonal degeneration. Neuropathy due to folate deficiency is characterized by sensorimotor neuropathy with mainly sensory deficits and electrophysiological characteristics of axonal neuropathy. It may occur in the context of subacute combined degeneration. Neuropathy due to niacin deficiency is a sensory-motor neuropathy with severe paresthesia and burning pain due to axonal degeneration. Vitamin E deficiency produces dysarthria, cerebellar ataxia, and peripheral neuropathy with loss of proprioception. Nerve conduction abnormalities are typical of a sensory neuronopathy pattern. In contrast to many vitamin deficiency neuropathies, one neuropathy due to vitamin toxicity has been reported: neuropathy due to pyridoxin toxicity. This neuropathy is classically a sensory ataxic neuropathy and sensory neuronopathy in the NCS. It develops usually after daily consumption of megadoses (2 to 6 g) of pyridoxin.

MAXIMS

1. Vitamin B12 deficiency neuropathy is characterized by sensory neuropathy. The main pathological change in peripheral nerve is axonal degeneration. In contrast, a central nervous system lesion is predominantly demyelinating.
2. Pyridoxin toxicity can produce sensory ataxic neuropathy and sensory neuronopathy in the nerve conduction.

REFERENCES

1. Schaumburg H, Kaplan J, Winderbank A, et al. Sensory neuropathy from pyridoxin abuse. N Engl J Med 1983;309:445–448.
2. Mayer RF. Peripheral nerve function in vitamin B12 deficiency. Arch Neurol 1965;13:355–361.

CASE 10

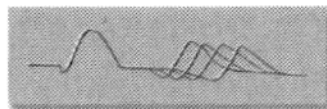

DIABETIC AMYOTROPHY OR CIDP?

CASE PRESENTATION

Two years ago, a 61 year-old man with a history of diabetes for 8 years developed sharp pains radiating from his back to his left lower abdomen. These pains resolved spontaneously. Sixteen months ago, he had a recurrence of his pain with radiation to the left thigh. Because of continuing worsening of pain, he was evaluated by a neurologist. EMG study revealed not only diabetic neuropathy but also possibly demyelinating neuropathy. He was treated initially with 150 mg/day Imuran without much benefit. Soon, he developed severe pain and weakness in his right thigh. Four months ago he underwent one course of IVIg with some improvement of pain and weakness lasting for 2 weeks. Another 1-day IVIg treatment a month later brought improvement of pain for only 2 to 3 days. His pain was partially controlled with large doses of narcotics. He was not able to cough well, had some problems emptying his bowels and bladder, and had not had a penile erection for 1 year. He had lost 75 pounds over the preceding year. The patient was currently not taking any medication for his diabetes. His glucose ranged from 120 to 180. Abnormal neurological findings were as follows: marked atrophy of the right quadriceps muscle; MRC strength of 2+ in the right iliopsoas, 4− in the right quadriceps, 4 in the right anterior tibialis, 4 in the left iliopsoas, and 5− in the left quadriceps muscles; decreased pin-prick sensation up to the knees; decreased position sense and absent vibration on the toes; decreased vibration on the ankles; patchy areas of decreased pin-prick sensation over the lower abdomen; and absent reflexes in the legs and decreased reflexes in the arms.

CASE ANALYSIS

This patient had a rather classic history of diabetic amyotrophy, beginning with lower thoracic radiculopathy that spread to the left thigh initially and finally to the right thigh. Severe pain, prominent thigh muscle atrophy, and marked weight loss are the typical features of diabetic amyotrophy: diabetic polyradiculoneuropathy. The major question was whether this patient had superimposed CIDP. Apparently, according to the referring neurologist, NCS had shown evidence of demyelination.

PLAN OF TESTING

1. NCS: To identify the nature of the neuropathy. This should include femoral nerve conduction.
2. Needle EMG: To identify polyradiculoneuropathy. Thus, this should include extensive paraspinal EMG testing.
3. Other tests: Spinal fluid evaluation to check for any immune abnormality. Muscle and nerve biopsies to detect any inflammatory or vasculitic changes.

ELECTROPHYSIOLOGICAL TESTS AND FINDINGS

NCS Findings (Table 9.14)

1. Absent CMAP in the right and left femoral nerves.
2. Slow motor NCV, absent F-waves, and low CMAP amplitudes in the peroneal and posterior tibial nerves with conduction block in the posterior tibial nerve and suggestive temporal dispersion in the peroneal nerves.
3. Absent CNAP in the sural nerve and slow sensory and mixed NCV and low CNAP amplitude in the median and ulnar nerves.
4. Prolonged terminal and F-wave latencies in the median and ulnar nerves with low CMAP amplitude in the median nerve and slow motor NCV in the ulnar nerve.

Needle EMG (Table 9.15; Fig. 9.9)

1. Fibrillation and PSWs in almost all tested paraspinal and proximal and distal leg muscles.
2. Some simple and polyphasic HALD MUPs in most tested limb muscles.
3. Reduced interference pattern in all tested limb muscles.

TABLE 9.14. Nerve Conduction Data in Case 10

	Latent/NCV (ms/m/s)	Amplitude (mV/μV)	Shape		Latent/NCV (ms/m/s)	Amplitude (mV/μV)	Shape
	Median	**Motor**	**Nerve**		**Peroneal**	**Motor**	**Nerve**
TL	4.0	4		TL	4.4	0.48	
E-W	50.0	4		FH-A	28.8	0.40	D
AX-E	56.8	4		PF-FH	45.4	0.35	D
F-wave	32.0			F-wave	NP		
	Ulnar	**Motor**	**Nerve**		**Post Tibial**	**Motor**	**Nerve**
TL	3.4	5.1		TL	5.2	1.3	
BE-W	42.8	5.1		PF-A	31.7	0.66	CB
AE-BE	36.6	5.1					
AX-AE	50.0	5.1					
F-wave	34.4			F-wave	NP		
	Median	**Sens/Mixed**	**Nerve**		**Sural**	**Sens**	**Nerve**
F-W	39.0	4		MC-A	NP		
W-E	47.2	5					
E-AX	54.4	8					
	Ulnar	**Sens/Mixed**	**Nerve**		**Femoral**	**Motor**	**Nerve**
F-W	34.2	2		Rt	NP		
W-E	46.1	5		Lt	NP		
E-AX	58.3	5					

Height: 182.9 cm.

ELECTROPHYSIOLOGICAL INTERPRETATION

Thoracolumbosacral polyradiculopathy with generalized and bilateral femoral neuropathy typical of diabetic amyotrophy and most likely secondary demyelination in the peroneal and posterior tibial nerves.

OTHER TEST FINDINGS

CSF showed a high protein (88 mg/dL) with increased IgG synthesis rate and increased total IgG level. No oligoclonal bands. Muscle biopsy showed mild denervation and nerve biopsy revealed severe end-stage neuropathy. No inflammatory cells were noted in either tissue.

FINAL DIAGNOSIS

Diabetic amyotrophy

TREATMENT AND FOLLOW-UP

Azathioprine was gradually tapered. Over the next 6 months, the patient experienced a lessening of pain and improvement in muscle strength to normal except for 4 MRC strength in the right iliopsoas muscle.

COMMENTS

Overall, the clinical features and EMG data are typical of diabetic amyotrophy in this case. Thus, we interpreted some evidence of demyelination in the peroneal and posterior tibial nerves as secondary demyelination rather than an expression of CIDP. Muscle and nerve biopsies did not show any evidence of inflammatory vasculopathy. Consequently, we did not treat this patient with continued immunotherapy and he improved, as expected in classic diabetic amyotrophy. An unanswered question is whether the increased IgG level and IgG synthesis in the spinal fluid were indicative of diabetic amyotrophy. It has been well known

TABLE 9.15. Needle EMG Data in Case 10

Muscle	Root	Nerve	Insertion Activity	Spontaneous Potentials				Motor Unit Potential				Interference	
				Fib	PSW	Fasc	CRD	Amplitude (mV)	Duration (ms)	Polyphasic Potential	HALD MUP	Pattern	Mean Amplitude (mV)
Rt L1-5, S1		L1-5, S1	+	++	++	−	−						
Iliopsoas	Femoral	L 2–4	+	++	++	−	−	1–6.0	8–20	+	+	RIP	5
Vast lat	Femoral	L3,4	+	+++	+++	−	−	1–5.5	6–20	+[a]	+	RIP	4
Gastroc	Post tibial	S1,2	+	−	−	++	−	1–4	6–14	N	−	RIP	4
Ant tibial	Peroneal	L4,5	+	++	++	−	−	0.5–6.5	10–20	+[a]	+	RIP	5
Lt T4–10		T4-10	+	++	++	−	−						
L1–4		L1–4	+	+	+	−	−						
Vast lat	Femoral	L3,4	+	+	+	−	−	0.5–7	10–22	+[a]	+	RIP	5

[a] Long-duration polyphasic MUPs.

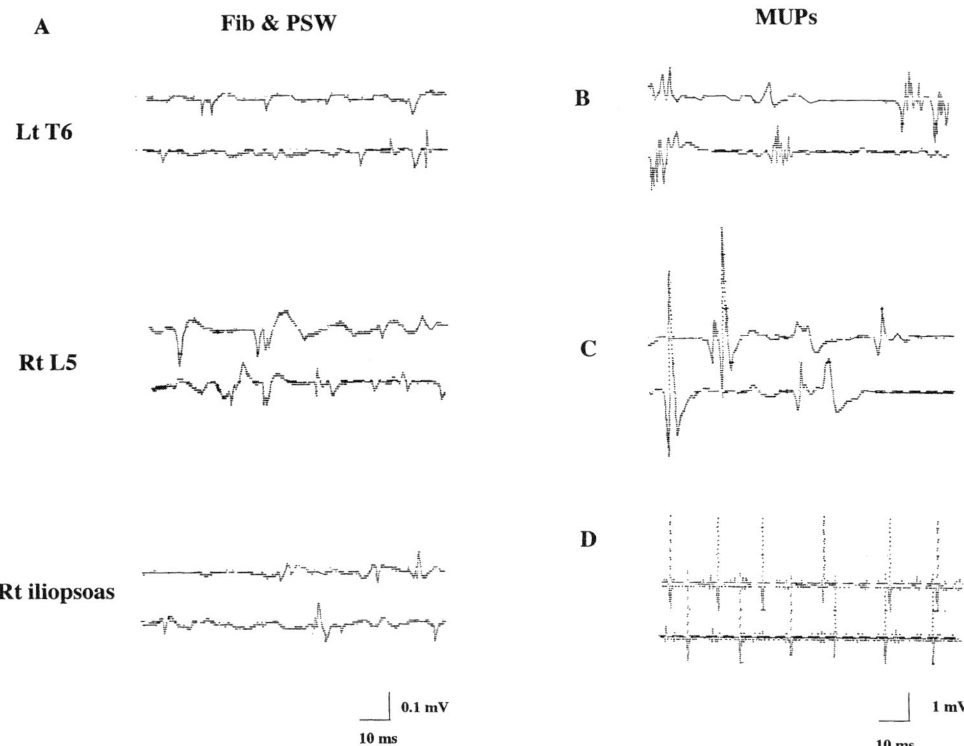

FIGURE 9.9. Some EMG tracings in the tested muscles. **A.** Fibrillations (*fib*) and PSWs in the various paraspinal and iliopsoas muscles. **B.** Polyphasic MUPs. **C.** HA MUPs. **D.** Discrete activity. Rt, right; Lt, left.

that CSF protein is high in diabetic amyotrophy, but we are not aware of any study on CSF IgG in this disorder.

Diabetic neuropathy is the most common known cause for peripheral neuropathy in the United States and is manifested by various clinical manifestations: painful ophthalmoplegia, diabetic polyradiculopathy, diabetic amyotrophy, symmetrical polyneuropathy, and autonomic neuropathy. Over the years, there has been a lot of controversy as to the exact pathology of diabetic neuropathy. At present, many believe that diabetic neuropathy is a primarily axonal neuropathy and that some evidence of demyelination may be present as a secondary process.

Diabetic amyotrophy is a syndrome consisting of unilateral or bilateral, but often asymmetrical, marked weakness and atrophy that primarily affect the pelvifemoral muscles and are accompanied by pain in the back and thighs. The patellar reflex is frequently decreased or absent, but sensation is little affected. This disorder is usually subacute in onset and occurs in middle-aged or elderly men with poorly controlled or previously unrecognized diabetes mellitus. Severe weight loss is a common concomitant disorder. The prognosis is favorable in that most patients improve within 6 to 18 months. Generalized peripheral neuropathy is documented by NCS in most patients and is a strong argument in favor of a metabolic cause for diabetic amyotrophy.

The femoral NCS is extremely useful in recognizing this condition. Prolonged distal latency of the femoral nerve (>6 ms) was noted in 67% of patients. Saphenous nerve conduction was abnormal in all the cases we studied (Oh SJ, 1997, unpublished data). The common nerve conduction abnormalities in the femoral and saphenous nerves are most helpful in differentiating this disorder from lumbar radiculopathy of other etiologies, in which the femoral nerve latency and saphenous nerve conductions are normal.

The needle EMG is invariably abnormal in diabetic amyotrophy. Fibrillations and PSWs are often detectable in the lumbar paraspinal muscles and in the quadriceps, iliopsoas, and adductors of the thigh muscles. In one series, fibrillations were present in the lumbar paraspinal muscles in over half the patients and often only in a single area. If more extensive paraspinal muscle searches are performed, most of these patients are likely to show evidence of active denervation in the paraspinal muscles, typically in multiple roots beyond the clinically suspected level. The MUPs in the limb muscles in diabetic amyotrophy are typical of acute or chronic denervation, depending on the duration of the lesion. When the reinnervation is active, small polyphasic MUPs are present and mimic myopathy. Usually, these polyphasic MUPs caused by reinnervation have normal duration. In many patients with diabetic amyotrophy, the needle EMG abnormalities are strictly unilateral, found only in the thigh muscles and often in the ipsilateral lumbar paraspinal muscles. However, in some patients, the EMG test shows abnormalities on the contralateral side and an extension of the lesion caudally to the L5-S1 roots in the symptomatic limbs.

The role of immunotherapy in diabetic neuropathy is not clearly defined as yet. Immunotherapy is clearly indicated in diabetic patients with CIDP or GBS. When the EMG data are not straightforward, Wilbourn suggested the following findings as favoring demyelinating neuropathy: sensory conduction responses that are normal in the lower extremities but are of low amplitude or unelicitable in the upper extremities; marked slowing of lower extremity motor NCV in the absence of abundant axon loss; and generalized, markedly slowed motor NCV with normal motor distal latencies or, conversely, normal motor NCV with very prolonged distal latencies. He stated that these features, which are sometimes seen in acquired demyelinating neuropathy, almost never occur with diabetic neuropathy. Immunotherapy is also indicated in diabetic patients with vasculitis proven by muscle or nerve biopsy. Krendal et al. showed "small vessel inflammatory vasculopathy" in 7 of 10 patients with diabetic amyotrophy and successfully treated these patients with immunotherapy. What remained unanswered is the role of immunotherapy in otherwise classic diabetic amyotrophy without vasculopathy or demyelinating neuropathy.

MAXIMS

1. The classic EMG findings in diabetic amyotrophy are polyradiculoneuropathy involving proximal limb muscles. Femoral nerve conduction is abnormal in 67% of cases and helpful in differentiating these cases from lumbar polyradiculopathy.
2. Immunotherapy is indicated in diabetic patients when acquired demyelinating neuropathy or vasculitic neuropathy are confirmed.

REFERENCES

1. Wilbourn AJ. The diabetic neuropathies. In: Brown WF, Bolton CF, eds. Clinical electromyography. Boston: Butterworth, 1987:330–364.
2. Krendal DA, Costigan DA, Hopkins LC. Successful treatment of neuropathies in patients with diabetes mellitus. Arch Neurol 1995;52:1053–1061.

CASE 11

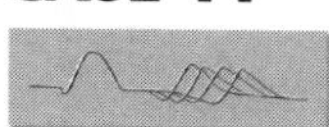

NUMBNESS OF THE HANDS FOLLOWED BY WALKING DIFFICULTY IN A 54-YEAR-OLD SMOKER

CASE PRESENTATION

A 54-year-old woman experienced numbness and tingling sensations in the first two fingers of both hands 7 months ago. This spread over her entire hands, and in 3 weeks she began to have trouble walking. She stated that the floor felt "funny" and her gait became wide based. In 4 months, her ambulation had become so poor that she required a walker and eventually she could not walk at all. For the past several months, she noticed that both upper extremities were getting weaker, and she also complained of intermittent diplopia. Past history was significant for tobacco abuse and a 10-pound weight loss. Previous workup included normal B12 and folate, heavy metal screen, normal serum protein electrophoresis, rheumatoid profile, and thyroid functions. NCS and EMG studies in the left upper and lower extremities were reported to be normal. MRI of the cervical cord was said to show two bulging discs.

Abnormal neurological findings included a right lateral rectus palsy, right lower facial weakness, 4 MRC strength in both arms, loss of vibration to the wrists and knees, impaired position sense on fingers and toes, areflexia, impaired finger-to-nose test when she closed her eyes, wide-based unsteady gait, and positive Romberg test. Pin-prick examination and muscle strength in her legs were normal. Another significant medical finding was many deformed joints.

CASE ANALYSIS

This patient was admitted to the hospital by an attending for a cervical myelogram. The chief neurology resident thought that the patient showed no evidence of a cervical cord lesion but appeared to have a peripheral neuropathy, although the cranial nerve findings did not fit well with this. He suggested two possibilities: vasculitic neuropathy because of many deformed joints that might be due to rheumatoid arthritis and paraneoplastic neuropathy because of the history of smoking and weight loss. Profound proprioception loss, ataxia, and areflexia are indicative of ataxic sensory neuropathy. Thus, clinically this patient had a subacute ataxic sensory neuronopathy with some motor weakness and cranial nerve findings.

PLAN OF TESTING

1. NCS: To confirm sensory neuronopathy.
2. Needle EMG: To confirm additional motor denervation.
3. Other studies: Spinal fluid evaluation including cytology, anti-Hu antibody, Sjögren's antibody, and nerve biopsy.

ELECTROPHYSIOLOGICAL TESTS AND FINDINGS

NCS Findings (Table 9.16)

1. Absent sensory and mixed CNAPs in all tested nerves.
2. Mild slowing in motor NCV in all tested nerves and mildly prolonged terminal latencies in three nerves.
3. Low CMAP amplitudes in peroneal and posterior tibial nerves.

Needle EMG. Relatively normal needle EMG findings in all tested muscles except the right flexor digitorum longus, with PSWs and increased polyphasic MUPs, and the right EDB muscle, with high-amplitude MUPs.

ELECTROPHYSIOLOGICAL INTERPRETATION

Sensory neuronopathy with minimal motor nerve involvement but without any diffuse denervation process in muscle.

OTHER TEST FINDINGS

CSF protein was 102 mg/dL with 9 cell/mm^3 and two oligoclonal bands. Anti-Hu antibody was positive. An extensive cancer workup showed nothing except paratracheal lymph nodes

TABLE 9.16. Nerve Conduction Data in Case 11

	Latent/NCV (ms/m/s)	Amplitude (mV/μV)		Latent/NCV (ms/m/s)	Amplitude (mV/μV)
	Median	**Motor N**		**Peroneal**	**Motor N**
TL	3.2	3	TL	4.3	5
E-W	50.0	3.2	FH-A	42.1	5
AX-E	63.4	3.2	PF-FH	53.1	5
F-wave	28.8		F-wave	49.2	
	Ulnar	**Motor N**		**Post Tibial**	**Motor N**
TL	2.2	5	TL	4.4	15
BE-W	50.0	5	PF-A	45.2	13
AE-BE	47.5	5			
AX-AE	58.3	5			
F-wave	29.6		F-wave	49.2	
	Median	**Sens/Mixed N**		**Sural**	**Sens N**
F-W	NP		MC-A	NP	
W-E	NP				
E-AX	NP				
	Ulnar	**Sens/Mixed N**		**Superficial Peroneal**	**Sens N**
F-W	NP		MC-A	NP	
W-E	NP				
E-AX	NP				
	Superficial Radial	**Sens N**			
W-F	NP				
	Lateral Antebrachial Cutaneous	**Sens N**			
	NP				

Height: 164.2 cm.

on the chest CT. Biopsy of these nodules confirmed small cell lung carcinoma. SSA and SSB Sjögren antibodies were negative.

FINAL DIAGNOSIS

Anti-Hu-positive paraneoplastic sensory neuronopathy with cranial neuropathy

TREATMENT AND FOLLOW-UP

The patient was treated with one course of IVIg, 80 mg of prednisone daily, and cisplatinum and VP-16 chemotherapy for cancer. Minimal improvement was noted in her sensory neuronopathy, but the patient died from cancer in 6 months.

COMMENTS

The NCS was the first finding indicative of paraneoplastic neuropathy in this patient. This led us to the search for occult carcinoma. Studies included CT of abdomen, GYN evaluation, mammogram, and chest CT. Needle biopsy of the paratracheal lymph nodes confirmed the diagnosis of small cell lung cancer in this patient. Anti-Hu antibody was later reported to be positive.

In a recent review, Graus and Rene classified paraneoplastic neuropathies into four separate groups according to their clinical features: motor neuropathy, sensory neuropathy, dysautonomic neuropathy, and sensorimotor neuropathy. Among these, sensory neuropathy has been known to be a classic paraneoplastic peripheral neuropathy and has been termed "paraneoplastic sensory neuronopathy." Although other malignancies have been reported, SCLC is the dominant malignancy in PSN. Anti-Hu antibody is positive in subacute sensory neuronopathy due to SCLC. The presence of the anti-Hu antibody not only suggests that sensory neuropathy is paraneoplastic but predicts that the underlying tumor will be SCLC. Thus, when anti-Hu antibody is positive, a diligent search for SCLC should be made, as was the case in our patient. Another syndrome associated with anti-Hu antibody is limbic encephalomyelitis. Even in PSN, pure sensory neuropathy as a sole clinical manifestation is relatively rare, and in most cases there are manifestations of other systemic involvement, reflecting widespread CNS, and peripheral nerve involvement in anti-Hu-positive syndrome. In our patient, motor and cranial nerves were involved. The pathological basis for PSN is sensory ganglionitis, thus producing prominent sensory loss of proprioception and sensory ataxia. CSF protein was elevated in 93% of these cases, with pleocytosis in 21%. Anti-Hu antibody is usually positive in CSF. As a sensory ganglionitis, PSN shows the classic pattern of sensory neuronopathy; sensory CNAPs are reduced or absent in the presence of normal motor nerve conduction and normal needle EMG findings. However, if the motor system is involved, motor nerve conduction may show axonal neuropathy and the needle EMG may show evidence of denervation, as in our patient. Anti-Hu antibody neuropathy does not respond well to immunotherapy or cancer therapy. In PSN either with or without anti-Hu antibody, there has not been a single report of improvement with therapy in two big series. The poor outcome in PSN is ascribed to irreversible neuronal damage that had already occurred before treatment was begun, and only a handful of cases of anti-Hu-positive neuropathy respond to immunotherapy. Among the various paraneoplastic syndromes, LEMS and paraneoplastic vasculitic neuropathy are known to be consistently responsive to therapies: immunotherapy and anti-cancer therapy in LEMS and immunotherapy in PVN. In other paraneoplastic syndromes, any clinical improvement with either immunotherapy or anti-cancer therapy has been exceptional.

MAXIMS

1. Anti-Hu antibody is positive in paraneoplastic sensory neuronopathy associated with SCLC.
2. The subacute sensory neuronopathy pattern is characterized by marked sensory nerve conduction (absent sensory CNAPs or markedly reduced CNAP amplitude) in the presence of relatively normal motor nerve conduction. This is typically observed in anti-Hu antibody neuropathy.

REFERENCES

1. Dilemma J, Graus F, Rosenblum MK, Posner JB. Anti-Hu-associated paraneoplastic encephalomyelitis/sensory neuropathy. A clinical study of 71 patients. Medicine 1992;71:59–72.
2. Graus F, Rene R. Paraneoplastic neuropathies. Eur Neurol 1993;33:279–286.

CASE 12

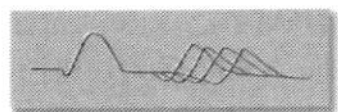

NUMBNESS IN THE LEFT FOOT FOLLOWED BY A SIMILAR PROBLEM IN THE RIGHT LEG OVER AN 8-MONTH PERIOD

CASE PRESENTATION

A 59-year-old male heavy smoker developed numbness on the bottom of his left foot 8 months ago. This symptom gradually worsened to involve his entire left foot, the lateral aspect of the left lower extremity, and his entire right foot. He also had symptoms of tingling and severe burning pain. His pain was incapacitating to the point that he became unable to keep his desk job. NCVs and EMGs by the referring neurologist showed findings indicative of a right S1 and a left L5 radiculopathy with active denervation. The patient had an MRI that was indicative of degenerative disc disease with some disc bulging. His significant laboratory finding was a high sedimentation rate of 60. The remainder of his workup for peripheral neuropathy was negative. Review of systems was negative for weight loss, fever, or any other systemic symptoms. Abnormal neurological findings were MRC strength of 4 in the left anterior tibialis, 3 in the left extensor hallucis longus, 4− in the right anterior tibialis, and 2 in the right extensor hallucis longus muscles, absent ankle reflexes, sensory loss on the entire right foot and over the left superficial peroneal nerve territory, and decreased vibration sense in both feet. Straight-leg raise was negative bilaterally. He had some difficulty with heel walking.

CASE ANALYSIS

The patient's initial symptoms, subsequent development, and asymmetrical neurological deficits were indicative of mononeuropathy multiplex, raising the possibility of vasculitic or multifocal motor and sensory demyelinating neuropathy. His high sedimentation rate favored vasculitic neuropathy. The absence of any systemic symptoms did not favor vasculitic neuropathy. Previous NCS/EMG and MRI findings were misleading. We had to repeat NCS and needle EMG studies to verify that he had peripheral neuropathy and perform muscle and nerve biopsy to confirm vasculitic neuropathy.

PLAN OF TESTING

1. NCS: To confirm the presence and nature of neuropathy.
2. Needle EMG: To see whether there is active denervation process.
3. Other tests: Complete blood count and sedimentation rate. Antineutrophile cytoplasmic antibody. Sural nerve biopsy.

ELECTROPHYSIOLOGICAL TESTS AND FINDINGS

NCS Findings (Table 9.17; Fig. 9.10)

1. Low CMAP amplitudes in the peroneal nerves and in the posterior tibial nerve with popliteal fossa stimulation.
2. Mild slowing in motor, sensory, and mixed NCV in all tested nerves.
3. Absent sensory CNAP in the sural nerves.

Needle EMG (Table 9.18)

1. Prominent fibrillations and PSWs, increased polyphasic MUPs, normal duration and amplitude MUPs, and reduced interference pattern in the right and left anterior tibialis and gastrocnemius and APB muscles.

ELECTROPHYSIOLOGICAL INTERPRETATION

Axonal peripheral neuropathy.

OTHER TEST FINDINGS

Normal complete blood count. Sedimentation rate was 95 mm/hr. Sural nerve biopsy confirmed vasculitic neuropathy. Normal antineutrophile cytoplasmic antibody.

TABLE 9.17. Nerve Conduction Data in Case 12

	Latent/NCV (ms/m/s)	Amplitude (mV/μV)		Latent/NCV (ms/m/s)	Amplitude (mV/μV)
	Median	**Motor N**		**Peroneal**	**Motor N**
TL	3.0	7.4	TL	5.5	0.15
E-W	48.2	6.3	FH-A	31.8	0.15
AX-E	44.8	7.6	PF-FH	44.4	0.15
F-wave	29.7		F-wave	NP	
	Ulnar	**Motor N**		**Post Tibial**	**Motor N**
TL	3.1	12.3	TL	4.6	5.5
BE-W	46.0	10.4	PF-A	38.5	3.2
AE-BE	31.2	8.5			
AX-AE	50.0	8.5			
F-wave	32.9		F-wave	59.0	
	Median	**Sens/Mixed N**		**Sural**	**Sens N**
F-W	37.5	21.9	MC-A	NP	
W-E	47.2	17.0			
E-AX	51.9	28.0			
	Ulnar	**Sens/Mixed N**		**Plantar**	**Sens N**
F-W	34.3	6.4	Medial		
W-E	41.5	33.0	Lateral		
E-AX	62.5	26.9			

Height: 171.5 cm.

FINAL DIAGNOSIS

Vasculitic neuropathy

TREATMENT AND FOLLOW-UP

The patient was treated with cyclophosphamide and prednisone. Despite bone marrow suppression due to cyclophosphamide, his neuropathy gradually improved during 2 years of treatment although some foot drop remained.

COMMENTS

Peripheral neuropathy is common in systemic necrotizing vasculitis. Systemic symptoms (malaise, weight loss, anorexia, and fever), multisystem involvement, and a high sedimentation rate are typical of this disorder. Mononeuropathy multiplex is said to be most typical of this disorder, but symmetrical or asymmetrical polyneuropathy is also common and mononeuropathy is less common. Systemic necrotizing vasculitis is seen in many diseases. Polyarteritis nodosa is a classic example of a systemic necrotizing vasculitis affecting small- and medium-sized arteries and producing systemic symptoms and multiple organ involvement. The predominantly involved organs are the peripheral nerves, kidneys, gastrointestinal tract, and liver. Needle EMG findings in this case are typical of axonal degeneration: prominent fibrillation and PSWs, increased polyphasic MUPs, and reduced recruitment of MUPs.

NCSs are vital to the workup of patients with systemic necrotizing vasculitis for two reasons. First, adequate nerve conduction tests can detect asymptomatic peripheral neuropathy. According to our series, one-third of patients had no clinical signs of peripheral neuropathy and neuropathy was detected by extensive NCSs. Second, abnormal sural nerve conduction is a prerequisite to the demonstration of vasculitis on biopsy of this nerve. According to our experience, in all 15 patients in whom the sural nerve conduction was abnormal, vasculitic neuropathy was diagnosed by sural nerve biopsy. A later study of 47 cases showed abnormal sural nerve conduction in all cases, and the diagnosis of vasculitis was confirmed in all but one case by the sural nerve biopsy. Thus, it is recommended that abnormal sural nerve

TABLE 9.18. Needle EMG Data in Case 12

				Spontaneous Potentials				Motor Unit Potential				Interference	
Muscle	**Root**	**Nerve**	**Insertion Activity**	**Fib**	**PSW**	**Fasc**	**CRD**	**Amplitude (mV)**	**Duration (ms)**	**Polyphasic Potential**	**HA MUP**	**Pattern**	**Mean Amplitude (mV)**
Lt vast lat	L3,4	Femoral	N	–	–	–	–	1–4	8–12	N	–	RIP	2
Ant tibial	L4,5	Peroneal	N	–	–	–	–	1–3	8–12	N	–	RIP	2
Gastroc	S1,2	Post tibial	+	++	++	–	–	1–2	8–12	+	–	DA	1
Peroneus longus	L5, S1	Peroneal	+	+	+	–	–	1–4	9–12	+	–	DA	1
Rt ant tibial	L4,5	Peroneal	+	++	+++	–	–	1–2	8–12	++	–	RIP	1
Peroneus longus	L5, S1	Peroneal	+	+	+	–	–	1–2	8–12	+	–	RIP	1
Gastroc	S1,2	Post tibial	+	+	++	–	+	1–3	8–12	+	–	RIP	1

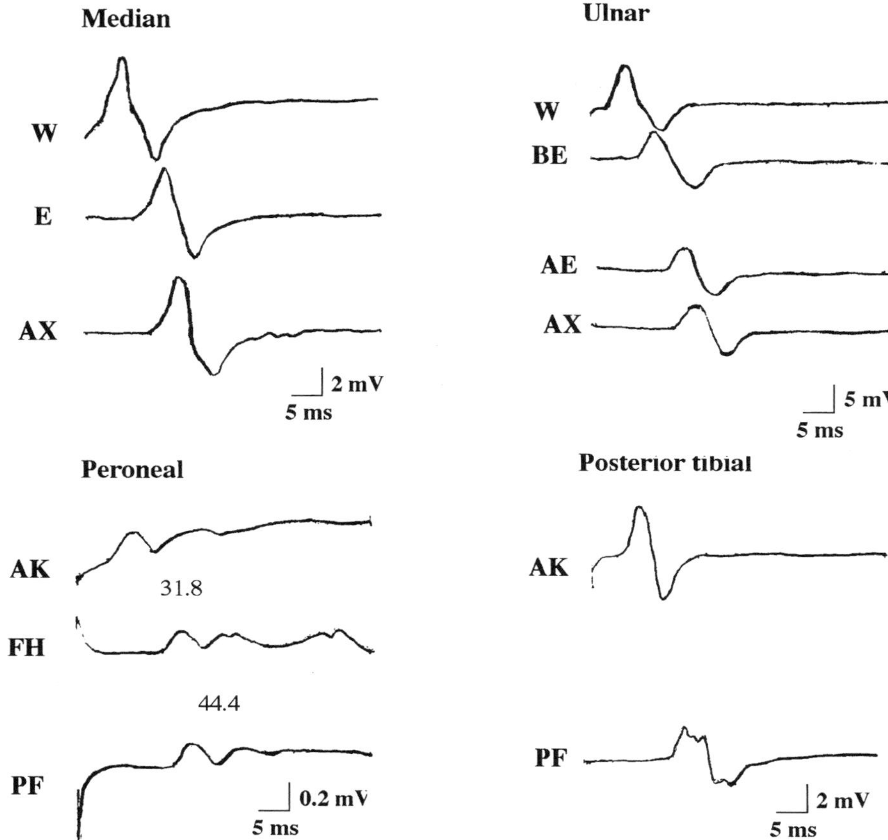

FIGURE 9.10. Motor nerve conduction in the various nerves. Low CMAP amplitude is noted in the peroneal nerve and posterior tibial nerve with popliteal fossa stimulation. Low CMAP and mild NCV slowing are typical of axonal degeneration. *W*, wrist stimulation; *E*, elbow stimulation; *AX*, axilla stimulation.

conduction should be used as a guide in the nerve biopsy. This certainly will enhance the diagnostic yield of sural nerve biopsy. Nerve conduction abnormalities in vasculitic neuropathies are typical of axonal degeneration. Vasculitic neuropathy is the best indication for the nerve biopsy, because it is a treatable disorder. The nerve biopsy shows a significantly higher diagnostic yield than the muscle biopsy. However, we do recommend nerve and muscle biopsies for vasculitis because the muscle biopsy may reveal more specific features of vasculitis when the nerve biopsy shows nonspecific perivascular inflammation.

MAXIMS

1. NCS can detect asymptomatic neuropathy in a substantial number of cases of vasculitis. Once asymptomatic neuropathy is found, the sural nerve biopsy can confirm the diagnosis of vasculitis.
2. Symmetrical or asymmetrical polyneuropathy does not rule out vasculitic neuropathy.

REFERENCES

1. Wees SJ, Sunwoo IN, Oh SJ. Sural nerve biopsy in systemic notarizing vasculitis. Am J Med 1981;71: 525–531.
2. Bouche P, Léger JM, Travers MA, Cathala HP, Castaigne P. Peripheral neuropathy in systemic vasculitis: clinical and electrophysiologic study of 22 cases. Neurology 1986;36:1598–1602.

CASE 13

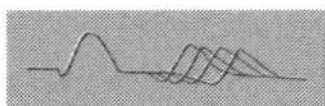

PROGRESSIVE ATAXIA FOR 1 YEAR IN A 17-YEAR-OLD BOY

CASE PRESENTATION

A 17-year-old high school senior was evaluated for progressive clumsiness in writing and difficulty in walking for 1 year. According to his mother, most of his movements were clumsy and his writing was illegible. No other neurological abnormality was noted. Family history was not productive, except that his mother had a high-arched foot. Examination showed no retinitis pigmentosa, nystagmus, or telangiectasia. Spine examination showed mild kyphoscoliosis. Reflexes were decreased in biceps and triceps, normal in the knees, and absent at the ankles. Plantar responses were extensor. Pin-prick perception was completely normal; vibration sense was decreased on ankles, toes, and fingers; and position sense was 50% impaired on the toes. There was mild pes cavus. Muscle strength was normal. A mild intention tremor was noted in finger-to nose and heel-to-knee testing. The patient clearly had an ataxic gait and was unable to do tandem gait. Spinal fluid was normal. Head CT was also normal. Serum VDRL was negative. Serum vitamins B12 and E were normal.

CASE ANALYSIS

Clinically, this patient had the typical constellation of Friedreich's ataxia: pes cavus, areflexia, position sense loss, plantar extensor reflexes, and ataxia. Differential diagnoses should include vitamin B12 deficiency and tabes dorsalis. In vitamin B12 deficiency, ataxia is due to proprioception loss, not to cerebellar dysfunction, and sensory complaints are prominent features. In tabes dorsalis, pain, visceral crises, and Argyll-Robertson pupils are common findings, and plantar reflexes are flexor.

PLAN OF TESTING

1. NCS: To confirm sensory neuronopathy.
2. Somatosensory evoked potential study: To document any central conduction defect.
3. Phytanic acid, vitamins B12 and E, and serum VDRL.

ELECTROPHYSIOLOGICAL TESTS AND FINDINGS

NCS Findings (Table 9.19)

1. Low amplitude of the sensory CNAP in the left sural, right median, and ulnar nerves.
2. Absent sensory CNAP in the right sural nerve.
3. Normal NCS in all tested mixed and motor nerves.

Somatosensory Evoked Potential (median nerve) (Fig. 9.11)

1. Absent N10 (Erb's potential) in the right and left somatosensory evoked potential(s).
2. Normal latencies to N14 (cervical potential) in the right and left somatosensory evoked potential(s).
3. Absent N20 (cortical potential) in the left somatosensory evoked potential and prolonged (8.45 ms) N14 to N20 interpeak latency in the right somatosensory evoked potential.

ELECTROPHYSIOLOGICAL INTERPRETATION

Sensory neuropathy with central conduction defect typical of Friedreich's ataxia.

OTHER TEST FINDINGS

Serum phytanic acid, vitamins E and B12, and VDRL were normal.

FINAL DIAGNOSIS

Friedreich's ataxia

TREATMENT AND FOLLOW-UP

Gradually, the patient's ataxia progressed, involving his speech and eye movements. Within 10 years, he became wheelchair bound due to marked truncal ataxia and severe ataxic gait.

TABLE 9.19. Nerve Conduction Data in Case 13

	Latent/NCV (ms/m/s)	Amplitude (mV/μV)		Latent/NCV (ms/m/s)	Amplitude (mV/μV)
	Median	**Motor N**		**Peroneal**	**Motor N**
TL	3.2	14.0	TL	4.0	5.5
E-W	59.0	12.0	FH-A	47.5	5.0
AX-E	53.0	10.0	PF-FH		
F-wave	27.6		F-wave	48.8	
	Ulnar	**Motor N**		**Post Tibial**	**Motor N**
TL	2.1	8.0	TL	3.4	17
BE-W	50.0	8.0	PF-A	43.8	17
AE-BE	71.4	8.0			
AX-AE	50.0	8.0			
F-wave	26.8		F-wave	46.4	
	Median	**Sens/Mixed N**	**Left**	**Sural**	**Sens N**
F-W	45.0	1.2	MC-A	NP	
W-E	52.7	10.0	**Right**	**Sural**	**Sens N**
E-AX	64.5	15.0		38.5	1.2
	Ulnar	**Sens/Mixed N**		**Plantar**	**Sens**
F-W	45.6	2.2	Medial		
W-E	53.2	10.3	Lateral		
E-AX	53.5	16.0			

Height: 166 cm.

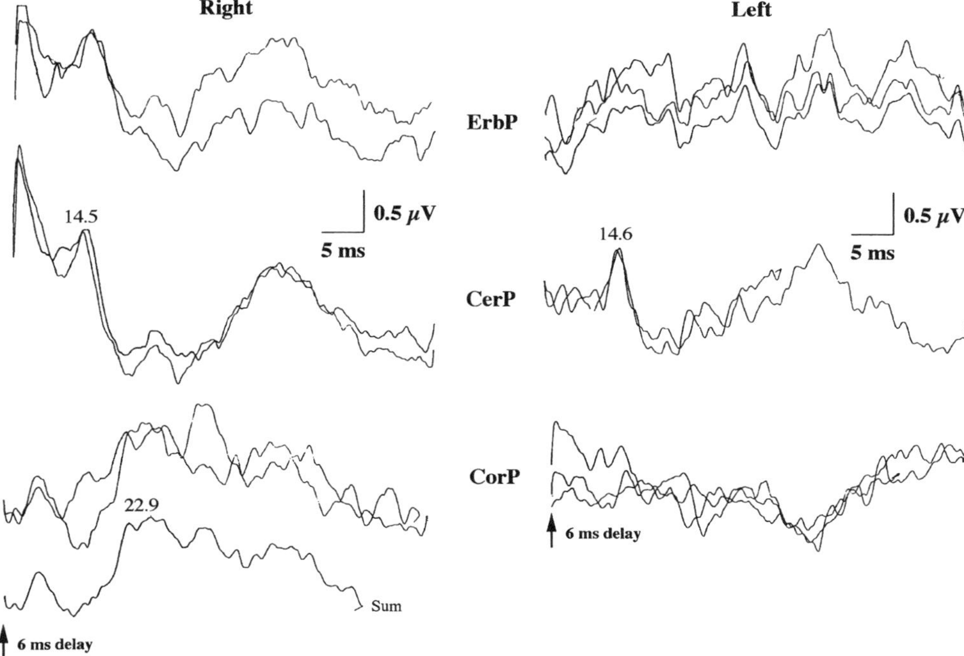

FIGURE 9.11. Right and left median somatosensory evoked potentials. Right SEP: absent N10 (Erb's potentials [ErbP]), normal latency to N14 and prolonged N14-N20 (cervical [CerP]-cortical potentials [CorP]) interpeak latency). Left SEP absent N10, normal latency to N14, and absent cortical potentials. These are indicative of peripheral and central conduction dysfunction typical of Friedreich's ataxia.

COMMENTS

Friedreich's ataxia, the most common form of spinocerebellar degeneration, is an autosomal-recessive disorder with an onset almost always before the age of 20 years. Clinically, it is characterized by ataxia, an absence of deep tendon reflexes, a loss of proprioceptive sensations in the extremities, extensor plantar responses, pes cavus, and kyphoscoliosis. Cardiomyopathy is also common. The disorder is due to a selective degeneration of large cells of the dorsal root ganglia, spinocerebellar tracts, posterior column, and pyramidal tracts. The characteristic nerve conduction abnormality in this disease is sensory neuronopathy; sensory or mixed nerve potentials are either absent or markedly reduced in amplitude, whereas the motor nerve conduction is normal or near normal. Other hereditary ataxias with sensory neuronopathy include ataxia telangiectasia and Bassen-Kornzweig syndrome. Vitamin E deficiency has been reported in some cases of Bassen-Kornzweig syndrome.

The somatosensory evoked potential study is extremely helpful in documenting central nervous system involvement in Freidreich's ataxia. The characteristic somatosensory evoked potential features are loss of amplitude of peripheral (N9, Erb's point) and cervical (N13) potentials without evidence of markedly delayed peripheral nerve conduction and dispersed and delayed cortical potentials (N20) with a prolongation of N20 onset-to-peak separation. These SEP changes can be explained by axonal degeneration of peripheral nerves and degeneration of the posterior column in the central nervous system. The pattern of somatosensory evoked potentials in Friedreich's ataxia is sufficiently characteristic to distinguish this condition from pure peripheral neuropathy without central nervous system involvement, degenerative central nervous system disease without peripheral nerve involvement, and multiple sclerosis.

MAXIMS

1. Sensory neuronopathy (marked sensory nerve conduction abnormalities in the presence of normal motor NCS) is the characteristic nerve conduction abnormality in Friedreich's ataxia.
2. The pattern of pure sensory neuronopathy is pathognomonic of a sensory neuronopathy involving the dorsal root sensory ganglia.

REFERENCES

1. Oh SJ, Halsey JH. Abnormality in nerve potential in Friedreich's ataxia. Neurology 1973;23:52–54.
2. McLeod JG. An electrophysiological and pathological study of peripheral nerves in Friedreich's ataxia. J Neurol Sci 1971;12:333–346.

CASE 14

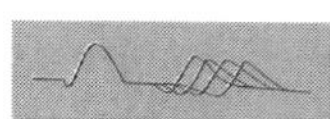

GLOBAL WEAKNESS AND SENSORY LOSS IN THE ENTIRE LEFT ARM IN A WORKER'S COMPENSATION CASE

CASE PRESENTATION

In 1983, a 33-year-old man apparently developed "complete paralysis" of the left arm without any pain after a tree fell on his left arm a year before at his job. With "weekly injections" from a physician, the weakness of his left arm gradually improved over an 8-month period. The referring neurologist found a severe polyneuropathy by the NCS and referred the patient for further evaluation. Abnormal neurological findings were as follows: absent knee and ankle reflexes, decreased biceps, triceps, and brachioradialis reflexes; MRC strength of 4 in the entire left arm muscles; analgesia over the entire left arm below the shoulder, absent position sense on the toes, decreased vibration sense on the wrists, fingers, and iliac bones, and absent vibration sense on the toes, ankles, and knees. He had minimal difficulty walking on his heels.

CASE ANALYSIS

Neurological examination in this Worker's Compensation case showed rather "functional" motor and sensory deficits as noted in many such patients, giving the impression that he did not have any organic neurological disease. The only reliable objective neurological deficit was decreased or absent reflexes. It was mandatory to repeat the NCS to verify the previously reported nerve conduction abnormalities.

PLAN OF TESTING

1. NCS: To see whether the previous test was genuine.
2. Needle EMG: To document any organic abnormalities.
3. Other tests: Nerve biopsy and other workup for neuropathy.

ELECTROPHYSIOLOGICAL TESTS AND FINDINGS

NCS Findings (Table 9.20; Fig. 9.12)

1. Slow motor NCV in the axilla-elbow segment and prolonged terminal latencies in median and ulnar nerves.
2. Conduction block in the left median nerve and dispersion phenomenon in the left ulnar nerve.
3. Prolonged terminal latencies and slow motor NCV in the peroneal and posterior tibial nerves.
4. Low CMAP amplitude in the left ulnar and peroneal nerves.
5. Mild slowing in sensory and mixed NCV and low CNAP amplitudes in the finger-elbow segments in the left median and ulnar nerves.
6. Mild slowing in sensory NCV in the sural nerves.

Needle EMG

Prominent fasciculation and HALD MUPs in all tested muscles.

ELECTROPHYSIOLOGICAL INTERPRETATION

Demyelinating neuropathy suggestive of acquired neuropathy.

OTHER TEST FINDINGS

Sural nerve biopsy showed tomaculous neuropathy. The remaining neuropathy workup was negative.

FINAL DIAGNOSIS

Hereditary neuropathy to pressure palsy

TABLE 9.20. Nerve Conduction Data in Case 14

	Latent/NCV (ms/m/s)	Amplitude (mV/μV)	Shape		Latent/NCV (ms/m/s)	Amplitude (mV/μV)
Left	**Median**	**Motor N**	**Nerve**		**Peroneal**	**Motor N**
TL	5.2	5.3		TL	7.5	4.5
E-W	57.7	2.7	CB	FH-A	39.5	3.4
AX-E	35.7	1.3	CB/D	PF-FH	37.5	3
F-wave	29.7			F-wave	58.8	
	Ulnar	**Motor**	**Nerve**		**Post Tibial**	**Motor N**
TL	4.3	2.2	D	TL	6.7	10
BE-W	54.2	2.1	D	PF-A	35.5	8
AE-BE	40.9	2.0	D			
AX-AE	36.2	2.0	D			
EB-AX						
F-wave	35.9			F-wave	67.5	
	Median	**Sens/Mixed**	**Nerve**		**Sural**	**Sens N**
F-W	29.3	5		MC-A	30.2	7
W-E	42.5	3				
E-AX	54.0	10				
	Ulnar	**Sens/Mixed**	**Nerve**		**Superficial Peroneal**	**Sens N**
F-W	23.5	2		MC-A		
W-E	38.3	5				
E-AX	43.7	10				

Height: 180.3 cm.

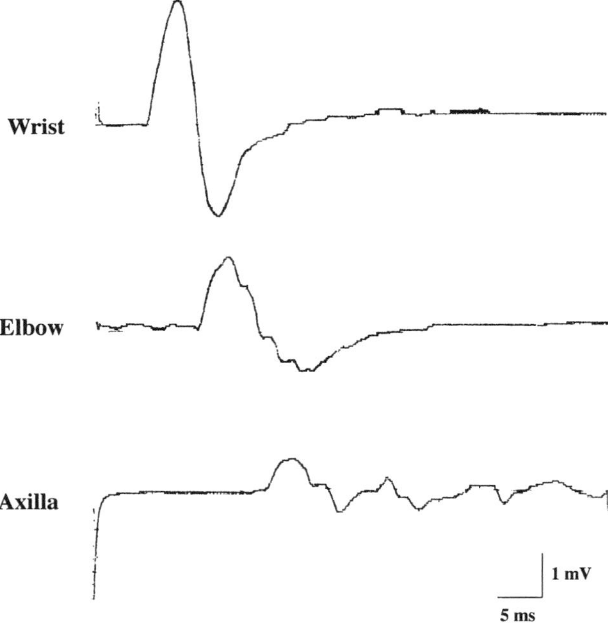

FIGURE 9.12. Left median nerve motor conduction. Conduction block is present in the elbow-wrist segment and the axilla-elbow segment. Temporal dispersion is also present in the CMAP with axilla stimulation.

TREATMENT AND FOLLOW-UP

After the diagnosis of tomaculous neuropathy was made, the patient told us that his father had been treated by us for CIDP. His father had an asymmetrical polyneuropathy with pes cavus and high CSF protein (170 mg/dL) and had been treated with prednisone with some improvement. His father's NCS showed nonuniform demyelinating neuropathy with conduction block and dispersion. A review of his biopsy showed tomaculous neuropathy. Over the next 6 months, his neuropathy resolved completely.

COMMENTS

Except for his "functional neurological deficits," our case was classic for HNNP: most likely a brachial plexus neuropathy after a minor injury, positive family history, tomaculous changes in the nerve biopsy, widespread nerve conduction abnormalities even in unaffected nerves, and gradual recovery. Tomaculous neuropathy is classically observed in two disorders: HNPP and recurrent brachial plexus neuropathy. As noted in this patient's father, polyneuropathy mimicking CIDP has been reported in a few cases.

HNPP is a rare disorder characterized by susceptibility to pressure palsies after relatively minor episodes of compression or ischemia, improvement of symptoms within weeks or months, frequent recurrence of pressure palsies, and autosomal-dominant inheritance. The disorder may present along with recurrent brachial plexus neuropathy. Tomacula, or ballooned internodal "sausages" caused by the formation of extra myelin lamellae and segmental demyelination are pathognomonic of this disorder. Electrophysiological findings in this disorder can be summarized as follows.

1. The electrophysiological hallmark is nonuniform mild demyelinating neuropathy with prolonged distal latency, which is out of proportion to NCV slowing, and focal neuropathy at the entrapment site. Focal neuropathy can be expressed as the slowest NCV or conduction block. This is in sharp contrast to the most classic hereditary neuropathy, HMSN type 1 (Charcot-Marie-Tooth [CMT] type 1), in which uniform demyelination neuropathy is the typical finding. These electrophysiological features should raise a "red flag" and lead to consideration of tomaculous neuropathy.
2. The classic pattern of nerve conduction abnormalities is the presence of focal nerve lesions in the clinically affected nerves superimposed on a generalized neuropathy affecting motor and sensory fibers in clinically unaffected nerves.
3. Nerve conduction abnormalities can be demonstrated in clinically unaffected relatives, possibly identifying individuals at risk of developing this disorder.

Recent studies concluded that HNPP is caused by a 1.5-Mb deletion in 17p11.2-p12, which spans the same region duplicated in most CMT1A patients. This region encompasses the PMP-22 gene, which is expressed on Schwann cells. Because 1.5-Mb deletion in 17p11.2-p12 has been observed in most HNPP patients, this DNA testing can now be used to detect HNPP in individual patients and in unaffected family members.

MAXIMS

1. Nerve conduction hallmarks for HNPP are nonuniform mild demyelinating neuropathy with prolonged distal latency that is out of proportion to slowing in NCV and focal neuropathy with superimposed generalized neuropathy.
2. DNA testing (1.5-Mb deletion in 17p11.2-p12) for HNPP can be used for the diagnosis of HNPP in affected individuals and in unaffected family members.

REFERENCES

1. Amato AA, Gronseth GS, Callerame KJ, Kagan-Hallet KS, Bryan WW, Barohn RJ. Tomaculous neuropathy: a clinical and electrophysiological study in patients with and without 1.5-MB deletions in chromosome 17p11.2. Muscle Nerve 1996;19:16–22.
2. Magistris MR, Roth G. Long-lasting conduction block in hereditary neuropathy with liability to pressure palsy. Neurology 1985;35:1639–1641.

CASE 15

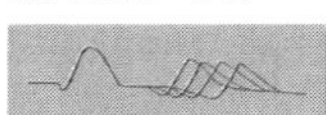

HAND SHAKING AS AN INITIAL MANIFESTATION OF HEREDITARY NEUROPATHY

CASE PRESENTATION

A 25-year-old woman first noticed tremors in her hands and feet at age 14. Her developmental history was normal. After the birth of a child at age 18, her tremors became worse and she began to have cramps in her toes and calf muscles. One year ago, she experienced decreased sensation in her toes and weakness of the legs, especially in dorsiflexion of her feet. In the past 2 years, she had two surgeries to remove bony spurs from her feet. Her tremors were worse under stress and when she attempted to write. Family history was interesting in that her mother was crippled with "claw hands" and weakness of the feet, her aunt possibly had a similar problem, and her 22-year-old brother had a tremor and weakness of the feet. Abnormal neurological findings were atrophy of intrinsic hand muscles; pes cavus without hammer toes; 4− MRC strength in anterior tibialis, peroneus, and posterior tibial muscles; absent patellar and ankle reflexes; decreased pin-prick sensation below the midcalf and midforearm; and a fine tremor in the hands on extension of the arms. Vibratory and position senses were normal. No thickened nerves were noted on palpation.

CASE ANALYSIS

It is interesting that the initial presentation of this patient's neuropathy was essential tremor. Essential tremor in the presence of neuropathy is always due to demyelinating neuropathy, either hereditary or acquired. Her essential tremor was soon followed by weakness of the legs. Examination confirmed the classic findings of chronic neuropathy: pes cavus and distal leg weakness. A strong family history clearly pinpointed the hereditary nature of her neuropathy. Pes cavus and an autosomal-dominant family history are strongly suggestive of HMSN (CMT). Considering the presence of essential tremor, we were dealing with HMSN type 1 (hypertrophic type of CMT or CMT 1), Roussy-Levy syndrome. Essential tremor is not observed in HMSN type 2 (neuronal type of CMT or CMT 2).

PLAN OF TESTING

1. NCS: To identify peripheral neuropathy and delineate the nature of peripheral neuropathy.
2. Needle EMG: To see whether the neuropathy was axonal or demyelination.
3. Other tests: Nerve biopsy to confirm HMSN type 1. Examine one other family member to confirm the hereditary nature of the neuropathy.

ELECTROPHYSIOLOGICAL TESTS AND FINDINGS

NCS Findings (Table 9.21; Fig. 9.13)

1. Absent sensory and mixed CNAPs in most tested nerves.
2. Markedly slow sensory and mixed NCVs in the median and ulnar nerves, respectively.
3. Markedly prolonged terminal latency and markedly slow motor NCV in all segments in all tested nerves.
4. No conduction block or dispersion phenomenon in any tested nerves.
5. Low CMAP amplitude in the ulnar, peroneal, and posterior tibial nerves.
6. Absent F-wave or markedly prolonged F-wave latencies.

Needle EMG Data in the Right Anterior Tibialis and Gastrocnemius Muscles

1. Fasciculations and discrete activity in both muscles.
2. Many HALD MUPs (amplitude, 1 to 7K; duration, 8 to 25 ms) are mixed with normal MUPs.
3. Rapidly firing MUPs; discrete activity (mean amplitude, 5 mV) on maximal contraction in both muscles.

TABLE 9.21. Nerve Conduction Data in Case 15

	Latent/NCV (ms/m/s)	Amplitude (mV/μV)		Latent/NCV (ms/m/s)	Amplitude (mV/μV)
	Median	**Motor N**		**Peroneal**	**Motor N**
TL	9.8	8.4	TL	9.9	0.5
E-W	24.2	7.6	FH-A	14.3	0.4
AX-E	38.4	7.4	PF-FH	21.6	0.4
F-wave	48.2		F-wave	NP	
	Ulnar	**Motor N**		**Post Tibial**	**Motor N**
TL	5.1	2.2	TL	11.9	1.2
BE-W	20.3	2.2	PF-A	15.6	1.1
AE-BE	24.2	2.2			
AX-AE	29.4	2.2			
F-wave	56.5		F-wave	NP	
	Median	**Sens/Mixed N**		**Sural**	**Sens N**
F-W	16.7	2.2	MC-A	NP	
W-E	NP				
E-AX	NP				
	Ulnar	**Sens/Mixed N**		**Plantar**	**Sens N**
F-W	NP	6.4	Medial		
W-E	21.9	3.2	Lateral		
E-AX	NP				

Height: 165.5 cm.

ELECTROPHYSIOLOGICAL INTERPRETATION

Uniform demyelinating motor and sensory polyneuropathy typical of HMSN type 1 (CMT 1A).

OTHER TEST FINDINGS

Nerve biopsy showed hypertrophic neuropathy with onion-bulb formation.

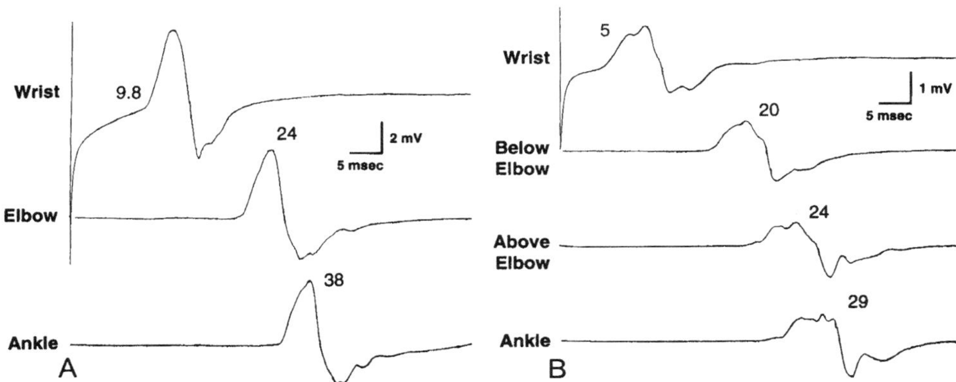

FIGURE 9.13. "Uniform slowing" typical of HMSN type 1. Conduction block and abnormal temporal dispersion are absent. **A.** Median nerve: NCVs between the segments are "not uniformly slow." **B.** Ulnar nerve: NCVs between the segments are "uniformly slow." Numbers on the left represent the terminal latencies in ms. Numbers on the right represent the NCVs.

FINAL DIAGNOSIS

HMSN type I (CMT 1A); Roussey-Levy syndrome

TREATMENT AND FOLLOW-UP

Two other members of the patient's family were evaluated. Both had HMSN type 1 with uniform demyelinating neuropathy, confirming the hereditary nature of this neuropathy. Over a 10-year period, no significant worsening was noted in the patient's lower leg strength and her tremor was well controlled with Inderal and valium.

COMMENTS

CMT disease is the most common hereditary neuropathy. It is inherited as an autosomal-dominant trait and is characterized clinically by pes cavus (highly arched feet) and marked atrophy of the feet and lower legs, resulting in a characteristic appearance sometimes described as "stork-leg" or "inverted champagne bottle leg." Weakness is seen predominantly in the peroneal muscle group, as a result of which the term "peroneal muscular atrophy" was coined for this disorder. CMT disease is slowly progressive.

CMT disease can be classified in two types: hypertrophic (onion-bulb formation) and neuronal. Although clinically it is not always possible to distinguish the type of neuropathy in an individual patient, the NCS has been of definite help in differentiating between the types. Median motor NCV 40 m/s in an affected individual is a magic number for the two groups: hypertrophic type < 40 m/s and neuronal type > 40 m/s. The pattern of NCV changes seems to be constant within a family.

In HMSN type 1 (CMT type 1; hypertrophic type CMT), marked and uniform slowing in motor NCV and marked abnormalities in sensory nerve conduction are the classic findings. The motor NCV is usually less than 60% of normal values: distal motor latencies averaging almost three times longer than normal, NCVs and CMAP amplitudes less than half of normal. Extreme slowing of the motor NCV (11.2 m/s) is reported in this disorder. In sensory nerve conduction, either the CNAP is absent or there is marked slowing of the sensory NCV. Marked slowing in NCV in this disorder is due to segmental demyelination characterized by onion-bulb formation in the nerves. In HMSN (CMT type 2; neuronal CMT), normal or near-normal motor NCV and normal or mildly abnormal sensory nerve conduction are typical findings. These nerve conduction changes are thought to be due to axonal degeneration of the nerves.

In HMSN type 1, NCV slowing is found in members of the family who show only minimal or no abnormalities on clinical examination. Thus, the NCS is helpful in detecting clinically unaffected carriers of the disease. A slowing of NCV precedes the onset of clinical symptoms and may even be present at birth. Thus, NCS is also valuable as a screening test in preclinical stages of the disease. It should be mentioned that the NCV may be normal during early childhood and become abnormal at a later time. A consensus of various studies suggests that 3 to 5 years of age may be optimal for the study of potentially affected children. Thus, if the motor NCV is normal after 5 years of age, the diagnosis of HMSN type 1 can safely be excluded in the tested child.

Attempts have been made to distinguish HMSN type 1 from acquired chronic demyelinating neuropathy. This distinction is important because some patients with acquired chronic demyelinating neuropathy may respond to steroid therapy or immunosuppressants. It is possible to make this distinction with the nerve conduction test. In HMSN type 1 (specifically in CMT1A), nerve conduction is slowed uniformly over all nerve segments and conduction block is not observed, whereas in chronic acquired demyelinating neuropathy, multifocal slowing of nerve conduction and conduction block are typical. Although this rule is generally correct, it should not be regarded as always accurate because two studies have shown exceptions in rare HMSN type 1 and uniform slowing may be observed in acquired CIDP.

Roussy-Levy syndrome resembles CMT in the following features: its familial nature, the prevalence of clubfoot, weakness and minimal atrophy of the distal extremity muscles, and some distal sensory loss. It differs from CMT because there is a static tremor of the hands.

TABLE 9.22. Contrasting Features in CMT1A and HNPP

	CMT1A	HNPP
Clinical features	Slowly progressive symmetrical polyneuropathy, pes cavus with hammer toes	Recurrent mononeuropathy or plexopathy; asymmetrical
Antecedent events	None	Minor nerve compression or trauma
NCS	Uniform demyelinating neuropathy with markedly slow NCV	Non-uniform demyelinating neuropathy with conduction block and dispersion phenomenon
Nerve biopsy findings	Onion bulb formation	Tomacula
Inheritance	Autosomal dominance	Autosomal dominance
Genetic marker	Duplication of 17p11.2-p12	Deletion in 17p11.2-p12

Dyck and Lambert classified this syndrome as type 1 HMSN because they concluded that Roussy-Levy syndrome is nothing more than CMT plus an essential tremor. Nerve biopsy showed hypertrophic neuropathy (numerous onion-bulb formations). Marked slowing of the motor NCV has been reported in this condition. We found that sensory and mixed CNAPs were absent in most patients with this disorder.

Recent studies in CMT disease have identified genetic heterogeneity. For example, HMSN type 1 is now divided into three types (CMT1A, CMT1B, CMT1C). In CMT1A, the most common type of HMSN type 1, the gene defect is known to be a 1.5-Mb tandem DNA duplication in 17p11.2-p1.12, which is the same region where DNA deletion was found in HNPP (Table 9.22). The CMT1A duplication has been identified in more than 70% of patients with CMT1. Given this high frequency, the detection of the CMT1A duplication is a useful molecular test in patients with inherited and sporadic peripheral neuropathies of unknown etiology because it is a biologic marker for the disease. This test can also be used for prenatal and preclinical diagnosis of CMT1A and for detection of carriers of the disease.

MAXIMS

1. A uniform demyelinating neuropathy pattern is the classic nerve conduction finding in CMT1A.
2. The CMT1A duplication test is a biologic marker for CMT1A. Thus, this can be used for diagnosis of CMT1A in symptomatic patients and for prenatal and preclinical diagnosis of CMT1A in asymptomatic individuals.

REFERENCES

1. Kuku DA, Parry GJ, Malamut R, Lupski JR, Garcia CA. Uniform slowing of conduction velocities in Charcot-Marie-Tooth polyneuropathy type 1. Neurology 1993;43:2664–2667.
2. Murakami T, Carcia CA, Teiter LT, Lupski JR. Charcot-Marie-Tooth disease and related inherited neuropathies. Medicine 1996;75:233–250.

CHAPTER 10

Anterior Horn Cell Diseases

Motor neuron disease (MND) refers to the heterogenous group of diseases caused by lesions in the anterior horn cells and pyramidal tracts. Thus, *the cardinal sign of MND is selective motor weakness and wasting without any sensory or cerebellar impairment.* Depending on the site of the lesions, MNDs are divided into amyotrophic lateral sclerosis (ALS), characterized by a combined disease process affecting the anterior horn cells and pyramidal tracts; progressive or spinal muscular atrophy, in which the disease process affects the anterior horn cells alone; and primary lateral sclerosis (PLS), caused by lesions in the bilateral pyramidal tracts.

AMYOTROPHIC LATERAL SCLEROSIS

ALS, more commonly known as Lou Gehrig's disease in the United States, is the most common form of MND. It is a primarily a disease of older adults who develop asymmetrical weakness and atrophy, most often initially in the hand muscles. The disease is slowly but relentlessly progressive, spreading to other limbs and bulbar muscles in a few months or years. As a form of MND, in this disease, weakness is classically painless and is the primary reason that the patient seeks medical help. *As important negative signs, there should not be any complaints of pain, definite sensory complaints, or symptoms of sphincter or ocular muscle involvement.* Muscle cramping on exertion is not an unusual complaint in this disorder.

Usually, 80% of patients die within 5 years of onset, but there are some who live longer than 10 years. I usually emphasize the latter fact in discussing the natural course of this disease with a patient at the time of diagnosis, giving the patient some hope.

Because ALS involves the lower and upper motor neurons together, the patient must have *a combination of upper and lower motor neuron (UMN and LMN) signs.* Fasciculations due to irritation of surviving anterior horn cells and their axons are the most distinctive sign in ALS, occurring early but disappearing in muscles that are no longer innervated. Widespread fasciculations differentiate ALS from myopathy or peripheral neuropathy. Thus, without either clinical or electromyographic (EMG) evidence of fasciculation, it is extremely difficult to make the diagnosis of ALS. Another prominent sign suggestive of ALS is increased reflexes in the presence of marked weakness and wasting due to an LMN lesion. However, this combination can be observed in the arms in cervical spondylotic myelopathy (CSM). It should be noted that even though UMN signs are common in ALS, the Babinski sign is seen in only 50% of cases and is due to weakness of the extensor hallucis longus muscles. Another helpful diagnostic sign of ALS is a distinct "spastic" dysarthria, caused by combined LMN and UMN bulbar involvement. In contrast to the nasal phonation classically observed in bulbar palsy, *dysarthria in ALS is characterized by forced guttural slurring as if the tongue were tightly stuck to the floor of the mouth.* It is worth listening to "ALS dysarthria" because it defies exact description.

The El Escorial ALS diagnostic criteria were created in 1990 to provide uniform guidelines for the diagnosis of ALS. Under the proposed scheme, the central and peripheral nervous system are divided into four regions: bulbar, cervical, thoracic, and lumbosacral. According to the El Escorial criteria, the diagnosis of ALS require the progression of disease for more than 6 months (although it is stated that two examinations should be conducted 6 months apart, this is rarely necessary with other diagnostic measures), the presence of signs of LMN degeneration by clinical or electrophysiological examination and of UMN degeneration by clinical examination in each of at least two regions (probable ALS) or in a total of three

TABLE 10.1. Diseases Mimicking ALS

Diseases	Definitive Tests for Exclusion
Cervical spondylotic myelopathy	MRI, CT myelogram
Myasthenia gravis	AChR antibody, repetitive nerve stimulation test
Multifocal motor neuropathy	Conduction block in NCS, GM1 antibody
CIDP (motor form)	Demyelination in NCS, high CSF protein
Inclusion body myopathy	Muscle biopsy, needle EMG
Thyroid myopathy	Thyroid profile, needle EMG
Parathyroid myopathy	Parathyroid hormone assay, needle EMG
Tandem cervical and lumbar stenosis	MRI, CT myelogram
Lymphoma	Serum protein immunoelectrophoresis by immunofixation high CSF protein, bone marrow study
Kennedy syndrome (X-linked bulbospinal muscular atrophy)	CAG repeat in androgen receptor antibody
HTLV 1 myelopathy	HTLV 1 antibody, CSF protein
Hexosaminidase-A deficiency (adult form)	Hexosaminidase-A enzyme assay

regions (definite ALS), and no other disease processes that could lead to UMN and LMN changes, as determined by the use of appropriate electrodiagnostic and neuroimaging techniques. In this connection, the electrophysiological and MRI studies become an essential part of the diagnostic workup in ALS.

In view of the relentless nature of ALS and the absence of any effective treatment, it is important to rule out other treatable diseases (Table 10.1). Disorders mimicking ALS include myasthenia gravis, inclusion body myopathy (IBM), cervical radiculopathy or spondylotic myelopathy, lumbar stenosis, multifocal motor neuropathy (MMN), chronic inflammatory demyelinating polyneuropathy (CIDP), hyperthyroid or parathyroid myopathies, paraneoplastic motor neuron syndrome, and hexosaminidase-A deficiency (adult form).

PROGRESSIVE (SPINAL) MUSCULAR ATROPHY

Progressive muscular atrophy (PMA) is a form of MND involving the LMN and comprising about 8% of cases. *There should not be any UMN signs in this condition.* PMA is slightly more common in men, with onset at an earlier age than the average age for ALS. In contrast to ALS, bulbar or respiratory involvement is rare. The most important difference from ALS is a slower course; most patients with PMA live for many years with slowly worsening limb weakness.

It is important to remember two clinical points. First, pure LMN manifestation can be an initial manifestation of ALS. *The appearance and rapid progression of UMN symptoms are usually the warning signs for ALS.* In some series, about 20% of ALS patients have LMN symptoms as the initial symptom. Second, PMA is a disorder in which MMN, IBM, and hexosaminidase-A deficiency must be ruled out, because these disorders mimic PMA more than ALS clinically. In this connection, the key tests to suggest these other disorders are the electrodiagnostic tests. PMA is different from adult-onset spinal muscular atrophy (SMA) in that a positive family history is lacking. Otherwise, there is no difference.

PROGRESSIVE BULBAR PALSY

Progressive bulbar palsy (PBP) is not a separate subset of MND but usually represents an early manifestation of ALS. In some series, it occurs in 15% of ALS patients. Early in the disease, it may be impossible to make a definite diagnosis of ALS in some patients because of the lack of limb involvement by either clinical or electrophysiological evaluation or muscle biopsy. Thus, this separate diagnosis is justified until a definite diagnosis of ALS can be reached. Clinically, PBP is characterized by a combination of pseudobulbar and bulbar palsy. *The classic speech of ALS patients, as described above, is the cardinal symptom and sign in this disorder.* A snout reflex, jaw jerk, and exaggerated gag reflexes are usual findings confirming the

UMN signs. The speech disorder is invariably followed by swallowing difficulty, resulting in frequent choking and difficulty disposing of saliva. Because of the danger of aspiration pneumonia and weight loss, the percutaneous gastrostomy and early tracheostomy may be life-saving devices in PBP. Bulbar palsy is usually considered a poor prognostic sign because of the shorter survival period compared with limb-onset ALS. Before confirming the diagnosis of PBP, a brain MRI is essential to rule out progressive supranuclear palsy or bilateral multiinfarct vascular diseases. The needle EMG study in the muscles innervated by the cranial nerves is essential in this disorder, and the EMG in the limb muscles is also necessary to document the extent of limb muscle involvement.

PRIMARY LATERAL SCLEROSIS

PLS is one extreme of MND with purely UMN symptoms. *There should not be any LMN signs in this disorder.* PLS is classically characterized by slowly progressive UMN symptoms and signs alone without any involvement of other long tracts. Because there are many central nervous system (CNS) diseases that present initially with pyramidal tract involvement alone, these disorders have to be ruled out. Thus, the diagnosis of PLS should be made by exclusion. It is also important to remember that some ALS patients first present with pyramidal signs with spastic paraplegia. In this group, the needle EMG either at the initial evaluation or during the course of follow-up is crucial in documenting LMN signs, making the diagnosis of ALS definite. PLS is slowly progressive, but many patients may expect a normal lifespan. There are two points to remember in this disorder: PLS can be an initial manifestation of other CNS diseases and PLS is quite different from ALS in its prognosis. In this sense, it is not a good idea to tell patients that they have MND, because they sometimes equate MND with ALS.

FAMILIAL SPINAL MUSCULAR ATROPHY

Five different groups of familial SMA are now well established. Their clinical, laboratory, and genetic findings are summarized in Table 10.2. Each subject is discussed further in connection with individual cases.

TABLE 10.2. Clinical and Needle EMG Feature of Familial Spinal Muscular Atrophy

Type	Onset	Unsupported Sitting	Clinical Feature	Fasciculation	CPK	Needle EMG	Survival	Inherit	Gene Defects
Type I (infantile) (Werdnig-Hoffman)	<6 mo	Never	Generalized "frog-leg position"	±[a]	Normal	Widespread fib and PSW Common spontaneous MUP discharge Normal MUP	<18 mo	AR	Deletion in SMN gene Prenatal carrier detection is extremely accurate
Type II (intermediate)	6–24 mo	+ in 25%	Usually generalized	+ in 33%[b]	Usually normal	Often fib and PSW Rare spontaneous MUPs Often HALD MUPs	>2 yr	AR	Deletion in SMN
Type III (juvenile) (Kugelberg-Welander)	>2–20 yr	Always	Usually proximal	+ in 50%	Often raised	Often fib, PSW, and fasciculation; HALD MUPs	Adulthood	AR	Deletion in SMN
Adult	>20 yr	Always	Usually proximal	+ +	Often raised	Often fib, PSW, and fasciculation; HALD MUPs	Adulthood	Usually AD	?
Kennedy disease	>30 yr	Always	Bulbospinal gynecomastia testicular atrophy impotence	+ + perioral/ facial tremor[a]	Usually high	Often fib, PSW, and fasciculation HALD MUPs Abnormal sensory nerve conduction	Adulthood	Sex-linked recessive	Androgen, receptor gene CAG repeat >40

[a] Fasciculation may be present in the wasted tongue.

[b] Tremor of fingers (minipolymyoclonus) in one of three cases. Tongue fasciculation may be present.

[c] Facial, particularly perioral fasciculation is characteristic, if not pathognomonic, of this disease.

AR, autosomal recessive; AD, autosomal dominant; SMN, survival motor neuron; CAG, nucleotide cytosine-adenine-guanine; fib, fibrillation.

CASE 1

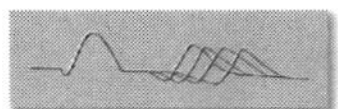

PAINLESS WEAKNESS OF BOTH ARMS FOR 6 MONTHS

CASE PRESENTATION

A 50-year-old right-handed woman had a 5- to 6-month history of weakness of both arms, left greater than right, without sensory complaints such as numbness, tingling, or pain. She reported no involvement of the legs, neck, or lower back. She had no episodes of double vision, swallowing or chewing difficulties, or changes in her voice. Symptoms had been slowly progressive over the preceding 6 months. She denied cramping or abnormal movements of the muscles. MRI of the cervical spine and cervical CT myelogram were normal. Spinal fluid protein was normal.

Abnormal neurological findings were scarce. The patient had 4 MRC strength in the right deltoid, 4- in the left deltoid, and 4+ in both biceps muscles. Reflexes were 1+ in biceps, 3+ in knee and ankle jerks. Fasciculation was observed in both deltoid muscles. Tone, sensory, and cerebellar findings were all normal, and no obvious atrophy or fasciculation was observed in any leg muscles. Plantar responses were flexor.

CASE ANALYSIS

The patient had a 6-month history of painless weakness confined to the C5 and 6 myotomes, suggesting a C5 and 6 lower motor neuron lesion. Considered together with hyperreflexia in the legs and pyramidal tract signs, weakness in the C5 and 6 myotomes clearly raised the possibility of cervical cord compression, but it was well ruled out by the normal MRI and CT myelogram. Myopathy confined to the arms was a definite possibility. However, usually in myopathy, the pelvic girdle muscles are also involved. MMN or a focal expression of MND also had to be ruled out.

PLAN OF TESTING

1. NCS: To rule out chronic demyelinating neuropathy or multifocal motor neuropathy.
2. Needle EMG: To confirm denervation process. This should include tests in the leg muscles.
3. Other tests: CPK and muscle biopsy to rule out myopathy or any disease that can mimic ALS.

ELECTROPHYSIOLOGICAL TESTS AND FINDINGS

NCS Findings

1. Low CMAP amplitude in the right and left median and left ulnar nerves.
2. Prolonged terminal latency, mildly slow motor NCV, and mild slowing in motor NCV in some segments of the right and left median nerves.
3. Low CMAP amplitude in the right peroneal nerve.
4. Normal sensory and mixed NCS in all tested nerves.

Needle EMG (Table 10.3 and Fig 10.1)

1. Increased insertion activity, fibrillations, and fasciculation in almost all tested muscles in both arms.
2. Normal or HA MUPs with reduced recruitment in almost all tested muscles.
3. Fibrillations, PSWs, and fasciculation in the cervical paraspinal muscles.
4. Fibrillations, PSW, fasciculation, normal MUP, and reduced interference pattern in the right and left anterior tibialis muscles.
5. Fasciculation, HA MUPs, and reduced recruitment in the left gastrocnemius and vastus lateralis muscles.

ELECTROPHYSIOLOGICAL INTERPRETATION

Widespread active and chronic denervation typical of anterior horn cell disease.

TABLE 10.3. Needle EMG Data in Case 1

				Spontaneous Potentials				Motor Unit Potential				Interference	
Muscle	**Root**	**Nerve**	**Insertion Activity**	**Fib**	**PSW**	**Fasc**	**Myotonia CRD**	**Amplitude (K)**	**Duration (ms)**	**Polyphasic Potential**	**HA MUP**	**Pat-tern**	**Mean Amplitude (K)**
Lt C6–8	C6-8		+	+	+	+	–						
Deltoids	C5,6	Axillary	+	+	+ + +	+	–	1–7	6–12	+	+	FIP	2
Biceps	C6,7	Musc cut	+	+	+ +	+	–	1–10	7–14	N	+ +	RIP	4
FDI	C7, T1	Ulnar	+	+ +	+ +	+ +	–	1–4	10–14	N	–	DA	4
Rt Deltoids	C5,6	Axillary	+	+	+ +	+	–	1–6	10–15	N	+	RIP	3
Biceps	C6,7	Musc cut	+	+	+ +	+	–	1–4	10–18	+	–	RIP	2
Triceps	C7	Radial	+	+	+ +	+	–	1–5.5	8–12	N	+	RIP	2
APB	C8, T1	Median	+	+	+ +	–	–	1–5	9–12	+	–	DA	1
Lt Ant Tibial	L4,5	Peroneal	+	+	+	+	–	0.5–3	8–13	N	–	RIP	2
Gastroc	S1,2	Post tibial	+	–	–	+	–	1–6	5–15	N	+	RIP	2
Vast lat	L3,4	Femoral	+	–	–	+	–	1–7	10–15	N	+	RIP	2
Rt Ant Tibial	L4,5	Peroneal	+	+	+	+	–	0.5–3	10–15	N	–	RIP	2

Fib, fibrillations; PSW, positive sharp wave; Fasc, fasciculations; HA, high amplitude; FIP, full interference pattern; Musc cut, musculocutaneous; N, normal; RIP, reduced interference pattern; DA, discrete activity; APB, abductor pollicis brevis; +, present or increased; –, absent.

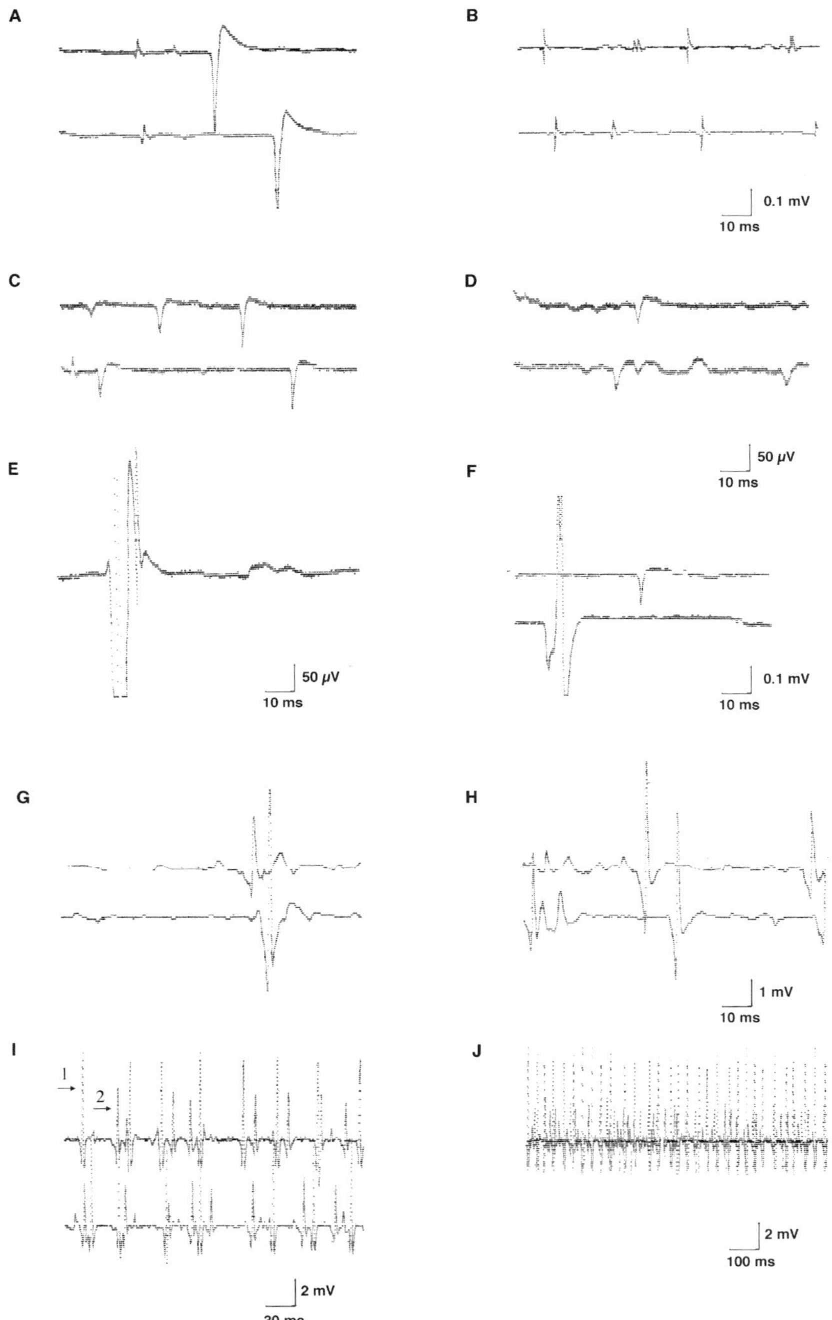

FIGURE 10.1. Widespread denervation process in the needle EMG. **A.** Fibrillations and PSW in the left deltoid muscle. **B.** Fibrillations in the right biceps muscle. **C.** Fibrillations and PSW in the left anterior tibialis muscle. **D.** PSW in the right anterior tibialis muscle. **E.** Fasciculations in the left deltoid muscle. **F.** Fasciculations and PSW in the right biceps muscle. **G** and **H.** Normal and HA MUPs in the right biceps muscle. **I.** Normal recruitment firing rate (27 Hz). *1*, MUP *1* and *2*, MUP 2. **J.** Reduced interference pattern.

OTHER TEST FINDINGS

Muscle biopsy showed prominent fascicular atrophy typical of ALS. CPK was normal.

FINAL DIAGNOSIS

ALS

TREATMENT AND FOLLOW-UP

After a discussion of the marginal benefits of riluzole, the patient decided to take this drug. There was slow but gradual progression of weakness in arms. No weakness in the legs or bulbar muscles was observed during the next year. The patient's main complaint was lack of energy, which is sometimes helped by pemoline.

COMMENTS

Fasciculation alone is not pathological and can be observed in normal individuals (benign fasciculation). Most patients who present with benign fasciculation are medical professionals who know something about the malignant implications of fasciculation in ALS. Classically, these patients complain of fasciculation in a few muscles without any demonstrable weakness or atrophy. With benign fasciculation, it is often difficult to see fasciculation during the brief examination period. In contrast, fasciculation in the weakened or atrophied muscles is pathognomonic of pathological fasciculation. It is common and classically widespread in ALS. Thus, one is hesitant to make a diagnosis of ALS without fasciculation in patient. Fasciculation is also seen in radiculopathy, MMN, CIDP, and hyperexcitable peripheral disorders.

Pathologically, the anterior horn cells and pyramidal tracts are classically involved in ALS. Thus, the diagnosis of ALS relies on the demonstration of UMN and LMN signs in the affected areas of the body: painless muscle weakness and wasting of muscles, fasciculation, and increased reflexes. The cervical area is most commonly the first involved area in ALS. Thus, the first disease to rule out is CSM, which is common in older individuals. It can mimic ALS because combined upper and motor neuron signs in the upper extremities is not uncommon due to the multilevel involvement in the cervical cord. The key findings in favor of CSM are sensory deficits and sphincter impairment, which are absent in ALS. The key findings for ALS are cranial nerve involvements and fasciculation in the leg muscles. An MRI of the cervical cord can easily rule out CSM.

The needle EMG is an essential diagnostic tool in ALS, where it must document active ongoing and chronic denervation in symptomatic and many asymptomatic muscles in widespread areas of the body. In this case, active denervation in both anterior tibialis muscles and chronic denervation in other leg muscles, which was not expected with UMN signs, clinched the diagnosis of MND. In typical cases, the electrophysiological findings of active and chronic denervation patterns are often asymmetrical and multifocal. To document the widespread denervation typical of ALS, abnormalities must be present in at least three muscles innervated by different nerves and spinal roots in at least three extremities; the head may be counted as one extremity. Thus, the needle EMG study in asymptomatic muscles and in muscles of the limbs with UMN signs is extremely critical in reaching a definite diagnosis of ALS. In the present case, it was particularly important to differentiate ALS from CSM or cervical cord compression in which the denervation process is confined to the upper extremities. However, when a patient has tandem cervical and lumbar stenosis together, it is almost impossible to differentiate ALS on the basis of the electrophysiological study alone. Fortunately, such combined cases are rare.

The selection of muscles for the needle EMG is an important consideration in evaluation of a patient suspected of having ALS because so many muscles must be examined. The following guidelines are helpful for this purpose: Because fibrillation and PSW are best observed in weak and atrophic muscles, it is best to first select muscles in the most clinically involved limbs, testing proximal and distal muscles innervated by different nerve roots and peripheral nerves; intrinsic hand muscles and anterior tibialis are likely to be involved first in ALS and should be examined first; it is very important to examine muscles in clinically uninvolved limbs or in limbs with upper motor neuron signs; and too much time should not be spent in attempting to determine whether abnormalities have a root or peripheral nerve distribution. Testing should progress from one limb to another limb or to the cranial muscles after abnormalities are found in three muscles with different innervation in one limb.

The most important and readily recognizable EMG abnormalities in ALS are fibrillation and PSWs. Without these, it is almost impossible to make a diagnosis of ALS, which represents the most rapidly developing form of MND. Fasciculation potentials are a particular significance in ALS because they are responsible for one of the physical signs characteristic of this condition and they are particularly prominent in most cases of ALS. The needle EMG is the only tool to demonstrate fasciculation from deep layers of muscles that are otherwise invisible to the naked eye. Fasciculations are generated primarily in the distal axons of motor units that are still intact; they therefore disappear in muscles that have lost all their innervation. CRD may also occur in ALS but are even more frequent in patients with SMA. Clearly, polyphasic MUPs are increased in ALS and, depending on the duration of disease, they are normal or increased in duration or amplitude.

Because of unstable end plates associated with ongoing degeneration and regeneration in ALS, varying MUP amplitudes may occur. This is a poor prognostic sign signifying ongoing disease. Clearly, MUPs are reduced during maximal contraction. In summary, the needle EMG in ALS is characterized by a combination of active and chronic denervation in widespread areas of the body.

MAXIMS

1. Fasciculation potentials without any other evidence of needle EMG denervation are not pathological.
2. Widespread denervation process in at least three limb muscles (tongue is listed as one limb) and motor neuronopathy are typical of ALS.

REFERENCES

1. Lambert EH. Electromyography in amyotrophic lateral sclerosis. In: Norris FH Jr, Kurland LT, eds. Motor neuron diseases: research on amyotrophic lateral sclerosis and related disorders. New York: Grune & Stratton, 1969:135–153.
2. Belxrud MD, Windebank AJ, Daube JR. Long-term follow-up of 121 patients with benign fasciculations. Ann Neurol 1993;34:622–625.

CASE 2

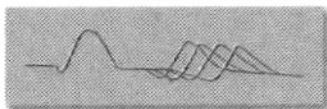

WEAKNESS SOON AFTER START OF PRAVASTATIN

CASE PRESENTATION

Soon after being placed on pravastatin for hypercholesterolemia, 10 months before the initial evaluation, the patient began to notice weakness of the legs. Her internist suspected cholesterol-lowering agent-induced myopathy on the basis of elevated CPK (400 units versus normal 250 units) and ordered a needle EMG. The EMG was reported to show "active myopathy," and a subsequent muscle biopsy was said to show "inflammatory myopathy." Even though pravastatin was discontinued after 3 months, her leg weakness worsened and soon spread to her arms. MRIs of the cervical and lumbar spine was normal. Despite surgery for carpal tunnel release, her hand weakness continued to worsen. She became unable to walk for more than 30 feet without shortness of breath and was no longer able to roll her hair. In addition, her voice became very weak with prolonged talking and she experienced occasional episodes of choking. Her speech was dysarthric. No tongue atrophy or fasciculation was observed; jaw jerk was present. Fasciculation was observed in deltoids, biceps, and quadriceps. Her arms and legs were weak, with MRC strength of 4 in proximal muscles and 3 in distal muscles. There was marked atrophy of the forearm and hand muscles and mild atrophy in the quadriceps. DTRs were 3 in the biceps, triceps and knee reflexes, and absent at the ankles. Plantar response was equivocal on the left with Babinski sign on the right. Vibration was decreased on the toes, but other sensory functions were normal.

CASE ANALYSIS

In view of the onset of weakness right after starting pravastatin, a 3-hydroxy-methylglutaryl coenzyme A (HMG-CoA) reductase inhibitor that reduces cholesterol biosynthesis, a drug-induced myopathy was rightly suspected, especially in view of her high CPK. Needle EMG and muscle biopsy were noted to support myopathy. However, discontinuation of the drug did not stop progression of her weakness. Neurological examination 10 months after onset clearly documented a widespread combination of LMN and UMN signs and pseudobulbar dysarthria typical of ALS. Needle EMG was expected to show widespread denervation process and muscle biopsy to reveal severe denervation.

PLAN OF TESTING

1. NCS: To rule out a demyelinating neuropathy, which can mimic MND.
2. Needle EMG: To document denervation process in widespread areas of the body and rule out myopathy.
3. Review of muscle biopsy: To confirm the findings of inflammatory myopathy.

ELECTROPHYSIOLOGICAL TESTS AND FINDINGS

NCS Findings (Table 10.4)

1. Low CMAP amplitudes in all tested nerves.
2. Mild slowing of motor NCV in the forearm segment of median nerve, peroneal, and posterior tibial nerves.
3. Absent F-waves in median and ulnar nerves and mildly prolonged F-wave latency in peroneal and posterior tibial nerves.
4. Prolonged terminal latency and slow sensory NCV over the finger-wrist and palm-wrist segments of the median nerve.
5. Slow motor NCV across the elbow, prolonged terminal latency, and slow sensory NCV with low CNAP amplitude over the finger-wrist segment in the ulnar nerve.

Needle EMG (Table 10.5)

1. Fibrillation, PSW, fasciculation, some HA MUPs, increased polyphasic MUPs, and reduced recruitment of MUPs in all tested muscles in three limbs and lumbar paraspinal muscles (Fig. 10.2).
2. Spontaneous MUP discharge in the right vastus lateralis and deltoid muscles (Fig. 10.3).
3. Some HALD MUPs in the right vastus lateralis and anterior tibialis muscles (Fig. 10.4).

TABLE 10.4. Nerve Conduction Data in Case 2

	Latent/NCV (ms/m/s)	Amplitude (mV/μV)		Latent/NCV (ms/m/s)	Amplitude (mV/μV)
Left	**Median**	**Motor N**	**Left**	**Peroneal**	**Motor N**
TL	**5.7**	**0.28**	TL	**7.4**	**0.8**
E-W	**46.5**	**0.24**	FHA	**41.7**	**0.62**
AX-E	65.5	**0.20**	PF-HF	50.0	**0.58**
F-wave	**NP**		F-wave	**54.5**	
	Ulnar	**Motor N**		**Post Tibial**	**Motor N**
TL	**3.0**	**2.6**	TL	3.4	1.5
BE-W	57.5	**2.2**	PF-A	**34.7**	**1.1**
AE-BE	**41.1**	**2.0**			
AX-AE	71.8	**2.0**			
F-wave	**NP**		F-wave	**57.2**	
	Median	**Sens/Mixed N**		**Sural**	**Sens N**
F-W	**35.0**	10.8	MC-A	41.3	16
P-W	**33.8**	17.2			
W-E	54.6	14.4			
E-AX	68.4	13.2			
	Ulnar	**Sens/Mixed N**		**Superficial Peroneal**	**Sens/Mixed N**
F-W	**36.1**	**7.6**	MC-A		
W-E	58.7	10			
E-AX	61.8	12			

Height: 165.1 cm.
TL, terminal latency; E, elbow; W, wrist; AX, axilla; AE, above elbow; BE, below elbow; F, finger; P, palm; MC, mid-calf; A, ankle; FH, fibular head; PF, popliteal fossa.

ELECTROPHYSIOLOGICAL INTERPRETATION

1. Widespread denervation in four different parts of the body typical of ALS.
2. Motor neuronopathy in all motor nerves.
3. Asymptomatic carpal tunnel syndrome and ulnar compression neuropathy at the elbow.

OTHER TEST FINDINGS

Muscle biopsy that we reviewed showed fascicular atrophy typical of anterior horn cell disease. There were a few muscle fibers undergoing phagocytosis, which was secondary to severe denervation. The inexperienced pathologist had interpreted "fascicular atrophy" as "inflammatory cells."

FINAL DIAGNOSIS

ALS

TREATMENT AND FOLLOW-UP

There was no serious laboratory abnormality except for mildly elevated CPK, which is more common than suspected in ALS. Once the diagnosis of ALS was made, the patient was started on riluzole. There has been a gradual progression in her weakness.

COMMENTS

Cholesterol-lowering agent-induced myopathy is a well-known drug-induced myopathy that is reversible with discontinuation of medication. In fact, myopathy, which is manifested as elevated CPK, rhabdomyolysis, and myoglobinuria, is the most serious side effect of these

TABLE 10.5. Needle EMG Data in Case 2

				Spontaneous Potentials				Motor Unit Potential				Interference	
Muscle	**Root**	**Nerve**	**Insertion Activity**	**Fib**	**PSW**	**Fasc**	**Myotonia CRD**	**Amplitude (K)**	**Duration (ms)**	**Polyphasic Potential**	**HALD MUP**	**Pat-tern**	**Mean amplitude (K)**
Rt Vast Lat	L3,4	Femoral	+	++	++	++[a]	–	2–7	8–38	+	+	RIP	2
Ant tibial	L4,5	Peroneal	+	+++	++	++	–	2–8	9–28	+	+	RIP	2
Gastroc	S1,2	Post tibial	+	+++	+++	–	–	1–6	8–22	+	+	RIP	2
Deltoid	C5,6	Axillary	+	++	+++	++*	–	1–5.5	6–18	+	+	RIP	2
Biceps	C5,6	Musc cut	+	++	+++	++	–	1–6	6–18	+	+	RIP	2
FDI	C8, T1	Ulnar	+	+++	++++	++	–	No	MUP				
Lt L3,4	L3,4	L3,4	+	+	++	–	–						
Lt Ant Tibial	L4,5	Peroneal	+	++	+++	++*	–	1–6	6–20	+	+	RIP	3
Vast lat	L3,4	Femoral	+	++	+++	++	–	1–6	6–16	+	+	DA	8

[a] Spontaneous MUP discharge.

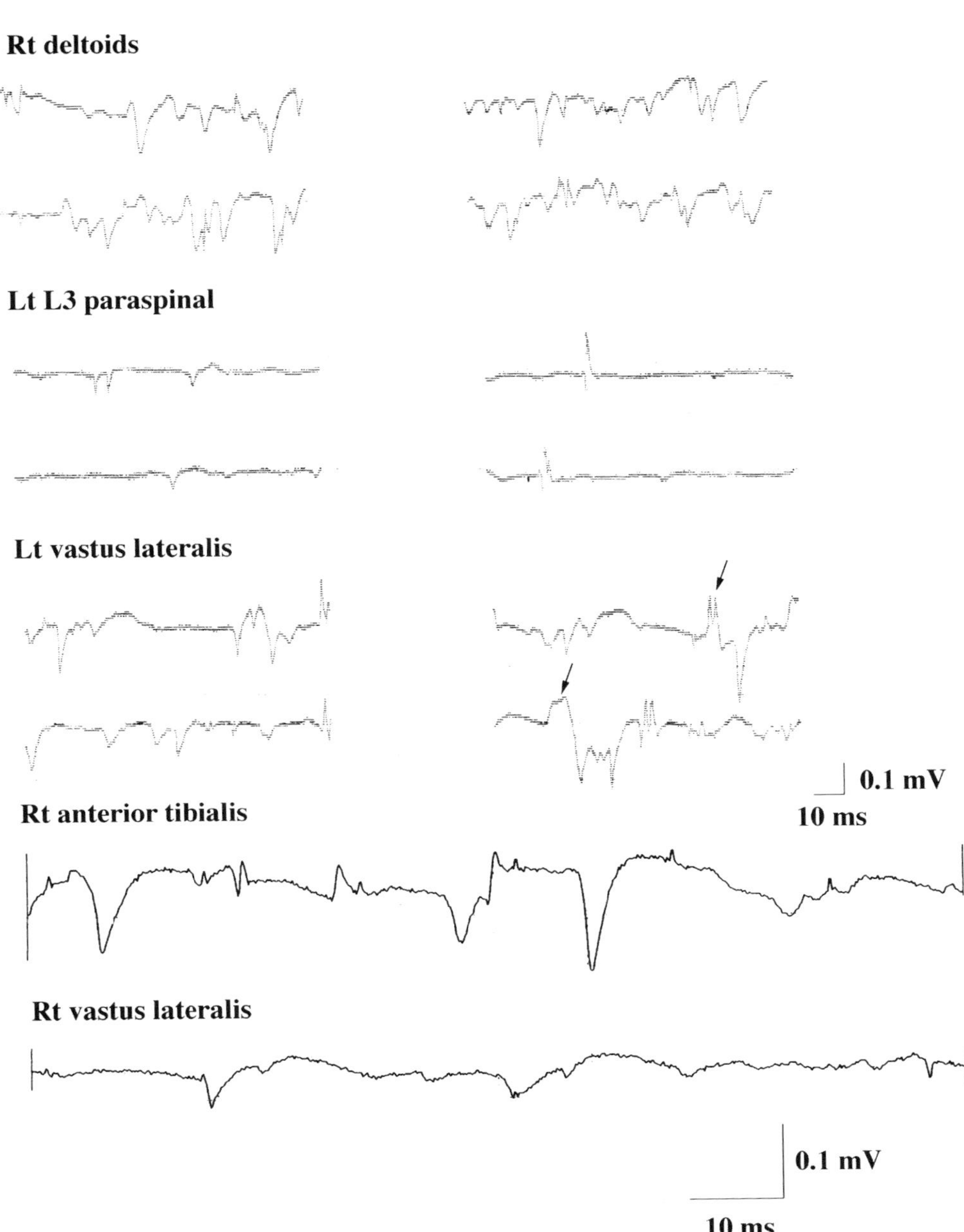

FIGURE 10.2. Fibrillations and PSW in various muscles in three different limbs. Fasciculations (*arrows*).

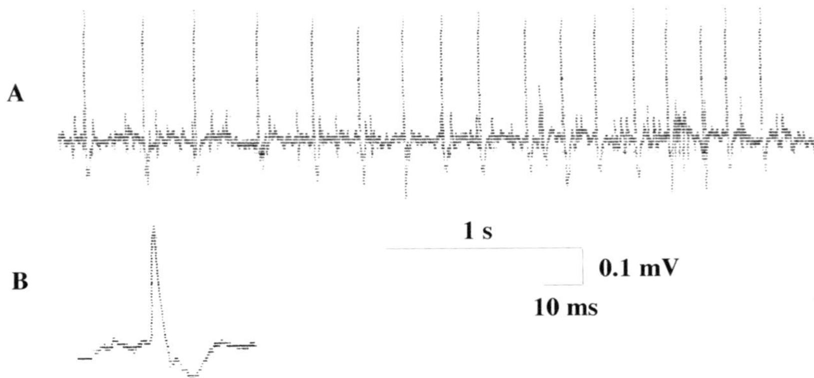

FIGURE 10.3. Spontaneous MUP discharges: relatively regular firing of MUPs at rest. Clinical significance of this is the same with fasciculation. **A.** Firing rate of spontaneous MUP discharges. **B.** Spontaneously firing MUPs.

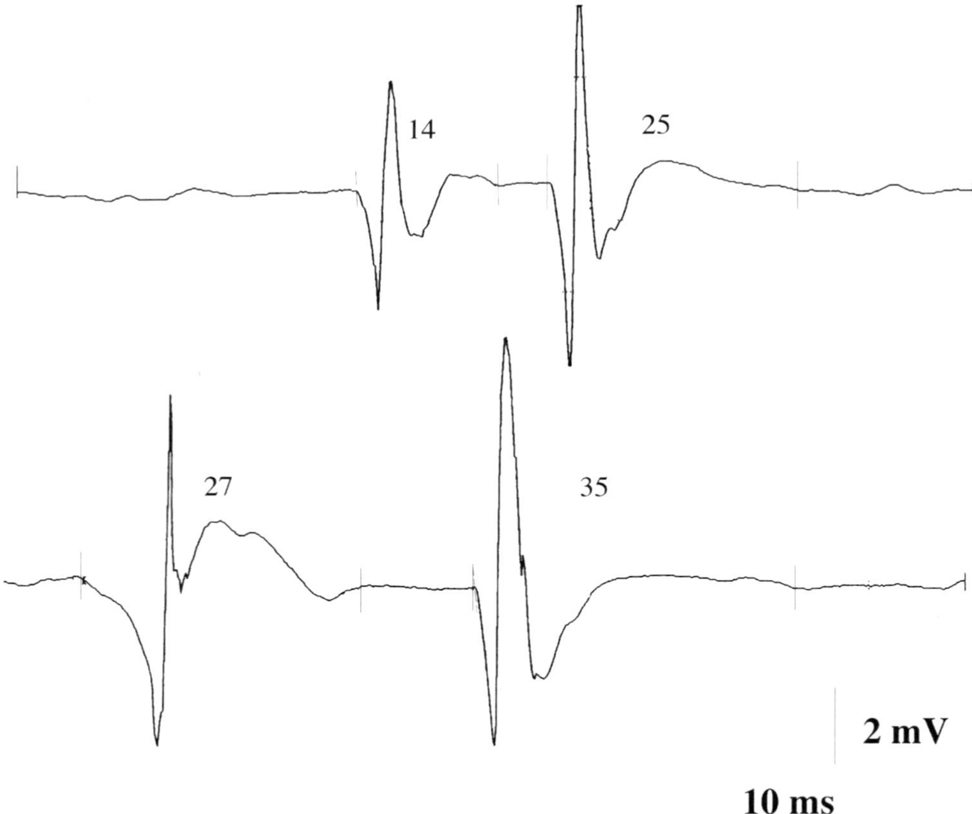

FIGURE 10.4. HALD MUPs. Numbers above the MUPs represent the duration of MUPs. One MUP with normal duration. All other MUPs have longer duration.

agents. This has been reported in almost all cholesterol-lowering agents, from niacin to lovastatin. These agents inhibit HMG-CoA reductase and reduce the blood concentration of low-density lipoproteins while raising that of high-density lipoproteins. Characteristically, the CPK is elevated and needle EMG shows a myopathic pattern. Muscle biopsy shows a nonspecific myopathy and mitochondrial myopathy in some cases. In view of this patient's mildly elevated CPK, drug-induced myopathy was suspected. Mildly elevated CPK is not uncommon (seen in 52 to 76% of cases) in ALS and is due to myopathic changes secondary to rapidly progressing denervation. CPK is highest in patients who have had the disease for 3 to 15 months. Thus, a mildly elevated CPK alone is not helpful in differentiation of ALS from myopathy.

An inexperienced electromyographer interpreted "fibrillation" as "active myopathy" without paying any attention to MUPs. Similarly, fasciculation may be interpreted as "lack of patient cooperation." Furthermore, an inexperienced pathologist interpreted "lots of cells" in small given areas (in fact, fascicular atrophy) as "inflammatory cells," making a diagnosis of inflammatory myopathy.

The typical nerve conduction pattern in ALS is a pure motor neuropathy of axonal type, reflecting pure motor neuronopathy. Most motor NCV values fall within normal limits in ALS. The amplitude of the CMAPs is low in some patients, in proportion to the wasting of muscles. Motor NCVs are slightly slowed in some patients but never fall below 70% of the lower limit of normal. This is what was observed in our case. The mild slowing is caused by selective loss of the larger, faster-conducting fibers with axonal degeneration after neuronal degeneration in the anterior horn. Slowing of conduction is proportional to the reduction of CMAP amplitude and to the degree of atrophy of the muscle. Sensory nerve conduction is normal in ALS. Thus, any sensory nerve conduction abnormality is due to a concomitant entrapment neuropathy, as noted in this case. The F-wave latencies may be slightly prolonged or absent in patients with ALS, as noted in our case, but not as prominently as in neuropathy or polyradiculopathy. One of the important roles of the NCS in ALS is to rule out CIDP or MMN, which can mimic MND and is characterized by demyelinating neuropathy. In ALS, the H-reflex was present in the gastrocnemius in almost all cases and in other muscles in 66 to 77% of ALS patients. This is expected in view of the neuronal hyperexcitability due to pyramidal tract involvement in ALS. Thus, the H-reflex test can be a valuable aid in differentiating ALS from SMA and polyneuropathy, in which the H-reflex is rarely observed in either muscle.

Riluzole (Rilutek), a glutamate antagonist, affects neurons by three mechanisms: by inhibiting excitatory amino acid release, by inhibiting events after stimulation of excitatory amino acid receptors, and by stabilizing the inactivated state of voltage-dependent sodium channels. This is the first drug that has been shown to have a modest effect on survival in patients with ALS. It has demonstrated neuroprotective activity in vivo and in vitro. Results from two randomized, double-blind, placebo-controlled trials in patients with ALS have demonstrated that riluzole can extend survival and/or time to tracheostomy. After 18 months, the relative risk of death or tracheostomy with riluzole 100 mg/day was reduced by 21%. Although riluzole slowed the rate of deterioration in muscle strength in the first trial, this was not confirmed in a second larger trial. Riluzole had no effect on any other functional or secondary variable. Gastrointestinal effects, anorexia, asthenia, circumoral paraesthesia, and dizziness were reported more frequently with riluzole than with a placebo. Elevated alanine aminotransferase levels, the most serious side-effect, were observed in 10.6% of patients treated with riluzole 100 mg/day versus 3.8% in those taking the placebo, leading to treatment withdrawal in 3.8% versus 2.1% of patients. This reaction usually occurs in the first 2 months of treatment. Treatment with 100 mg/day gave the best risk-benefit ratio. Granulocytopenia was reported in a few patients. Thus, the complete blood count and liver function must be monitored monthly in the first 3 months.

MAXIMS

1. The typical nerve conduction pattern in ALS is a pure motor neuronopathy: low CMAP amplitude, normal or slightly slow motor NCV, and normal sensory NCS.
2. Mildly elevated CPK is observed in 52 to 76% of cases with ALS and in cases of shorter duration.

REFERENCES

1. Bryson HM, Fulton B, Benefield P. Riluzole. A review of its pharmacodynamic and pharmacokinetic properties and therapeutic potential in amyotrophic lateral sclerosis [review]. Drugs 1996;52: 549–563.
2. Achari AN, Anderson MS. Serum creatine phosphokinase in amyotrophic lateral sclerosis. Neurology 1974;24:834–837.

CASE 3

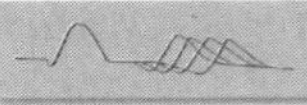

PROGRESSIVE DYSARTHRIA FOR 8 TO 12 MONTHS IN A MIDDLE-AGED WOMAN

CASE PRESENTATION

A 55-year-old right-handed woman presented with an 8- to 12-month history of progressively worsening slurred speech, especially for words beginning with the letters C and L. In addition, she complained of difficulty moving her tongue that caused her to drag out her words, excessive saliva, but no difficulty with drooling or swallowing. There was no regurgitation of food through the nose, no double vision, paresthesia or weakness in the upper or lower extremities, bladder disturbances, or gait difficulties. On examination, her speech was thick and slurred as if her tongue was tightly fixed to the bottom of her mouth. However, her tongue was in the midline and move quite well, with some fasciculations but no atrophy. Her palate moved well and gag reflex was intact. Jaw jerk was brisk. She had normal muscle strength in the arms and legs, and no fasciculation was observed. Tone was also normal. DTRs were brisk in the upper extremities and exaggerated in the lower limbs with downgoing plantar responses. There was no ankle clonus. Hoffman sign was positive. Nerve conduction and EMG studies performed by the referring neurologist were reported as normal. MRI of the brain was normal, but MRI of the cervical spine showed evidence of mild osteophytes.

CASE ANALYSIS

This patient had had progressive dysarthria for 8 to 12 months. Progressive dysarthria without any other bulbar involvement in a patient of this age usually represents a "CNS" disease, including MND. In this case, her dysarthria was typical of that observed in ALS: a combination of pseudobulbar and bulbar palsy. Brisk jaw jerk, brisk DTRs, and fasciculation of the tongue were compatible with MND, but these findings were not enough to make the diagnosis of ALS on clinical grounds. The needle EMG would be critical in this case to document widespread denervation and definite LMN signs, thus confirming the diagnostic suspicions.

PLAN OF TESTING

1. Needle EMG: To document widespread denervation. This test should include the tongue muscle.
2. NCS: To rule out any demyelinating neuropathy, which can mimic MND.

ELECTROPHYSIOLOGICAL TESTS AND FINDINGS

NCS Findings

Normal motor and sensory NCS in all tested nerves.

Needle EMG (Table 10.6)

1. Increased insertion activity and fibrillations or PSW in the right biceps, anterior tibialis, and genioglossus muscles.
2. Fasciculations in the right deltoid, biceps, and genioglossus muscles (Fig. 10.5).
3. Reduced interference pattern in all tested muscles.
4. MUPs with 1 to 5 K amplitude in the right genioglossus muscle.

ELECTROPHYSIOLOGICAL INTERPRETATION

Widespread denervation process in three scattered areas of the body, typical of anterior horn cell disease.

TABLE 10.6. Needle EMG Data in Case 3

				Spontaneous Potentials				Motor Unit Potential				Interference	
Muscle	**Root**	**Nerve**	**Insertion Activity**	**Fib**	**PSW**	**Fasc**	**Myotonia CRD**	**Amplitude (K)**	**Duration (ms)**	**Polyphasic Potential**	**HA MUP**	**Pattern**	**Mean Amplitude (K)**
Rt Genioglossus		CN XII	+	+	–	++	–	1–5	8–12	N	–	RIP	3
Deltoid	C5,6	Axillary	+	±	–	+	–	0.5–4	8–15	N	–	RIP	2
Biceps	C6,7	Musc cut	+	–	+	+	–	0.5–2.5	8–12	N	–	RIP	1
Vast lat	L3,4	Femoral	+	–	–	±	–	0.5–4	8–12	N	–	RIP	2
Ant tibial	L4,5	Peroneal	+	–	+	±	–	0.5–4	8–14	N	–	RIP	2

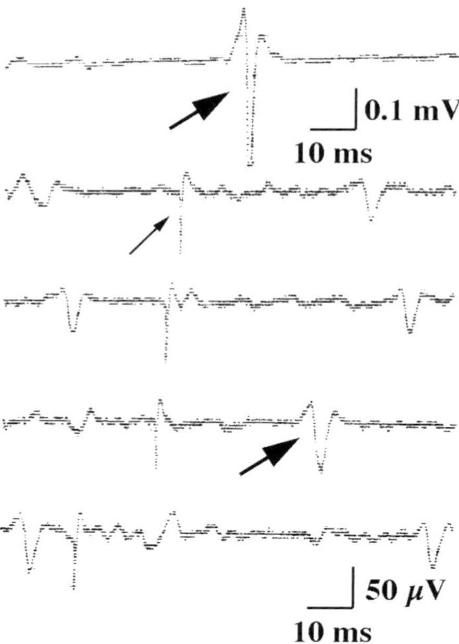

FIGURE 10.5. Fasciculations (*thick arrows*) and fibrillations (*thin arrows*) in the genioglossus muscle.

FINAL DIAGNOSIS

Chronic bulbar palsy as a variety of ALS

TREATMENT AND FOLLOW-UP

Muscle biopsy from the right biceps showed minimal denervation. In 1 year, she needed PEG placement because of severe swallowing difficulty and developed the classic findings of ALS. She died in 2 years due to respiratory failure.

COMMENTS

There are two approaches to the needle EMG in the tongue muscle. One is to insert the needle into the genioglossus muscle from below the chin. This method does not require any anesthetic agent but does provide better relaxation. Another method is to insert the needle into the hypoglossal muscle through the tongue. I prefer to anesthetize the tongue with novocaine gel before needle insertion. One major problem with EMG testing of the tongue muscle is the difficulty of muscle relaxation. There is no single method I can recommend for best relaxation of the hypoglossal muscle, and it is often almost impossible to relax the tongue muscles completely. Thus, recognition of fibrillations and PSW has to be aided with an audioamplifier. Another point to remember in the needle EMG is that MUPs in the tongue muscle are shorter and smaller than those in the limb muscles, sometimes mimicking SASD MUPs. Thus, 4 to 5 mV MUPs for this muscle are definitely abnormal and indicative of chronic denervation.

The needle EMG in the tongue, masseter, and facial muscles is critical for diagnosis of ALS for two reasons. One is the necessity of documenting widespread denervation process in three limb muscles, with the cranial muscles, including the tongue muscle, being considered as one "limb." Another reason is to document denervation process above the neck. When the differentiation between ALS and cervical disease is clinically difficult, the presence of fibrillations and PSWs in the tongue muscles clearly rules out cervical disease. Thus, the needle EMG in cranial muscles, including the tongue, is an important test in the workup of patients suspected of having ALS.

MAXIMS

1. The needle EMG in the cranial muscles, including the tongue, is critical for the diagnosis of ALS to document widespread denervation process and differentiate ALS from cervical diseases.
2. MUPs from the cranial muscles, including the tongue muscles, are usually shorter in duration and smaller in amplitude than those from the limb muscles.

REFERENCES

1. Daube JR. Electrophysiologic studies in diagnosis and prognosis of motor neuron disease. Neurol Clin 1985;3:473–493.

CASE 4

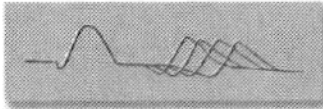

PROGRESSIVE PROXIMAL MUSCLE WEAKNESS FOR 20 YEARS

CASE PRESENTATION

An 83-year-old woman noted gradually progressive proximal muscle weakness, especially in the lower extremities, for the past 20 years. Because of frequent falls, she sought neurological attention. She reported difficulty rising from a chair and climbing stairs and also noted that her left hand had become weak in the past year, causing her to drop items. She denied any paresthesia or bowel or bladder incontinence. An EMG performed 15 years previously had revealed no evidence of neuropathy or myopathy but "subtle suggestion of denervation." Her CPK was normal. A muscle biopsy 3 years ago revealed end-stage atrophy. MRI of the lumbosacral spine was negative. Spinal fluid evaluation was normal.

Abnormal neurological findings included atrophy of bilateral APB, hand intrinsic and quadriceps muscles, MRC strength of 3+ in deltoids, 4+ in the hand intrinsics, 4 in iliopsoas and quadriceps, and 5− in hamstrings muscles. The patient had decreased vibratory sensation on the toes and diffuse areflexia, but no fasciculation was noted of the tongue or extremities. She used a quad-cane because of her unsteady gait.

CASE ANALYSIS

A 20-year history of painless proximal muscle weakness without any sensory deficits and relative proximal muscle weakness are suggestive of myopathy. In chronic myopathy, areflexia is not an unusual finding due to fibrosis of the muscle itself. Decreased vibration on the toes is normal for this age. However, her CPK was normal. Other diagnostic possibilities included chronic denervation process such as CIDP or SMA.

PLAN OF TESTING

1. NCS: To rule out CIDP.
2. Needle EMG: To determine myopathy or chronic denervation.
3. RNS test: To rule out LEMS.
4. Other tests: CPK, muscle biopsy, and serum autoantibody.

ELECTROPHYSIOLOGICAL TESTS AND FINDINGS

NCS Findings

1. Normal sensory and mixed NCS.
2. Low CMAP amplitude in the median, peroneal, and posterior tibial nerves. Otherwise, normal.
3. No conduction block was observed.

Needle EMG (Table 10.7 and Fig. 10.6)

1. A few fibrillations, PSWs, and fasciculation potentials in most muscles tested.
2. CRD in a few muscles tested.
3. HALD MUPs and reduced interference pattern in most muscles tested.

RNS Test in the ADQ and FCU Muscles. Normal

TABLE 10.7. Needle EMG Data in Case 4

				Spontaneous Potentials				Motor Unit Potential				Interference	
Muscle	**Root**	**Nerve**	**Insertion Activity**	**Fib**	**PSW**	**Fasc**	**CRD**	**Amplitude (K)**	**Duration (ms)**	**Polyphasic Potential**	**HALD MUP**	**Pattern**	**Mean Amplitude (K)**
Lt Ant Tibial	L4,5	Peroneal	+	–	–	++	–	2–8	16–28	N	++	DA	6
Gastroc	S1,2	Post tibial	+	+	+	++	+	2–10	12–35	N	++	DA	4
Vast lat	L3,4	Femoral	+	+	+	++	–	2–20	14–24	N	++	DA	6
Rt Vast Lat	L3,4	Femoral	+	+	+	++	+	1–3	10–15	N	–	DA	4
Ant tibial	L4,5	Peroneal	+	+	+	++	–	2–10	14–22	N	++	RIP	4
Rt L3-5, S1	L3-5S1		+	+	+	+	+						
Deltoid	C5,6	Axillary	+	+	+	+	–	1–6	10–20	N	+	RIP	3
APB	C8	Median	+	+	–	+	–	1–6	10–20	N	+	DA	3

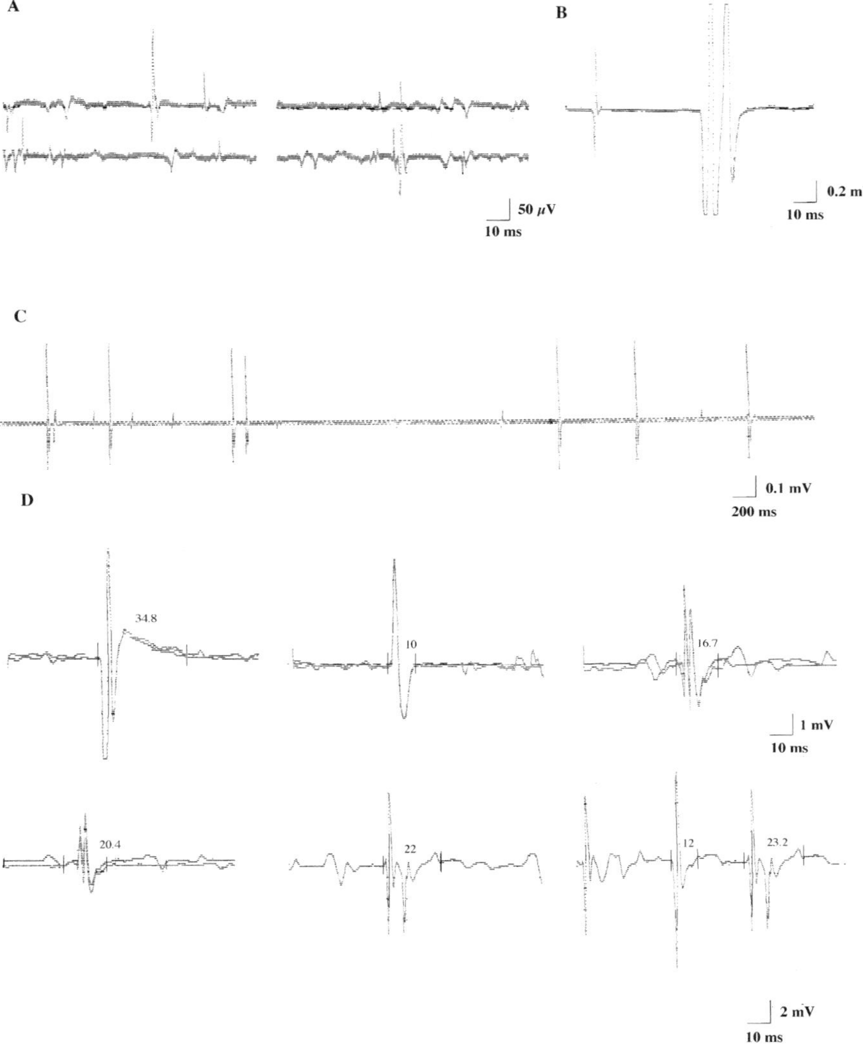

FIGURE 10.6. **A.** Fibrillations and PSW. **B.** Fasciculations. **C.** Irregular firing of fasciculations. **D.** HALD MUPs and HA MUPs. Numbers above the MUPs represent the duration of MUP.

ELECTROPHYSIOLOGICAL INTERPRETATION

Widespread chronic denervation typical of anterior horn cell lesions.

OTHER TEST FINDINGS

Normal CPK. Severe denervation with fibrosis in muscle biopsy. Asialo GM1 antibody was positive at 6400 titer. Other autoantibodies were normal.

FINAL DIAGNOSIS

Adult-onset proximal SMA

TREATMENT AND FOLLOW-UP

Because of the positive asialo GM1 antibody, this patient received a full course of IVIg treatment together with azathioprine treatment. No benefit was observed. There has been a slow progression of disease.

COMMENTS

Adult-onset SMA is a heterogenous group of diseases. All have a more benign course than ALS, with the patient often surviving 20 or more years after onset in adult life. In all cases of adult-onset SMA, except for X-linked spinobulbar muscular atrophy, bulbar muscles are spared. For this reason, SMA should be separated from ALS when it is discussed as a form of MND. Most cases of adult-onset SMA are either sporadic or autosomal recessive in inheritance, although rare autosomal-dominant SMA has been reported. Four main types are recognized: chronic proximal SMA, distal SMA, scapuloperoneal SMA, and spinal bulbar muscular atrophy. Chronic proximal SMA resembles limb-girdle muscular dystrophy. Onset ranges from 15 to 60 years. Muscle weakness is slowly progressive and predominantly involves the proximal arms and legs. Eventually, distal weakness occurs, but bulbar involvement is unusual. Some forms of autosomal-recessive SMA have been mapped to chromosome 5q. Rare adult-onset, autosomal-dominant SMA with onset beginning as late as 65 years of age has been reported. Distal SMA is characterized by predominant distal muscle weakness and atrophy, resembling the neuronal form of Charcot-Marie-Tooth disease. An additional type of autosomal-dominant SMA with a scapuloperoneal distribution has been described with onset at age 70. X-linked spinal bulbar muscular atrophy is caused by a mutation in the androgen receptor gene (Table 10.2). Onset of weakness usually begins in the third to seventh decade of life. The presence of an X-linked inheritance of androgen insufficiency (gynecomastia, impotence, infertility) in combination with LMN abnormalities should lead to the correct diagnosis. Facial and particularly perioral fasiculations are highly characteristic, if not pathognomonic, of this disease, being present in more than 90% of cases. Elevated CPK is common. In this disorder, the mutation is characterized by increased size of a polymorphic tandem CAG repeat within the first exon of the androgen receptor gene. This now can be used for definitive diagnosis and carrier detection. Despite the absence of sensory symptoms, sensory CNAPs are frequently low in amplitude or absent in this disorder. This electrophysiological feature distinguishes this disorder from other MNDs.

The needle EMG test is also critical for the diagnosis of adult-onset SMA. It is typically characterized by chronic denervation process. In fact, SMA represents the pivotal disease that typically shows chronic denervation process in the needle EMG. Although all electrophysiological abnormalities in ALS are observed in SMA, there are important quantitative differences between the two disorders. In SMA, fibrillations, PSWs, and fasciculations are less prominent, whereas CRDs are more common as compared with ALS. In SMA, HALD MUP is the cardinal finding in the needle EMG, without which the diagnosis is untenable. Sometimes, HALD MUPs are mixed with SASD MUPs, representing a secondary myopathic change. Because of this mixed pattern in the needle EMG and the insidious progressive weakness, atrophy, and areflexia, SMA has often been confused with IBM. Usually, in IBM, fibrillation and PSW are more prominent findings. Polyphasic MUPs are less common than in ALS and may include separate, time-locked components called "satellites" in SMA. Variation of MUP amplitude is not observed in SMA because of mature end-plate status. NCS of motor and sensory nerve fibers are normal. CMAPs are not as low as those in ALS and are often normal.

MAXIMS

1. In X-linked spinobulbar muscular atrophy, sensory CNAPs are low in amplitude or absent. This electrophysiological feature distinguishes this disorder from other MNDs.
2. In SMA, HALD MUPs are the needle EMG hallmark; fibrillation, PSW, and fasciculation potentials are scarce and less prominent.

REFERENCES

1. Pouget J, Azulay JP, Bille-Turc F, Sangla I, Serratrice GT. The diagnosis of amyotrophic lateral sclerosis [review]. Adv Neurol 1995;68:143–52.
2. Harding AE, Thomas PK, Baraitser M, Bradbury PG, Morgan-Hughes JA, Ponsford JR. X-linked recessive bulbospinal neuronopathy: a report of ten cases. J Neurol Neurosurg Psychiatry 1982;45: 1012–1019.

CASE 5

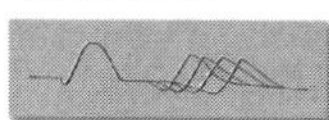

DIFFICULTY CLIMBING STAIRS IN THE FATHER OF A 9-YEAR-OLD PATIENT WITH SMA TYPE II

CASE PRESENTATION

This 41-year-old man was the father of a child with SMA type II. During childhood, he had some difficulty running, was always behind other children in athletic development, and at age 30 had begun to notice some difficulties, especially in climbing stairs. There had been gradual but steady progression over the years, to the point that he was now unable to climb stairs without supporting himself with both hands or to get up from the floor without help. There had been no pain nor heart problems in the past. The patient's son, now 9 years old, was diagnosed with SMA type II at the age of 4 years by biopsy. The family history was strongly positive.

Abnormal neurological findings were MRC strength of 4 in neck flexor, deltoids, biceps, and iliopsoas muscles; 2 in anterior tibialis; mild atrophy in the upper arms; prominent pes cavus; and diminished DTRs. Other upper and lower extremity muscles were normal in strength. The patient was unable to do any knee bends and could not get up from a chair without support. He could walk on his toes but not on his heels due to footdrop. No scoliosis or fasciculation was noted.

CASE ANALYSIS

Although the history suggested a childhood developmental delay, his symptoms were not obvious until age 30, when he began to notice some difficulty in climbing stairs. Family members had been thought to have "muscular dystrophy" until the patient's son was diagnosed with SMA type II. On the basis of the distribution of affected muscles, the diagnosis of scapulohumeroperoneal syndrome can be made. A thorough needle EMG study is critical to distinguish SMA from myopathy.

PLAN OF TESTING

1. NCS: To rule out neuropathy as a cause of scapuloperoneal syndrome.
2. Needle EMG: To find myopathy or chronic denervation.
3. Other tests: CPK and muscle biopsy.

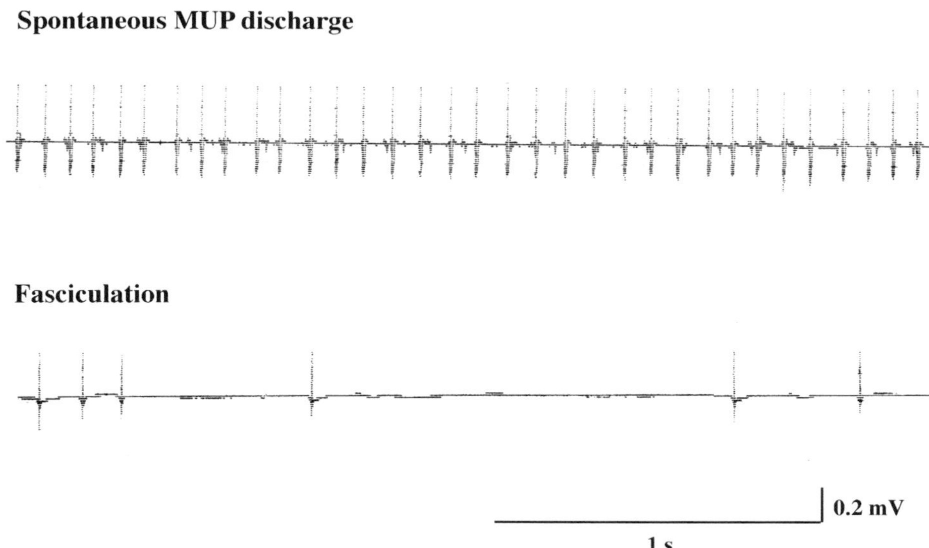

FIGURE 10.7. The difference between the spontaneous MUP discharge and fasciculations is obvious: regular firing rate in spontaneous MUP discharges and irregular firing rate in fasciculations.

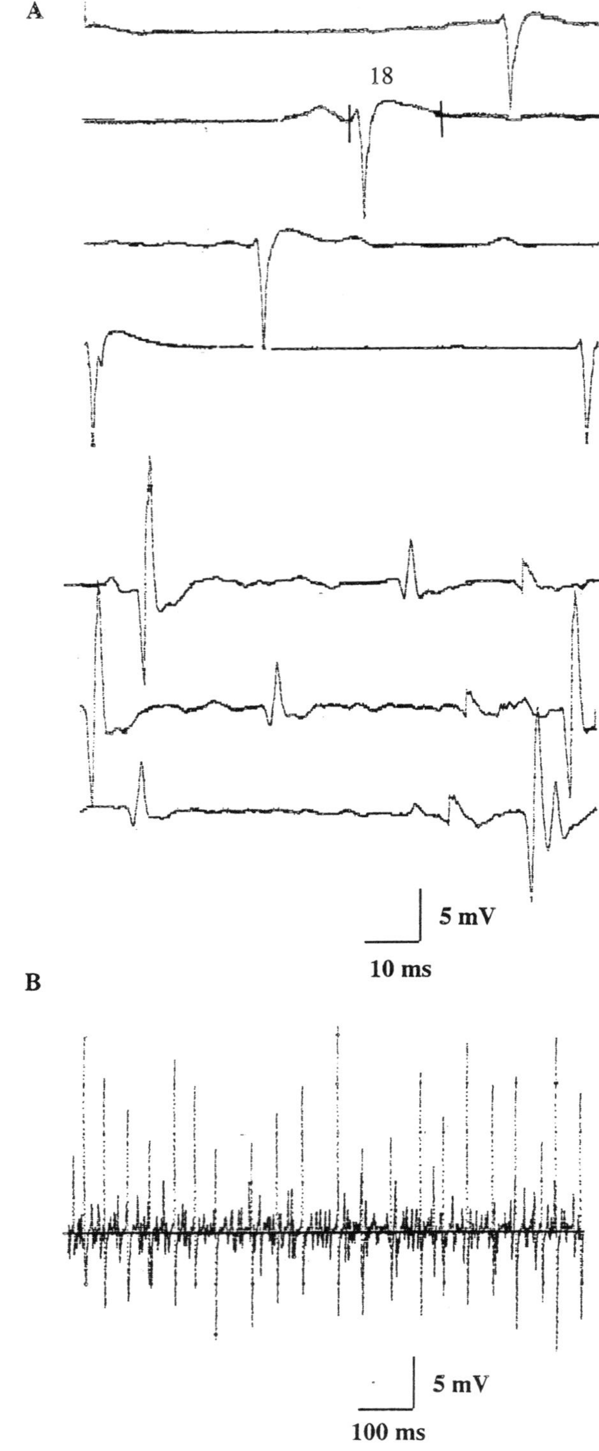

FIGURE 10.8. **A.** HA and HALD MUPs in the anterior tibialis muscle. **B.** Discrete activity on maximal contraction.

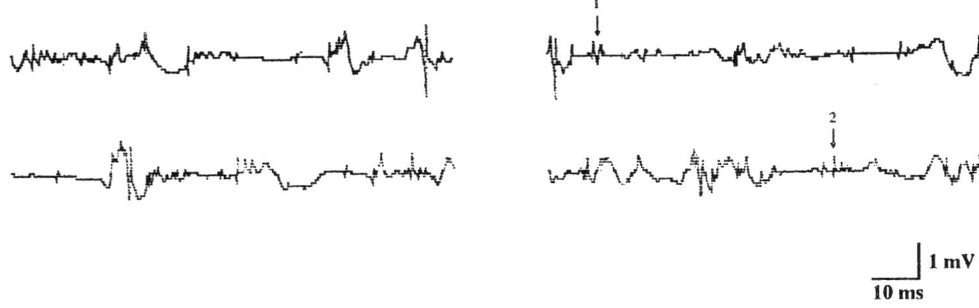

FIGURE 10.9. Many SASD MUPs from different sites in the same muscle in which HALD MUPs are present.

ELECTROPHYSIOLOGICAL TESTS AND FINDINGS

NCS Findings

Normal motor NCS and sensory and mixed NCS except for reduced CMAP in the peroneal nerves.

Needle EMG (Table 10.8 and Fig. 10.7 to 10.9)

1. Fasciculation in the anterior tibialis muscle and spontaneous MUP discharges in the vastus lateralis muscles.
2. Many HALD or HA MUPs and poor recruitment of MUPs on maximal contraction.
3. SASD MUPs in some areas of deltoid muscle.

ELECTROPHYSIOLOGICAL INTERPRETATION

Chronic denervation with some myopathic pattern, more typical of SMA. IBM must be ruled out.

OTHER TEST FINDINGS

CPK was 356 units (normal up to 250). Muscle biopsy in the deltoid muscle showed prominent type I fiber grouping with fascicular atrophy and many plump nuclei in one area and a few muscle fibers undergoing floccular change.

FINAL DIAGNOSIS

Scapuloperoneal SMA

TREATMENT AND FOLLOW-UP

There has been no obvious progression in the neurological examination during a 5-year follow-up period. However, the patient stated that he had more difficulty in walking.

COMMENTS

SPS refers to the heterogenous group of diseases clinically characterized by selective weakness and wasting in the shoulder-girdle muscles and distal lower leg weakness. SPS can be divided into four main groups: muscular dystrophy, spinal muscular atrophy, peripheral neuropathy, and others. Others include mitochondrial myopathy, IBM, nemalin myopathy, minicore myopathy, polymyositis, and Pompe's disease, according to our experience. Most varieties of SPS are inherited by autosomal-dominant pattern, although sporadic or autosomal-recessive cases have been reported.

Scapuloperoneal muscular dystrophy represents a familial myopathy in a scapuloperoneal distribution. Symptoms may begin either in the shoulder girdle or distal leg muscles around 20 years of age. The disease is relatively benign with slow progression. CPK is mildly elevated. Needle EMG shows a myopathic pattern. Muscle biopsy shows nonspecific chronic myopathy.

TABLE 10.8. Needle EMG Data in Case 5

				Spontaneous Potentials				Motor Unit Potential				Interference	
Muscle	Root	Nerve	Insertion Activity	Fib	PSW	Fasc	Myotonia CRD	Amplitude (K)	Duration (ms)	Polyphasic Potential	HALD MUP	Pattern	Mean Amplitude (K)
Rt Deltoid	C5,6	Axillary	N	–	–	–	–	0.5–6	2.8–15	+	±	RIP	2
Ant tibial	L4,5	Peroneal	N	–	–	+[a]	–	3–20	10–30	N	+	DA	5
Vast lat	L3,4	Femoral	N	–	–	+	–	1–10	8–20	N	+	DA	8

[a] Spontaneous MUP discharge at rest.

Emery-Dreyfuss muscular dystrophy resembles scapuloperoneal muscular dystrophy but has a sex-linked recessive inheritance pattern, prominent contracture of elbows and neck. Cardiomyopathy also distinguishes it from scapuloperoneal muscular dystrophy.

The symptoms of scapuloperoneal spinal atrophy always begin in the lower legs. Onset of disease is between ages 30 and 50 years. It is usually inherited in an autosomal-dominant pattern and progresses slowly over the years. CPK may be elevated, as noted in our case. The needle EMG shows a pattern of chronic denervation. Sometimes, a few SASD MUPs may be present, especially in mildly involved muscles. Muscle biopsy clearly shows chronic denervation with some muscle fibers undergoing myopathic change.

Scapuloperoneal neuropathy (Davidenkow's syndrome) usually begins with weakness in the lower legs in either childhood or adult years. The motor deficit is classically accompanied by stocking-glove sensory loss and is slowly progressive. NCS clearly shows a slow motor NCV with absent sensory CNAPs. Needle EMG reveals a chronic denervation pattern. The nerve biopsy findings are indicative of neuropathy.

Except when there is a definite sensory loss in scapuloperoneal neuropathy, there are no clinical features to distinguish muscular dystrophy from SMA. The most important diagnostic test is the needle EMG. Usually in clinical practice, the needle EMG is the first sign suggestive of spinal muscular atrophy. Among the needle EMG abnormalities, HALD MUPs are the key findings. In SMA, HALD MUPs are unmistakable, because they are extremely high, not uncommonly attaining 20 mV, as in this case. Unfortunately, many inexperienced electromyographers do not pay any attention to MUPs and may miss the diagnosis of SMA. It should be noted that in some cases of SMA, a few pockets of SASD MUPs may be present as noted in this case, confusing the interpretation. When a mixed pattern is observed, it is always wise to consider the possibility of inclusion body myopathy.

MAXIMS

1. SMA, muscular dystrophy, and peripheral neuropathy can be causes for scapuloperoneal syndromes.
2. HALD MUPs are the key needle EMG finding in SMA.

REFERENCES

1. Kaeser HE. Scapuloperoneal syndrome. In: Vinken PJ, Bruyn GW, eds. Handbook of clinical neurology. Amsterdam: North-Holland Publishing, 1975;22:57–65.
2. Riser J, Arnold T, Oh SJ. The clinical spectrum of scapuloperoneal syndrome. Neurology 1988; 38(Suppl 1):340.

CASE 6

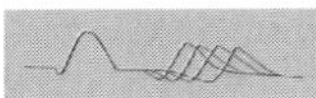

NO IMPROVEMENT AFTER CERVICAL LAMINECTOMY FOR A 27-YEAR-OLD MAN WITH LEFT ARM WEAKNESS FOR 3 YEARS

CASE PRESENTATION

A 27-year-old man's problems had started about 3 years previously when he noticed weakness and loss of muscle mass in the left upper extremity. The year before, a C5-6 and C6-7 cervical discectomy with locking-plate internal fixation was performed on the basis of CT myelogram. After surgery, he had transient recovery of his left arm strength. Over the past 6 weeks, however, his weakness and atrophy progressed. The patient did not have pain or other neurological symptoms.

Abnormal neurological findings were wasting of the left upper arm, forearm, and small muscles of the hand, with the most prominent atrophy in the triceps, fasciculations in the left triceps, and brachioradialis; MRC strength of 4− in the left triceps, 4 in the left forearm extensor and flexor, and 3 in the left hand intrinsic muscles; absent DTRs in the left biceps and triceps; and diminished DTRs in the right biceps and triceps. No mass was palpable over the left brachial plexus area.

CASE ANALYSIS

This patient had slowly progressive, painless, focal weakness and atrophy of the left upper extremity for 3 years that were confined to C6, 7, 8 and T1 myotomes. Diagnostic possibilities included multiple cervical radiculopathies, CSM, MMN, or lower brachial plexus neuropathy, benign focal amyotrophy, and a focal expression of anterior horn cell disease. The last possibility was less likely in view of the absence of UMN signs, and both anterior horn cell disease and CSM were ruled out for this reason.

PLAN OF TESTING

1. NCS: To rule out brachial plexus neuropathy and MMN.
2. Needle EMG: To confirm denervation process in the involved limb. This study should also include the needle EMG in the opposite arm and one leg.
3. Review of MRI of the cervical cord and brachial plexus before the surgery.

ELECTROPHYSIOLOGICAL TESTS AND FINDINGS

NCS Findings (Table 10.9 and Fig. 10.10)

1. Low CMAP amplitude in the left ulnar nerve with prolonged F-wave latency.
2. Pseudoconduction block in the right ulnar nerve due to Martin-Grüber anastomosis.
3. Normal NCS in the left and right median motor, sensory, and mixed nerve conductions.
4. Normal NCS in the left and right radial motor and sensory nerve conductions.

Needle EMG (Table 10.10)

1. Fibrillations and PSW in the left triceps, extensor carpi radialis, flexor carpi radialis, APB, and FDI muscles.
2. Fasciculations in the left deltoid and extensor carpi radialis and in bilateral FDI and APB muscles.
3. HALD or HA MUPs in all tested muscles in the upper extremities.
4. Normal needle EMG findings in the left vastus lateralis, anterior tibialis, and gastrocnemius muscles.

ELECTROPHYSIOLOGICAL INTERPRETATION

1. Chronic denervation in the right and left C6-8 T1 innervated myotomes with active denervation in the left C6-8 T1 innervated muscle.
2. Martin-Grüber anastomosis in the right forearm.

OTHER TEST FINDINGS

MRI of the cervical cord showed hemiatrophy of the left side at the C6 and 7 levels. No obvious disc or cord compression was observed. MRI of the left brachial plexus showed normal findings.

TABLE 10.9. Nerve Conduction Data in Case 6

	Latent/NCV (ms/m/s)	Amplitude (mV/μV)		Latent/NCV (ms/m/s)	Amplitude (mV/μV)	Others
Left	**Ulnar**	**Motor N**	**Right**	**Ulnar**	**Motor**	**Nerve**
TL	3.2	**4.1**		2.1	11.0	
BE-W	52.2	**3.8**		54.7	**3.3**	**PCB**
AE-BE	45.8	**3.8**		41.6	**3.3**	
AX-AE	62.5	**3.8**		63.8	**3.3**	
EB-AX	89.5	**3.4**				
F-wave	**32.0**			24.8		
	Ulnar	**Sens/Mixed N**		**Ulnar**	**Sens/Mixed**	**Nerve**
F-W	44.2	10		42.5	26.4	
W-E	52.0	18		58.0	10	
E-AX	53.3	17.2		54.7	13.0	
AX-EB	60.0	18.0				

Height: 162 cm.
PCB, pseudo-conduction block due to Martin-Grüber anastomosis; SG, spiral-groove; W-F, wrist-forearm.

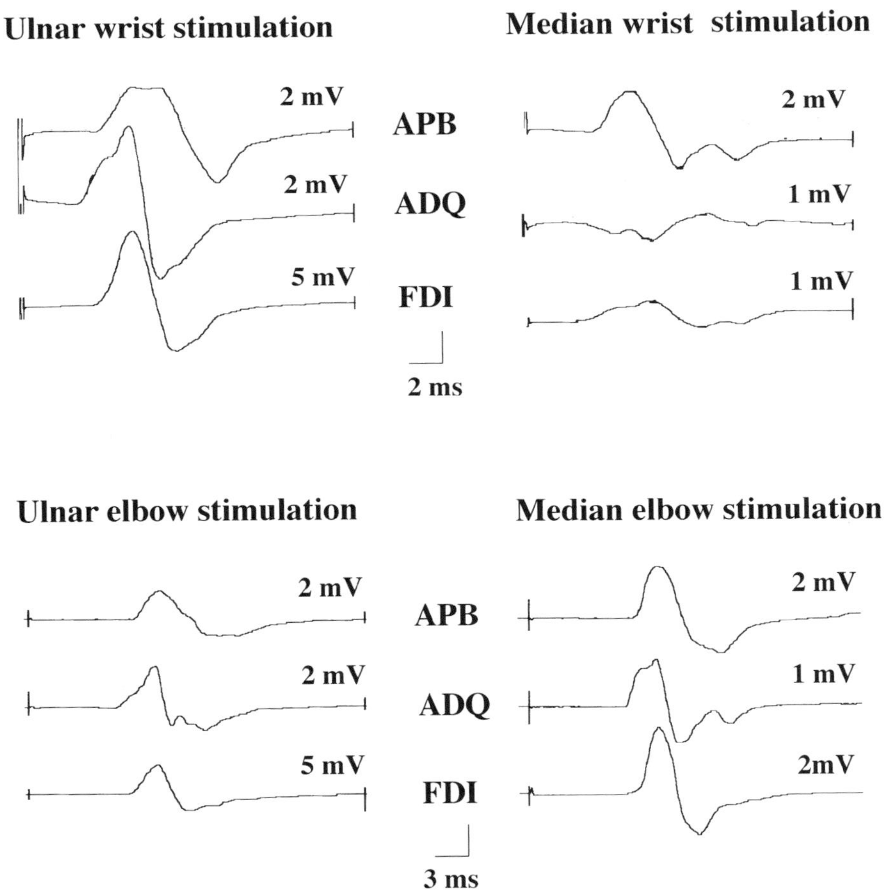

Ulnar wrist stimulation

Median wrist stimulation

2 mV APB 2 mV

2 mV ADQ 1 mV

5 mV FDI 1 mV

2 ms

Ulnar elbow stimulation

Median elbow stimulation

2 mV APB 2 mV

2 mV ADQ 1 mV

5 mV FDI 2mV

3 ms

FIGURE 10.10. Apparent conduction block in the right ulnar nerve between elbow and wrist due to Martin-Grüber anastomosis (MGA) to the ADQ and FDI muscles, which is clearly shown here. On the other hand, MGA to the APB muscle is not clear.

TABLE 10.10. Needle EMG Data in Case 6

Muscle	Root	Nerve	Insertion Activity	Spontaneous Potentials: Fib	PSW	Fasc	Myotonia CRD	Motor Unit Potential: Amplitude (K)	Duration (ms)	Polyphasic Potential	HA MUP	Interference: Pattern	Mean amplitude (K)
Lt C5-8 Paraspinal	C-8		N	–	–	–	–						
Biceps	C6	Musc cut	N	–	–	–	–	1.5–6	6–10	N	+	FIP	3
Deltoids	C5,6	Axillary	+	–	–	+	–	1–6	10–16	+	++	RIP	3
Triceps	C7	Radial	+	++	++	–	–	2–8	6–16	N	++	DA	4
ECR	C6	Radial	+	+	+	+	–	2–8	8–20	N	++[b]	DA	6
FCR	C7	Median	+	–	++	–	–	1–7	6–15	N	+	DA	4
APB	C8, T1	Median	+	+	+	+	–	1–8	7–13	N	+	RIP	6
FDI	C8, T1	Ulnar	+	+	–	+	–	10–13	5–10	N	+	DA	5
Rt Biceps	C6	Musc cut	N	–	–	–	–	0.5–6	6–18	+	+[b]	FIP	2.5
Triceps	C7	Radial	N	–	–	–	–	0.5–7	6–15	N	+	FIP	2.5
FDI	C8, T1	Ulnar	N	–	–	+	–	0.5–8	6–16	N	+	FIP	3
APB	C8, T1	Median	N	–	–	+	–	0.5–6	6–18	N	+[b]	FIP	3

[a] Normal needle EMG findings in the left vastus lateralis, anterior tibialis, and gastrocnemius muscles.

[b] HALD MUP

FINAL DIAGNOSIS

Benign focal amyotrophy

TREATMENT AND FOLLOW-UP

During the next 5-years, there was no obvious progression of atrophy or weakness in the left arm.

COMMENTS

In this case, it was difficult to rule out MMN on clinical grounds, and the NCS were essential in this regard. There was a 70% reduction of CMAP amplitude in the forearm segment in the right ulnar nerve, suggesting an apparent conduction block. A genuine conduction block even in the asymptomatic arm could be a key finding in support of the diagnosis of MMN. Before interpreting the above finding as definite evidence of conduction block, we had to rule out Martin-Grüber anastomosis in this segment, because Martin-Grüber anastomosis can mimic conduction block. Martin-Grüber anastomosis was studied systematically with the recording electrodes in three muscles (APB, ADQ, and FDI) and with stimulation at the wrist and elbow of the ulnar and median nerves. By calculating the CMAP amplitudes with wrist and elbow stimulation between the ulnar and median nerves, the contribution of nerve fibers through median-ulnar anastomosis can be estimated. By this systematic study, we confirmed that this patient had Martin-Grüber anastomosis to the ADQ and FDI muscles. The responses in the ADQ and FDI muscles with median nerve stimulation at the elbow were noteworthy: 2.5 mV CMAP in the ADQ and 7 mV CMAP in the FDI muscle, which were not present with median nerve stimulation at wrist. These were critical findings indicative of Martin-Grüber anastomosis to these muscles. This apparent conduction block is called a pseudoconduction block.

Benign focal amyotrophy (monolemic amyotrophy) is a benign disorder of the anterior horn cells characterized by slowly progressive muscle weakness and wasting involving one limb disproportionally more than the other. It usually involves the upper extremities. The age of onset ranges from 2 to 30 years with most patients between the ages of 18 and 22. The disorder affects more men than women. The disease produces insidious weakness, atrophy, and fasciculations in one limb, usually involving the intrinsic muscles of the hands and the forearm flexors and extensors more so than more proximal muscles. Reflexes are normal or reduced. NCS are usually normal except for a motor neuronopathy pattern (reduced CMAP, prolonged motor and F-wave latencies, and slight slowing in motor NCV) in severe cases. Needle EMG shows chronic and active denervation process in the involved muscles. The most common MRI abnormality is a focal, unilateral atrophy in the lower cervical cord as noted in our case. The clinical course of this illness is usually one of progression for 1 to 2 years followed by relative stabilization thereafter. One autopsy reported anterior horn cell shrinkage and necrosis, degeneration of large and small nerve cells, and mild gliosis of spinal cord segments C5 through T1, particularly marked at the C7 and 8 levels. This entity is never associated with UMN signs.

MAXIMS

1. Benign focal amyotrophy (monolemic amyotrophy) represents "benign focal spinal muscular atrophy" predominantly involving, usually unilaterally, the lower cervical cord.
2. Motor neuronopathy in the involved limb is the classic nerve conduction pattern in benign focal amyotrophy.

REFERENCES

1. Donofrio PD. Monomelic amyotrophy. Muscle Nerve 1994;17:1129–1134.
2. Biondi A, Dormont D, Weitzner I, Bouche P, Chaine P, Bories J. MR imaging of the cervical cord in juvenile amyotrophy of distal extremity. AJNR 1989;10:264–268.

CASE 7

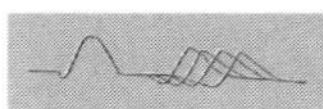

PROGRESSIVE LEG WEAKNESS AND GAIT DIFFICULTY FOR 6 MONTHS

CASE PRESENTATION

A 74-year-old man had progressive leg weakness and gait difficulty for 6 months. This was associated with weight loss (44 pounds). There was no numbness, pain, sphincter, or speech problems and no family history of cancer or neurological diseases.

Abnormal neurological findings were oromandibular dyskinesia, atrophy of both thighs, and fasciculations in arm, calf, and thigh muscles. MRC strength was 4 − in the right iliopsoas and 4 in the left iliopsoas muscles. Reflexes were 3 + at the knees, 1 + at the ankles, and normal in the arms. There was no Babinski sign. The patient was not able to stand up from a seated position without using his arms.

Blood tests by the referring neurologist showed microcytic anemia (hemoglobin 11.4 g/dL and MCV 77 fl), albumin 3.4 g/dL, high GGT (78 IU/L), and erythrocyte sedimentation rate (121 mm/hr).

CASE ANALYSIS

This patient had progressive painless weakness, weight loss, and a constellation of LMN and UMN signs, which were strongly suggestive of ALS. In fact, the patient was referred to the UAB for a second opinion on this diagnosis. The initial impression was, in fact, that he had ALS. In view of the poor prognosis of this disease, it was essential to rule out any other possible treatable neurological diseases, including paraneoplastic MND. This was especially true in view of the high GGT and ESR in this case.

PLAN OF TESTING

1. NCS: To rule out demyelinating neuropathy.
2. Needle EMG: Three-limb study to document widespread denervation process.
3. Other tests: Repeat some of the abnormal laboratory tests, cerebrospinal fluid, muscle biopsy, and workup for treatable MND and occult carcinoma.

ELECTROPHYSIOLOGICAL TESTS AND FINDINGS

NCS Findings

Normal motor and sensory nerve conductions in all tested nerves in one arm and leg.

Needle EMG (Table 10.11 and Fig. 10.11)

1. Fibrillations, PSW, fasciculations, and high-amplitude MUPs in the right anterior tibialis and gastrocnemius muscles.
2. Fasciculations and high-amplitude MUPs in the left anterior tibialis, gastrocnemius, and first interosseous muscles.
3. Increased polyphasic MUPs and reduced interference pattern in the right and left vastus lateralis and medialis and iliopsoas muscles.
4. Fasciculation in the right and left vastus medialis and lateralis, left deltoid and biceps muscles.

ELECTROPHYSIOLOGICAL INTERPRETATION

Widespread chronic denervation process and focal acute denervation in the right L5 and S1 innervated muscles, which were compatible with MND.

OTHER TEST FINDINGS

1. Normal CSF, including MS profile or oligoclonal bands and immunoelectrophoresis of serum protein.
2. CT myelogram showed posterior osteophytes in the cervical region without cord compression.
3. Muscle biopsy of the right anterior tibialis muscle showed type I fiber grouping and type II fiber atrophy.

TABLE 10.11. Needle EMG Data in Case 7

				Spontaneous Potentials				Motor Unit Potential				Interference	
Muscle	**Root**	**Nerve**	**Insertion Activity**	**Fib**	**PSW**	**Fasc**	**Myotonia CRD**	**Amplitude (K)**	**Duration (ms)**	**Polyphasic Potential**	**HA MUP**	**Pattern**	**Mean Amplitude (K)**
Rt and lt L3-5, S1			N	–	–	–	–						
Rt and lt vast lat	L3,4	Femoral	N	–	–	+	–	0.5–4	10–15	+	–	RIP	1.5
Rt and lt vast med	L3,4	Femoral	N	–	–	+	–	0.5–3	8–12	+	–	RIP	1
Rt and lt iliopsoas	L2,3	Femoral	N	–	–	–	–	0.3–3.5	6–12	+	–	RIP	1
Rt ant tibial	L4,5	Peroneal	+	+ +	+	+	–	1–7	8–15	+	+	DA	5
Gastroc	S1,2	Post tibial	+	+	+ +	+ +	–	1–8	8–16	+	+ +	DA	6
Lt ant tibial	L4,5	Peroneal	+	–	–	+	–	1–6	6–15	N	+	RIP	5
Gastroc	S1,2	Post tibial	+	–	–	+ +	–	0.7–7	7–14	N	+	RIP	5
FDI	C8, T1	Median	+	–	–	+ +	–	1–9	8–17	+	+ +	DA	7

* Needle EMG findings in the left biceps and deltoid muscles except some fasciculations.

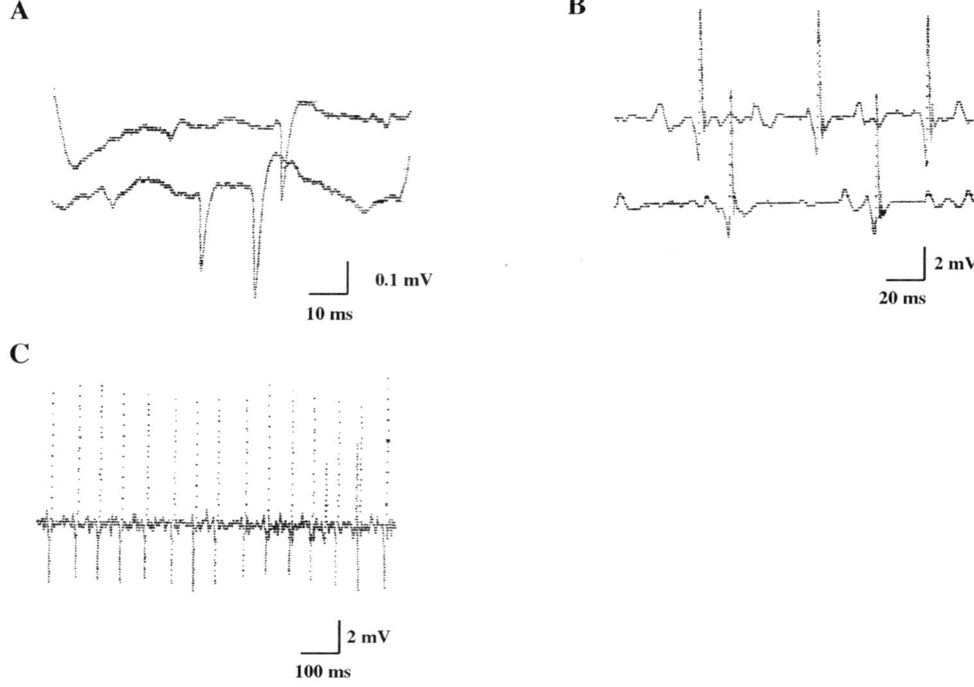

FIGURE 10.11. A. PSW. **B.** HALD MUP. **C.** Discrete activity.

4. Abnormal ultrasound and abdominal-pelvic CT showed a fatty liver and a 10-cm diameter mass of the hilum of the right kidney. A radical nephrectomy revealed moderately differentiated renal cell carcinoma.

FINAL DIAGNOSIS

Paraneoplastic MND and renal cell carcinoma

TREATMENT AND FOLLOW-UP

Within 6 months after nephrectomy, the patient could do a deep-knee bend. Atrophy and fasciculations were gone. Reflexes were unchanged. EMG showed improvement: high-amplitude MUPs (up to 22 mV), but no fibrillations, PSW, or fasciculations. All other abnormal laboratory findings became normal.

COMMENTS

Clinically, this patient had MND, but laboratory abnormalities suggested the possibility of a "symptomatic" MND syndrome. This led us to do the workup for occult carcinoma, which revealed renal cell carcinoma. Elevated ESR, high serum GGT and alkaline phosphatase, hypoalbuminemia, hypercalcemia, anemia, and fatty liver are paraneoplastic manifestations of renal cell carcinoma.

MND can, on rare occasions, be a paraneoplastic manifestation of cancer. Although the issue of whether cancer is the cause of the MND has not been settled, there have been cases of MND that improved with tumor treatment, providing evidence that the cancer caused the MND. These patients had cancer with wasting, fasciculations, weakness, far worse motor than sensory signs, no bowel or bladder involvement, and stabilization or improvement of weakness after cancer treatment. Cancers involved were renal cell carcinoma, lung carcinoma, thymoma, lymphoma, and Waldenström's macroglobulinemia. No clinical abnormality can differentiate treatable paraneoplastic MND from the classic MND. A few patients had other paraneoplastic, but nonneurologic, manifestations. None had dementia or ataxia. A few had abnormal sensory examinations. CSF was usually normal. Atypical laboratory findings, more than the neurological examination, were key in recognition of occult cancer.

Occasionally, a motor neuronopathy occurs in patients with lymphoma and can be the presenting feature. Thus, serum protein immunoelectrophoresis by immunofixation should also be obtained. The presence of a monoclonal gammopathy and elevated spinal protein should lead to an aggressive workup for lymphoma. Recently, a few cases of a rapidly progressive MND and anti-Hu antibodies were reported, strengthening evidence for the paraneoplastic nature of MND. However, these patients had signs and symptoms that suggested involvement of other areas of the nervous system beyond MND. An UMN syndrome initially resembling PLS and breast cancer has also been reported.

Forsythe et al. recommended the following guidelines for the search for cancer in an MND setting. First, patients in whom the MND is a fragment of an encephalomyelopathy syndrome should be examined for anti-Hu antibodies and, if these are positive, suspected of harboring SCLC. Second, examination of bone marrow should be considered in patients with an LMN syndrome or in patients with ALS if there is an M-protein by immunofixation electrophoresis, CSF protein content greater than 75 mg/dL, clinical or laboratory evidence of lymphoproliferative disease (adenopathy, abnormal chest film, high ESR, anemia, or leukocytosis), or if the neurological disorder is atypical (age $<$ 40 years, slow progression). Finally, women who have a UMN syndrome resembling PLS should undergo mammography to rule out breast carcinoma.

Other treatable diseases that can mimic MND include thyrotoxicosis and hyperparathyroidism, which can result in muscle weakness, fasciculations, and hyperreflexia. Therefore, serum calcium parathyroid hormone levels and thyroid function tests should be obtained in all patients with a MNS. Rarely, exposure to inorganic or organic mercury and lead intoxication may mimic ALS.

MAXIMS

1. MND can be a paraneoplastic manifestation of cancer. These cancers include renal cell carcinoma, lung carcinoma, thymoma, and lymphoma.
2. MND with monoclonal gammopathy and a high CSF protein suggest the possibility of lymphoproliferative disease. Thus, bone marrow evaluation should be done.

REFERENCES

1. Evans BK, Fagan C, Arnold T, Dropcho EJ, Oh SJ. Paraneoplastic motor neuron disease and renal cell carcinoma: improvement after nephrectomy. Neurology 1990;40:960–962.
2. Forsythe PA, Dalmau J, Graus F, Cwik V, Rosenblum MK, Posner JB. Motor neuron syndromes in cancer patients. Ann Neurol 1997;41:722–730.

CASE 8

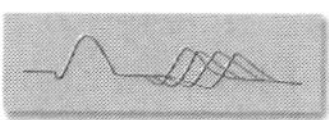

RENEWED WEAKNESS, FATIGUE, AND MUSCLE PAIN IN A PATIENT WITH PREVIOUS POLIO

CASE PRESENTATION

A 40-year-old man had poliomyelitis at age 5, which left him quadriplegic and requiring a mechanical respirator for 6 months. Gradually he recovered and at age 15 only had minor difficulty with his left leg. He led a normal life until about 1 year ago, when he began to notice extreme fatigue and pain in the left calf muscle. During the previous few months he had also noted weakness in the left leg. Abnormal neurological findings were a shorter left leg with atrophy in the calf, left footdrop, absent right triceps, and left patellar reflexes and MRC strength of 4 in the right deltoid and forearm extensor muscles, 3 in the right forearm flexor, 0 in the left anterior tibialis, and 4 in the left gastrocnemius muscle. Sensory examination was normal. No fasciculation was noted. Straight leg raising sign was absent.

CASE ANALYSIS

This patient with a history of poliomyelitis developed subacute weakness, fatigue, and pain in the previously involved muscles and pure LMN signs on examination. The clinical history suggested neurological worsening of the left leg. Thus, the clinician was obligated to rule out any new focal diseases, such as a lumbar disc or stenosis. The absence of any sensory deficit and the complaints of extreme fatigue were two findings against the possibility of focal disease. On the other hand, extreme fatigue and muscle pain are two cardinal symptoms of postpolio syndrome.

PLAN OF TESTING

1. NCS: To rule out focal entrapment neuropathy.
2. Needle EMG: To document chronic denervation and look for acute denervation in the left paraspinal and leg muscles.

ELECTROPHYSIOLOGICAL TESTS AND FINDINGS

NCS Findings

1. Low CMAP amplitude in the left peroneal nerve.
2. Otherwise normal NCS in the right median and ulnar nerves and left peroneal, posterior tibial, and sural nerves.

Needle EMG (Table 10.12 and Fig. 10.12)

1. HA MUPs in the tested muscles in the right upper and left lower extremities except for the right deltoid and left medial gastrocnemius muscles.
2. Long-duration MUPs in the right triceps and left medial gastrocnemius muscles.
3. RIP or DA in all tested muscles except for the right anterior tibialis muscle.
4. No fibrillation or PSW in any tested muscles.

ELECTROPHYSIOLOGICAL INTERPRETATION

Multifocal chronic denervation process compatible with either postpolio syndrome or a recovered polio state. There was no electrophysiological evidence of active denervation process.

OTHER TEST FINDINGS

MRI of the lumbosacral cord was normal.

FINAL DIAGNOSIS

Postpolio syndrome

TREATMENT AND FOLLOW-UP

During a 5-year follow-up period, there was a gradual increase in weakness in the left leg that required an ankle-foot orthosis. The patient's fatigue was improved with pyridostigmine

TABLE 10.12. Needle EMG Data in Case 8

				Spontaneous Potentials				Motor Unit Potential				Interference	
Muscle	**Root**	**Nerve**	**Insertion Activity**	**Fib**	**PSW**	**Fasc**	**Myotonia CRD**	**Amplitude (K)**	**Duration (ms)**	**Polyphasic Potential**	**HA MUP**	**Pat-tern**	**Mean Amplitude (K)**
Rt Deltoid	C5,6	Axillary	N	–	–	–	–	1–3	10–15	N	–	RIP	1.5
Triceps	C7	Radial	N	–	–	–	–	5–8	10–19	N	+	DA	6
EDC	C7	Radial	N	–	–	–	–	2–12	10–15	N	++	RIP	6
FDI	C8, T1	Ulnar	N	–	–	–	–	2–8	10–14	N	+	RIP	4
Vast lat	L3,4	Femoral	N	–	–	–	–	4–14	10–17	N	++	RIP	8
Ant tibial	L4,5	Peroneal	N	–	–	–	–	1–8	10–15	N	+	FIP	4
Lt Vast Lat	L3,4	Femoral	N	–	–	–	–	1–6	10–16	N	+	DA	3
Ant tibial	L4,5	Peroneal	N	–	–	–	–	No	MUP				
Med gastroc	S1,2	Post tibial	N	–	–	–	–	1–3	10–19	N	–	DA	2

EDC, extensor digitorum communis.

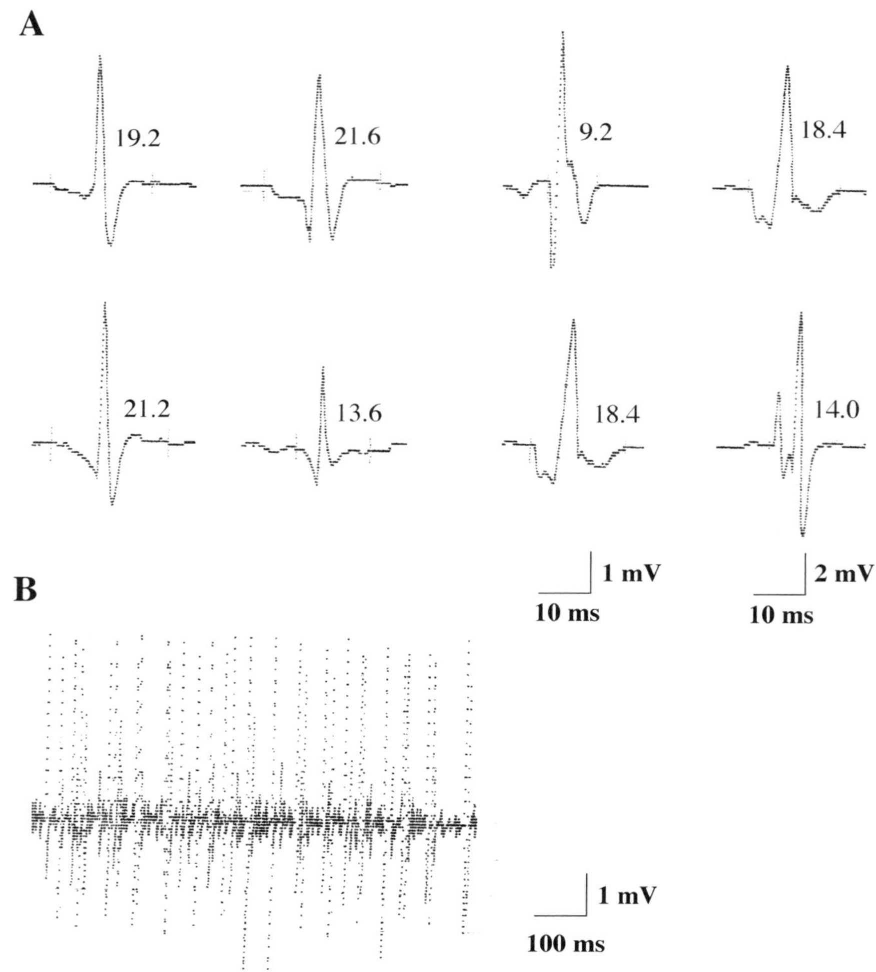

FIGURE 10.12. A. HA and HALD MUPs. **B.** Discrete activity on maximal contraction. Numbers above MUP represent the duration of MUP.

30 mg four times a day, and his pain was controlled with butarbital. At present, on many occasions, he has to teach his classes from a wheelchair.

COMMENTS

Postpolio syndrome is now a well-recognized entity. The diagnosis of postpolio syndrome is made entirely on the basis of clinical findings, mostly by exclusion of other diseases, which can mimic the disorder. Typically, patients have a well-documented history of poliomyelitis followed by a symptom-free interval of 20 to 40 years before the onset of renewed weakness and atrophy, fatigue, and myalgia. New muscle weakness usually involves previously affected muscles that have fully or partially recovered and is asymmetrical. Fatigue is a universal phenomenon that probably precedes muscle weakness and typically represents a lack of energy and stamina that improves after a brief period of rest. Myalgia represents deep muscle aching and is often mixed with arthralgias. Fasciculation may be observed but is less frequent than that seen in ALS. Two known risk factors for postpolio syndrome are poliomyelitis after 10 years of age and severe poliomyelitis (quadriplegia and use of a respirator). Although no laboratory test is diagnostic, confirmation of postpolio syndrome should be substantiated by

EMG evidence of past denervation. Studies showed that no difference in NCS, needle EMG, or EMG were found between patients with postpolio syndrome and "recovered polio patients" without postpolio syndrome. In short, there is no distinctive electrophysiological features typical of postpolio syndrome. However, NCS/EMG studies are valuable in ruling out other diseases such as entrapment neuropathy or radiculopathy, which can occur in previous polio patients.

MAXIMS

1. There are no characteristic EMG findings indicative of postpolio syndrome. Needle EMG shows a chronic denervation pattern.
2. Postpolio syndrome is characterized by renewed muscle weakness, extreme generalized fatigue, and muscle pain in previous polio patients.

REFERENCES

1. Dalakas MC. The postpolio syndrome as an evolved clinical entity. Definition and clinical description. Ann N Y Acad Sci 1995;753:68–80.
2. Cashman NR, Maselli R, Wollman L, Roos R, Simon R, Antel JP. Late denervation in patients with antecedent paralytic poliomyelitis. N Engl J Med 1987;1317:7–12.

CASE 9

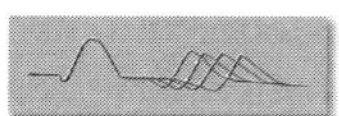

FAMILIAL ALS WITH A 2-YEAR HISTORY OF ARM AND LEG WEAKNESS AND HYPERREFLEXIA IN A 46-YEAR-OLD WOMAN

CASE PRESENTATION

A 46-year-old right-handed woman was diagnosed with familial ALS and encouraged to enroll in an experimental drug trial at another medical center. The patient's cousin, a physician, encouraged her to seek a second opinion for this diagnosis. Two years previously, the patient had severe pain in her back after lifting a heavy child. Since then, she began to experience problems climbing stairs and needed to hold on to the railing. She also noted that she was dragging her left toe and frequently stumbling. For 1 year, she had been having infrequent falls and difficulty using her hands to type. She had noticed muscle twitching in her legs and occasionally in her arms. She underwent an EMG by a local neurologist who documented fibrillations and PSW in all tested muscles in both arms and legs. Spinal fluid was normal, including multiple sclerosis profile. GM1 and MAG were normal. Immunofixation protein immunoelectrophoresis was normal. Heavy metals and porphyrins were also normal. MRI of the brain was remarkable only for several small white-matter abnormalities in the distal corona radiata. Family history was remarkable for her father, who died at age 50 after a 10-year history of ALS and whose symptoms had begun with walking difficulty.

Abnormal neurological findings were atrophy of the distal lower extremities and intrinsic hand muscles, mild pes cavus, diffuse hyperreflexia with normal ankle reflexes, MRC strength of 4 in the deltoids, hand intrinsics, and finger extensor muscles, 4+ in the iliopsoas, 4− in the right anterior tibialis, 4 in the left anterior tibialis, 4 in bilateral peroneus muscles, and difficulty walking on her heels.

No Babinski sign was noted, but Hoffman sign was positive on the left. Fasciculation was absent. Sensory examination was completely normal.

CASE ANALYSIS

This patient had a 2-year history of progressive weakness of the arms and legs, objective atrophy and weakness of arm and leg muscles, diffuse hyperreflexia, and widespread fibrillations and PSW on the needle EMG study. These findings were typical of MND. It seemed that the diagnosis of familial ALS was certain. Mild pes cavus and the absence of fasciculations were somewhat unusual. In some ALS cases, fasciculations are only detected with the needle EMG, because they are present deep in muscles. Thus, the absence of fasciculation by examination does not rule out ALS.

PLAN OF TESTING

1. NCS: To rule out demyelinating neuropathy.
2. Needle EMG: To confirm widespread denervation and to rule out any myopathy.
3. Other tests: CPK and muscle biopsy and MRI of the cervical cord to rule out cervical cord compression such as CSM.

ELECTROPHYSIOLOGICAL TESTS AND FINDINGS

NCS Findings

1. Low CMAP amplitude in the median, ulnar, and peroneal nerves.
2. Otherwise normal motor, sensory, and mixed nerve conduction.

Needle EMG (Table 10.13 and Figs. 10.13–10.14)

1. Increased insertion activity, fibrillation, PSW, and increased polyphasic MUPs in all tested muscles.
2. Fasciculation potentials in the left FDI, right anterior tibialis, and gastrocnemius muscles.
3. HALD, MUPs, and SASD MUPs in the bilateral anterior tibialis and left gastrocnemius muscles.
4. HA MUPs in the right gastrocnemius muscle.
5. RIP in the left anterior tibialis and bilateral gastrocnemius muscles.

TABLE 10.13. Needle EMG Data in Case 9

				Spontaneous Potentials				Motor Unit Potential				Interference	
Muscle	**Root**	**Nerve**	**Insertion Activity**	**Fib**	**PSW**	**Fasc**	**Myotonia CRD**	**Amplitude (K)**	**Duration (ms)**	**Polyphasic Potential**	**HALD MUP**	**Pat-tern**	**Mean Amplitude (K)**
Lt Deltoids	C5,6	Axillary	+	+ + +	+ + +	−	−	0.5–2	6–12	+	−	FIP	2
Biceps	C6,7	Musc cut	+	+ +	+ + +	−	−	0.3–2	6–12	+	−	FIP	2
FDI	C8, T1	Ulnar	+	+ + + +	+ + + +	+	+	0.5–4	6–12	+	−	FIP	2
Vast lat	L3,4	Femoral	+	+ +	+ +	−	−	0.5–4	6–12	+	−	FIP	2
Lt Ant Tibial	L4,5	Peroneal	+	+ + + +	+	−	−	0.3–5.5	3–20	+	+	RIP	1
Gastroc	S1,2	Post tibial	+	+ + + +	+ +	+	−	0.5–4	4–28	+	LD	RIP	2
Rt Ant Tibial	L4,5	Peroneal	+	+ +	+ +	−	+	0.5–3	4–23	+	LD	FIP	2

LD, long-duration MUP.

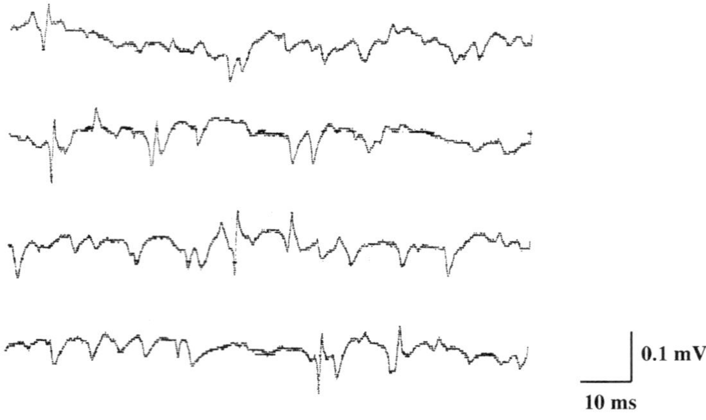

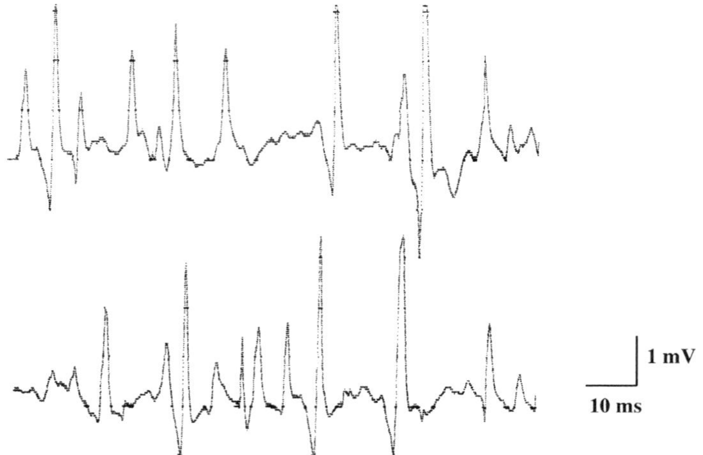

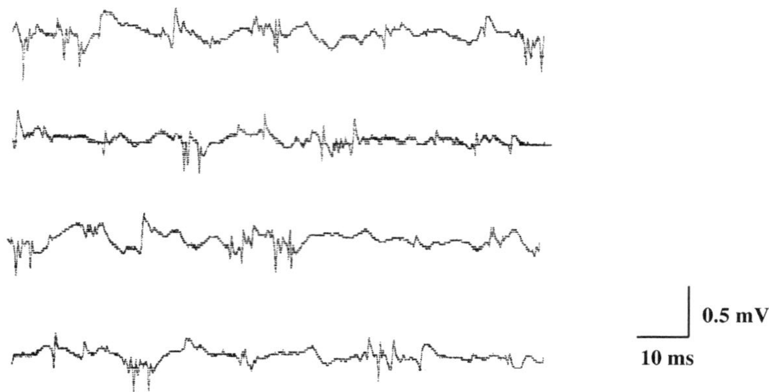

FIGURE 10.13. Needle EMG findings in the left anterior tibialis muscle.

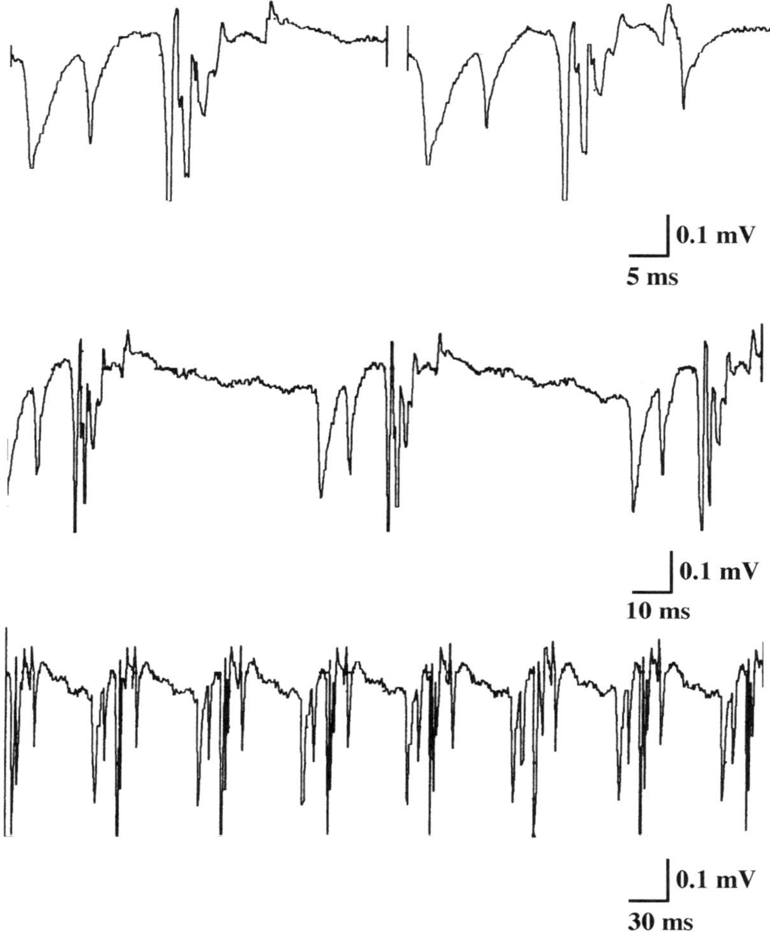

FIGURE 10.14. CRDs at different sweeps in the biceps muscle. Notice no waxing or waning of amplitude or frequency of the potentials.

ELECTROPHYSIOLOGICAL INTERPRETATION

Widespread denervation process mixed with localized myopathic process was found, which is compatible with MND with secondary myopathic process or IBM.

OTHER TEST FINDINGS

Muscle biopsy showed a typical IBM characterized by many fibers with rimmed vacuoles, increased endomysial connective tissue, groupings of many angular fibers, and few endomysial inflammatory cells.

FINAL DIAGNOSIS

IBM

TREATMENT AND FOLLOW-UP

In view of the father's diagnosis of ALS, we thought about the possibility of familial IBM in this case. Fortunately, an autopsy had been performed on the father. A review of the autopsy slides confirmed that her father had classic ALS showing degeneration in anterior horn cells and pyramidal tracts. Thus, this case represents ALS in the father and sporadic IBM in the daughter. Follow-up evaluation in 1 year did not show any progression of disease.

COMMENTS

ALS is classically the disease of UMNs and LMNs. Thus, the pyramidal tract is invariably involved in the disease. Without UMN involvement, the diagnosis of ALS is untenable. However, a positive Babinski sign, which is pathognomonic of UMN impairment, is not always present because of lower motor involvement in the extensor hallucis longus muscles. The Babinski sign has been observed in 75% of cases. Hyperreflexia alone is not a definite sign of UMN disease, as seen in this patient. In her case, diffuse hyperreflexia must have been "normal" for her. Hyperreflexia has also been reported in chronic demyelinating neuropathy.

Most cases of ALS are sporadic, with approximately 5 to 10% being familial. In most of these cases, the pattern of inheritance is autosomal dominant. Familial ALS is clinically indistinguishable from sporadic ALS. However, the mean age of onset for familial ALS is 46 years, approximately 10 years earlier than for sporadic patients. Twenty percent of cases of autosomal-dominant familial ALS are linked to chromosome 21q21 and are associated with mutations in a copper-zinc binding superoxide dismutase (*SOD1*) enzyme gene. This enzyme detoxifies the superoxide anion, a free radical formed as a byproduct of aerobic metabolism. Abnormal function of superoxide dismutase could cause accumulation of free radicals and initiate lipid and protein peroxidation and DNA damage. This observation led to a hypothesis that excessive formation of free radicals damages motor neurons in ALS. A further finding in support of this hypothesis is that transgenic mice, which express mutant forms of human superoxide dismutase, developed a disease somewhat similar to ALS.

IBM can be confused with ALS, as noted in this case, and more often with SMA. This is because of the progressive painless atrophy and weakness of muscles without any sensory loss and areflexia in older individuals. In addition, needle EMG findings can be confusing, as seen here. Prominent fibrillations and PSW in almost all muscles tested in this case could be interpreted as an indication of denervation to the inexperienced electromyographer. Fibrillations and PSW are present in almost all cases of IBM. MUPs have to be carefully analyzed. MUPs can be of SASD, HALD, and normal in IBM. In fact, when there is a mixed pattern of SASD and HALD, IBM should be the first diagnostic consideration, because these are the typical findings in one-third of the cases of IBM.

MAXIMS

1. Familial ALS is indistinguishable clinically from sporadic ALS except for its earlier onset. In 20% of familial ALS cases, mutation of in the superoxide mutase (*SOD1*) gene was found.
2. Inclusion body myopathy can mimic MND clinically and electrophysiologically.

REFERENCES

1. Joy JL, Oh SJ, Baysal AL. Electrophysiological spectrum of inclusion body myositis. Muscle Nerve 1990;13:949–951.
2. Siddique T, Nijhawan D, Hentati A. Molecular genetic basis of familial ALS. Neurology 1996;47: 27–35.

CASE 10

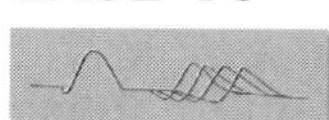

CONDUCTION BLOCK IN A CASE WITH WIDESPREAD FASCICULATION AND MUSCLE WEAKNESS

CASE PRESENTATION

A 78-year-old man with a history of coronary artery disease had been in good health until 11 months ago, when he noticed that he was unable to hold items in his left hand. Since then, there had been a gradual increase in weakness in his left arm. After extensive evaluation 4 months ago, he had undergone left ulnar transposition surgery without any improvement. At approximately the same time he began to notice difficulty with his feet, with his feet slapping the floor when he walked, dragging of the left toe, and stumbling over objects. He denied any speech, swallowing, bowel or bladder problems, or any sensory symptoms including numbness and tingling. He did complain of muscle twitching, particularly in the left arm and leg, and also of frequent muscle cramps. He had dyspnea on exertion and shortness of breath. A neurologist observed widespread fasciculation, muscle weakness and atrophy, and well-preserved reflexes. CPK was 539. A total myelogram and CT and MRI of the spine were negative, according to the patient, except for a spur in his neck. EMG/NCS showed widespread denervation process and fasciculation with motor neuropathy. The patient was sent for a second opinion for the diagnosis of ALS.

Abnormal neurological findings were MRC strength of 4 in the left wrist flexor, left hand intrinsics, left ilipsoas, and right anterior tibialis, 4+ in the right iliopsoas and left gastronomists, 2 in the left anterior tibialis, decreased vibration to the ankles bilaterally, decreased proprioception in the right toes, atrophy in the left forearm and hand, widespread fasciculations across the back and in all four extremities, normal biceps, triceps and patellar reflexes, and absent ankle reflexes. Plantar responses were equivocal. No increased tone or spasticity was noted. He was not able to heel or toe walk.

CASE ANALYSIS

This patient had many of the clinical features typical of ALS: progressive motor weakness for 11 months, widespread fasciculation, asymmetrical weakness and atrophy, and relatively well-preserved reflexes. In fact, a resident physician thought that this patient had classic ALS. EMG/NCS findings and elevated CPK were all typical findings of ALS. The minor sensory abnormalities could be due to aging. On the other hand, every finding in this case can also be explained by CIDP.

PLAN OF TESTING

1. NCS: To rule out demyelinating neuropathy.
2. Needle EMG: To document widespread denervation process.
3. Other tests: CSF, sural nerve, and muscle biopsies. Serum autoantibody test.

ELECTROPHYSIOLOGICAL TESTS AND FINDINGS

NCS Findings (Table 10.14 and Fig. 10.15)

1. No CMAP in the median nerve and low CMAP amplitude in other nerves.
2. Prolonged terminal latencies in ulnar and peroneal nerves.
3. Slow motor NCV in the ulnar nerve.
4. Moderately slow motor NCV in all tested nerves in the legs.
5. Conduction block and abnormal dispersion phenomenon in posterior tibial nerves.
6. Absent H-reflex and F-wave in most tested nerves.
7. Low CNAPs and slow sensory and mixed NCVs.

Needle EMG (Table 10.15)

1. Fibrillation, PSW, fasciculation, and CRD in many tested muscles.
2. HA MUPs in some tested muscles.
3. Reduced recruitments of MUPs in all tested muscles.

ELECTROPHYSIOLOGICAL INTERPRETATION

Demyelinating neuropathy with secondary axonal change.

TABLE 10.14. Nerve Conduction Data in Case 10

	Latent/NCV (ms/m/s)	Amplitude (mV/μV)	Others		Latent/NCV (ms/m/s)	Amplitude (mV/μV)	Others
	Median	**Motor**	**Nerve**		**Peroneal**	**Motor**	**Nerve**
TL	**NP**			TL	**7.0**	**0.74**	
E-W	**NP**			FH-A	**26.0**	**0.54**	
AX-E	**NP**			PF-FH	**33.3**	**0.5**	
F-wave	**NP**			F-wave	**78.8**		
	Ulnar	**Motor**	**Nerve**	**Left**	**Post Tibial**	**Motor**	**Nerve**
TL	4.0	3		TL	4.8	**0.69**	
BE-W	45.8	2.5		PF-A	**28.9**	**0.14**	**CB**
AE-BE	42.8	2.0		F-wave	**68.4**		
AX-AE	52.2	2.0		H-reflex	**NP**		
EB-AX	42.1	1.52					
F-wave	NP						
	Median	**Sens/Mixed**	**Nerve**	**Right**	**Post Tibial**	**Motor**	**Nerve**
F-W	36.7	10		TL	4.8	0.92	
W-E	37.3	5		PF-A	27.3	0.84	**Disp**
E-AX	52	5		F-wave	73.6		
				H-reflex	NP		
	Ulnar	**Sens/Mixed**	**Nerve**		**Sural**	**Sens**	**Nerve**
F-W	35.0	3		MC-A	36.1	**4.4**	
W-E	39.3	5					
E-AX	44.4	2					
AX-EB	45.2	3.9					

OTHER TEST FINDINGS

1. CSF: no cell; protein was 78 mg/dL with oligoclonal bands.
2. Nerve biopsy showing demyelinating neuropathy.

FINAL DIAGNOSIS

Multifocal motor and sensory demyelinating neuropathy

TREATMENT AND FOLLOW-UP

This patient was treated with high-dose prednisone and IVIg initially. Gradually, his neuropathy improved. He needed 20 mg of prednisone every other day to maintain his improved status.

COMMENTS

In this case, initially the diagnosis of ALS was suspected rightly on the basis of progressive widespread motor weakness and fasciculation, EMG evidence of denervation, and relatively well-preserved reflexes. If we discounted the minimal vibratory and proprioception loss as aging phenomena, it was impossible to make a distinction between ALS and CIDP or multifocal motor and sensory demyelinating neuropathy on clinical grounds alone in this case. In view of the onset of symptoms from the left hand, asymmetrical motor and sensory deficits, and demyelinating nerve conduction findings, the most accurate diagnosis in this case was multifocal motor and sensory demyelinating neuropathy rather than MMN.

MMN can mimic ALS. This entity is characterized by slowly progressive asymmetric pure motor weakness, conduction block in the motor nerve conduction, high GM_1 antibody titer,

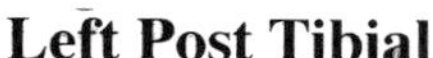

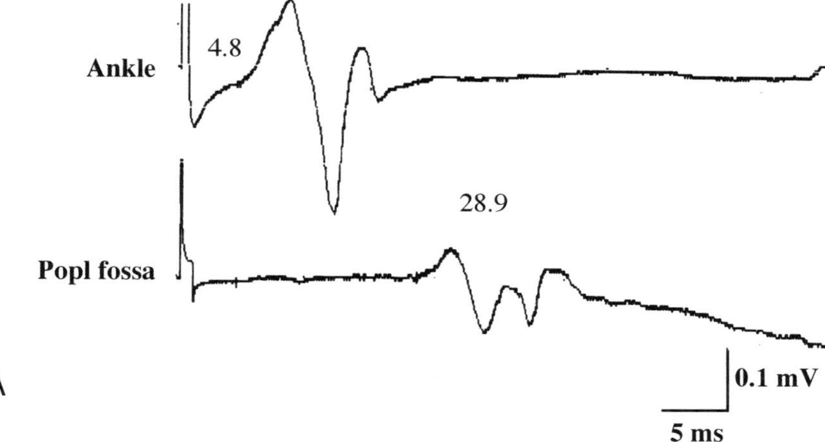

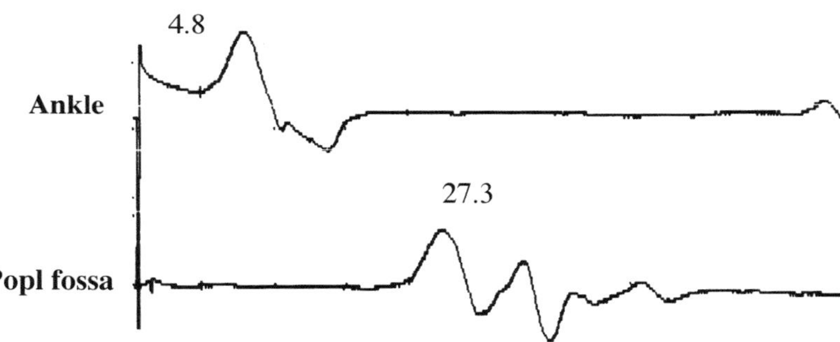

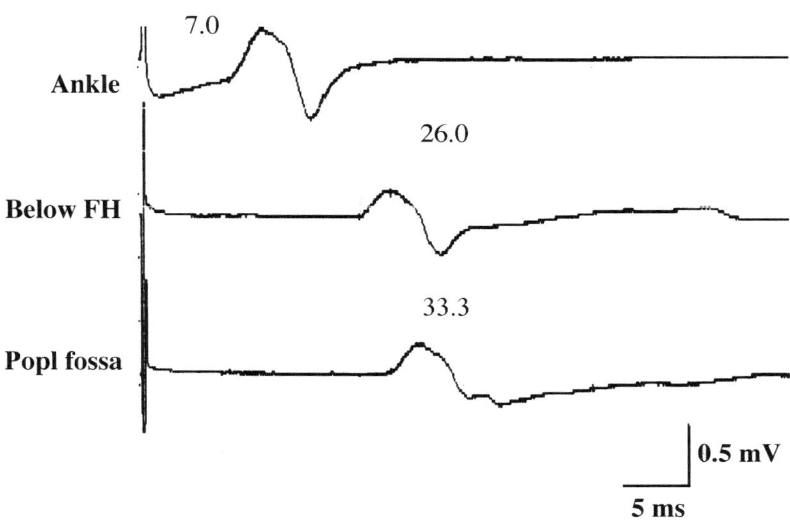

FIGURE 10.15. **A.** Conduction block in the left posterior tibial nerve. **B.** Temporal dispersion at the popliteal fossa in the right posterior tibial nerve. **C.** Slow NCV in the right peroneal nerve. Numbers above the responses indicate the terminal latencies and NCV.

TABLE 10.15. Needle EMG Data in Case 10

				Spontaneous Potentials				Motor Unit Potential				Interference	
Muscle	**Root**	**Nerve**	**Insertion Activity**	**Fib**	**PSW**	**Fasc**	**CRD**	**Amplitude (K)**	**Duration (ms)**	**Polyphasic Potential**	**HA MUP**	**Pat-tern**	**Mean Amplitude (K)**
Lt Ant Tibial	L4,5	Peroneal	+	+ + +	+ +	–	–	1–4	5–10	N	0	DA	2
Gastroc	S1,2	Post tibial	+	+ + + +	+ + +	–	–	1–17	6–20	N	+ + +[a]	DA	13
Vast lat	L3,4	Femoral	+	+	+	+ + +	–	1–5	6–11	N	0	RIP	3
Rt Vast Lat	L3,4	Femoral	+	+	+ +	+	–	1–10	6–13	+	+ +	DA	8
Ant tibial	L4,5	Peroneal	+	+ + +	+ + + +	–	–	1–6	6–16	+	+	RIP	4
Gastroc	S1,2	Post tibial	+	+ +	+ + +	–	+	1–5.5	6–13	N	+	RIP	4
Lt Deltoid	C5,6	Axillary	+	+	+ +	+ +	–	1–5	6–11	N	0	FIP	3
Biceps	C6	Musc cut	+	+	+ +	+ + +	+	1–5	6–9	N	0	FIP	3
Pron teres	C6,7	Median	+	+ +	+	+	–	1–5	6–12	+	0	RIP	4

[a] HALD MUP.

and response to cyclophosphamide and intravenous gamma globulin. In 25% of MMN cases, the reflexes were preserved, and in 46% of cases, fasciculation was present. In this disorder, conduction block was noted in all cases and is now considered to be the most important diagnostic criterion.

The pure motor form of CIDP can also mimic ALS. We have reported three cases of CIDP with symmetrical motor weakness, fasciculation, and well-preserved reflexes. Otherwise, these patients had all the diagnostic features of CIDP, including high spinal fluid protein, demyelination in the NCS, and good response to steroid treatment. Serum GM_1 antibody was absent in the tested cases. Because MMN and CIDP are treatable with immunotherapies, it is important to do an extensive NCS to rule out demyelinating neuropathy in all patients suspected of having ALS.

Multifocal motor and sensory demyelinating neuropathy is an entity recently reported by us. These patients have the clinical pattern of motor and sensory mononeuropathy multiplex, electrophysiological evidence of demyelination including conduction block, and segmental demyelination in the sural nerve biopsy, high CSF protein in 60% of cases, and a good response to steroid treatment in 80% of cases. Clinically, except for definite sensory deficits, multifocal motor and sensory demyelinating neuropathy is not too different from MMN. Unlike MMN, however, multifocal motor and sensory demyelinating neuropathy is characterized by a shorter course, sensory deficits and sensory nerve conduction abnormalities, absence of GM_1 antibody in most tested cases, and good response to steroid. Most likely, multifocal motor and sensory demyelinating neuropathy represents a variant of CIDP and a link between CIDP and MMN.

MAXIMS

1. MMN and CIDP can mimic ALS. To rule out these treatable demyelinating neuropathies, an extensive NCS is a must in every case of ALS.
2. Conduction block is the most important diagnostic finding for MMN.

REFERENCES

1. Parry G, Clarks S. Multifocal acquired demyelinating neuropathy masquerading as motor neuron disease. Muscle Nerve 1988;11:103–107.
2. Oh S. The "amyotrophic lateral sclerosis form" of chronic demyelinating polyneuropathy. Am Neurol 1990;28:269.

CHAPTER 11

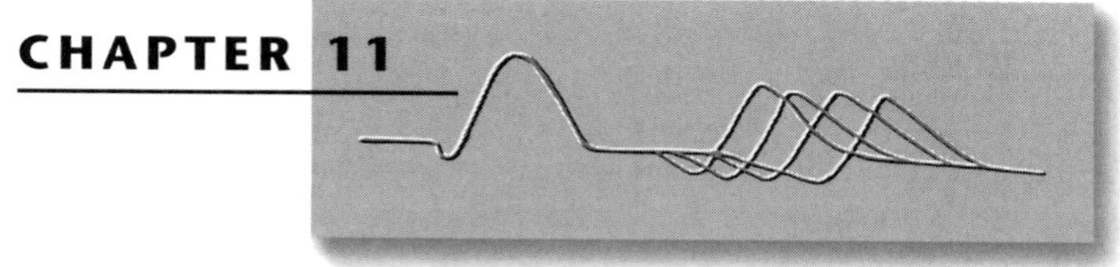

Myopathies

Myopathies are diseases of muscle, usually characterized clinically by symmetrical muscle weakness and wasting and histologically by structural damage of the muscle fibers. In about two-thirds of adult cases of myopathies, the patients have an acquired treatable myopathy. Polymyositis is the most common form of treatable adult myopathy. In children, the reverse is true: about one-third of these patients have treatable myopathies. Benign congenital myopathies are the major group of myopathies in children.

CLINICAL FEATURES OF MYOPATHIES

As in other lower motor neuron disorders, *muscle weakness is the most important clinical feature of myopathy*. Thus, the first step in the diagnosis of myopathy is to rule out other lower motor neuron diseases (Table 11.1). Because of the predominant involvement of proximal muscles in myopathy, patients have difficulty raising their arms above their shoulders, rising from a chair, climbing stairs, and doing deep knee bends. These are the most helpful symptoms suggestive of proximal muscle weakness. Because of pelvic girdle muscle weakness, the patients with myopathy have Gowers sign ("climbing up one's own trunk with the arms when rising from a supine to an erect position) and waddling gait. Invariably, no sensory abnormality or reflex change is present in myopathy. These are the most important points in differentiating myopathy from neuropathy or anterior horn cell disorders.

Atrophy of muscle follows the prolonged muscle weakness and is much more prominent in patients with lower motor neuron lesions. Thus, muscle atrophy is commonly seen in chronic myopathy. "Pseudohypertrophy" is a term used to describe a hypertrophied muscle caused by prominent fibrosis of muscle. Pseudohypertrophy of the calf muscle is commonly associated with Duchenne or Becker dystrophy. Muscle tenderness is less commonly seen in myopathy but is not an uncommon finding in polymyositis.

Myasthenia, an exertional weakness or easy fatigability, is a typical clinical feature of the neuromuscular transmission disorders such as myasthenia gravis.

Myotonia, a difficulty of relaxation after contraction of muscle, is a sine qua non in myotonic syndrome. It is commonly demonstrated as grasp or percussion myotonia in patients with myotonic syndrome, who usually complain of "stiffness." Myotonia is classically aggravated by cold and eased by "warming up exercises."

DIAGNOSIS OF THE ETIOLOGY OF MYOPATHY

Family History

A positive family history is very helpful in the diagnosis of progressive muscular dystrophy, myotonic dystrophy, and familial periodic paralysis. The mode of inheritance is important in genetic counseling. Sex-linked recessive inheritance is the characteristic pattern seen in Duchenne and Becker dystrophy. Autosomal-dominant inheritance is the characteristic pattern seen in myotonic dystrophy and familial periodic paralysis.

Age at Onset

This is helpful in suggesting the etiology. A general rule is that adult-onset myopathy is acquired and treatable and that childhood-onset myopathy is nonacquired and nontreatable.

TABLE 11.1. Differential Features in Various Neuromuscular Diseases

	Anterior Horn Cells	Peripheral Nerves	Neuromuscular Junctions	Muscles
Disease entity	Motor neuron diseases	Peripheral neuropathy	Myasthenia gravis	Myopathy
Predilected involvement	Widespread	Distal part	Proximal part/oculobulbar area	Proximal part
Sensory involvement	Absent	Usually present	Absent	Absent
Reflexes	Weak/absent	Weak/absent	Normal	Normal
Other helpful signs	Fasciculation		Myasthenic symptoms	
Serum muscle enzymes	Normal	Normal	Normal	Increased
Nerve conduction study	Normal	Slow nerve conduction	Normal	Normal
Needle EMG findings	Duration of motor unit potentials (MUP) is increased. Fibrillation and PSWs in distal muscles over widespread areas. Similar findings in both anterior horn cells and peripheral nerve diseases.		Normal or decreased MUP duration	Decreased MUP duration
Repetitive nerve stimulation test	Normal	Normal	Decremental response	Normal
Muscle biopsy	Denervation process	Denervation process	Nonspecific	Myopathy

A myopathy presenting at birth is usually nonprogressive and benign (e.g., congenital myopathy). A myopathy presenting in early or late childhood is usually progressive (e.g., progressive muscular dystrophy).

History of Nonprogression, Remission, or Progression

Remission is often observed in myasthenia gravis, periodic paralysis, and polymyositis. Nonprogression is typically seen in many congenital myopathies and are thus termed benign congenital myopathies. These include nemalin myopathy, central core disease, fiber-type disproportion syndrome, myotubular myopathy, and mitochondrial myopathy. Recognition of these entities is important in future planning for individual patients. Progression is a typical feature of muscular dystrophy.

System Review

A typical skin rash is almost pathognomonic of polymyositis. Rheumatoid features are suggestive of collagen vascular diseases and of polymyositis. Signs indicative of endocrine disorders are suggestive of endocrine myopathy.

Chief Site of Involvement

As stated above, myopathy is characterized by the predominant involvement of proximal muscles. However, there are a few exceptions. Myotonic dystrophy and distal dystrophy are characterized by predominant distal muscle weakness and wasting. Generalized muscle weakness is commonly seen in floppy infant syndrome, periodic paralysis, and myotonia congenita.

DIAGNOSTIC PROCEDURES

Laboratory investigation is essential in confirming the diagnosis of myopathy and in identification of the etiology of myopathy. The main diagnostic procedures important in myopathy are laboratory studies, the electromyography (EMG) study, and the muscle biopsy.

Laboratory Studies

Creatine phosphokinase (CPK), SGOT, aldolase, and lactic dehydrogenase are called "muscle enzymes" (Table 11.2). Their elevation reflects the degree of active muscle fiber necrosis. An increase in muscle enzymes is due to increased permeability of enzymes from the damaged or diseased muscle cells. Among these enzymes, the most sensitive is CPK. Remember that there are many other nonmyopathic causes of elevated CPK: simple muscle contusion, myocardial infarction, intramuscular injection, hypothyroidism, and chronic alcoholism. Thus, these common causes of elevated CPK should be ruled out. Fractionation of CPK is not necessary in the work-up of myopathy because the MB fraction is a small component compared with the MM component in CPK in myopathy. The serial determination of muscle enzymes is an important objective measure in the follow-up evaluation of patients with myopathy. This is especially true in polymyositis because the enzyme improvement precedes the clinical improvement by a few weeks. In Duchenne dystrophy, the determination of CPK has been used in carrier detection because many carriers show a mild CPK elevation, but this has been replaced by the more specific DNA deletion test in the blood. Also, in this disease, CPK is known to be elevated long before the clinical onset, with the highest value noted in the early stage of disease. A gradual decrease in CPK is observed as the disease progresses. Thus, CPK is useful in detection of asymptomatic cases among siblings of patients with confirmed diagnosis. On the other hand, there are myopathies with normal CPK. These include myasthenia gravis, periodic paralysis, steroid myopathy, and many benign congenital myopathies. Normal CPK is an important feature in differentiating steroid myopathy from polymyositis.

The serum potassium level at the peak of an attack of periodic paralysis determines the

TABLE 11.2. Basic Laboratory Tests for Causes of Obscure Myopathy

Test	Diagnostic Possibilities
Muscle enzymes	
CPK (isoenzyme CPK MM)	More specific for myopathy
SGOT, aldolase, LDH	Less specific for myopathy
Rheumatology profile	
ANA and rheumatoid factor	SLE, rheumatoid arthritis
Sjögren antibody	Sjögren disease
Anti-Jo antibody	Polymyositis with interstitial lung disease
Antinuclear cytoplasmic antibody	Wegener's granulomatosis
CBC, sedimentation rate	Collagen vascular diseases, systemic diseases, dysproteinemia, leukemia, lymphoma
Renal functions	Myopathy associated with chronic renal failure
Immunoglobulins	Monoclonal gammapathy
Electrolytes	
Potassium	Hypokalemic myopathy; periodic paralysis; aldosteronism
Calcium, phosphorus	Hypophosphatemic myopathy; hyperparathyroid myopathy; tetany
Magnesium	Magnesium-induced myasthenia
Sodium	Corticosteroid myopathy
Endocrine tests	
T_3, T_4, and TSH	Hypo- or hyperthyroid myopathy
Plasma cortisol in AM and PM	Myopathy due to corticosteroids
Parathyroid hormone	Parathyroid myopathy
Myoglobinuria	Massive necrosis of muscles, metabolic myopathy, paroxysmal myoglobinuria or alcoholic myopathy
Acetylcholine receptor antibody	Myasthenia gravis
Voltage-gated calcium channel antibody	LEMS

type of periodic paralysis and suggests the treatment of choice. There are three types of periodic paralysis in which serum potassium is either decreased, increased, or normal.

Myoglobinuria is suspected when the red blood cells are not detected by urinalysis and "red urine" is positive on the dipstick for heme pigment. Serum color is normal in myoglobinuria. This is associated with crush syndrome, certain drugs and viral infections, alcoholism, and some metabolic myopathies. CPK is invariably markedly elevated. Periodic myoglobinuria is a reason to suspect metabolic myopathies. Myoglobinuria is an important cause of acute tubular necrosis of the kidney, producing acute renal failure.

The acetylcholine receptor antibody is diagnostic of myasthenia gravis when it is definitely positive. Thus, it should be checked in any myopathy patient when the etiology is unclear. Serological tests for rheumatoid diseases are an integral part of the work-up for myopathy. When any test is positive, it strongly suggests the possibility of polymyositis because in one-third of patients, polymyositis is associated with other collagen vascular diseases. Anti-Jo antibody is often positive in patients with polymyositis and interstitial lung disease. Myopathy is seen in hypothyroidism and hyperthyroidism. Thus, the thyroid profile should be a routine test in the work-up for myopathy of unknown type.

EMG Studies

The needle EMG is the most important diagnostic procedure in myopathy. This test is essential for confirmation of myopathy by differentiating myopathy from neuropathy and of myotonia. In myopathy, the classic EMG finding is the small-amplitude, short-duration (SASD) MUP. This is due to loss of functioning muscle fibers in a single motor unit resulting from muscle fiber necrosis. Myotonic response, which is easily detected by the needle EMG because of the high-frequency repetitive discharge of either biphasic spikes or positive waves with fluctuating frequency or amplitude, is associated with a characteristic "dive-bomber sound." Myotonic potentials are a sine qua non in myotonic syndromes.

Myasthenic response is tested by the repetitive nerve stimulation (RNS) test (Jolly test) and is characterized by a decremental response of the compound muscle action potential (CMAP) with repetitive nerve stimulation at various rates. This response is classically noted in the neuromuscular transmission disorders such as myasthenia gravis. In myasthenia gravis, the decremental response is seen at the low rate of stimulation (2 to 5 Hz), whereas normal or decremental response is observed at the high rate of stimulation (20 to 50 Hz) and the CMAP amplitude is normal. In contrast, a low CMAP amplitude, a decremental response at the low rate of stimulation, and an incremental response at the high rate of stimulation are the triad diagnostic of the Lambert-Eaton myasthenic syndrome, which is commonly associated with small cell carcinoma of the lung. The nerve conduction study (NCS) is essential in ruling out peripheral neuropathy in the work-up of patients suspected with myopathy.

Muscle Biopsy

Muscle biopsy is essential in the diagnosis of myopathy. This procedure should not be considered lightly because a definite diagnosis should be made with a single muscle biopsy. Because myopathy involves proximal muscles predominantly, the biopsy of a proximal muscle such as deltoid, biceps, and quadriceps is most suitable. A nontouch technique should be used in excision of the muscle. As a routine, the biopsied muscle is stained for histological and histochemical examination on frozen and paraffin sections. In certain cases, the electron microscope study is essential in reaching a definite diagnosis.

A specific diagnosis of systemic diseases can be reached by muscle biopsy in sarcoidosis, vasculitis (periarteritis nodosa), and trichinosis. Muscle is an important tissue for biopsy in sarcoidosis because of its frequent involvement in this disease. Although vasculitis can be diagnosed by muscle biopsy when present, the nerve biopsy is the preferred method of diagnosis in vasculitis because of the more frequent involvement of nerve. Muscle biopsy can confirm histologically the specific diagnosis in certain myopathies like McArdle's disease, polymyositis, glycogen-storage myopathy, lipid myopathy, mitochondrial myopathy, nemalin myopathy, central core disease, and fiber type disproportion syndrome. A definite diagnosis of specific types of muscular dystrophies can be made by assay of the deficiency of specific muscle

TABLE 11.3. Molecular Genetics and Muscle Membrane Protein Defects in Muscular Dystrophies

Muscular Dystrophies	Gene Locations	Protein Defects
X-linked recessive		
Duchenne dystrophy	Xp21	Dystrophin
Becker dystrophy	Xp21	Dystrophin
Emery-Dreifuss	Xq28	Emerin
Autosomal recessive		
LGMD 2 C (SCARMD)	13q12	Gamma sarcoglycan
LGMD 2 D	17q21	Alpha sarcoglycan (adhalin)
LGMD 2 E	4q?	Beta sarcoglycan
Congenital MD with leukodystrophy	6q 2	Merosin

LGMD, limb-girdle muscular dystrophy; SCARMD, severe childhood autosomal-recessive muscular dystrophy.

membrane proteins (Table 11.3), such as the dystrophin assay in Duchenne and Becker dystrophy. In certain myopathies, biochemical analysis will clinch the definite diagnosis. These include Pompe's disease (acid maltase deficiency) and phosphofructokinase deficiency. The muscle biopsy can also distinguish myopathy from denervation process, although the specific cause of myopathy or denervation may not be diagnosed. Myopathy is characterized by muscle fiber necrosis: floccular change, phagocytosis, and regeneration. On the other hand, denervation is characterized by fascicular atrophy, angular fibers, target fibers, and fiber type grouping. Muscle biopsy can also identify nonspecific abnormalities such as type II fiber atrophy.

CASE 1

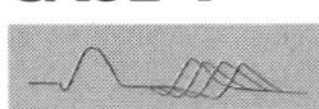

WALKING DIFFICULTY IN A DIABETIC PATIENT AFTER A FALL 1 YEAR BEFORE

CASE PRESENTATION

A 75-year-old diabetic woman began to have weakness of the legs, with trouble climbing stairs, a year before examination. Seven months ago, she had surgery for a right hip fracture after a fall. Since then, her weakness had become gradually worse. For the past 6 months, she was in a wheelchair and then developed swallowing difficulty and a strangling feeling in her throat in the past 2 months. She lost 100 pounds in the past 7 months. Her internist diagnosed diabetic amyotrophy.

Abnormal neurological findings included MRC strength of 4− in neck extensor, 1 in deltoids and biceps, 3 in triceps, wrist extensors and flexors, 4 in hand grip, 1 in iliopsoas, and 4 in hamstrings and anterior tibialis muscles. She also demonstrated mild atrophy in her upper arms and thighs, hyperesthesia to pinprick below the ankles and on her fingers, absent vibration on the toes and slightly decreased vibration on the ankles, and absent reflexes.

CASE ANALYSIS

This patient had slowly progressive generalized weakness with more proximal muscle involvement for 1 year and recent swallowing difficulty. Examination showed mild peripheral neuropathy and proximal muscle weakness. Because she had diabetes mellitus, her physician thought that she had diabetic amyotrophy in addition to diabetic neuropathy. The patient had prominent weight loss, one of the characteristics of diabetic amyotrophy. What was lacking in this patient for diabetic amyotrophy was pain. Shoulder girdle muscle weakness is unheard of in diabetic amyotrophy. Other diseases to be ruled out were CIDP and polymyositis with superimposed diabetic peripheral neuropathy.

PLAN OF TESTING

1. NCS: To confirm peripheral neuropathy and identify further whether it was demyelinating.
2. Needle EMG: To identify whether the patient had myopathy or denervation process.
3. CPK and muscle biopsy: To confirm what was found on the needle EMG.
4. Cancer work-up.

TABLE 11.4. Nerve Conduction Data in Case 1

	Latent/NCV (ms/m/s)	Amplitude (mV/μV)		Latent/NCV (ms/m/s)	Amplitude (mV/μV)
	Median	**Motor N**		**Peroneal**	**Motor N**
TL	4.8	1.8	TL	7.9	0.6
E-W	43.1	1.4	FH-A	37.2	0.6
AX-E			PF-FH	67.0	0.4
F-wave	NP		F-wave	NP	
	Ulnar	**Motor N**		**Post-Tibial**	**Motor N**
TL	3.9	3.1	TL	5.2	3.9
BE-W	42.0	2.8	PF-A	42.2	3.0
AE-BE	38.0	2.2			
F-wave	NP		F-wave	NP	
	Median	**Sens N**		**Sural**	**Sens N**
F-W	33.2	3.3	MC-A	32.2	2.2
	Ulnar	**Sens N**		**Plantar**	**Sens N**
F-W	27.2	1.4	Medial		

Height, 167 cm.

TL, terminal latency; W, wrist; E, elbow; BE, below elbow; AE, above elbow; F, finger; FH, fibular head; A, ankle; PF, popliteal fossa; MC, mid-calf; NP, no potential.

ELECTROPHYSIOLOGICAL TESTS AND FINDINGS

NCS Findings (Table 11.4)

1. Prolonged terminal latency, mild slowing in motor NCV, and low CMAP amplitude in all tested nerves.
2. Low sensory CNAP amplitude and mild slowing in sensory NCV in all tested nerves.
3. Prolonged F-wave latency or no potential in all tested nerves.

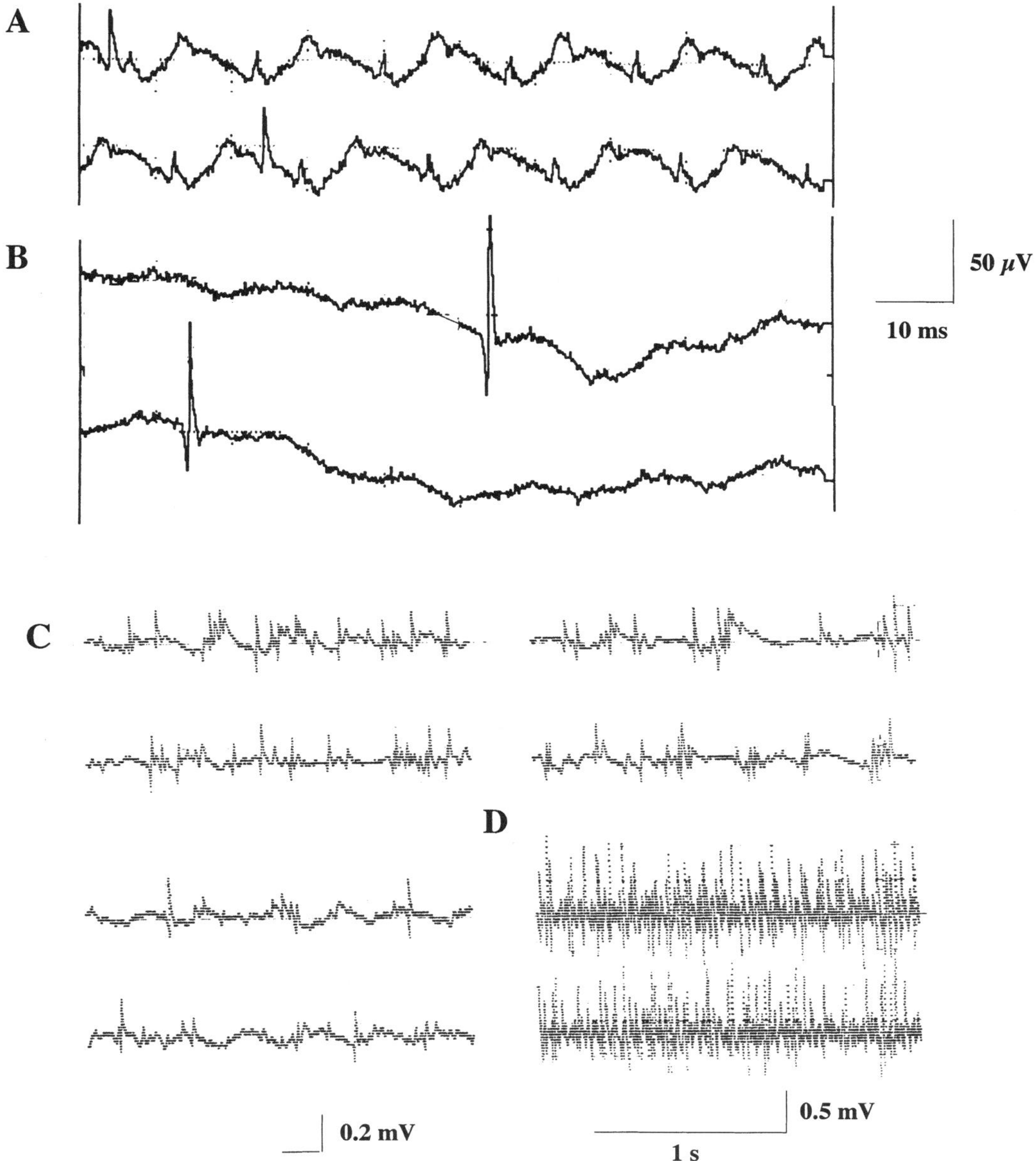

FIGURE 11.1. A. Fibrillations with 60-Hz artifacts. **B.** Fibrillations. **C.** Many obvious SASD MUPs. **D.** Normal interference pattern.

TABLE 11.5. Needle EMG Data in Case 1

				Spontaneous Potentials				Motor Unit Potential			Interference	
Muscle	**Root**	**Nerve**	**Insertion Activity**	**Fib**	**PSW**	**Fasc**	**CRD**	**Amplitude (K)**	**Duration (ms)**	**Polyphasic Potential**	**Pattern**	**Mean Amplitude (K)**
Left deltoids	C5,6	Axillary	+	+	+	−	−	0.3–0.6	2–8	++	FIP[a]	0.5
Biceps	C6,7	Musc cut	+	++	++	−	+	0.2–0.5	2–6	++	FIP[a]	0.5
Vast lat	L3,4	Femoral	+	+	+	−	+	0.3–1.5	3–8	++	FIP	1.3

[a] Early recruitment.

Fib, fibrillations; PSW, positive sharp wave; Fasc, fasciculations; CRD, complex repetitive discharge; −, absent; +, present or increased; FIP, full interference pattern.

Needle EMG (Table 11.5; Fig. 11.1)

1. Fibrillations and PSWs in all tested muscles and CRDs in two tested muscles.
2. Many simple and polyphasic SASD MUPs and early recruitment.

ELECTROPHYSIOLOGICAL INTERPRETATION

Active myopathy typical of polymyositis and peripheral neuropathy.

OTHER TEST FINDINGS

Muscle biopsy showed findings indicative of polymyositis: perivascular or endomysial infiltration of inflammatory cells and many muscle fibers undergoing phagocytosis, regeneration, and floccular changes. Laboratory findings were a normal CPK, a high sedimentation rate (12 mm/hr), and positive rheumatoid factor. Cancer work-up was negative.

FINAL DIAGNOSIS

Polymyositis

TREATMENT AND FOLLOW-UP

This patient was treated with IVIG and high-dose steroids. Gradually, there was improvement, and she could walk with support in 3 months. However, she needed high-dose daily steroids to maintain her improved state, which aggravated her diabetes.

COMMENTS

This patient had biopsy-proven severe polymyositis in the presence of normal CPK and some systemic symptoms and laboratory data. Polymyositis is the most common acquired myopathy in adults. In any patient with adult-onset myopathy, polymyositis has to be ruled out. Unfortunately, there is no single laboratory test to diagnose polymyositis. CPK is the most helpful test, being elevated in 95% of cases. Rheumatological profiles are abnormal only in about one-third of patients. Jo autoantibody is positive in one-third of patients with polymyositis and more commonly in patients with interstitial lung disease. Thus, a definite diagnosis of polymyositis is based on the muscle biopsy, which typically shows muscle fiber necrosis and inflammatory cells.

Motor and sensory nerve conductions are usually normal in polymyositis. If peripheral neuropathy is present, other collagen vascular diseases have to be considered as diagnostic possibilities. In polymyositis, muscles are often affected in a patchy distribution. Proximal muscle groups are affected more than distal muscles. Therefore, the needle EMG should be performed in different areas within one muscle, and proximal muscles, including paraspinal muscles, should be examined.

The cardinal needle EMG finding in polymyositis is an active myopathy pattern: fibrillation, PSWs, CRDs, and SASD MUPs. Fibrillation and PSWs are observed in 60 to 100% and a "myopathic MUP pattern" is seen in 89 to 100% of patients with polymyositis/dermatomyositis. Fibrillation and PSWs were reported in 100% of cases in a study that included paraspinal muscles. CRDs are also common in polymyositis. The classic MUPs in polymyositis are simple or polyphasic SASD MUPs. They recruit early and are excessive in number with minimal effort.

The high frequency of abnormal spontaneous potentials is a striking finding in polymyositis. Fibrillation potentials and PSWs are commonly observed in denervated muscles. These potentials have been reported in 15 to 18% of patients with various primary myopathies and are due to "hyperirritable muscle membrane" caused by active muscle fiber necrosis. Thus, this spontaneous activity is present in the active stage of disease and disappears with clinical improvement. In the chronic inactive stage of disease, these potentials are absent. Thus, the presence of fibrillations and PSWs can be used as an index of disease activity. SASD MUPs remain unchanged in the chronic stage. An increased proportion of long-duration, high-amplitude, polyphasic MUPs were reported in chronic polymyositis by Mechler. Personally, I have not observed this phenomenon and I would not be surprised to learn that such patients have inclusion body myopathy rather than polymyositis.

MAXIMS

1. Fibrillations and PSWs are observed commonly in polymyositis.
2. Fibrillations and PSWs should not be called "denervation potentials" because they are also observed in myopathies.

REFERENCES

1. Streib EW, Wilbourn AJ, Mitsumoto H. Spontaneous electrical muscle fiber activity in polymyositis and dermatomyositis. Muscle Nerve 1979;2:14–18.
2. Bucthal F, Rosenfalck P. Spontaneous electrical activity of human muscle. EEG Clin Neurophysiol 1966;20:321–336.
3. Pinelli P. Muscle action potentials in polymyostis. Neurology 1953;3:424–436.

CASE 2

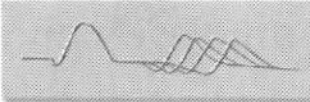

A 3-MONTH HISTORY OF RASH AND "TIREDNESS OF ARMS" IN AN 8-YEAR-OLD GIRL

CASE PRESENTATION

A previously healthy 8-year-old girl presented with a 3-month history of rash over her arms, trunk, legs, and face without any history of treatment with antibiotics or drugs. She did not complain of joint pain, ulcers, or weakness of the arms or legs. However, she did complain of her arms being tired when she carried books at school. She had a low grade fever of 99 to 100 F. Examination showed a heliotrophic eye rash, "butterfly distribution" of erythematous macular rash over the face and the anterior portion of the chest, and raised excoriated erythematous plaques over the extensor surface of the elbows, fingers, and knees. Examination in the EMG laboratory showed 4+ strength in the deltoids and 5− strength in the iliopsoas muscles. She could do knee bends without difficulty. Reflexes were normal.

CASE ANALYSIS

The pediatrician thought the rashes were characteristic of systemic lupus erythematosus or dermatomyositis. A detailed examination clearly showed that this patient had proximal muscle weakness, pointing to a diagnosis of dermatomyositis. In fact, this patient had the classic features of childhood dermatomyositis: heliotrophic eye rash, Grotton's sign, systemic symptoms (low-grade fever and a high erythrocyte sedimentation rate), an elevated CPK, and proximal muscle weakness.

PLAN OF TESTING

1. NCS: To find any associated neuropathy.
2. Needle EMG: To confirm muscle involvement.
3. ESR, ANA, rheumatoid factor, and CPK.

ELECTROPHYSIOLOGICAL TESTS AND FINDINGS

NCS Findings. Normal motor and sensory NCS in all tested motor and sensory nerves.

Needle EMG Findings in the Deltoid Muscle (Fig. 11.2)

1. Prominent fibrillations and PSWs (+ + +) at rest in the deltoid.
2. Many simple and polyphasic SASD MUPs: durations are 2.8 to 10 ms; amplitude, 0.2 to 1 mV; increased polyphasic MUPs.
3. Early recruitment of MUPs and full interference pattern with mean 0.5-mV amplitude.

ELECTROPHYSIOLOGICAL INTERPRETATION

Active myopathy typical of dermatomyositis.

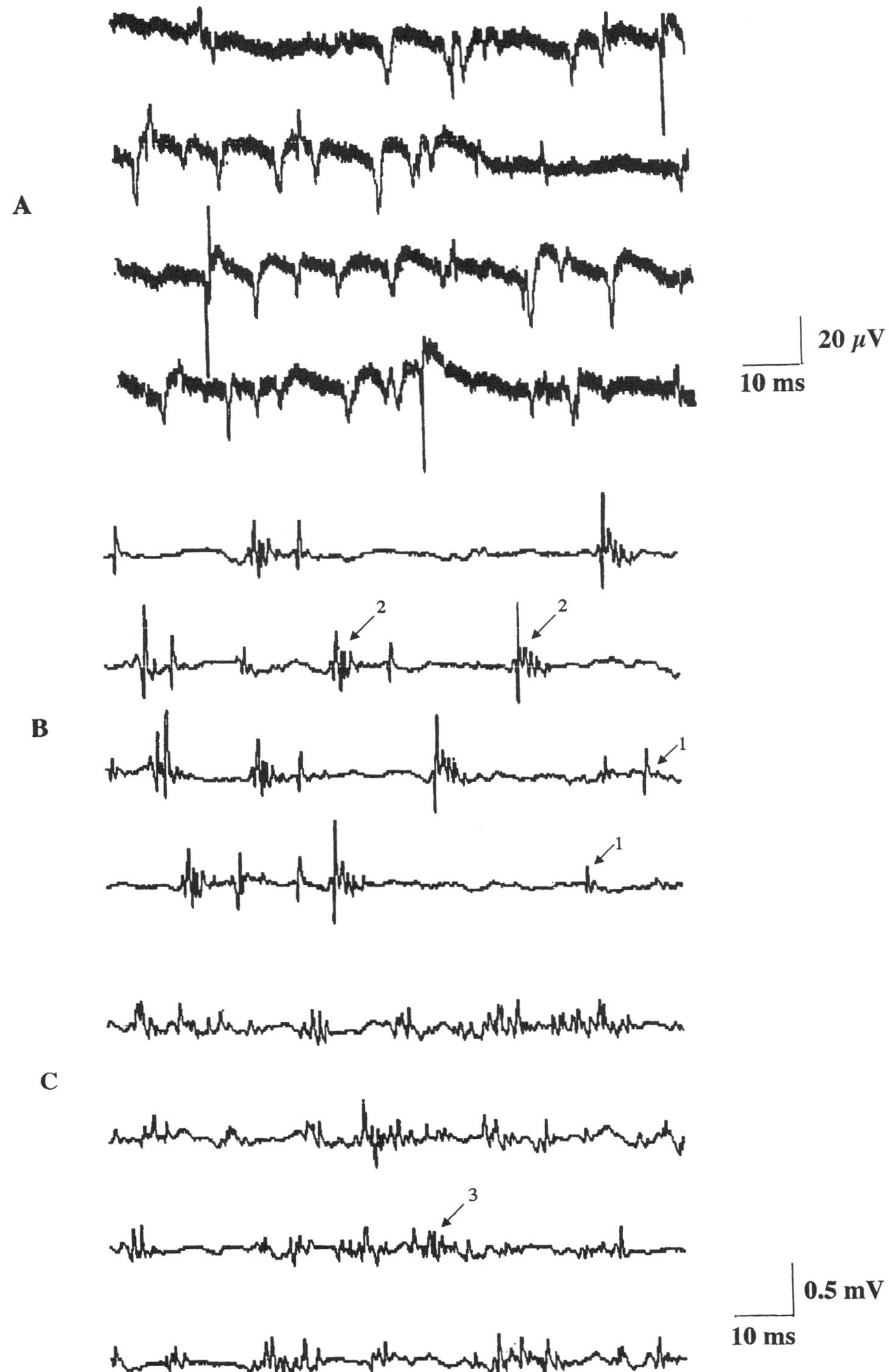

FIGURE 11.2. A. Fibrillations and PSWs. **B.** SASD MUPs (*arrow 1*) and normal duration polyphasic MUPs (*arrow 2*). **C.** Many SASD MUPs with polyphasic MUP (*arrow 3*).

OTHER TEST FINDINGS

Laboratory studies showed normal ANA titer, elevated CPK (636 unit versus normal, 215), AST (77 versus normal 45), and LDH (1111 versus normal 450) enzyme levels and high ESR (40 mm/hr). Muscle biopsy showed the classic feature of perifascicular atrophy typical of dermatomyositis.

FINAL DIAGNOSIS

Dermatomyositis

TREATMENT AND FOLLOW-UP

The patient was treated with a high dose of steroids with gradual improvement.

COMMENTS

Dermatomyositis is a distinct form of inflammatory myopathy. Unlike polymyositis, this disorder is thought to be due to microvascular insult. It has a highly specific histological feature, perifasicular "atrophy" (muscle fiber necrosis), and immune deposits in blood vessels. Heliotrophic rash and Grotton's sign in patients with proximal muscle weakness are diagnostic of dermatomyositis because these skin changes are almost pathognomonic. Similar skin changes have been reported only in two cases of sarcoid myopathy. In the past, childhood dermatomyositis was thought to be more severe than adult polymyositis because of severe subcutaneous calcinosis, contracture of joints, and gastrointestinal complications. This is no longer true with judicious steroid treatment, which is as effective as in adult polymyositis. In childhood dermatomyositis or polymyositis, systemic symptoms such as mild fever and generalized malaise are not unusual. Thus, systemic symptoms together with proximal muscle weakness are highly diagnostic of polymyositis.

Polymyositis can be manifested as a paraneoplastic syndrome of occult carcinoma in 16% of patients with polymyositis. This association is strong in men over 60 years of age who have dermatomyositis. Thus, cancer work-ups are needed in this high-risk group.

MAXIMS

1. Proximal muscle weakness and systemic symptoms in children are indicative of polymyositis.
2. Perifascicular atrophy is pathognomonic of dermatomyositis.

REFERENCES

1. Lakhanspal S, Bunch TW, Ilstrup DM, Melton LJ. Polymyositis-dermatomyositis and malignant lesions: does an association exist? Mayo Clin Proc 1986;61:645–653.
2. Pachman LM. Juvenile dermatomyositis. Pediatr Clin North Am 1986;33:1097–1117.

CASE 3

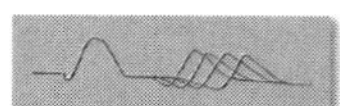

"DROPPED HEAD" (ANTEROCOLLIS) IN A 65-YEAR-OLD MAN

CASE PRESENTATION

Three months before examination, a 65-year-old man noticed that he could not hold his head erect and that it tended to droop forward. He initially had pain in the back of the neck and upper shoulders, but this had resolved. If he concentrated very hard, he could hold his head up for a short period of time, but then it continued to droop again. He had difficulty swallowing solid food, but swallowing became easier if he held his head up. He lost 10 to 15 pounds because of swallowing difficulty. He had no other neurological complaints such as diplopia, voice change, or fatigue. Cervical spine x-ray showed mild arthritis in his neck. The patient was sent for evaluation for botulinum toxin (Botox) injections for treatment of "anterocollis." He had a right Bell's palsy 10 years before, left lung resection in the 1950s secondary to tuberculosis, and hypertension. No neuromuscular disease was reported in the family. Examination showed a rather thin man with moderate right facial weakness. Muscle strength was 4 MRC in neck extensor, 5− strength in neck flexor, 5− in deltoids and iliopsoas muscles. There was no fatigability in proximal muscles. Reflexes were normal. He walked with neck drop.

CASE ANALYSIS

This patient was sent for Botox treatment for anterocollis. However, examination clearly showed that his main problem was head drop. Subtle proximal muscle weakness in this patient suggested the possibility of myasthenia gravis and myopathy. Myasthenia gravis was less likely in view of the absence of fatigue, exertional fatigability, and ocular signs.

PLAN OF TESTING

1. Needle EMG: To confirm myopathy in the paraspinal muscles and proximal muscles.
2. NCS: To rule out a peripheral neuropathy as the cause for his "dropped-head syndrome."
3. RNS test: To rule out myasthenia gravis.
4. Acetylcholine receptor antibody, CPK, and muscle biopsy: To identify the nature of myopathy, a muscle biopsy in the C7 and C8 paraspinal muscles.

ELECTROPHYSIOLOGICAL TESTS AND FINDINGS

NCS Findings. Normal NCS in all of tested nerves.

Needle EMG (Table 11.6; Fig. 11.3)

1. Prominent fibrillation and PSWs in the right C5-8 paraspinal muscles and many SASD MUPs in the right C7 and C8 paraspinal muscles.
2. Normal needle EMG findings in all other tested proximal muscles.

RNS Test Findings. Normal in the ADQ, FCU, and trapezius muscles.

ELECTROPHYSIOLOGICAL INTERPRETATION

Active myopathy.

OTHER TEST FINDINGS

All pertinent laboratory tests for myopathy were negative. CPK was 206 (normal, <250). Muscle biopsy from the trapezius muscle was normal. However, biopsy of a deeper cervical paraspinal muscle showed polymyositis.

FINAL DIAGNOSIS

Dropped-head syndrome due to polymyositis

TREATMENT AND FOLLOW-UP

The patient was treated with prednisone with gradual improvement in strength of neck and proximal muscles and in swallowing.

TABLE 11.6. Needle EMG Data in Case 3

Muscle	Root	Nerve	Insertion Activity	Spontaneous Potentials				Motor Unit Potential				Interference	
				Fib	PSW	Fasc	CRD	Amplitude (mV)	Duration (ms)	Polyphasic Potential	HA MUP	Pattern	Mean Amplitude (mV)
Rt C5-6			+	+	+	–	–						
C7-8			+	+++	++	–	+	0.3–1	3–10	+			
T1			+	+	+	–	–						
Lt deltoid	C5,6	Axillary	N	–	–	–	–	0.5–3.5	6–12	N	0	RIP	2
Biceps	C6,7	Musc cut	N	–	–	–	–	0.5–2.5	6–12	N	0	RIP	3
Iliopsoas	L3,4	Femoral	N	–	–	–	–	0.5–3	6–12	N	0	FIP	3
Vast lat	L3,4	Femoral	N	–	–	–	–	0.5–3	6–13	N	0	FIP	2

HA, high amplitude; RIP, reduced interference pattern; N, normal.

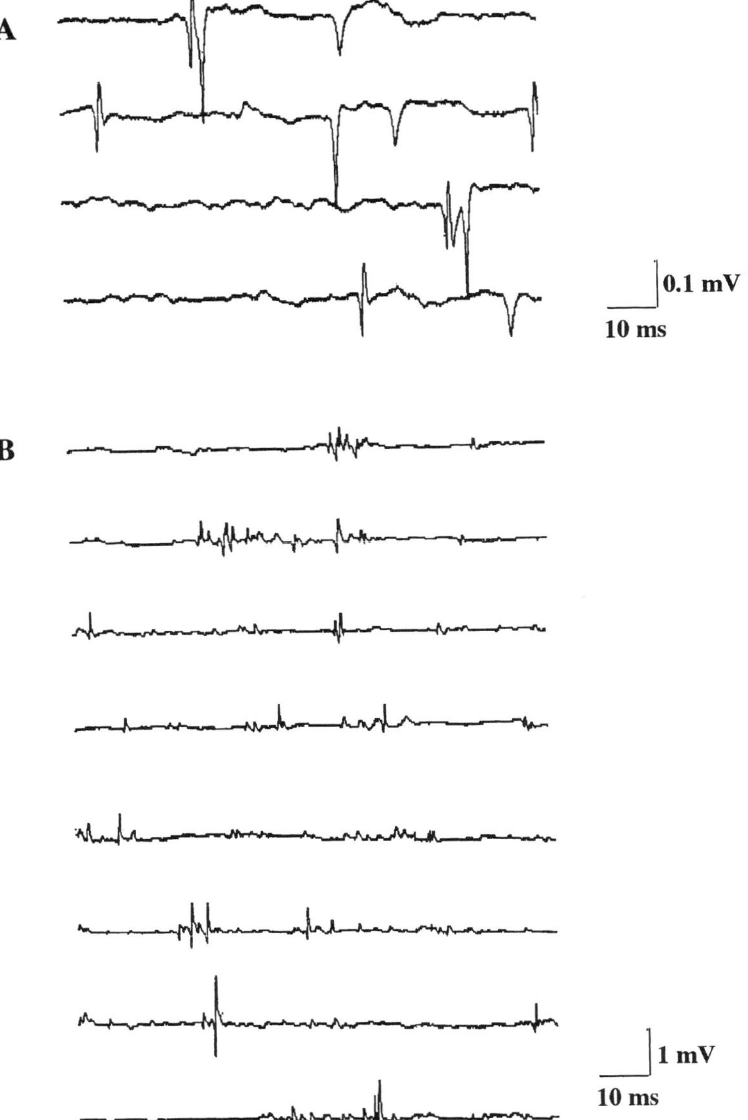

FIGURE 11.3. Needle EMG in cervical paraspinal muscles. **A.** Fibrillations and PSWs. **B.** All MUPs are short in duration (2 to 4 ms). Many SASD MUPs but some MUPs with normal amplitude.

COMMENTS

Head drop alone is an extremely unusual finding in neuromuscular diseases. It is not uncommon to see head drop as an expression of generalized weakness in myasthenia gravis and amyotrophic lateral sclerosis. Causes for dropped-head syndrome alone include "minicore" myopathy, facioscapular humeral muscular dystrophy, and chronic inflammatory demyelinating polyneuropathy. We have seen cases of mitochondrial myopathy and of denervation due to cervical spondylotic myelopathy that were confirmed by the biopsy of neck muscles.

The needle EMG can be used as a guide in selection of muscle for muscle biopsy. The muscle that showed the most prominent abnormality should be selected for muscle biopsy.

In this case, proximal muscles that were commonly involved did not show any EMG abnormality. Thus, the biopsy was performed in cervical paraspinal muscles. Superficial muscle (trapezius) was normal. Deep paraspinal muscle showed definite evidence of inflammatory myopathy, emphasizing the importance of biopsy of an involved muscle. This patient had focal myositis confined to the extensor neck muscles.

MUPs in the paraspinal muscles are generally shorter and smaller than MUPs in the limb muscles. Thus, one has to be careful in interpreting MUPs in paraspinal muscles. A prominent myopathic EMG pattern must be present to interpret the findings as myopathic.

MAXIMS

1. PSWs and fibrillation in paraspinal muscles are not necessarily indicative of radiculopathy. These have also been observed in active myopathy.
2. The most common causes for dropped-head syndrome are amyotrophic lateral sclerosis and myasthenia gravis.

REFERENCES

1. Suzrez G, Kelly JJ. The dropped head syndrome. Neurology 1992;42:1625–1627.

CASE 4

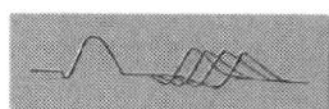

DELTOID AND BICEPS MUSCLE WEAKNESS DUE TO C5 AND 6 RADICULOPATHY?

CASE PRESENTATION

A 48-year-old man was referred to us for muscle biopsy for the evaluation of slowly progressive bilateral arm and shoulder weakness for 2 years. The weakness had progressed to the point that the patient was unable to lift his arms above his head. He denied any history of sensory loss, pain, cramping, dysphagia, dysarthria, or visual disturbance. There was no family history of neurological disease. His past medical history was significant only for asthma and hypertension.

The primary care physician obtained a needle EMG that was reported to show bilateral C5 and C6 radiculopathy. NCS was reported to be normal. MRI of the cervical cord was completely normal. RF was positive at 1 : 1280, ANA was negative, CPK was 273 units (normal, 250), and ESR was 8. Thyroid function tests, electrolytes, and complete blood count were normal. A telephone consultation with the neurologist raised the possibility of motor neuron disease. Thus, a muscle biopsy was requested.

Examination in the biopsy room showed that abnormal neurological findings were 1 MRC strength in the deltoids, 3 strength in the supra- and infraspinatus muscles, and 4 strength in the iliopsoas bilaterally, with mild atrophy in the deltoid and supraspinatus muscles. There was no skin rash or fasciculation. Deep tendon reflexes were present and symmetrical bilaterally. Plantar responses were flexor.

CASE ANALYSIS

Bilateral cervical polyradiculopathy diagnosed on the first needle EMG was based on the presence of fibrillations and PSWs. This had raised the question of cervical stenosis, but MRI of the cervical cord did not confirm this. Thus, at this point, the question of motor neuron disease was raised. A mildly elevated CPK is compatible with motor neuron disease. There was no fasciculation or upper motor neuron signs suggestive of motor neuron disease. Clinically, this patient had acquired subacute proximal muscle weakness without reflex abnormalities, suggesting an acquired myopathy until proven otherwise. We had to persuade the patient to have a limited needle EMG in one muscle because of his refusal to undergo another painful needle EMG test.

PLAN OF TESTING

1. Repeat Needle EMG: To confirm the diagnostic impression.
2. Muscle biopsy: To confirm myopathy and identify the causes of myopathy.

ELECTROPHYSIOLOGICAL TESTS AND FINDINGS

Needle EMG in the Right Deltoid Muscle (Fig. 11.4). Many small-amplitude (0.5 to 3.0 mV), short-duration (3.5 to 6.0 ms), MUPs along with PSWs, fibrillation potentials, CRDs (+ + +), and full interference pattern (1 mV) and early recruitment of MUPs.

ELECTROPHYSIOLOGICAL INTERPRETATION

Active myopathy typical of polymyositis.

OTHER TEST FINDINGS

Muscle biopsy showed marked endomysial inflammation and several noncaseating granulomas diagnostic of sarcoid myopathy. Serum ACE level was 62 (normal range, 8 to 52). Chest x-ray was normal. Chest CT showed bilateral granulomas and two mediastinal lymph nodes (2.5 × 2 cm).

FINAL DIAGNOSIS

Sarcoidosis with muscle and pulmonary involvement

TREATMENT AND FOLLOW-UP

The patient was begun on high-dose prednisone (80 mg/day) that had to be reduced secondary to hyperglycemia and development of diabetes. The patient was then treated with a lower

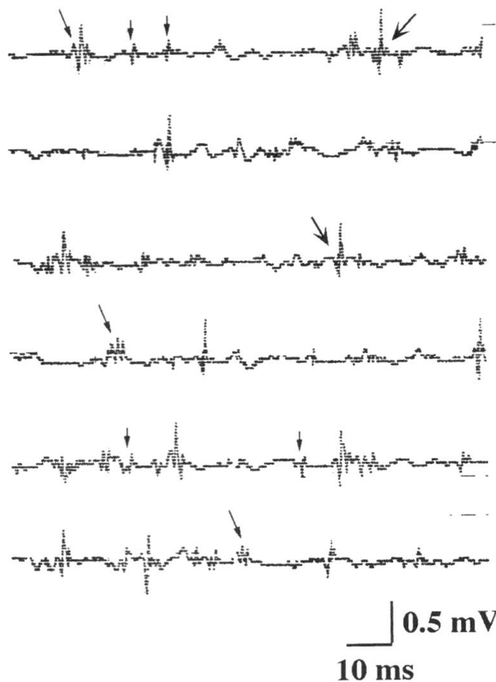

FIGURE 11.4. Many simple SASD MUPs (*downward pointed arrows*) and polyphasic SASD MUPs (*side-pointed arrows*).

dose of prednisone (10 mg/day) along with Imuran (150 mg/day) with slow but definite improvement.

COMMENTS

This case teaches two lessons to the serious electromyographer: an incorrectly performed EMG can misdirect the diagnostic work-up and fibrillation and PSWs are not pathognomonic of denervation. On the basis of clinical findings of weakness in deltoid and biceps muscles, the first electromyographer thought of C5 and C6 radiculopathy but never considered a myopathy and thus did not pay any attention to MUPs. This is one of the most common errors made by inexperienced electromyographers: the failure to recognize "SASD MUPs." Fibrillations and PSWs are not pathognomonic of denervation process as noted in this case, in which they were expressions of active myopathy. Fibrillations and PSWs are usually indicative of denervation process but are also observed in active myopathy and in myotonia. Fibrillations and PSWs are common in inflammatory myopathy.

Sarcoidosis may present as myopathy without other features of sarcoidosis, as noted in this case. Muscle involvement in sarcoidosis can be asymptomatic. Overall, neurological involvement occurs in about 5% of patients with sarcoidosis, and about 7 to 12% of these patients have a myopathy. Muscle biopsy shows characteristic noncaseating granulomas in 20 to 70% of sarcoidosis patients without any muscular symptoms. Asymptomatic muscle involvement in sarcoidosis has been found almost exclusively in the early stages of disease. Symptomatic involvement of muscle is only found in the chronic stage and presents as a focal (palpable nodule) or symmetrical myopathy. Two patients with skin rash typical of dermatomyositis were also reported in sarcoidosis. Sarcoidosis is one of the few diseases in which muscle biopsy can make a definite systemic diagnosis, the others including vasculitis and trichinosis. Muscle biopsy is preferred in sarcoidosis, whereas nerve biopsy is preferred in vasculitis.

MAXIMS

1. Fibrillations and PSWs are not pathognomonic of denervation process.
2. A definite diagnosis of sarcoidosis can be diagnosed by muscle biopsy, which shows classic noncaseating granuloma.

REFERENCES

1. Silverstein A, Siltzbach LE. Muscle involvement in sarcoidosis. Arch Neurol 1969;21:235–241.
2. Stjernberg N, Cajander S, Truedsson H, Uddenfeldt P. Muscle involvement in sarcoidosis. Acta Med Scand 1981;209:213.

CASE 5

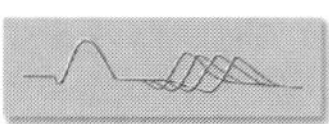

MOTOR NEURON DISEASE, POLYRADICULOPATHY, OR POLYMYOSITIS IN A 67-YEAR-OLD MAN WITH INSIDIOUS WEAKNESS OF THIGHS FOR 3 YEARS

CASE PRESENTATION

This 67-year-old man was very healthy until about 3 years ago, when he began to notice weakness in his left leg. This had clearly been getting more severe and was noted in his right leg as well. No pain, tingling, or numbness was associated with the weakness. The patient had difficulty getting up from a couch, fell occasionally because of weakness, but was still able to drive a school bus. He had no difficulty swallowing and no change in his voice.

He had surgery for a ruptured lumbar disc 3 years previously. EMG by the referring neurologist showed "active denervation" in all muscles tested. Apparently, polyphasic MUPs were increased and maximal contraction showed poor recruitment. The impression was anterior horn cell disease, polyradiculopathy, or inflammatory myopathy. Blood tests showed elevated CPK with values of 1892 and 1299 units. Lumbar CT myelogram showed extensive degeneration of facet disease and disc disease without herniation or significant spinal stenosis.

Neurological examination showed normal muscle strength in the upper extremities and in the right iliopsoas and quadriceps, bilateral hamstring, and gastrocnemius muscles. Muscle strength in the left iliopsoas was 4 (MRC scale); left quadriceps was 2, left anterior tibialis was 3, and right anterior tibialis 4. Ankle and knee jerks were absent bilaterally. Biceps reflexes were 1+ and triceps reflexes were absent on the right and 1+ on the left. Moderate atrophy was noted in his left thigh. No fasciculation was noted. The patient was able to walk on his right toes but not on the left. The remainder of the examination was normal.

CASE ANALYSIS

This patient had subacute, progressive, asymmetrical, painless weakness and atrophy of leg muscles and areflexia. Differential diagnoses included multifocal motor neuropathy, benign focal amyotrophy, focal myopathy, and amyotrophic lateral sclerosis presenting as focal weakness and wasting. Clinically, amyotrophic lateral sclerosis was less likely in view of the absence of upper motor neuron signs and fasciculation. On the other hand, elevated CPK is not an unusual finding in the rapidly progressing amyotrophic lateral sclerosis patient. The first electromyographer was not able to distinguish myopathy from anterior horn cell disease, most likely because of the mixed pattern of MUPs and prominent abnormal spontaneous potentials.

PLAN OF TESTING

1. NCS: To rule out multifocal motor neuropathy.
2. Needle EMG: To assess whether this was an anterior horn cell process or primary myopathy.
3. Muscle biopsy.

TABLE 11.7. Needle EMG Data in Case 5

				Spontaneous Potentials				Motor Unit Potential				Interference	
Muscle	**Root**	**Nerve**	**Insertion Activity**	**Fib**	**PSW**	**Fasc**	**CRD**	**Amplitude (K)**	**Duration (ms)**	**Polyphasic Potential**	**HALD MUP**	**Pattern**	**Mean Amplitude (K)**
Lt ant tibial	L4,5	Peroneal	+	+++	+++	−	+	0.3–8	4–26	++	+	RIP	5
Gastroc	S1,2	Post tib	+	+	+	−	−	0.3–2	3–16	++	−	RIP	1
Vast lat	L3,4	Femoral	+	+≠	+≠	−	−	0.66 0.12–1.33	8.4[a] 3.4–20.0	45%	+[b]	RIP	0.5
Deltoid	C5,6	Axillary	−	−	−	−	−	0.5–2	6–12	N	−	FIP	1.5
Rt ant tibial	L4,5	Peroneal	++	++	−	−	+	0.3–6	3–20	+	+	RIP	1
Lt L3-5, S1 paraspinal			N	−	−	−	−						

[a] Quantitative MUPs with a concentric needle. All other tests are performed with monopolar needle. Normal duration is 14.0 ms.

[b] Long-duration MUPs.

HALD, high-amplitude long-duration.

ELECTROPHYSIOLOGICAL TESTS AND FINDINGS

NCS Findings. NCS in the left peroneal, posterior tibial, and sural nerves were all normal.

Needle EMG (see Fig. 5.25; Table 11.7)

1. Fibrillation, PSW, and increased polyphasic MUPs in all tested muscles in both legs.
2. CRDs in the right and left anterior tibialis muscles.
3. SASD MUPs mixed with HALD MUPs in the right and left anterior tibialis muscles.
4. A few long-duration MUPs in the left vastus lateralis muscle.
5. Significant decrease in mean duration of MUPs in the left vastus lateralis muscle.
6. Normal needle EMG in deltoid muscles.

ELECTROPHYSIOLOGICAL INTERPRETATION

Active myopathy with a few long-duration MUPs highly suggestive of inclusion body myopathy.

OTHER TEST FINDINGS

Sedimentation rate and thyroid and rheumatoid profiles were normal. CPK was 800 units (four times normal). Muscle biopsy from the left vastus lateralis showed many fibers with rimmed vacuoles, some endomysial inflammatory cells, many angular fibers, and some increase in the endomysial connective tissue, which are typical of inclusion body myositis.

FINAL DIAGNOSIS

Inclusion body myopathy

TREATMENT AND FOLLOW-UP

Despite treatment with azathioprine, insidious progression was noted in the left leg. Even 7 years after the initial diagnosis, the patient was ambulatory with no weakness of the arm muscles.

COMMENTS

In view of the mixed pattern on the needle EMG, it was not apparent whether we were dealing with myopathy or not. Thus, we decided to do a quantitative MUP analysis, which was indicative of myopathy. Thus, the quantitative EMG study was the crucial study indicative of myopathy in this patient.

Inclusion body myositis is one of three major forms of inflammatory myopathy. It is characterized by rimmed vacuoles, filamentous inclusions, slowly progressive proximal and/or distal weakness, prominent muscle atrophy, high incidence of hyporeflexia, male predominance, and poor response to corticosteroids. Some investigators have claimed that this is the most common form of inflammatory myopathy in older patients. A recent study showed that the rimmed vacuoles contain congophilic amyloid substance. The most common clinical form is proximal myopathy, but it can present variously as generalized myopathy, distal myopathy, scapuloperoneal myopathy, or focal myopathy. Thus, inclusion body myositis can mimic motor neuron disease, polymyositis, or myasthenia gravis. CPK is usually minimally elevated. One has to suspect inclusion body myopathy if "polymyositis" patients do not respond to steroid therapy. Prominent atrophy with areflexia in myopathy is strongly suggestive of inclusion body myopathy.

In the needle EMG, the most prominent findings are fibrillations and PSWs observed in almost all cases. A mixed pattern of HALD MUPs ("neurogenic pattern") and SASD MUPs ("myopathic") accompanied by abnormal spontaneous activity is highly suggestive of inclusion body myopathy. Unfortunately, this pattern is seen in only one-third of cases, the most common pattern being SASD MUPs together with fibrillation and PSWs, similar to that of polymyositis.

MAXIMS

1. When an active myopathy pattern is found mixed with a neurogenic pattern, inclusion body myopathy is the first diagnostic choice.

2. Rimmed vacuoles as the predominant feature on the muscle biopsy are diagnostic of inclusion body myopathy.

REFERENCES

1. Joy JL, Oh SJ, Baysal AL. Electrophysiological spectrum of inclusion body myositis. Muscle Nerve 1990;13:949–951.
2. Lozt BP, Engel AG, Nishino H, Stevens JC, Litchy WJ. Inclusion body myositis: observations in 40 patients. Brain 1989;112:727–747.

CASE 6

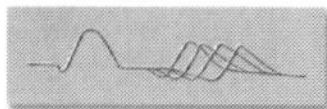

NONPROGRESSIVE WEAKNESS SINCE INFANCY

CASE PRESENTATION

A 21-year-old right-handed college student was evaluated for weakness of the legs since childhood. Apparently she had some mild weakness as an infant and was evaluated at 6 weeks of age. As she grew older, her motor milestones were slightly delayed so that she walked later than her siblings. When the patient was 10 years of age, the family moved to a two-story home and she began to notice difficulty walking up and down stairs. She had rare falls as a result of her weakness and was aware of cramping in her muscles on exertion that was usually relieved by rest. Occasionally, her exercise was limited by these muscle cramps. The family history was entirely unremarkable.

Neurological examination showed 4/MRC strength in neck flexion, deltoids, triceps, biceps, wrist extensors, iliopsoas, quadriceps, and hamstrings muscles. Deep tendon reflexes were 1 +. Sensory testing was entirely normal. CPK was normal.

CASE ANALYSIS

Onset in infancy, nonprogression, normal CPK, and proximal myopathy suggest a benign congenital myopathy. Certainly, spinal muscular atrophy type III should be ruled out by needle EMG study. Muscle biopsy is needed to confirm the type of congenital myopathy.

PLAN OF TESTING

1. Needle EMG in the proximal muscles: To confirm myopathy and rule out spinal muscular atrophy.
2. NCS: To rule out peripheral neuropathy.
3. Muscle biopsy.

ELECTROPHYSIOLOGICAL TESTS AND FINDINGS

NCS Findings. Normal NCS in all tested nerves.

Needle EMG (Table 11.8; Fig. 11.5)

1. Significant decrease in mean duration of MUPs in deltoid muscles.
2. Some SASD MUPs in the right biceps, vastus lateralis and medialis muscles.

ELECTROPHYSIOLOGICAL INTERPRETATION

Inactive myopathy.

OTHER TEST FINDINGS

Muscle biopsy showed central cores.

FINAL DIAGNOSIS

Central core disease

TABLE 11.8. Needle EMG Data in Case 6

				Spontaneous Potentials				Motor Unit Potential			Interference	
Muscle	**Root**	**Nerve**	**Insertion Activity**	**Fib**	**PSW**	**Fasc**	**Myotonia CRD**	**Amplitude (K)**	**Duration (ms)**	**Polyphasic Potential**	**Pattern**	**Mean Amplitude (K)**
Rt deltoids	C5,6	Axillary	N	–	–	–	–	0.34	7.3	15.3%	FIP	1
Biceps	C6	Musc cut	N	–	–	–	–	0.5–2	3–12	N	FIP	2
Vast lat	L3,4	Femoral	N	–	–	–	–	0.5–2	4–15	N	RIP	1.5
Vast med	L3,4	Femoral	N	–	–	–	–	0.5–2	4–15	N	FIP	1.7

[a] Concentric needle in deltoids. All other muscles are tested with monopolar needle. Normal duration is 10.7 ms.

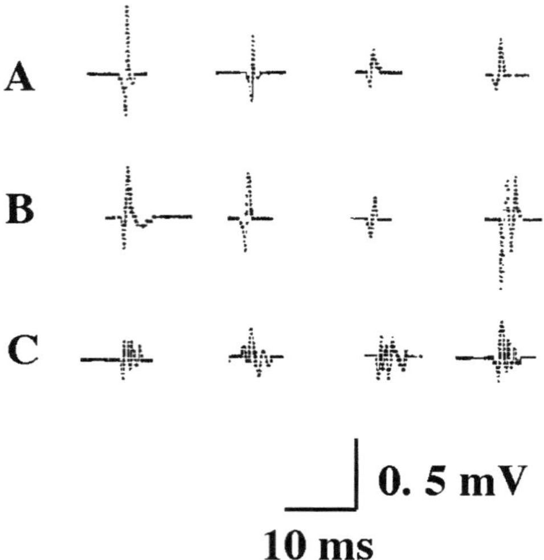

FIGURE 11.5. Twelve MUPs. **A** and **B**. Simple short-duration MUPs. **C.** Polyphasic SASD MUPs.

TREATMENT AND FOLLOW-UP

The patient was advised that CCD might predispose her to malignant hyperthermia if she ever required general anesthesia and that the anesthesiologist should be informed of her diagnosis. Moreover, she was advised to have a medical alert for malignant hyperthermia. Her muscle cramping was relieved quite well by quinine sulfate.

COMMENTS

CCD was described in 1956 as the first congenital myopathy. This became a historical landmark in myology, demonstrating the value of careful histological evaluation of muscle. It is an autosomal-dominant disorder with variable expression. Thus, patients may present in infancy or later in life, depending on the severity of the illness. Benign proximal myopathy is the most common manifestation. Congenital hip dislocation is the most common skeletal abnormality. Compared with other congenital myopathies, CCD has little or no involvement of ocular or bulbar muscles or muscle atrophy. Serum CPK is normal or slightly elevated. Needle EMG shows myopathic pattern without any abnormal spontaneous potential or a normal pattern in mild cases. Muscle biopsy is the key test for diagnosis of CCD, showing type 1 fiber predominance and central cores.

A high association with malignant hyperthermia is well known in this disease. In fact, the gene for CCD has been linked to chromosome 19q13.1, the same gene for malignant hyperthermia. Recognition of CCD is extremely important to prevent malignant hyperthermia during general anesthesia. Other diseases associated with malignant hyperthermia are Deborough-King syndrome (nonprogressive myopathy, short stature, webbed neck, and pectus carcinatum), Duchenne dystrophy, and myotonic dystrophy. Malignant hyperthermia is a rare and potentially lethal disorder. This condition is usually triggered by exposure to halogenated inhalational anesthetics, halothane, and the depolarizing muscle relaxant succinylcholine during general anesthesia. During or after general anesthesia, patients may develop muscular rigidity, hyperthermia, tachycardia, lactic acidosis, and rhabdomyolysis. In severe cases, ventricular fibrillations, disseminated intravascular coagulopathy, and hypoxemia develop and patients die because of these complications. Treatment of malignant hyperthermia includes discontinuation of triggering drugs, hyperventilation with oxygen, hypothermia measures to reduce body temperature, and rapid intravenous dantrolene injection. Dantrolene sodium is the specific therapy for malignant hyperthermia. The EMG study is not helpful for diagnosis of malignant hyperthermia. The primary diagnostic test for malignant hyperthermia is the in vitro caffeine and halothane contraction test on biopsied muscle. A concentration of halothane and caffeine too low to affect normal muscles produces contracture in a specimen obtained from the patient. The DNA test is limited by a low sensitivity at this time. To screen family members for malignant hyperthermia, the CPK has been simple and helpful; it is elevated in 70% of affected individuals. Thus, elevated CPK in a close relative to known malignant hyperthermia patients is considered diagnostic of MH until proven otherwise. For others, the in vitro contraction test is needed for this purpose.

MAXIMS

1. The possibility of malignant hyperthermia has to be discussed with patients with CCD because of high association.
2. Dantrolene sodium is the specific treatment for malignant hyperthermia.

REFERENCES

1. Bodensteiner JD. Congenital myopathies. Muscle Nerve 1994;17:131–144.
2. Kaus SJ, Rockoff MA. Malignant hyperthermia. Pediatr Clinic North Am 1994;41:221–237.

CASE 7

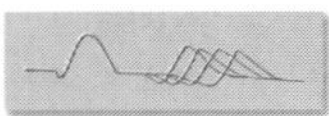

MYOCLONIC SEIZURE, HEARING LOSS, ATAXIA, AND MUSCLE WEAKNESS IN A FAMILY

CASE PRESENTATION

A 36-year-old woman developed a first episode of lapse of consciousness induced by dazzling light at a disco 5 years before examination. Electroencephalogram showed some seizure activity. Since then, she had frequent jerking spells without loss of consciousness that were well controlled with clonazepam. The patient also noticed progressive weakness of the limb and neck muscles, difficulty swallowing, nasal voice, and hearing difficulty. Past history was noncontributory except that she had been relatively thin all her life. Family history was positive in that her mother and sister had died at ages 52 and 22, respectively with a similar disease. Her younger sister had hearing loss. Examination showed an extremely thin woman with marked atrophy of the temporalis and masseter muscles and all limb muscles. Abnormal neurological findings were nasal speech, neural hearing loss, 3 MRC strength in proximal limb muscles, 4 in distal limb muscles, and diffuse hyperreflexia without Babinski toe signs. Her gait was ataxic and tandem walking was difficult.

CASE ANALYSIS

This patient had the constellation of myoclonic seizure, hearing loss, cerebellar ataxia, and predominant proximal muscle weakness, which is diagnostic of myoclonic epilepsy-ragged red fibers. When her mother and sister had been evaluated, the diagnosis was not easy, because MERRF had not yet been described. In her mother, we had suspected hyperthyroid myopathy on clinical grounds (she did have mild hyperthyroidism), but muscle biopsy showed mitochondrial myopathy. A few years after this, the patient's sister was found to have severe myoclonic seizure and ataxia, hearing loss, and mitochondrial myopathy. A few months after we saw her sister, the term mitochondrial encephalomyopathy was introduced.

PLAN OF TESTING

1. Needle EMG: To confirm myopathy.
2. NCS: To see whether peripheral nerve is involved.
3. Other tests: CPK, serum carnitine level, muscle biopsy, and blood DNA study.

ELECTROPHYSIOLOGICAL TESTS AND FINDINGS

NCS Findings. Normal motor and sensory NCS.

Needle EMG (Table 11.9; Fig. 11.6)

1. Many SASD MUPs with early recruitment.
2. Significant decrease in the mean duration of MUPs in the deltoid muscle.

ELECTROPHYSIOLOGICAL INTERPRETATION

Nonactive myopathy.

OTHER TEST FINDINGS

Serum carnitine and lactic acid levels were normal.

FINAL DIAGNOSIS

MERRF

TREATMENT AND FOLLOW-UP

The patient's seizures were well controlled with clonazepam. However, her myopathy gradually progressed, although she continued to be independently ambulatory at age 47. Her younger sister came to the clinic a few years later with myoclonic seizures, mild proximal muscle weakness, and neural hearing loss. Muscle biopsy showed mitochondrial myopathy.

TABLE 11.9. Needle EMG Data in Case 7

				Spontaneous Potentials				Motor Unit Potential			Interference	
Muscle	**Root**	**Nerve**	**Insertion Activity**	**Fib**	**PSW**	**Fasc**	**CRD**	**Amplitude (mV)**	**Duration (ms)**	**Polyphasic Potential**	**Pattern**	**Mean Amplitude (mV)**
Rt biceps	C6	Musc cut	N	–	–	–	–	0.3–0.9	2.8–6	+	FIP[a]	0.75
Deltoids	C5,6	Axillary	+	–	–	–	–	0.32	7.5[b]	45%	FIP[a]	0.6

[a] With early recruitment.

[b] With concentric needle, normal duration, 11.1 ms.

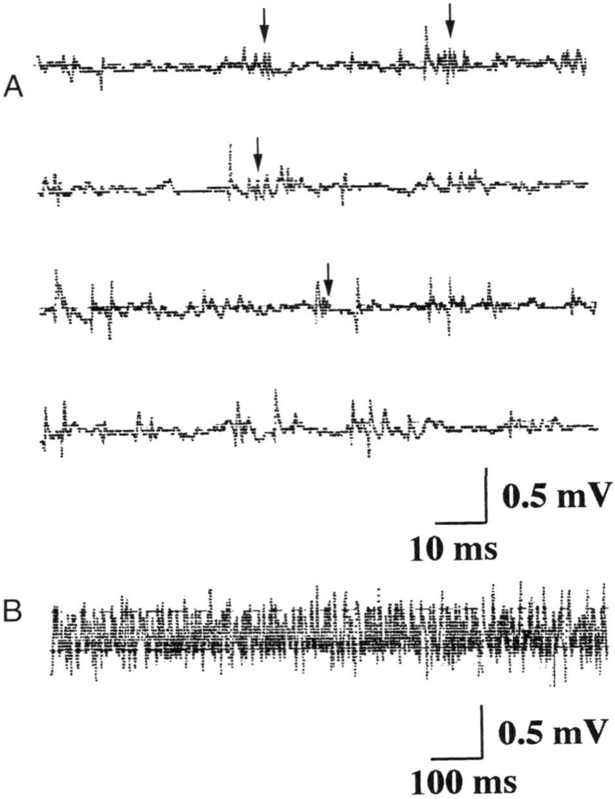

FIGURE 11.6. **A.** Many simple SASD MUPs and polyphasic SASD MUPs (*arrow*). **B.** Normal interference pattern.

COMMENTS

Since the introduction of mitochondrial myopathy under the terms megaconial and pleoconial myopathy in 1966, several distinct syndromes have been described and their gene defects identified. These include Luft disease, PEO, Kearns-Sayre syndrome, MERRF, MELAS, and MNGIES (Table 11.10). These different syndromes have one common characteristic: mitochondrial myopathy, identified by "ragged red fibers" in the muscle biopsy. Except for Luft disease, which is marked by a hypermetabolic state due to hyperactive mitochondrial activity, these syndromes have a hypometabolic state. The diagnosis of various syndromes is made by the constellation of findings as noted in our case. DNA testing can further identify each syndrome. In MERRF, a point mutation, an adenine-to-guanine transition at mt DNA at 8344, within a conserved region of the $tRNA^{Lys}$ gene, is thought to be a characteristic finding, observed in 90% of cases. In our case, a novel point mutation was found.

The needle EMG in mitochondrial myopathy shows a classic myopathic pattern: SASD MUPs. There has been a report of peripheral neuropathy in a few patients with mitochondrial myopathy. Some of them had demyelinating neuropathy.

At this time, no effective treatment is available for mitochondrial myopathy. Coenzyme Q and high-dose vitamin cocktails (vitamins C, riboflavin, thiamine, and K1) have been tried with varying results in individual cases. A low serum carnitine level has been reported in mitochondrial myopathies and, when found, oral carnitine was prescribed.

TABLE 11.10. Clinical Features and Genetic Defects of Various Mitochondrial Myopathy Syndromes[a]

Syndromes	Cardinal Clinical Features	Genetic Defects
PEO	Progressive external opthalmoplegia; nonfluctuating; diplopia is lacking	Maternal inheritance
Kearns-Sayre syndrome	PEO, retinitis pigmentosa, heart block, high CSF protein	Single mtDNA deletions; family history lacking
MERRF	Myoclonus, ataxia, seizure, weakness	Point mutation of tRNA lysine; non-Mendelian maternal inheritance
MELAS	Stroke-like syndromes (hemiparesis, hemianopsia, and cortical blindness), episodic vomiting	Point mutation of tRNA leucine; family history (+)
MNGIE	Neuropathy, gastrointestinal dysautonomia with intestinal pseudo-obstruction, leukodystrophy	Not known

[a] Ragged red fibers are present in all cases. Short stature, dementia, spongy degeneration of brain, sensory neural hearing loss, and lactic acidosis may be present.

MAXIMS

1. The presence of ragged red fibers in the muscle biopsy is pathognomonic of mitochondrial myopathy.
2. The needle EMG in mitochondrial myopathy shows a classic myopathic pattern.

REFERENCES

1. Dimauro S, Bonilla E, Zeviani M, Nakagawa M, De Vivo DC. Mitochondrial myopathies. Ann Neurol 1985;17:521–538.
2. Griggs RC, Mendell JR, Miller RG. Mitochondrial myopathies. In: Evaluation and treatment of myopathies. Philadelphia: FA Davis, 1995:294–317.

CASE 8

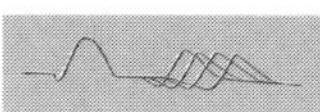

WEAKNESS OF LEGS, EXTREME FATIGUE, AND MYALGIAS FOR 5 YEARS IN A 54-YEAR-OLD WOMAN

CASE PRESENTATION

A 54-year-old woman had weakness in the legs for 5 years. More recently, she noted wasting of the right calf and pain in the right knee. During the evaluation, the rheumatologist found that her CPK was elevated at 900 units. The patient also complained of extreme fatigue and myalgia in the lower legs. Her fatigue was aggravated by exertion and helped by rest. Myalgia was improved by nonsteroidal anti-inflammatory agents. Abnormal neurological findings were mild bilateral ptosis and mild weakness of facial muscles, 5 − strength in deltoid and iliopsoas muscles; 4 in hamstrings, 2 in anterior tibialis, 4 − in gastrocnemius, 0 in right peroneus and 1 in left peroneus muscles. There was obvious atrophy in the right calf muscle. Reflexes were normal except for absent ankle jerks. She had bilateral mild pes cavus. Family history was negative.

CASE ANALYSIS

This patient's clinical history and findings presented challenging diagnostic problems. In view of her pes cavus, distal muscle weakness and atrophy, and mildly elevated CPK, three possibilities were considered: Hereditary motor sensory neuropathy type II (neuronal type of Charcot-Marie-Tooth disease), distal myopathy (Welander's disease), and the distal form of inclusion body myopathy. Mild ptosis, facial weakness, and extreme fatigue raised the possibility of myasthernia gravis, but her elevated CPK was a strong point against this.

PLAN OF TESTING

1. NCS: To rule out HMSN type II.
2. Needle EMG: To identify myopathy or denervation process.
3. Other tests: Acetylcholine receptor antibody and muscle biopsy.

ELECTROPHYSIOLOGICAL TESTS AND FINDINGS

NCS Findings. Normal except for bilateral CTS.

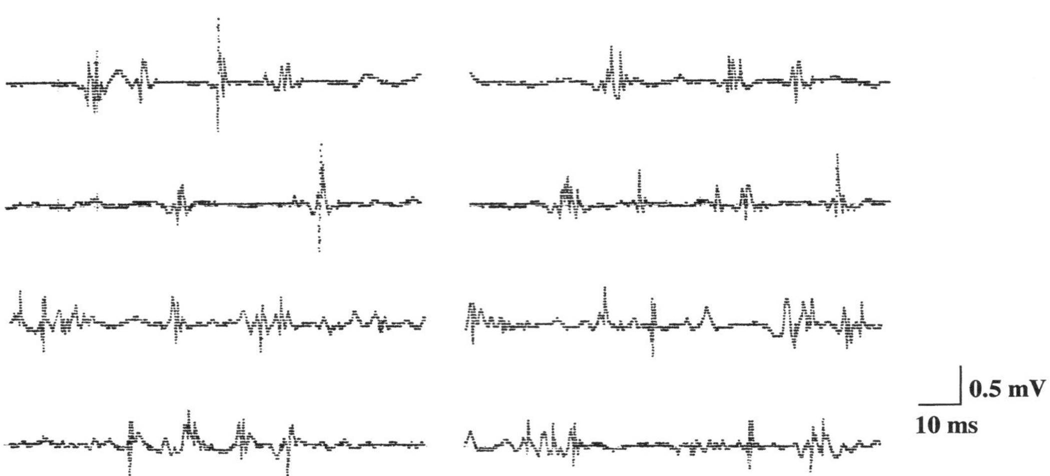

FIGURE 11.7. Many simple and polyphasic SASD MUPs.

TABLE 11.11. Needle EMG Data in Case 8

				Spontaneous Potentials				Motor Unit Potential				Interference	
Muscle	**Root**	**Nerve**	**Insertion Activity**	**Fib**	**PSW**	**Fasc**	**Myotonia CRD**	**Amplitude (K)**	**Duration (ms)**	**Polyphasic Potential**	**SASD MUP**	**Pattern**	**Mean Amplitude (K)**
Lt ant tibial	L4,5	Peroneal	N	–	–	–	–	0.5–1.5	3–8	++	++	FIP	1.5
Vast lat	L3,4	Femoral	+	–	+	–	–	0.5–2	8–12	N	–	FIP	1
Deltoid	C5	Axillary	N	–	–	–	–	<0.5	3–7	++	++	FIP	1

Needle EMG (Table 11.11; Fig. 11.7)

1. PSWs in the vastus lateralis muscles.
2. Many SASD MUPs in all of tested muscles.

RNS Test Findings. Normal test in the abductor digiti quinti and FCU muscles.

ELECTROPHYSIOLOGICAL INTERPRETATION

Active myopathy and bilateral CTS.

OTHER TEST FINDINGS

Normal AChR antibody. CPK was 616 units. Normal serum free and total carnitine levels. Normal serum lactic acid. Muscle biopsy from the anterior tibialis muscle showed mitochondrial myopathy.

FINAL DIAGNOSIS

Adult-onset mitochondrial myopathy

TREATMENT AND FOLLOW-UP

The patient was treated with coenzyme Q without any benefit. She was treated with high-dose riboflavin, thiamin, and vitamin C. Her fatigue was symptomatically relieved with pyridostigmine and premoline. There was no progression over a 10-year follow-up period.

COMMENTS

MEERF, MELAS, Kearns-Sayre syndrome, progressive external ophthalmoplegia, and congenital mitochondrial myopathy are well-known syndromes. However, adult-onset mitochondrial myopathy is relatively unknown. Clearly, there have been a few case reports of adult-onset mitochondrial myopathy, as well as a recent report of late-onset mitochondrial myopathy in individuals over 60 years old. Authors proposed that this is the most common form of myopathy in that age group. Late-onset mitochondrial myopathy is characterized by proximal weakness, normal or mildly elevated CPK, and many ragged red fibers in the muscle biopsy. According to these authors, the needle EMG was not very helpful because it showed normal findings in many cases. According to our experience, this is not true. The needle EMG study showed a myopathic pattern in almost all patients in whom we performed the study. We also found that myalgia and easy fatigability are common complaints in these cases. Thus, many patients were suspected of having polymyositis or myasthenia gravis. To us, the triad of myopathy, myalgia, and extreme fatigue in the adult is highly suggestive of mitochondrial myopathy. A low serum carnitine level was found in many cases of mitochondrial myopathy, and oral carnitine was successfully used. Thus, it is worthwhile to check serum carnitine level in patients with mitochondrial myopathy.

MAXIMS

1. A myopathic EMG pattern is extremely helpful in identification of adult-onset mitochondrial myopathy.
2. Myopathy, myalgia, and extreme fatigue are three common complaints in adult-onset mitochondrial myopathy.

REFERENCES

1. Oh SJ, Smith KKE. Diverse clinical syndromes associated with adult-onset mitochondrial myopathy. Ann Neurol 1993;34:270–271.
2. Johnston W, Karpati G, Carpenter S, Arnold D, Shoubridge A. Late-onset mitochondrial myopathy. Ann Neurol 1995;37:16–23.

CASE 9

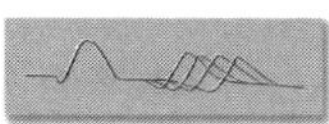

NUMBNESS IN THE HANDS AND PROXIMAL MUSCLE WEAKNESS FOR 3 YEARS

CASE PRESENTATION

A 27-year-old white woman complained of fatigue, numbness in the hands, painful muscle cramps, and proximal muscle weakness for 3 years. Proximal muscle weakness was characterized by difficulty raising her arms above the shoulders and getting up from a chair. Hand numbness was worse at night. Review of systems showed cold intolerance, hair loss, and weight gain. Abnormal neurological findings were 4+ MRC strength in the shoulder and pelvic girdle muscles, absent ankle jerks, somewhat enlarged gastrocnemius muscles, decreased knee jerks, decreased pin-prick sensation below the ankles, and positive Tinel's sign at the wrist on the median nerve. No muscle atrophy was observed. General examination showed a ''puffy'' expressionless face, sparse hair, and rough dry skin.

CASE ANALYSIS

This patient had somewhat different complaints from classic myopathy patients: fatigue, numbness in the hands, and pain. Neurological examination showed carpal tunnel syndrome, proximal weakness, and mild peripheral neuropathy. This constellation of symptoms and signs suggested two possibilities: collagen vascular disease and hypothyroidism. In this regard, the review of systems and general examination became important. In this patient, the classic features of myxedema were present. Careful examination of muscle stretch reflexes showed "hung-up reflexes" in knee jerks. These findings were enough to pinpoint the etiology of myopathy in this patient: hypothyroidism.

TABLE 11.12. Nerve Conduction Data in Case 9

	Latent/NCV (ms/m/s)	Amplitude (mV/μV)		Latent/NCV (ms/m/s)	Amplitude (mV/μV)
	Median	**Motor N**		**Peroneal**	**Motor N**
TL	6.1	10.9	TL	5.1	6.5
E-W	48.5	10.5	FH-A	41.3	6.0
AX-E	46.6	10.0	PF-FH		
	Ulnar	**Motor N**		**Post Tibial**	**Motor N**
TL	2.7	12.0	TL	5.0	10.0
BE-W	48.9	12.0	PF-A	39.7	9.0
AE-BE	53.9	12.0			
AX-AE	57.5	12.0			
			H-reflex	36.6	0.4
			Ankle T-reflex	NP	
	Median	**Sens/Mixed N**		**Sural**	**Sens/Mixed N**
F-W	20.7	8.0	MC-A	43.5	6.0
W-E	48.2	8.0			
E-AX	50.0	12.0			
	Ulnar	**Sens/Mixed N**		**Superficial Peroneal**	**Sens/Mixed N**
F-W	40.4	5.0	MC-A		
W-E	49.1	8.0			
E-AX	48.4	13.0			

Leg length, 39 cm.

PLAN OF TESTING

1. NCS: To confirm carpal tunnel syndrome and peripheral neuropathy.
2. Needle EMG: To confirm myopathy.
3. Thyroid profile: To confirm hypothyroidism.

ELECTROPHYSIOLOGICAL TESTS AND FINDINGS

NCS Findings (Table 11.12)

1. Slow sensory NCV in the finger-wrist segment and prolonged terminal latency in both median nerves.
2. Prolonged latency in the left H-reflex and absent right H-reflex.
3. Mildly slow motor NCV in the median, ulnar, and posterior tibial nerves.
4. Low CNAP amplitude below elbow in the median and ulnar nerves.
5. Slow mixed NCV in the forearm segment in the median and ulnar nerves.

Needle EMG (Table 11.13; Fig. 11.8)

1. Minimal fibrillation, PSWs, and CRDs in the tested muscles.
2. Significant decrease in mean duration of MUPs in the right deltoid muscle.
3. Many SASD MUPs in the other tested muscle.

RNS Test Findings. Normal in the ADQ and FCU muscles.

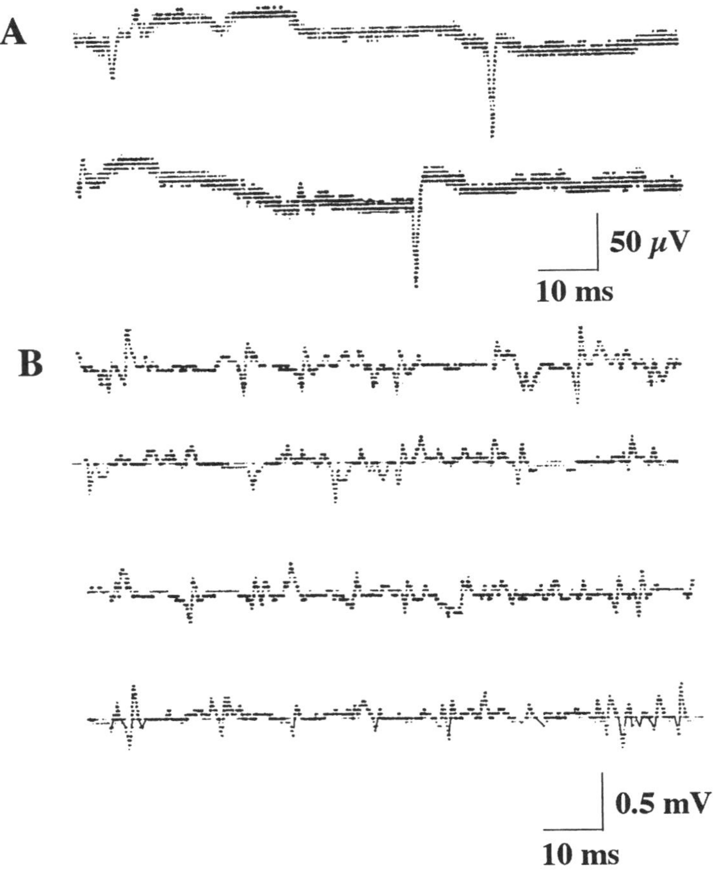

FIGURE 11.8. A. PSWs. **B.** Many SASD MUPs.

TABLE 11.13. Needle EMG Data in Case 9

				Spontaneous Potentials				Motor Unit Potential			Interference	
Muscle	**Root**	**Nerve**	**Insertion Activity**	**Fib**	**PSW**	**Fasc**	**CRD**	**Amplitude (K)**	**Duration (ms)**	**Polyphasic Potential**	**Pattern**	**Mean Amplitude (K)**
Rt deltoid	C5,6	Axillary	+	+	+	−	±	0.331[a]	5.74	13%	FIP	0.75
Biceps	C6	Musc cut	−	−	−	−	−	0.5–1.2	4–12	N	RIP	1.0
Vast lat	L3,4	Femoral	+	+	+	−	+	0.5–1.5	4–12	N	RIP	1.0

[a] Concentric needle. Monopolar needle in all other muscles. Normal duration is 11.4 ms.

ELECTROPHYSIOLOGICAL INTERPRETATION

Peripheral neuropathy with superimposed bilateral carpal tunnel syndrome and active myopathy.

OTHER TEST FINDINGS

CPK: 1250 units (normal 250). Extremely high TSH and low T_4 levels.

FINAL DIAGNOSIS

Hypothyroid myopathy

TREATMENT AND FOLLOW-UP

With thyroid replacement, the patient's myxedema and myopathy were improved in 6 months. In 2 years, she had a healthy baby. Before treatment, she had been married for 5 years and had not had a baby.

COMMENTS

Among the various endocrine myopathies, hypothyroid myopathy is an exception in regard to CPK, as it is the only endocrine myopathy with elevated CPK. Most other endocrine myopathies show a normal CPK. Two muscular syndromes are associated with hypothyroidism: hypothyroid myopathy and myasthenia gravis. Over one-third of hypothyroid patients have proximal muscle weakness, usually without atrophy. The CPK is elevated in about 90% of hypothyroid patients, most of whom do not have overt myopathy. The needle EMG documented a "myopathic pattern" in 70% of unselected hypothyroid patients. Most patients with severe hypothyroid myopathy have frank myxedema on examination and subclinical or clinical peripheral neuropathy, including carpal tunnel syndrome as seen in this patient. In patients with hypothyroid myopathy, several characteristic clinical features are diagnostically useful. They are prolonged muscle stretch reflexes, myoedema, painful cramp or stiffness, and hypertrophy of the muscles. DTRs in hypothyroidism are characteristically prolonged, especially during relaxation of the tendon reflexes. This gives rise to the characteristic "hung-up" ankle jerks in 80% of patients with hypothyroidism. Thus, when they are observed, they are diagnostic of hypothyroidism. Myoedema is a "mound or ridging of the muscle" on percussion. Myoedema is different from myotonia in that "depression" is noted in myotonia upon percussion. Hypothyroidism has been found in up to 6% of myasthenia gravis patients. The clinical and biochemical changes with hypothyroid myopathy are reversible when treated with replacement thyroid hormones.

MAXIMS

1. Hypothyroidism is one of the causes of asymptomatic CPK-emia.
2. "Hung-up reflexes" are diagnostic of hypothyroidism.

REFERENCES

1. Layzer RB. Neuromuscular manifestation of systemic disease. Philadelphia: FA Davis, 1984:79–126.
2. Rao SN, Katiyar BC, Nair KR, Misra S. Neuromuscular status in hypothyroidism. Acta Neurol Scand 1980;61:167–177.

CASE 10

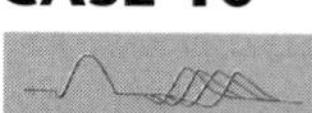

TINGLING SENSATION ON THIGHS AND HANDS FOLLOWED BY WEAKNESS FOR 3 DAYS

CASE PRESENTATION

Two days before admission, a 50-year-old woman experienced a "tingling sensation" on her thighs and hands followed by weakness in the legs and arms in the next several hours. The next day she was completely paralyzed. She had been treated with chlorothalidone (Hygroton) 50 mg daily and a low-salt diet for 2 months for hypertension. Her blood pressure was 140/85 mm. Neurological examination showed a bedridden woman due to flaccid muscle paralysis with sparing of facial, ocular, bulbar, and respiratory muscles. Proximal muscles were 0–1 MRC score and distal muscles were 2–3. Triceps, brachial, and ankle reflexes were absent, but biceps and patellar reflexes were weakly present. Plantar responses were flexor. No abnormality was noted in the cranial nerves or sensory functions. There had not been any antecedent event.

CASE ANALYSIS

This patient developed rather acute flaccid paralysis and decreased reflexes preceded by tingling sensation in a rather typical history of Guillain-Barré syndrome. Thus, until proven otherwise, the diagnosis of GBS should be made. However, it is always wise to consider other causes for acutely evolving weakness, such as tick paralysis, hypokalemic myopathy, myasthenia gravis, botulism, and cervical cord compression. Cervical cord compression was easily ruled out by the lack of a sensory level and upper motor neuron signs in the legs. Myasthenia gravis and botulism were less likely in view of the absence of oculobulbar involvement. Tick paralysis was ruled out by a lack of any history of tick bite and failure to find any ticks on examination.

PLAN OF TESTING

1. NCS: To confirm or rule out the diagnosis of GBS.
2. Needle EMG: To confirm or rule out myopathy.
3. CPK: To exclude myopathy.
4. CSF: To confirm the diagnosis of GBS.

ELECTROPHYSIOLOGICAL TESTS AND FINDINGS

NCS Findings. Normal motor and sensory nerve conductions in all tested nerves.

Needle EMG (Table 11.14)

1. Fibrillations and PSWs.
2. Many SASD MUPs with early recruitment.

ELECTROPHYSIOLOGICAL INTERPRETATION

1. Active myopathy.
2. No evidence of demyelinating neuropathy.

OTHER TEST FINDINGS

Normal cerebrospinal fluid findings. CPK, 1025 units (normal, 125). Serum K, 2.7 mEq/dL. All other electrolytes were normal. Muscle biopsy showed a classic vacuolar myopathy.

FINAL DIAGNOSIS

Hypokalemic myopathy

TREATMENT AND FOLLOW-UP

This patient was an avid user of milk of magnesia for constipation. Hypokalemia was induced by the therapeutic dose of chlorothalidone and abuse of laxatives in this patient. With a slow infusion of potassium, her weakness gradually improved in 5 days.

TABLE 11.14. Needle EMG Data in Case 10

				Spontaneous Potentials				Motor Unit Potential			Interference	
Muscle	**Root**	**Nerve**	**Insertion Activity**	**Fib**	**PSW**	**Fasc**	**Myotonia CRD**	**Amplitude (K)**	**Duration (ms)**	**Polyphasic Potential**	**Pattern**	**Mean Amplitude (K)**
Rt deltoid	C5,6	Axillary	+	++	++	–	–	0.3–1	3–10	++	RIP[a]	0.5
Biceps	C6	Musc cut	+	++	+	–	–	0.3–1	2–10	++	RIP[a]	0.5
FDI	C8T1	Ulnar	N	–	–	–	–	0.5–1.5	6–12	+	RIP	1
Vast lat	L3,4	Femoral	+	++	+	–	–	0.3–1	4–10	++	RIP[a]	0.75
Ant tibial	L4,5	Peroneal	+	+	+	–	–	0.5–1.5	4–10	++	RIP	1

[a] Early recruitment.

COMMENTS

Hypokalemia is the most common electrolyte abnormality that produces muscle weakness. A common cause of hypokalemia is the use of diuretics and chronic diarrhea (often associated with laxative abuse) and chronic renal tubular acidosis. The classic clinical feature of hypokalemic myopathy is painless proximal myopathy. When severe, it can produce generalized muscle paralysis, myoglobinuria, and vacuolar myopathy. Loss of DR, as seen in this patient, is one of the classic findings seen in severe hypokalemic myopathy and hypokalemic periodic paralysis during attacks, provoking a mistaken diagnosis of GBS. CPK is elevated reflecting the degree of severity of disease. Vacuolar myopathy is the most typical muscle biopsy finding in hypokalemia. Usually, there is no storage material identified in the vacuoles. EMG shows the classic myopathic pattern. If rhabdomyolysis is severe, the EMG shows evidence of active myopathy (fibrillation or PSW), as noted in this patient.

MAXIMS

1. Hyporeflexia is observed in severe hypokalemic myopathy. Thus, hypokalemic myopathy can mimic GBS.
2. The classic muscle biopsy finding in hypokalemia is vacuolar myopathy without any storage material in vacuoles.

REFERENCES

1. Knochel JF. Neuromuscular manifestations of electrolyte disorders. Am J Med 1982;72:521–534.

CASE 11

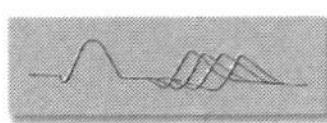

MUSCLE ACHING AND "COCA COLA-COLORED URINE" AFTER HEAVY EXERCISE

CASE PRESENTATION

One week before admission, a 16-year-old boy developed muscle aches, nausea, vomiting, and "coca cola-colored urine" after 2 hours of weight lifting. The patient was admitted to the hospital. Blood pressure was 150/86. Admission laboratory studies were as follows: serum creatinine, 1.9 mg%; BUN, 20 mg%; LDH, 16,000 units; SGOT, 2000 units; CPK, 20,000 units; 3 + protein; 3+ blood; no obvious red blood cells in urinalysis. Blood gases showed mild acidosis. He soon developed acute renal failure with diminished urinary output and with rising BUN and serum creatinine. The patient was given hemodialysis. Past history was interesting in that he had "recurrent exertional hematuria" with elevation of SGOT and LDH since 10 years of age. He had normal IVP and retrograde pyelogram. He had one 13-year-old sister who developed muscle cramps in her arm on exertion.

Physical examination was normal except for a blood pressure of 200/100 and muscle tenderness here and there. Normal reflexes and sensory, motor, and cerebellar functions were observed. A 1-minute exercise test consisting of a strong hand grip on a tennis ball under ischemia (above 200 blood pressure over the upper arm) induced muscle stiffness in the forearm that lasted for 5 minutes.

CASE ANALYSIS

This patient's presentation was rather classic in that initially myoglobinuria was mistaken for hematuria. If it had been hematuria, a simple microscopic urinalysis should show numerous red blood cells. In retrospect, this patient had a rather classic history of recurrent myoglobinuria. He was admitted to the hospital for acute renal failure due to massive myoglobinuria. Exercise-induced muscle aching and myoglobinuria are strongly suggestive of glycogen storage myopathy. The positive ischemic exercise test strengthened this clinical impression.

PLAN OF TESTING

1. Needle EMG: To assess the degree of muscle damage or detect permanent myopathy.
2. RNS test for prolonged period: 20-Hz stimulation for 60 seconds to induce clinical contracture of muscle.
3. Lactic acid ischemic exercise test: To identify glycogen storage myopathy.
4. Muscle biopsy: To confirm the exact enzyme deficiency of glycogen storage myopathy.

ELECTROPHYSIOLOGICAL TESTS AND FINDINGS

`Needle EMG.` Rare fibrillations and PSWs with normal MUP in the deltoid, biceps, and vastus lateralis muscles.

`RNS Test Findings` ***(Fig. 11.9).*** RNS at the rate of 20 Hz for 1 minute showed 48% decremental response. During this procedure, the patient's forearm and hand became "stiffened" with pain that persisted for 15 minutes.

ELECTROPHYSIOLOGICAL INTERPRETATION

1. Hyperirritable muscle membrane without any definite evidence of myopathy.
2. RNS test typical of McArdle's disease.

OTHER TEST FINDINGS

Ischemic exercise showed no rise in the lactic acid. Muscle biopsy showed absence of glucose phosphorylase staining, confirming the diagnosis of McArdle's disease.

FINAL DIAGNOSIS

McArdle's disease

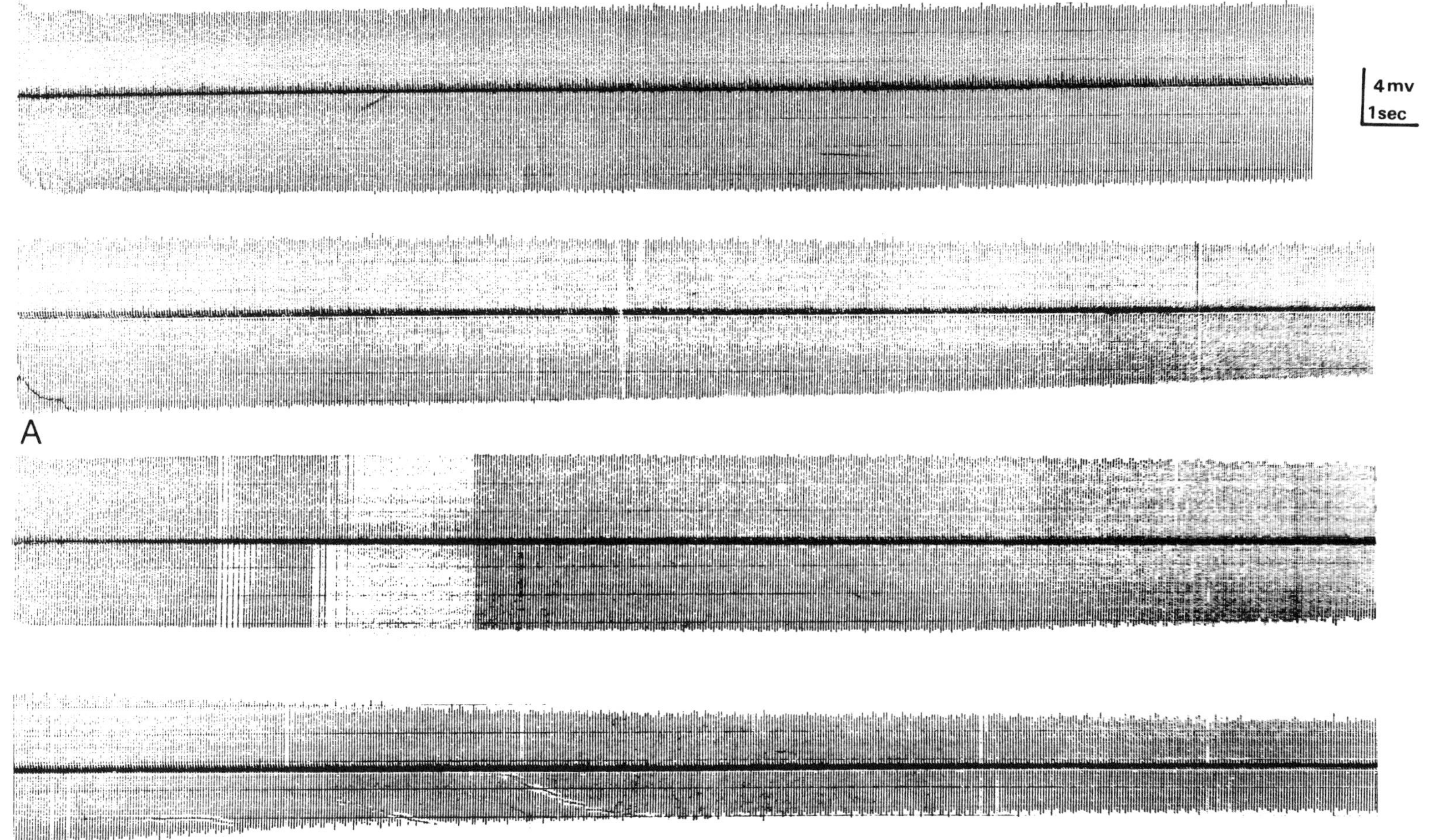

FIGURE 11.9. RNS response at 20-Hz stimulation for 60 s in McArdle's disease. **A.** Normal subject: 25.4% decremental response is noted. **B.** Patient with McArdle's disease: 47.5% decremental response is noted. This is accompanied by the sustained painful contracture of forearm muscles.

TREATMENT AND FOLLOW-UP

The patient was treated with hemodialysis with gradual improvement. Thereafter, he learned the limitation of his exercise endurance and did not experience any more episodes of acute renal failure. Muscle biopsy from his sister also confirmed McArdle's disease.

COMMENTS

It is not uncommon that myoglobinuria is misdiagnosed as "hematuria," as noted in this patient. This is because the "benzene dip test" for hematuria is positive for myoglobinuria. The simplest but most important clue for myoglobinuria is the absence of red blood cells in the urinalysis. Another helpful finding is an elevated CPK.

There are many causes for myoglobinuria, including trauma, viral infection, and drugs. Rare causes for myoglobinuria are metabolic myopathies. One practical way of approaching myoglobinuria is to see whether the patient has had recurrent myoglobinuria. One episode of myoglobinuria does not require muscle biopsy because most causes are due to causes other than metabolic myopathies. Recurrent myoglobinuria needs aggressive diagnostic work-up because it is often due to metabolic myopathy. Among the metabolic myopathies, McArdle's disease is the most common. Because the enzyme deficiency is only identifiable by biochemical assay, it is important to get an extra piece of muscle in the biopsy for the biochemical analysis.

Exercise intolerance with myalgia and painful stiffness in the exercised muscles are the cardinal manifestations of McArdle's disease and are usually present since adolescence. Classically, symptoms are precipitated by brief, sustained, high-intensity exercise, such as carrying heavy books between classes or sprinting. When severe, painful "stiffened or contracted muscles" are observed and myoglobinuria follows.

About 25% of patients develop renal failure and one-third of patients develop a fixed myopathy. The second-wind phenomenon, defined as improved exercise tolerance after a brief rest after an initial appearance of myalgia and muscle stiffness with light exercise, is common in this disease.

Diagnosis is strongly suggested by the abnormal decremental response on the RNS test for 1 minute at 20-Hz stimulation. This is invariably accompanied by sustained muscle contracture when the stimulation is given at the elbow. Needle EMG may show normal findings to an "active myopathy pattern," depending on the activity of muscle damage. Needle EMG in a stiffened muscle at the time of an acute attack is silent because it represents "rigor mortis," true contracture of muscle.

MAXIMS

1. "Hematuria" without identifiable red blood cells in urinalysis is indicative of myoglobinuria.
2. Silent electrical activity is typical of the needle EMG finding in the stiffened muscle during an attack in McArdle's disease.

REFERENCES

1. Rowland LP, Lovelace RE, Schottland DL, et al. The clinical diagnosis of McArdle's disease. Identification of another family with deficiency of muscle phosphorylase. Neurology 1966;16:93–100.
2. Penn AS. Myoglobinuria. In: Engel AG, Franzini-Armstrong C, eds. Myology, 2nd ed. New York: McGraw-Hill, 1994:1679–1696.

CASE 12

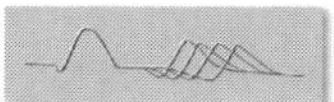

RESPIRATORY FAILURE AND ELEVATED CPK IN AN ADULT

CASE PRESENTATION

A 38-year-old man was admitted to the hospital with the chief complaints of shortness of breath, increasing episodic lethargy, and generalized muscular weakness. The patient had never been active in athletics in childhood and in the preceding few years had difficulty climbing stairs. During hospitalization, he was found to have hypoventilation associated with neuromuscular disease (Po_2 34, Pco_2 114), heart failure associated with cardiomegaly, diabetes mellitus with exogenous obesity, and pneumonia.

Neurological examination showed no obvious atrophy of muscles, no sensory or cerebellar abnormality, no myasthenic or myotonic response. Deep tendon reflexes were 1+ in biceps and triceps; knee jerks were absent and ankle jerks were positive. Muscle strength examination showed weakness of the neck flexor, deltoid, and iliopsoas muscles. Marked waddling gait was noted. Tensilon and neostigmine IM injections did not show any improvement in his neurological status. Studies revealed increased CPK (345 units) and aldolase (13).

CASE ANALYSIS

This patient was admitted to the MICU with respiratory failure and was found to have cardiomegaly and muscle weakness. Myasthenia gravis was ruled out clinically by negative Tensilon and neostigmine tests.

Neurological examination suggested the possibility of myopathy. The history also suggested myopathy since childhood. Thus, it was less likely that we were dealing with polymyositis. Respiratory failure as an initial manifestation is unheard of in polymyositis. We had to rule out GBS and amytrophic lateral sclerosis, but these were less likely in view of the early childhood onset of the disorder.

PLAN OF TESTING

1. NCS: To rule out peripheral neuropathy as a cause of respiratory failure.
2. Needle EMG: To differentiate myopathy from denervation process.
3. RNS test: To rule out myasthenia gravis or LEMS.
4. Muscle biopsy.

ELECTROPHYSIOLOGICAL TESTS AND FINDINGS

NCS Findings. Normal NCS in all tested nerves.
Needle EMG (Table 11.15; Fig. 11.10)

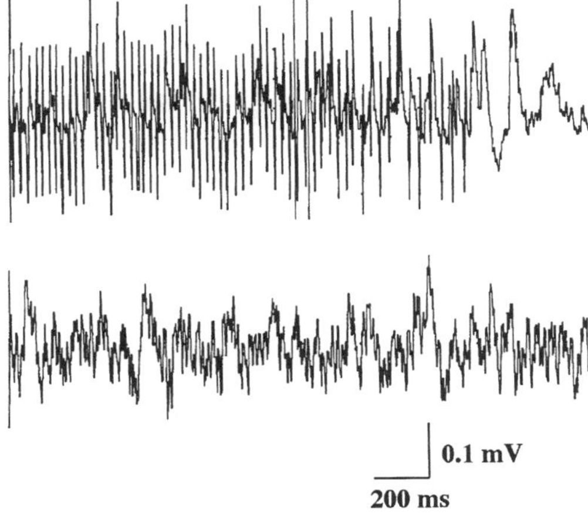

FIGURE 11.10. Two tracings of genuine myotonic potentials in a case with adult form of acid maltase deficiency.

TABLE 11.15. Needle EMG Data in Case 12

				Spontaneous Potentials				Motor Unit Potential				Interference	
Muscle	**Root**	**Nerve**	**Insertion Activity**	**Fib**	**PSW**	**Fasc**	**Myotonia**	**Amplitude (K)**	**Duration (ms)**	**Polyphasic Potential**	**Giant MUP**	**Pattern**	**Mean Amplitude (K)**
Rt deltoid[a]	C5,6	Axillary	+	++	++	−	+	0.78	8.1	50%	0	FIP	1
Biceps[a]	C6	Musc cut	+	+	+	−	+	0.91	7.1	25%	0	FIP	1
Vast lat	L3,4	Femoral	+	+	+	−	+	0.3–1.5	3–10	+	0	FIP	1

[a] Concentric needle. Normal duration for deltoid is 9.1 ms and for biceps, 10.8 ms.

1. Fibrillation, PSWs, and myotonic potentials.
2. Significant decrease in mean duration of MUPs in the deltoid and biceps muscles.
3. SASD MUPs in other tested muscles.

RNS Test Findings. Normal in the RNS tests on the ADQ and FCU muscles.

ELECTROPHYSIOLOGICAL INTERPRETATION

Myotonic myopathy typical of the adult form of acid maltase deficiency.

OTHER TEST FINDINGS

Muscle biopsy was performed and showed "vacuolar myopathy" with PAS and acid phosphatase-positive materials, indicative of lysosomal glycogen-storage myopathy. Biochemical assay of muscle showed a marked decrease (8% of normal) in acid maltase.

FINAL DIAGNOSIS

Acid maltase deficiency

TREATMENT AND FOLLOW-UP

Because of the difficulty in weaning this patient off the ventilator, a permanent tracheostomy was performed with intermittent connection to the ventilator. The patient was still alive 20 years after the diagnosis.

COMMENTS

The three most common neuromuscular diseases accompanied by respiratory failure are myasthenia gravis, GBS, and amyotrophic lateral sclerosis. These account for 95% of cases. Other rarer disorders in which respiratory failure may occur include Duchenne dystrophy, polymyositis, the adult form of acid maltase deficiency, inclusion body myopathy, and myotonic dystrophy. Thus, it is important to rule out the first three diseases before considering a rare disease.

There are three distinct forms of acid maltase deficiency: the infant form (Pompe's disease), the childhood form, and the adult form. In Pompe's disease, cardiomyopathy and tongue and liver enlargement are common. Invariably, the patient dies before 2 years of age. In the childhood form, organomegaly is variable and the patient dies before 19 years of age. In the adult form of Pompe's disease, the most characteristic presentation is respiratory failure, as noted in this patient. It is slowly progressive, but the prognosis is much better than in the other forms.

EMG findings in acid maltase deficiency are rather characteristic: genuine myotonic potentials without clinical myotonia and a myopathic EMG pattern, as noted in this patient. Genuine myotonic potentials have been reported in a few cases of inclusion body myopathy and polymyositis, and acid maltase deficiency is one disease that shows this abnormality consistently.

MAXIMS

1. The most typical presentation in the adult form of acid maltase deficiency is "respiratory failure."
2. Three common neuromuscular causes for respiratory failure are GBS, amyotrophic lateral sclerosis, and myasthenia gravis.

REFERENCES

1. Engel AG, Gomez MR, Seybold ME, Lambert EH. The spectrum and diagnosis of acid maltase deficiency. Neurology 1973;23:95–106.

CASE 13

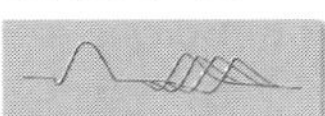

PROXIMAL MUSCLE WEAKNESS AND ELEVATED CPK IN A PATIENT WITH SJÖGREN'S DISEASE

CASE PRESENTATION

A 72-year-old woman with a history of Sjögren's syndrome, temporal arteritis, and hypertension had a 3-year history of weakness. Weakness was noted first in her arms, and she had difficulty raising her arms above her shoulders to do her hair. Over the preceding 8 months she also had problems climbing stairs. She denied any difficulty with chewing or swallowing. CPK was elevated at 208 and 200 units (normal, 140). Sjögren's anti-SS-A was 1:400 but anti-SS-B was negative. ANA (speckled pattern) was positive at 1:160. Sedimentation rate was normal. She had been treated with plaquenil 400 mg/day for 4 years, prednisone (initially 60 mg/day and then 8 mg), and methotrexate 20 mg/week. EMG and NCSs performed elsewhere demonstrated right L3-4 and S1 radiculopathy and a mild sensory neuropathy affecting both the right arm and the right leg. Examination showed a very thin and chronically ill-appearing woman with small muscle bulk throughout, 4+ strength in deltoid and 4 strength in iliopsoas muscles bilaterally, decreased pin prick in the distal upper and lower extremities, and 1+ DTRs.

CASE ANALYSIS

Neurological findings were suggestive of chronic myopathy and sensory neuropathy. In view of the history of Sjögren's syndrome and mild elevation of CPK, polymyositis was a definite possibility. The combination of polymyositis and neuropathy raises the possibility of vasculitis in the setup of collagen vascular diseases. Sedimentation rate was normal. Other possibilities should include drug-induced myopathy (steroid and plaquenil). In steroid-induced myopathy, CPK is usually normal.

PLAN OF TESTING

1. NCS: To confirm neuropathy.
2. Needle EMG: To identify myopathy.
3. Other tests: CPK and muscle biopsy to confirm myopathy and identify the cause of myopathy.

ELECTROPHYSIOLOGICAL TESTS AND FINDINGS

NCS Findings

1. Slow sensory NCV in the finger-wrist segment and prolonged terminal latency in the median nerve.
2. Slow sensory NCV in the sural nerve and low CMAP in the peroneal nerve.

Needle EMG (Table 11.16; Fig. 11.11)

1. PSWs and frequent SASD MUPs in the right deltoid muscle.
2. Fibrillations, PSWs, and CRD, and frequent SASD MUPs in the right biceps and vastus lateralis muscles.

ELECTROPHYSIOLOGICAL INTERPRETATION

Active myopathy and mild distal sensory neuropathy.

OTHER TEST FINDINGS

CPK was 1528 U/L. Muscle biopsy in the deltoid showed vacuolar myopathy without any inflammatory cells, consistent with chloroquine-induced myopathy.

FINAL DIAGNOSIS

Plaquenil-induced myopathy

TREATMENT AND FOLLOW-UP

With discontinuation of plaquenil, the patient showed gradual improvement in her muscle strength, confirming plaquenil-induced myopathy.

TABLE 11.16. Needle EMG Data in Case 13

				Spontaneous Potentials				Motor Unit Potential			Interference	
Muscle	**Root**	**Nerve**	**Insertion Activity**	**Fib**	**PSW**	**Fasc**	**CRD**	**Amplitude (K)**	**Duration (ms)**	**Polyphasic Potential**	**Pattern**	**Mean Amplitude (K)**
Rt deltoid	C5,6	Axillary	+	−	+	−	−	0.3–2.5	2–6	+	FIP	1
Biceps	C6	Musc cut	+	+	−	−	+	0.3–1	3–6	+	FIP	0.5
Vast lat	L3,4	Femoral	+	+	+	−	+	0.3–1	3–6	+	FIP	0.75

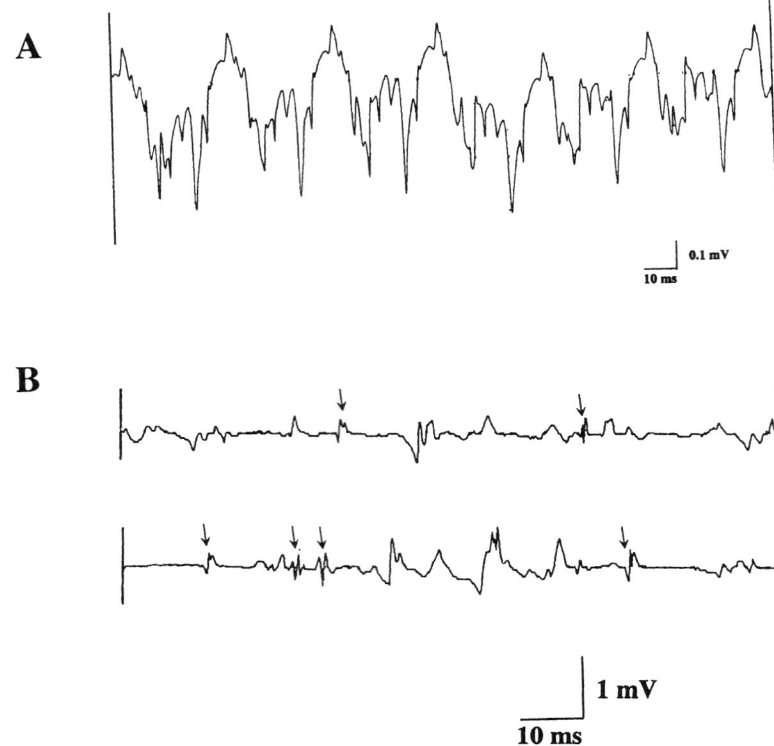

FIGURE 11.11. **A.** CRDs. **B.** SASD MUPs (*arrows*) mixed with normal duration MUPs.

COMMENTS

In this case, the needle EMG findings were indicative of active myopathy, which is typical of polymyositis. Also considering her elevated CPK, polymyositis was the most likely diagnosis until muscle biopsy showed vacuolar myopathy typical of chloroquine-induced myopathy.

Chloroquine, an antimalarial drug, is known to be toxic to the liver, skeletal and cardiac muscles, and came to be widely used for long-term treatment of many collagen vascular diseases since 1950. Shortly thereafter in 1963, a characteristic toxic reaction was reported in seven patients who had been taking the drug in doses of 250 to 500 mg daily for several months. Uniformly, these patients developed a slowly progressive myopathy that began in the legs and then involved the arms and even the face if the drug was not discontinued. Tendon reflexes were markedly reduced or absent and there was no sensory involvement. Biopsy of the affected muscles disclosed varying degrees of vacuolar degeneration involving as much as 50% of the muscle fibers. This disorder was slowly but completely reversible after discontinuation of the drug. Heart and skeletal muscles were involved in a few patients. Myocardial lesions were found similar to those in skeletal muscle. This drug is known to be toxic to liver and skeletal and cardiac muscles. Muscle biopsy classically shows vacuolar myopathy.

Steroids are the drugs most commonly known to induce myopathy. Considering the frequent use of steroids in medical practice, steroid-induced myopathy is extremely rare. The classic scenario of steroid-induced myopathy is that this is suspected in patients with collagen vascular diseases who are on steroids for long periods and develop proximal muscle weakness. According to my experience, even in this classic scenario, often the original disease is more responsible for myopathy than the steroid. Among steroids, fluorinated steroid is more likely to produce steroid-induced myopathy. The needle EMG is extremely helpful in differentiating steroid myopathy from polymyositis; fibrillations and PSWs are not present in steroid myopathy, but are seen in polymyositis.

MAXIMS

1. In steroid myopathy, CPK is normal and abnormal spontaneous potentials are absent.
2. Chloroquine myopathy is characterized by vacuolar myopathy in the muscle biopsy.

REFERENCES

1. Whisnant JP, Espinosa RE, Kierland RR, Lambert EH. Chloroquine neuromyopathy. Proc Mayo Clin 1963;38:501–513.
2. Hughes JT, Esiri M, Osbury JM, Whitty CW. Chloroquine myopathy. QJ Med 1971;63:85–93.

CASE 14

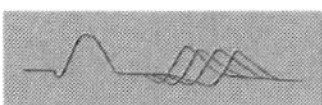

EPISODIC MUSCLE WEAKNESS IN A 28-YEAR-OLD MAN

CASE PRESENTATION

A 28-year-old man had episodic generalized muscle weakness for 8 years. Family history revealed that his father and sister had similar episodes. Episodic weakness occurred mostly in the morning, usually once or twice in a month, lasting 1 to 12 hours. When severe, he could not move his arms and legs at all but talked and breathed normally. The only known precipitating factors were a large evening meal and pickled cucumbers. Neurological examination between attacks was completely normal, but during attacks he had MRC strength of 3 in the proximal muscles and 4 in the distal muscles. Reflexes were absent during the attacks.

CASE ANALYSIS

Episodic generalized weakness is the classic feature in two diseases: myasthenia gravis and periodic paralysis. The patient's history was typical of familial periodic paralysis in view of the autosomal-dominant inheritance pattern, the sparing of oculobulbar and respiratory muscles during the attacks, absent reflexes during attacks, and normal neurological examination between attacks. The duration and severity of the attacks suggested hypokalemic periodic paralysis.

PLAN OF TESTING

1. Needle EMG: To document myopathic patterns of MUPs and check for myotonic potentials during attacks.
2. Other tests: Serial serum potassium and CPK during and between attacks.
3. Thyroid profile.

ELECTROPHYSIOLOGICAL TESTS AND FINDINGS

Needle EMG During Attacks (Table 11.17)

1. Decreased insertional activity and difficulty in obtaining decent MUPs (a relative electrophysiological silence) in the biceps muscle.
2. Minimal PSWs, significant decrease in the mean duration of MUPs, increased polyphasic MUPs, and normal interference pattern in the APB muscle.
3. Decreased insertional activity and significant decrease in the mean duration of MUPs, increased polyphasic MUPs, and normal interference pattern in the rectus femoris muscle.
4. No myotonic potentials in any tested muscles.

TABLE 11.17. Needle EMG Data in Case 14

				Spontaneous Potentials				Motor Unit Potential			Interference	
Muscle	**Root**	**Nerve**	**Insertion Activity**	**Fib**	**PSW**	**Fasc**	**Myotonia CRD**	**Amplitude (K)**	**Duration (ms)**	**Polyphasic Potential**	**Pattern**	**Mean Amplitude (K)**
1/3/73												
Lt biceps[a]	C5,6	Musc cut	–	–	–	–	–	[b]	[b]	[b]	[b]	[b]
APB	C8, T1	Median	N	+ +	–	–	–	0.42	8.5	14%	RIP	0.6
9/14/73												
Rectus femoris[c]	L3,4	Femoral	–	–	–	–	–	0.55	6.4	25	RIP	0.4
Triceps	C7	Radial	–	–	–	–	–	0.5–1.5	6–12	N	RIP	1.25

[a] MRC 3 strength.
[b] MUPs are difficult to elicit.
[c] MRC 4 strength.
APB, abductor pollicis brevis.

TABLE 11.18. RNS Test Data in Case 14

1/5/71	ADQ
CMAP (mV)	3.0
CMAP Ex (%)	
2 Hz (%)	0
5 Hz (%)	+31
50 Hz (%)	+40
5 Hz PT 0 (%)	+40[a]
5 Hz PT 4 m (%)	+19[b]

[a] CMAP after 50-Hz stimulation for 1 second.

[b] CMAP amplitude 4 minutes after 50-Hz stimulation. Post-tetanic facilitation in the CMAP amplitude lasted up to 4 minutes.

PT, post-tetanic; ADQ, abductor digiti quinti.

RNS Test During Attacks (Table 11.18)

1. Low CMAP.
2. Incremental response at low rate of stimulation.
3. Post-tetanic facilitation in the CMAP amplitude up to 4 minutes after tetanic stimulation.

ELECTROPHYSIOLOGICAL INTERPRETATION

Inactive myopathy compatible with hypokalemic periodic paralysis.

OTHER TEST FINDINGS

Serum K and CPK were normal between attacks. During attacks, serum K was decreased to 2.0 mEq/dL, confirming the diagnosis of hypokalemic periodic paralysis. CPK during attacks was elevated to 2.5 times normal. Thyroid profile was normal.

FINAL DIAGNOSIS

Familial hypokalemic periodic paralysis

TREATMENT AND FOLLOW-UP

The patient's attacks were treated with oral loading of potassium in the hospital. Attacks were prevented with a combination of daily KCl oral intake and 750 mg Diamox a day.

COMMENTS

In this case, the absence of myotonic potentials during attacks clearly ruled out potassium-sensitive periodic attacks with myotonia. The relative silence and myopathic pattern of the needle EMG were typical of periodic paralysis during attack. RNS responses were compatible with the responses typically observed in patients with periodic paralysis (see below). In retrospect, the prolonged exercise test, which was not reported at the time of the RNS test in this patient, would have given us the same information.

Unless a patient has fixed myopathy, the needle EMG in classic periodic paralysis is normal between attacks. During attacks, reduced recruitment of MUPs and myopathic pattern are the classic EMG pattern. Ultimately, the muscle becomes completely silent. With recovery, the number of MUPs increases until normal MUPs with full interference pattern are achieved. EMG abnormalities are similar in all types of periodic paralysis with one exception. In patients with potassium-sensitive periodic paralysis and myotonia, myotonic discharges are present early during attacks and are of diagnostic importance.

During attacks, the CMAP amplitude is markedly reduced. The CMAP amplitude is correlated with the degree of weakness. It increases progressively with HRS or during intermittent HRS. There are usually an early/fast and a late/slow phase of facilitation. This phenomenon is most likely due to a local membrane event resulting in recruitment of muscle fibers, which explains the beneficial influence of exercise in aborting or postponing attacks of periodic paralysis. During rest the CMAP amplitude falls again.

The prolonged exercise test may show diagnostically helpful abnormalities in the CMAP. The CMAP is recorded from the ADQ muscle with supramaximal stimulation in the RNS test. At least three control CMAPs are recorded at 1-minute intervals. Then the patient contracts maximally the ADQ muscle for 2 to 5 minutes, with a brief rest (3 to 4 seconds) every 15 seconds. CMAPs are recorded at 1-minute intervals during exercise and recovery. In controls, only minimal changes in CMAP amplitude occur; the amplitude may increase up to 27% immediately after exercise and decrease by 30% after 5 minutes of recovery. In periodic paralysis, a greater than normal increase (0 to 300%) in CMAP was observed immediately after exercise and the subsequent decline in CMAP amplitude was maximal during the first 20 minutes after the exercise and was greater than normal. Abnormal exercise tests have been observed in 70% of patients, regardless of the type of periodic paralysis. Thus, this test does not help to distinguish between different types of periodic paralysis but is helpful in diagnosis of periodic paralysis.

MAXIMS

1. Myotonic discharges in early phase of attacks are diagnostic of potassium-sensitive periodic paralysis with myotonia.
2. "Electrophysiological silence" is observed in severely paralyzed muscles in periodic paralysis.

REFERENCES

1. Campa JF, Sanders DB. Familial hypokalemic periodic paralysis. Arch Neurol 1974;31:110–115.
2. McMantis PG, Lambert EH, Daube JR. The exercise test in periodic paralysis. Muscle Nerve 1986; 9:704–710.

CASE 15

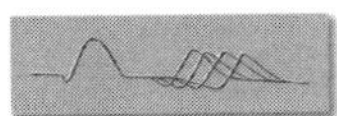

WHAT TO DO WITH ASYMPTOMATIC CPK-EMIA?

CASE PRESENTATION

A 57-year old woman in apparently good health attempted to donate blood 2 years ago and was refused on the grounds that she had elevated liver enzymes. She was asymptomatic at that time. Approximately 1 year later, she developed intermittent swallowing difficulties, which she described as feeling that the food was hanging in her throat, and required multiple swallows to get it down. She saw several doctors for this problem and had a barium swallow that was normal. Eight months ago when a routine blood test found elevated CPK, she was told that she was having a heart attack and needed to come into the hospital. At that time, she still had no symptoms. She underwent coronary angiography that showed 30 to 50% partial blockage of three vessels. She was in the hospital for 5 weeks, although her ECGs were normal. On discharge, she was referred to a gastroenterologist for her swallowing difficulty. Laboratory tests showed CPK of 984 with MB fraction of 146.3, LDH of 391, SGOT 60, SGPT 67, and normal total bilirubin. The gastroenterologist thought that the patient might have a myopathy and referred her to us for evaluation. The patient felt as though her legs had been getting weaker, particularly when she tried to climb steps, and she had frequent falls. Laboratory work-ups included a normal ASO titer, negative C-reactive protein and rheumatoid factor, TSH 4.5 (slightly elevated), ESR of 22, cholesterol of 237, triglycerides of 17~, SGOT of 47, LDH of 225, CPK of 406 (MB fraction of 56) and 984 (MB fraction 146.3) on two occasions. Neurological examination was normal except for 5− strength in the right iliopsoas muscle.

CASE ANALYSIS

This case represents a rather typical history of a patient with idiopathic CPK-emia. Because of asymptomatic elevated SGOT and SGPT, hepatitis was suspected. When CPK was found to be elevated, the patient was hospitalized for "myocardial infarction" despite a normal ECG. An astute internist suspected that her intermittent swallowing difficulty, subtle complaint of weakness in the legs, and elevated CPK were due to myopathy. Certainly her difficulty climbing stairs suggested proximal leg weakness, and the presence of subtle weakness in the right iliopsoas muscle confirmed myopathy.

PLAN OF TESTING

1. Needle EMG: To document myopathy.
2. Muscle biopsy: To confirm the diagnosis.

ELECTROPHYSIOLOGICAL TESTS AND FINDINGS

Needle EMG (Table 11.19; Fig. 11.12)

1. Increased insertional activity, fibrillations, PSWs, many SASD MUPs (some polyphasic MUPs) in almost all tested muscles.
2. CRDs in the right vastus lateralis, medial gastrocnemius, and iliopsoas muscles.

ELECTROPHYSIOLOGICAL INTERPRETATION

Active myopathy typical of polymyositis.

OTHER TEST FINDINGS

Muscle biopsy from the vastus lateralis confirmed the diagnosis of polymyositis.

FINAL DIAGNOSIS

Polymyositis

TREATMENT AND FOLLOW-UP

In view of the patient's subtle weakness in the right iliopsoas muscle and other significant complaints, she was treated with 40 mg prednisone a day. Her findings were completely normal within 2 months.

TABLE 11.19. Needle EMG Data in Case 15

				Spontaneous Potentials				Motor Unit Potential			Interference	
Muscle	**Root**	**Nerve**	**Insertion Activity**	**Fib**	**PSW**	**Fasc**	**CRD**	**Amplitude (K)**	**Duration (ms)**	**Polyphasic Potential**	**Pattern**	**Mean Amplitude (K)**
Rt vast lat	L3,4	Femoral	+	+ + +	+	–	+	0.3–2.2	3–11	+	FIP	1.5
Med gastroc	S1,2	Post tibial	+	+ + +	+ +	–	–	0.3–2.5	5–10	N	RIP	2
Iliopsoas	L2,3	Femoral	+	+ + +	+	–	+ +	0.3–1.5	2–10	+	FIP	1.5
Deltoid	C5,6	Axillary	N	–	–	–	–	0.6–1.5	2.8–10	N	FIP	1
Biceps	C6,7	Musc cut	+	+ +	+ +	–	–	0.4–1	3–10	N	FIP	1

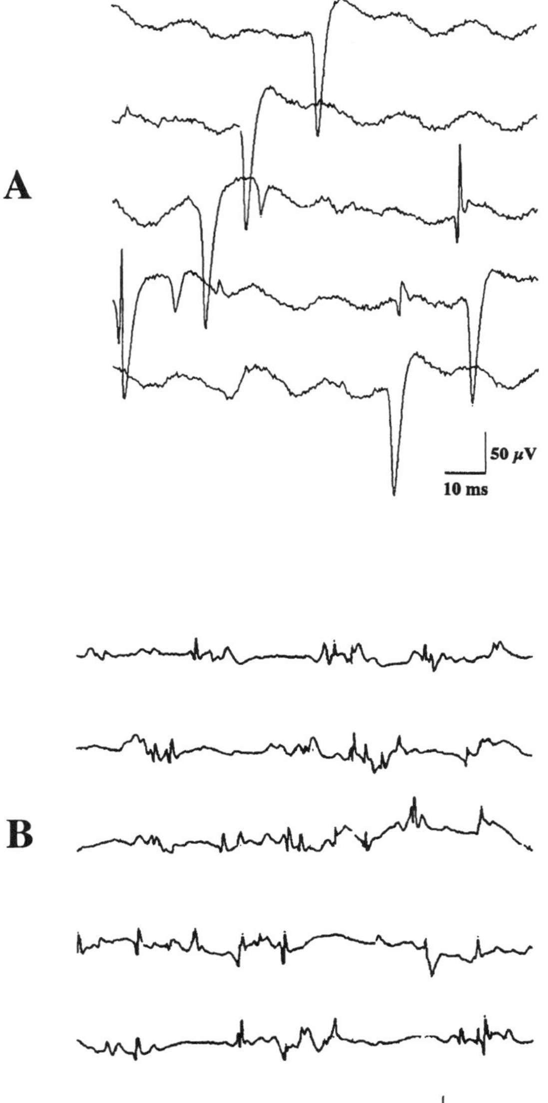

FIGURE 11.12. A. Fibrillations and PSWs. **B.** many SASD MUPs.

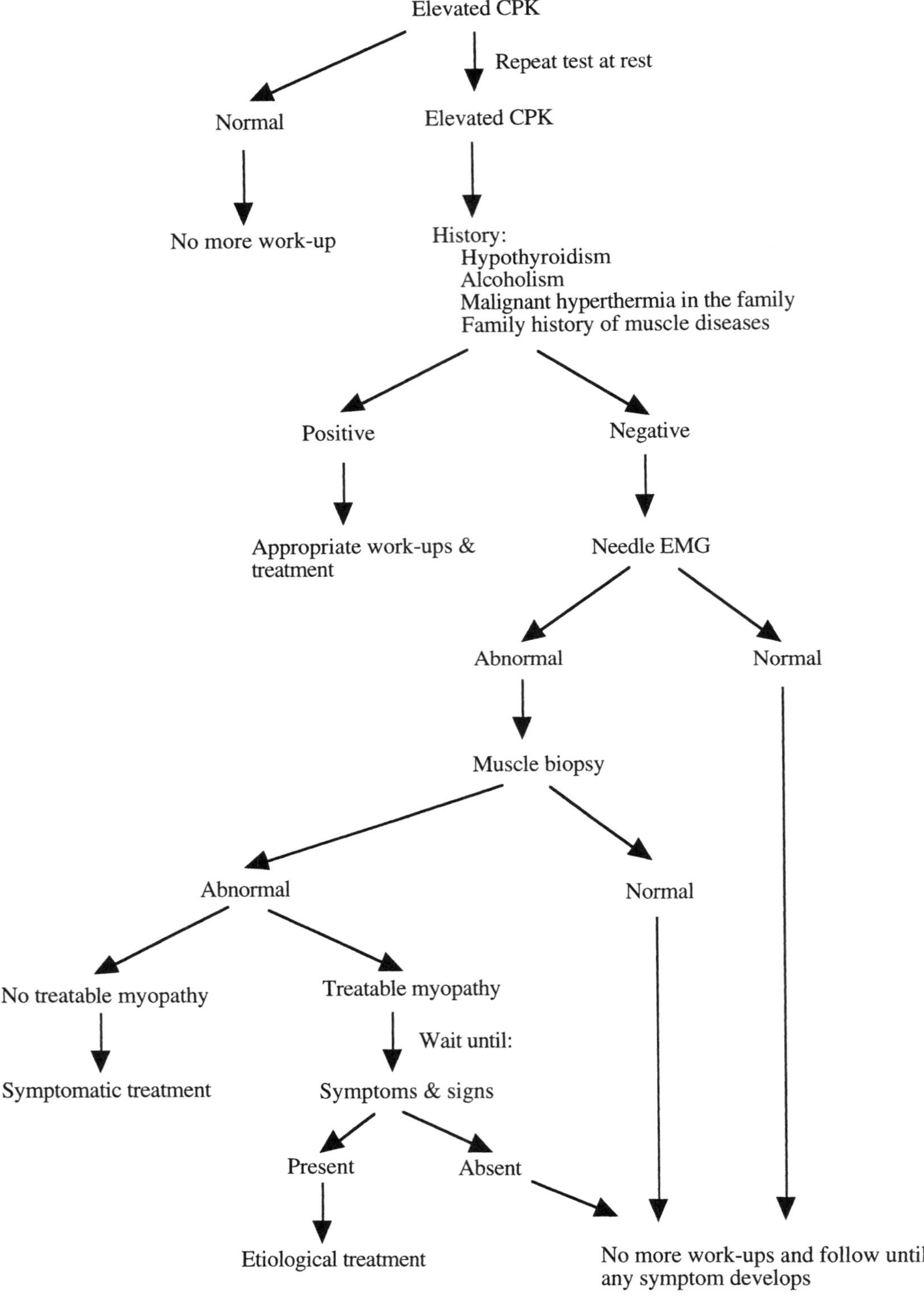

FIGURE 11.13. Algorithm for the work-up for asymptomatic CPK-emia.

COMMENTS

Because of the wide availability of CPK testing as a panel of blood chemistry, asymptomatic elevated CPK is often detected these days. As seen in this patient, this finding can lead to clinically inappropriate diagnoses and subsequent unnecessary diagnostic procedures. Hyper-CPK-emia has to be documented more than once before embarking on any diagnostic work-ups. When confronted with asymptomatic hyper-CPK-emia, multiple causes that can cause asymptomatic hyper-CPK-emia should be ruled out first: hypothyroidism, chronic alcoholism, carrier state of progressive muscular dystrophy or malignant hyperthermia, and heavy exercise (Fig. 11.13). Once these have been excluded, it is important to pursue the possibility of benign congenital myopathy by obtaining a detailed developmental history. This information often provides clinicians with a hint that they are dealing with benign congenital myopathy, which is one of most common causes of asymptomatic hyper-CPK-emia. Our approach is to follow these patients with a careful neurological examination to detect any subtle deficit such as that seen in this patient. At that point, a needle EMG is recommended. If the needle EMG is abnormal, a muscle biopsy should be done. The two most common causes for asymptomatic hyper-CPK-emia are benign congenital myopathy and polymyositis. If the needle EMG is normal, no further work-up is recommended. Treatment is instituted when clinical symptoms and signs are noted.

MAXIMS

1. Two common myopathies associated with asymptomatic hyper-CPK-emia are polymyositis and congenital myopathy.
2. When the needle EMG is abnormal in patients with asymptomatic hyper-CPK-emia, there is a better chance of confirming myopathy on the muscle biopsy.

REFERENCES

1. Joy JL, Oh SJ. Asymptomatic hyper-CPK-emia: an electrophysiologic and histopathologic study. Muscle Nerve 1989;12:206–209.
2. Joy JL, Riser JB, Oh SJ. Rational approach to asymptomatic creatine kinase elevation. Ala J Med Sci 1988;25:147–150.

CHAPTER 12

Myotonic Diseases

Myotonia, a difficulty of relaxation after muscle contraction, is a sine qua non in myotonic disorder. It is commonly demonstrated as grasp myotonia (a form of action myotonia) or percussion myotonia in patients with myotonic disorder. Percussion myotonia is best shown by tapping the hyperthenar and forearm extensor muscles or the tongue with a reflex hammer. "Napkin-ring sign" (dimpling) on the edge of the tongue is a classic sign of myotonia and can be demonstrated by tapping the tongue between two tongue depressors. Myotonia is usually described as "stiffness" or "cramp" by patients. It is typically aggravated by cold or by prolonged rest with the body in a fixed posture and eased by "warm-up exercises." When myotonia is induced by cold alone, it is termed paramyotonia. When myotonia worsens with warm-up exercises, it is called "paradoxical myotonia." Paradoxical myotonia is best demonstrated by five or six closures of the eyelids and is the most prominent finding in paramyotonia congenita.

Myotonic response is easily detected by needle electromyography (EMG) because of the high-frequency repetitive discharge of either biphasic spikes or positive waves with fluctuating frequency or amplitude. This is associated with a characteristic "dive-bomber sound." Myotonic potentials are a sine qua non in myotonic disorders.

Myotonia is due to the sustained firing of muscle potentials even after contraction ceases. The main abnormality in the myotonic fibers appears to be partial depolarization and spontaneous oscillation in the transmembrane potential. Recent in vitro studies have pointed toward sodium and chloride channels as the source of the defect in myotonia (e.g., Thomsen's myotonia congenita as a chloride channel disease and hyperkalemic periodic paralysis and paramyotonia congenita as sodium channel diseases). Recent molecular genetic studies have shown that myotonic dystrophy is a "trinucleotide (CTG) repeat expansion disease" and that a blood test can identify myotonic dystrophy.

There are three major myotonic entities that are inherited (Table 12.1). Myotonia congenita is a relatively benign nonprogressive disorder characterized by generalized myotonia alone. Thus, treatment of myotonia with drugs is most satisfying. The classic form of myotonia congenita is Thomsen's disease, which is inherited as autosomal dominant. The Becker form of myotonia congenita is inherited as autosomal recessive and is sometimes called autosomal-recessive generalized myotonia. Paramyotonia congenita is characterized by a prolonged myotonic response and flaccid paralysis induced by cold and often associated with potassium-sensitive (hyperkalemic) periodic paralysis.

Proximal myotonic myotonia is the most recently recognized entity characterized by late-onset, autosomal-dominant inheritance, generalized myotonia with proximal muscles weakness, and benign course. Unlike myotonic dystrophy, systemic signs, with the exception of cataracts, and CTG repeat expansion are missing in this condition.

On the other hand, myotonic dystrophy is a progressive disorder characterized by myotonia, distal myopathy, and systemic involvement. Because of systemic involvement, other organ dysfunction may present itself as the initial symptom of myotonic dystrophy. In this disorder, the main complaint is muscle weakness rather than myotonia. Thus, treatment of myotonia with drugs is less satisfying. Neonatal or infantile myotonic dystrophy is inherited from a mother with myotonic dystrophy and often present as "floppy infant syndrome." It is not easy to document clinical or electrophysiological myotonia at birth in neonatal or infantile myotonic dystrophy. Thus, it is important to examine the mother when suspecting this disor-

TABLE 12.1. Clinical Features of Various Myotonic Syndromes

	Myotonic Dystrophy (Steinert)	PROMM	Myotonia Congenita of Thomsen	Myotonia Congenita of Becker[a]	Paramyotonia Congenita[b]
Age of onset	Late adolescence	Late: 20–40 yr	Infancy to early child	Late childhood	First decade
Autosomal inheritance	Dominant	Dominant	Dominant	Recessive	Dominant
Myopathy (weakness)	Face, eyes, distal limb muscles	Proximal leg muscles	None	Rare	Very rare
Muscle pain	None	Prominent	None	None	None
Hypertrophy of muscle	None	None	Frequent	Frequent in legs	None
Myotonia	Hands, forearm, tongue	Hands, thighs	Generalized	Generalized	Paradoxical; eye
Associated findings	Cataract Cardiac arrthymia Frontal balding Testicular atrophy Mental retardation	(+) (±)	None	None	None
Gene defect	Chromosome 19; CTG expansion affecting a protein kinase disorder	Unknown; no CTG expansion	Chromosome 7; skeletal muscle Cl channel	Chromosome 7; skeletal muscle Cl channel	Chromosome 17; skeletal muscle Na channel

[a] Autosomal-recessive generalized myotonia.
[b] Sometimes associated with hyperkalemic periodic paralysis.

der in floppy infant syndrome because the full-blown features of myotonic dystrophy are usually obvious in the mother.

Myotonia is most effectively treated with quinine, quinidine, diphenylhydantion (Dilantin), procainamide, tocainamide, and mexiletine, which stabilize the irritable myotonic membrane. These medications are most effective in myotonia congenita but less effective in myotonic dystrophy. Among these, mexiletine is the most effective and popular antimyotonic agent. Dilantin is the safest drug for myotonia in myotonic dystrophy because of its least deleterious effect on myotonic cardiomyopathy.

In myotonic diseases, anticholinesterase agents should be avoided because they aggravate myotonia. Malignant hyperthermia is known to occur more frequently in myotonic dystrophy, and this possibility has to be considered when general anesthesia is contemplated. Thus, local or regional anesthesia is preferred whenever possible. When general anesthesia must be used, all precautions for malignant hyperthermia, including avoidance of succinylcholine and halothane, should be taken; a combination of nitrous oxide/oxygen and an agent such as enflurane or isoflurane is recommended. If muscle relaxation is necessary during anesthesia, a short-acting, nondepolarizing agent such as atracurium or vecuronium is preferable.

Acquired myotonic myopathy has been associated with some older cholesterol-lowering agents: clofibrate and dizaocholesterol. Myotonic potentials are present in the needle EMG without any clinical myotonia. Newer cholesterol-lowering agents are known to produce elevated CPK and myopathy but not myotonic myopathy. A few cases of paraneoplastic myotonia have been described. Again, myotonic potentials were seen in the needle EMG without any demonstrable clinical myotonia in association with cancer. Myotonic potentials disappeared with cancer treatment.

CASE 1

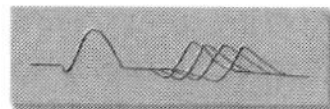

PROGRESSIVE BILATERAL FOOT DROP FOR 12 YEARS

CASE PRESENTATION

A 28-year-old man was evaluated by a neurologist for slowly progressive weakness of the legs for 12 years. The neurologist quickly observed steppage gait due to the bilateral foot drop as the patient entered the examining room. Further examination showed weakness of the hands and areflexia in knee and ankle jerks. No sensory or cerebellar abnormality was observed. Under the presumptive diagnosis of peripheral neuropathy, the patient was sent to the EMG laboratory for confirmation of diagnosis. A resident physician confirmed the findings and performed an NCS, which showed normal findings except for absent H-reflexes. Needle EMG in the anterior tibialis and gastrocnemius muscle showed fibrillations and PSW, CCRD, and normal MUPs. The resident presented this patient under the diagnosis of axonal peripheral neuropathy.

CASE ANALYSIS

After listening to the resident's presentation, the senior electromyographer was ready to accept his conclusion until he entered the EMG examination room. The patient was a gaunt, somewhat dull-appearing man with an elongated face, frontal balding, and wasted temporal muscles. His speech was nasal, and he had bilateral ptosis and facial weakness. When asked to check the patient's grasp, the resident demonstrated marked grasp myotonia. Further, there was percussion myotonia in the hyperthenar and tongue muscles and 4+ MRC strength in the anterior tibialis muscles.

PLAN OF TESTING

1. NCS: To rule out peripheral neuropathy.
2. Needle EMG: To confirm myotonia and myopathy.
3. CPK: To judge the degree of active muscle necrosis.
4. ECG: To check for any serious cardiac dysrhythmia.

ELECTROPHYSIOLOGICAL TESTS AND FINDINGS

NCS Findings. Normal motor and sensory NCS except for absent H-reflexes.

Needle EMG (Table 12.2)

1. Prominent myotonic discharge in the right APB muscle (Figs. 12.1 and 12.2).
2. Increased insertional activity, PSW, and fibrillation potentials in the right APB and deltoid muscles.
3. Many small-short MUPs in the right deltoid muscle.

ELECTROPHYSIOLOGICAL INTERPRETATION

Myotonic myopathy typical of myotonic dystrophy.

OTHER TEST FINDINGS

Normal CPK and ECG findings.

FINAL DIAGNOSIS

Myotonic dystrophy

TREATMENT AND FOLLOW-UP

Over the next few years, there was a gradual progression of weakness in the anterior tibialis muscles.

COMMENTS

Myopathy is characterized by proximal muscle weakness. However, there are two myopathies marked by distal muscle weakness: myotonic dystrophy and distal myopathy. Classically in these disorders, the distal weakness precedes the proximal weakness. Thus, it is not unusual

TABLE 12.2. Needle EMG Data in Case 1

				Spontaneous Potentials				Motor Unit Potential				Interference	
Muscle	Root	Nerve	Insertion Activity	Fib	PSW	Fasc	Myotonic Potential	Amplitude (K)	Duration (ms)	Polyphasic Potential	SASD MUP	Pattern	Mean Amplitude (K)
Rt ant tibial	L4,5	Peroneal	++	+	+	−	±	0.5–2	6–15	N	−	RIP	1
Gastroc	S1,2	Post tibial	++	+	+	−	±	0.5–2	8–16	N	−	RIP	1
APB	C8, T1	Median	+++	+	+	−	++++	[a]					
Deltoids	C5,6	Axillary	++	+	+	−	±	0.3–2	4–10	+	+	RIP	2

[a] Because of prominent myotonic potentials, the analysis of MUP was not possible.

Fib, fibrillations; PSW, positive sharp wave; Fasc, fasciculations; +, present or increased; −, absent; N, normal; RIP, reduced interference pattern; APB, abductor pollicis brevis.

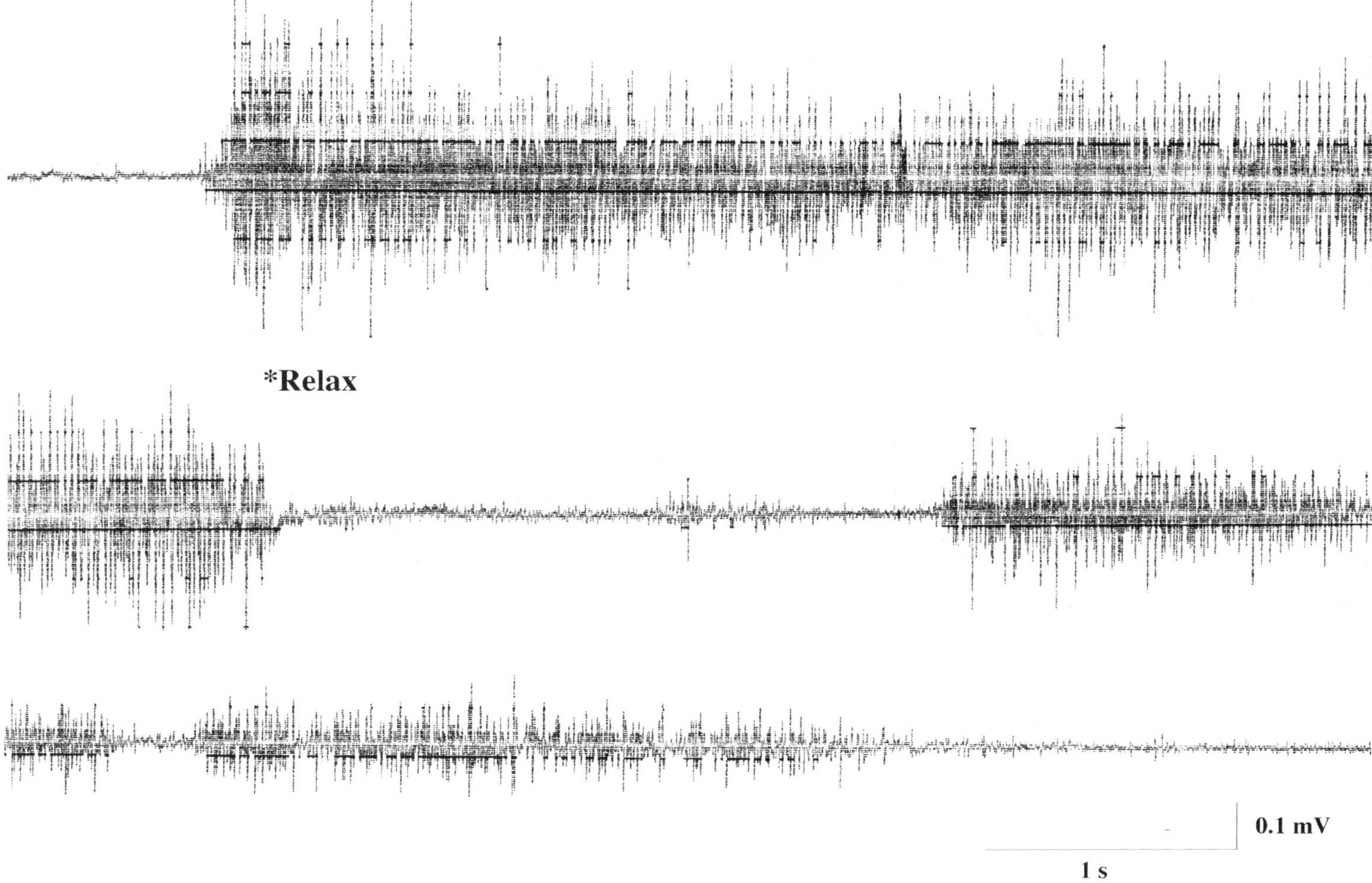

FIGURE 12.1. Needle EMG recording of action myotonia in the abductor pollicis brevis (APB) muscle. Difficulty of relaxation of APB muscle due to myotonic potentials is obvious here. It takes 10 seconds finally to relax APB muscle. Normally, there should be a flat line after relaxation. **Contract**, the subject is asked to contract APB minimally. **Relax**, the subject is asked to relax APB muscle.

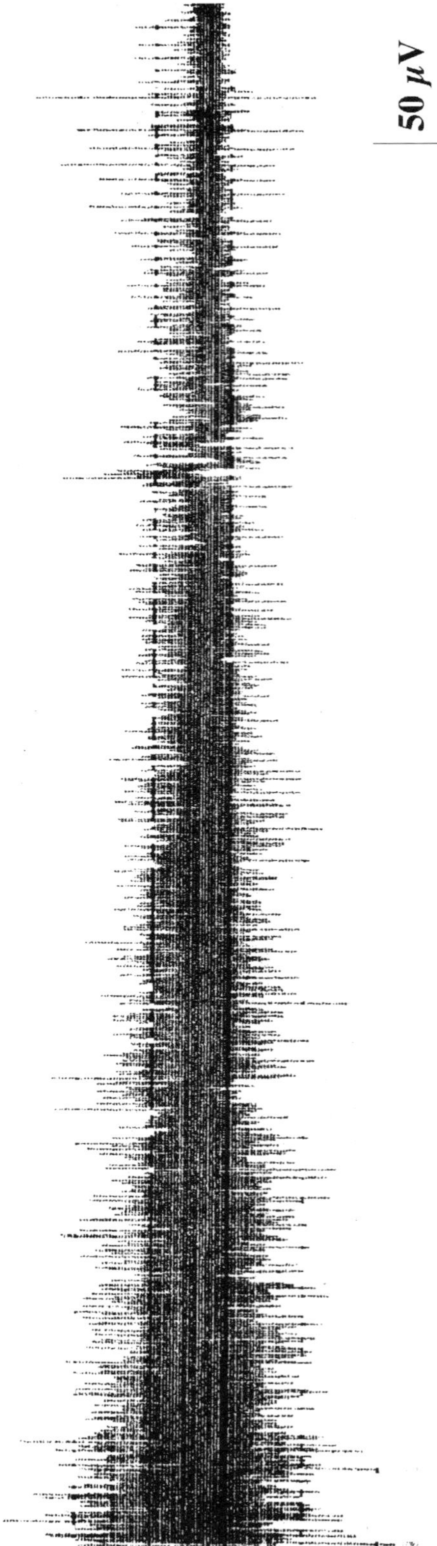

FIGURE 12.2. Needle EMG recording of percussion myotonia in the APB muscle. Myotonic potentials induced by tapping the muscle. Notice waxing and waning of amplitude and frequency of myotonic potentials.

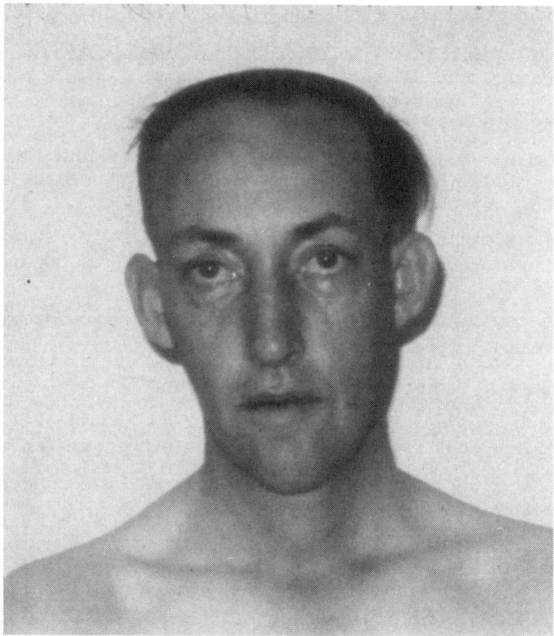

FIGURE 12.3. Typical facial features in myotonic dystrophy: narrow, elongated face with frontal balding and atrophy of the sternocleidomastoid.

for a patient with myotonic dystrophy to present with steppage gait as the initial symptom and for a motor neuropathy to be suspected, as noted in this case.

One of the clinical hallmarks of myotonic dystrophy is a characteristic "long, hatched, expressionless face" with frontal balding, ptosis, and wasting of temporalis, masseter, and sternocleidomastoid muscles. Such an appearance is pathognomonic of myotonic dystrophy (Fig. 12.3). There is no other disease that mimics the face of myotonic dystrophy. Speech is classically nasal in phonation because of bulbar muscle weakness.

Myotonia is defined as the sustained contraction of muscle caused by spontaneous repetitive depolarization of the muscle membrane. Among myotonic disorders, myotonic dystrophy is the classic example. The diagnosis of myotonic dystrophy is made by the characteristic facial appearance and the presence of myotonia in the limb muscles. Both percussion myotonia and grasp myotonia can be easily demonstrated. The best muscles for percussion myotonia are the thenar, wrist extensor, and tongue muscles. Grasp myotonia is easily tested by grip release after a firm handshake. As the disease progresses, myotonia becomes difficult to detect because of muscle wasting.

MAXIMS

1. A "long, hatched, expressionless face" with frontal balding and wasting of temporalis muscles is pathognomonic of myotonic dystrophy.
2. Myotonic dystrophy is one of two myopathies characterized by distal weakness.

REFERENCES

1. Moxley RT III. The Myotonias: their diagnosis and treatment. Comp Ther 1996;22:8–21.
2. Streib EW. Differential diagnosis of myotonic syndromes. Muscle Nerve 1987;10:603–615.

CASE 2

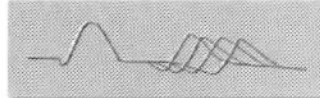

SON WHO HAD SYMPTOMS IDENTICAL TO THOSE OF HIS FATHER

CASE PRESENTATION

An 18-year-old man was brought to the MDA Clinic by his father who had an established diagnosis of myotonic dystrophy for evaluation of difficulty in relaxation of hand-grip for 4 years. This problem was somewhat worse during the winter and relieved by repeated exercise (warming-up phenomenon). There was no other complaint of weakness. A brother and sister were symptom free at the time. Abnormal neurological findings were a thin, elongated face with mild frontal balding, mild bilateral ptosis, mild facial weakness, nasal speech, 4 MRC strength in neck flexor with atrophy of sternocleidomastoid muscle, percussion myotonia in thenar and forearm extensor muscles, and grasp myotonia. There was no evidence of cardiomyopathy or cataracts at this time.

CASE ANALYSIS

The father suspected that his son had myotonic dystrophy, because he recognized that his son's symptoms were identical to those he had himself experienced at the onset of his disease. His complaints were classic for myotonia, which is aggravated by cold and relieved by warm-up exercises. Even at this early stage, there were mild but typical facial features and myotonia. Thus, the diagnosis of myotonic dystrophy was relatively easy.

PLAN OF TESTING

1. Needle EMG: To confirm myotonic myopathy.
2. Short-exercise test: To document postexercise depression, which is typically observed in myotonic syndrome.

ELECTROPHYSIOLOGICAL TESTS AND FINDINGS

Needle EMG (Table 12.3)

1. Fibrillation potentials, PSW, myotonic discharges (Figs. 12.4 and 12.5).
2. SASD MUPs in the left deltoid and APB muscles. (Fig. 12.6)

Short-Exercise Test Findings. Postexercise response was a 33.7% decrease in the CMAP immediately after 10 seconds of exercise (Fig. 12.7)

ELECTROPHYSIOLOGICAL INTERPRETATION

Myotonic myopathy typical of myotonic dystrophy

OTHER TEST FINDINGS

CPK was 199 units (normal). ECG was normal at the initial examination.

FINAL DIAGNOSIS

Myotonic dystrophy

TREATMENT AND FOLLOW-UP

The patient had a good response of myotonia with phenytoin 250 mg/day. During a 15-year follow-up period, he has not shown much change except an ECG abnormality of right ventricular conduction delay.

COMMENTS

Myotonic potentials are the most specific potentials in the needle EMG. If they are recognized by the needle EMG, the patient is considered to have myotonic disorder until proven otherwise. Myotonic potentials are characterized by spontaneous potentials with waxing and waning amplitude and frequency and the classic "dive-bomber sounds." Thus, it is much easier and more reliable to identify myotonic potentials by their sound than by visual aids. These sounds are easily induced by needle insertion and movement, muscle tapping, or minimal voluntary contraction of muscles. If a single myotonic potential is firing at the slower rate, it may sound

TABLE 12.3. Needle EMG Data in Case 2

				Spontaneous Potentials				Motor Unit Potential				Interference	
Muscle	**Root**	**Nerve**	**Insertion Activity**	**Fib**	**PSW**	**Fasc**	**Myotonic Potential**	**Amplitude (K)**	**Duration (ms)**	**Polyphasic Potential**	**SASD MUP**	**Pattern**	**Mean Amplitude (K)**
Rt APB	C8, T1	Median	+	++	++	–	+++	0.3–2	3–14	N	+	FIP	1
Deltoid	C5,6	Axillary	+	+	+	–	+++	0.3–1.5	3–14	+	+	FIP	1.5

FIP, full interference pattern.

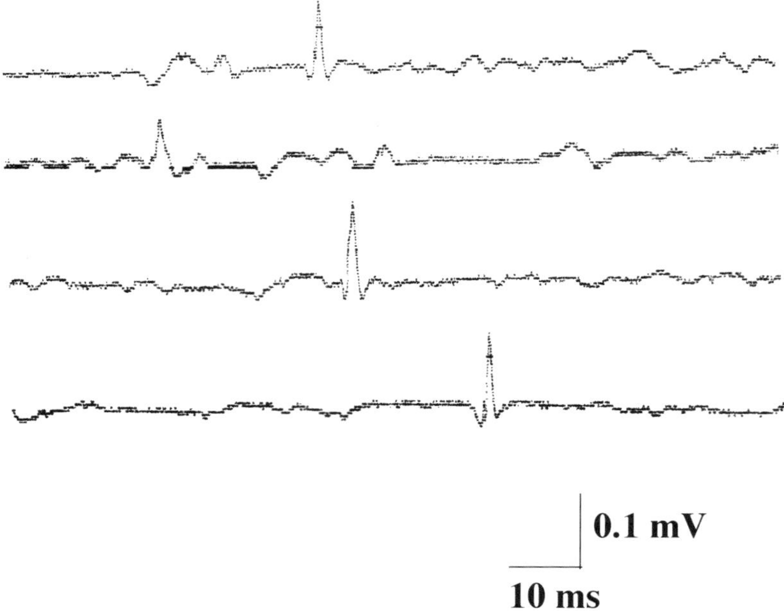

FIGURE 12.4. A few fibrillations in the ABP muscle with myotonia.

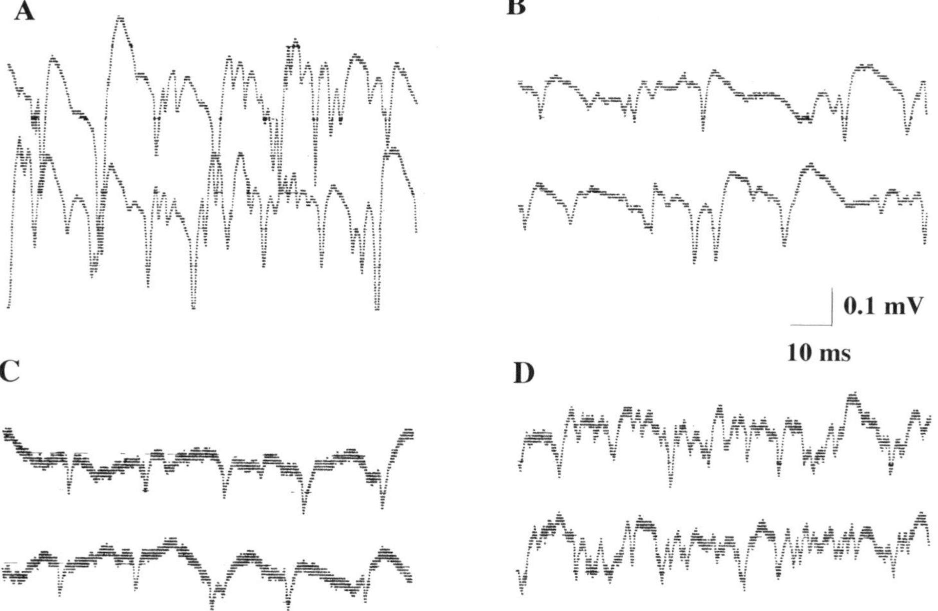

FIGURE 12.5. A. Myotonic potentials characterized by waxing and waning of MUP amplitude and frequency together with varying shape. **B.** Myotonic potentials mimicking PSW. **C.** PSW. **D.** Myotonic potentials.

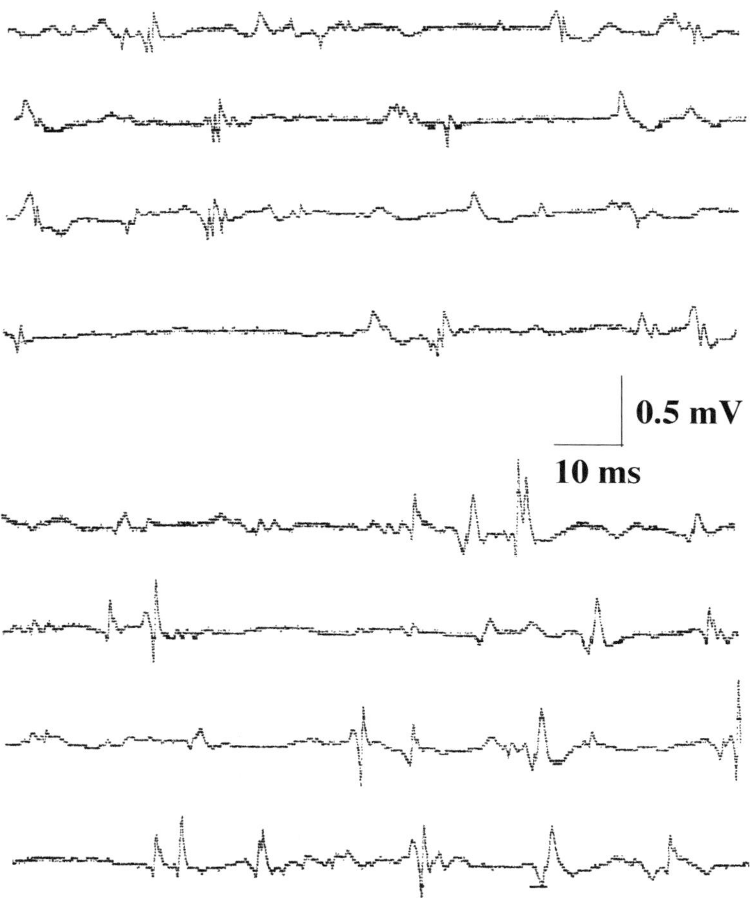

FIGURE 12.6. Many SASD MUPs in the deltoid muscle, typical myopathic MUP pattern in myotonic dystrophy.

and look like fibrillations or PSW. Until waxing and waning of amplitude and frequency are documented with more discharges of potentials, it is impossible to distinguish fibrillation or PSW from myotonic potentials. Myotonic potentials are the EMG hallmarks of myotonia and are invariably associated with clinical myotonia, such as grasp or percussion myotonia. Without myotonic potentials, the diagnosis of clinical myotonia is not justifiable.

In myotonic dystrophy, myotonic potentials are present in all clinically affected cases and most prominent in the distal hand and facial muscles. Not uncommonly, myotonic potentials are absent in proximal muscles and restricted to one or a few muscles. Because EMG myotonia is not present in all muscles, the examination has to include distal and proximal muscles and the facial muscles before it is concluded that EMG myotonia is absent. Although myotonic potentials are seen in newborns affected with congenital myotonic dystrophy, these are frequently absent before the age of 10 years and their frequency then increases progressively with age. MUPs in myotonic dystrophy are typical of myopathy: short-duration MUPs, increased polyphasic MUPs, and early recruitment. These changes are best detected in the forearm extensor and anterior tibialis muscles.

Another simple electrophysiological test for myotonia is postexercise depression (PED), the depression of CMAP amplitude immediately after 10 seconds of exercise as noted in our case. A mean decrease of 62% in the CMAP amplitude in three cases of myotonia congenita

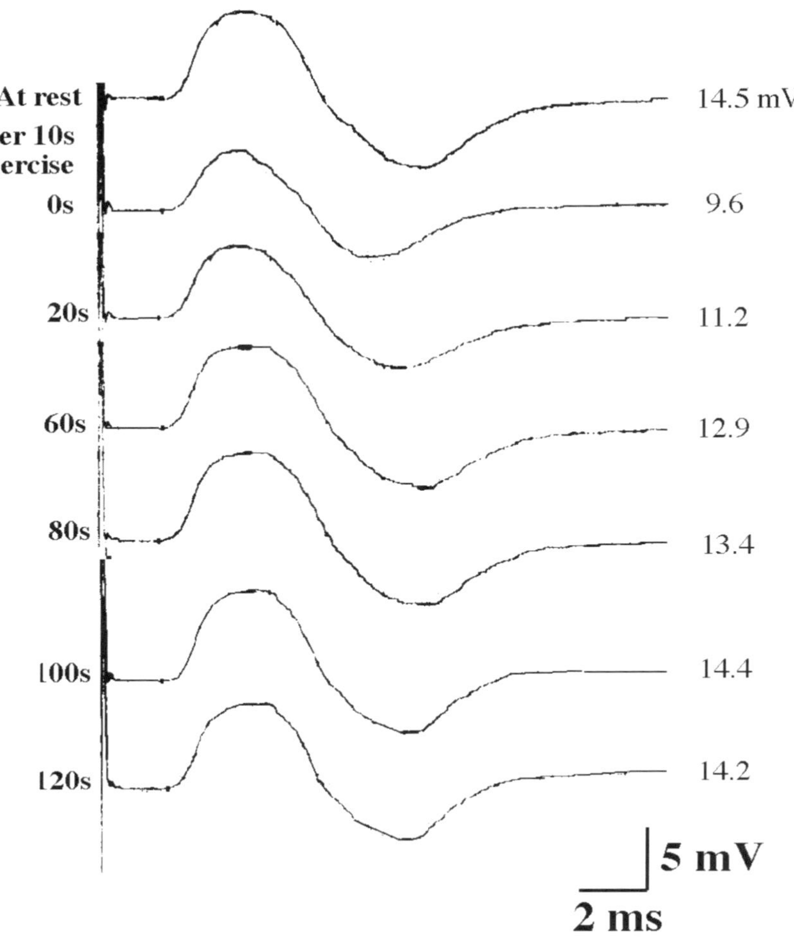

FIGURE 12.7. Postexercise depression typical of myotonic syndromes; 34% decrease of the CMAP amplitude immediately after 10 seconds of exercise, with return to the pre-exercise amplitude in 100 seconds.

and of 39% in 18 cases of myotonic dystrophy was observed. This PED lasted for more than 20 seconds. PED is due to a transient decrease in muscle fiber excitability and represents the well-known exercise-induced paresis after rest seen in myotonic patients. Streib used this test as an objective means of documenting improvement with tocainamide. We found this test useful in testing the severity of myotonia.

MAXIMS

1. In myotonic dystrophy, myotonic discharges are present in all clinically affected cases and the MUPs are typically short in duration in affected muscles.
2. A dramatic decrease in the CMAP amplitude after 10 seconds of exercise (PED) is typical of myotonia.

REFERENCES

1. Streib EW, Sun SF. Distribution of electrical myotonia in myotonic muscular dystrophy. Ann Neurol 1983;14:80–82.
2. Streib EW, Sun SF, Yarkowsky T. Transient paresis in myotonic syndromes: a simplified electrophysiologic approach. Muscle Nerve 1986;5:719–723.

CASE 3

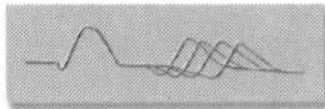

CARDIAC ARREST DURING CATARACT SURGERY

CASE PRESENTATION

In the late 1970s, a 28-year-old man was undergoing cataract surgery in the operating room under general anesthesia. During the surgery, the patient suddenly developed cardiac arrest and was immediately revived with a defibrillator and appropriate medications. ECG after recovery documented a second-degree block with a heart rate of 50 per minute. A cardiology consultant observed a thin man with "nasal tongue." A neurology consultation was requested.

CASE ANALYSIS

This patient presented an interesting constellation of problems: cataract, unexpected anesthetic complications, and "nasal tongue." This combination is strongly suggestive of myotonic dystrophy. In fact, the neurology consultant recognized an elongated face with nasal phonation and frontal balding and elicited without any trouble percussion and grasp myotonia. No weakness or wasting of muscles was apparent.

PLAN OF TESTING

Needle EMG: To confirm myotonic disorder.

ELECTROPHYSIOLOGICAL TESTS AND FINDINGS

`Needle EMG.` Fibrillations, PSW, myotonic discharges, and normal MUP in the right APB muscle and anterior tibialis muscles (Fig. 12.8).

ELECTROPHYSIOLOGICAL INTERPRETATION

Myotonic disorder compatible with myotonic dystrophy.

FINAL DIAGNOSIS

Myotonic dystrophy with cardiomyopathy

TREATMENT AND FOLLOW-UP

A detailed history showed that many family members had unexplained sudden death. Subsequent examination of family members confirmed that many had myotonic dystrophy inherited by an autosomal-dominant pattern. A cardiac pacemaker was implanted in this patient because of the second degree atrioventricular block.

COMMENTS

This patient developed cardiac arrest under general anesthesia due to the common cardiomyopathy associated with myotonic dystrophy. Diagnosis of myotonic dystrophy was not made until this serious complication was encountered during simple cataract surgery.

Unlike other muscular dystrophies, myotonic dystrophy patients invariably have systemic manifestations. Among the various systemic signs, cardiomyopathy, cataracts, and testicular atrophy are most common. In this patient, cataracts were the initial manifestation of myotonic dystrophy and sudden cardiac complication followed. Cataracts are common in patients with myotonic dystrophy. Most can be seen by direct ophthalmoscope. Slit-lamp examination of the eyes reveals cataracts in about 90% of cases. Cardiac involvement is common in myotonic dystrophy. ECG abnormalities are seen in 90% of patients. Bradycardia and first-degree heart block are common. Because of the frequency of cardiac complications, a yearly ECG checkup is recommended in these patients. Sudden death, probably due to progressive heart block, is well recognized as a common cause of death in this disorder. Serious complications of myotonic dystrophy include complete heart block and sudden death. A pacemaker can be a life saver when the patient has unexplainable syncope or when second-degree heart block is demonstrated by Holter monitoring.

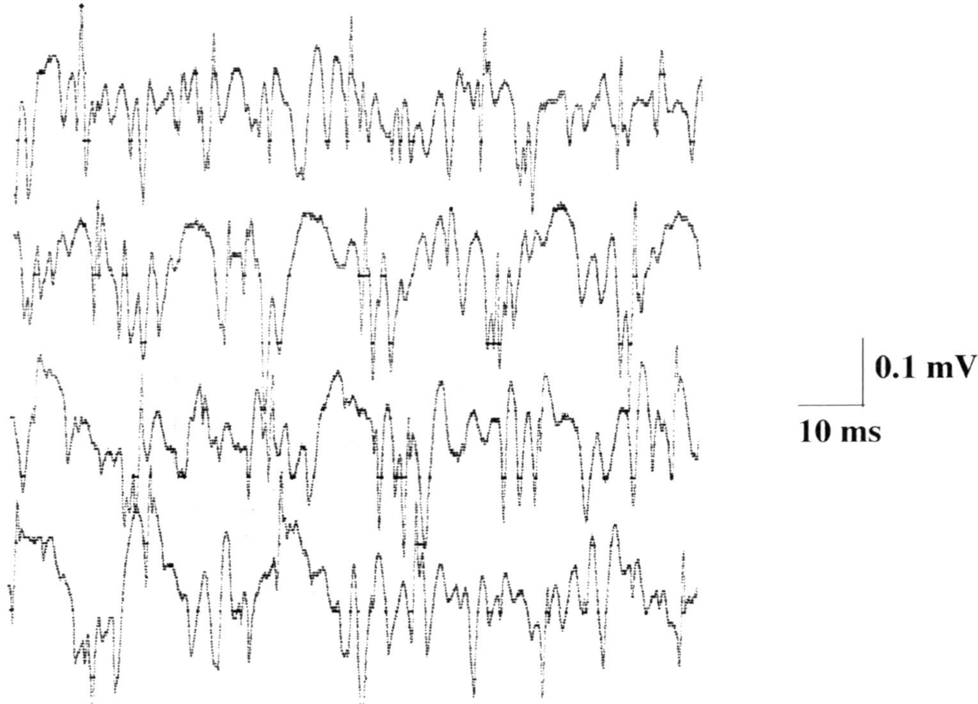

FIGURE 12.8. Waxing and waning of frequency, amplitude, and shape of myotonic potentials is responsible for "dive-bomber" sounds.

For myotonic dystrophy patients, the chance for anesthesia complication is higher. A susceptibility to malignant hyperthermia should be considered in patients with central core disease, Duchenne dystrophy, myotonic dystrophy, and Denborough and King syndrome (nonprogressive congenital myopathy, short-stature, congenital anomalies such as webbed neck and pectus carinatum). Malignant hyperthermia is a rare but potentially lethal disorder characterized by widespread muscle rigidity, hyperthermia, myoglobinuria, metabolic acidosis, and ventricular tachycardia. Because halogenated inhalational anesthetics and succinylcholine are two known agents inducing malignant hyperthermia, these agents should be avoided in patients with myotonic dystrophy. Balanced anesthesia (narcotics, barbiturates, and nitrous oxide) is safe for myotonic dystrophy patients. Also, anticholinesterase should be avoided because it exacerbates myotonia. If muscle relaxation is necessary during anesthesia, a short-acting depolarizing agent is recommended.

MAXIMS

1. Implantation of a cardiac pacemaker is the most important and helpful therapy in myotonic dystrophy. Thus, identification of significant cardiac abnormality is the most important part of the follow-up evaluation in myotonic dystrophy patients.
2. Patients with central core disease, Duchenne dystrophy, myotonic dystrophy, and Denborough and King syndrome are susceptible to malignant hyperthermia.

REFERENCES

1. Phillips MF, Harper PS. Cardiac disease in myotonic dystrophy. Cardiovasc Res 1997;33:13–22.
2. Russell SH, Hirsch NP. Anaesthesia and myotonia. Br J Anaesth 1994;72:210–216.

CASE 4

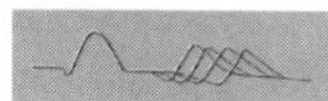

"DISTAL MUSCULAR DYSTROPHY" IN A FEMALE

CASE PRESENTATION

An 18-year-old woman with weakness in the hands for 2 years was now complaining of increasing weakness in her legs and frequent falling episodes. Her falls were due to tripping over her feet. She denied any such difficulty in childhood. She was a slightly obese lady with normal speech and cerebral function and normal reflexes and sensations. She had 4 MRC strength in neck flexor, 4 in the wrist extensors and flexors, 3 in the anterior tibialis, and 3+ in the gastrocnemius muscles. No obvious atrophy or fasciculations were observed. CPK reported by the referring neurologist was 513 units. Muscle biopsy was interpreted as "nonspecific myopathy" by the pathologist on the basis of a large number of muscle fibers with increased central nuclei. The patient was referred to the MDA Clinic under the diagnosis of "distal muscular dystrophy." Her mother denied any history of neuromuscular disease. Her 9-year-old brother had "cerebral palsy" since birth and was in a wheelchair.

CASE ANALYSIS

This patient complained of subacute distal muscle weakness of juvenile onset. In view of her high CPK, muscle biopsy was performed that showed nonspecific myopathy. Thus, the diagnosis of distal muscular dystrophy was made. The diagnostic possibilities in this patient should include spinal muscular atrophy, neuronal type of Charcot-Marie-Tooth disease, distal inclusion body myopathy, and myotonic dystrophy. Thus, the neurological examination should include demonstration of percussion and grasp myotonia, which confirmed the diagnosis in this patient.

PLAN OF TESTING

1. Needle EMG: To confirm myotonic myopathy.
2. Review of muscle biopsy: To rule out evidence of other myopathies, such as "rimmed vacuoles" or muscular dystrophy.

ELECTROPHYSIOLOGICAL TESTS AND FINDINGS

Needle EMG (Table 12.4)

1. Prominent myotonic discharges, increased insertional activity and PSW in the right deltoid, biceps, abductor pollicis brevis, and anterior tibialis muscle.
2. A significant decrease in the mean duration of MUPs in anterior tibialis muscle (Fig. 12.9).

ELECTROPHYSIOLOGICAL INTERPRETATION

Myotonic myopathy typical of myotonic dystrophy.

OTHER TEST FINDINGS

A review of the muscle biopsy showed type I fiber atrophy and many fibers with central nuclei typical of myotonic dystrophy. No rimmed vacuoles or muscle fiber necrosis was noted.

FINAL DIAGNOSIS

Myotonic dystrophy

TREATMENT AND FOLLOW-UP

Even though the patient's mother denied any neuromuscular disease in the family or any neuromuscular complaints, myotonia was easily detected on grasp and percussion. Her ECG was normal. She was tried with dilantin and quinine sulfate without any benefit. Ankle-foot-orthosis for footdrop helped her walking.

COMMENTS

In this case, the neurologist's focus was on the mildly elevated CPK, which is an exception in myotonic dystrophy. In myotonic dystrophy, CPK is usually normal, and a CPK higher

TABLE 12.4. Needle EMG Data in Case 4

				Spontaneous Potentials				Motor Unit Potential			Interference	
Muscle	**Root**	**Nerve**	**Insertion Activity**	**Fib**	**PSW**	**Fasc**	**Myotonic Potential**	**Amplitude (K)**	**Duration (ms)**	**Polyphasic Potential**	**Pattern**	**Mean Amplitude (K)**
Rt deltoids	C5, 6	Axillary	+	–	+	–	+	0.5–3	8–15	N	FIP	2
Biceps	C6	Musc cut	+	–	+ +	–	+	1–4	8–15	N	FIP	2
APB	C8, T1	Median	+	–	+ +	–	+ + +	1–3	8–15	N	FIP	2
Lt ant tibial	L4,5	Peroneal	+	–	+	–	+ +	0.352	7.2[a]	10%	FIP	1

[a] Normal duration of MUP: 10.5 ms.

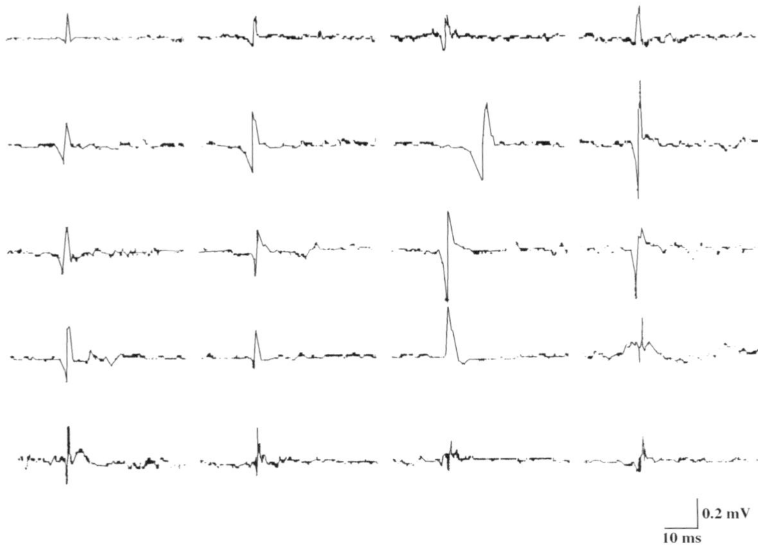

FIGURE 12.9. Twenty MUPs in the anterior tibialis muscle in myotonic dystrophy. Notice many SASD MUPs.

than 1000 units is extremely unusual. Thus, mildly elevated CPK does not rule out myotonic dystrophy. It is always wise to consider the possibility of myotonic disorder in case of myopathy when muscle biopsy is relatively normal.

In female patients, facial features typical of myotonic dystrophy are not prominent, especially in the early stage as seen in this patient. In obese patients, muscle atrophy is not obvious either. As in this case, the presentation of myotonic dystrophy is weakness of muscle. Thus, it is not easy to make the diagnosis of myotonic dystrophy if it is not already suspected. On many occasions, family history is not clearcut, as seen here. No obvious atrophy or myotonic facial features were observed in the mother, but she clearly had percussion and grasp myotonia, which was not a disabling factor.

Most likely, the patient's brother had congenital myotonic dystrophy rather than cerebral palsy. Congenital myotonic dystrophy occurs in 25% of infants of affected mothers. This form is more severe with generalized hypotonia, bulbar weakness (difficulty feeding, swallowing, and breathing), mental retardation, and often clubfoot. A tented upper lip due to weakness of the orbicularis oris muscle is a universal feature. Clinical myotonia is not obvious at birth. Thus, it is important to examine the mother rather than the "floppy infant" when congenital myotonic dystrophy is suspected. In all cases of congenital myotonic dystrophy, the mother is the parent affected. In affected infants, the CTG repeat size tends to be large, but the explanation for the maternal transmission of this severe form of myotonic dystrophy is not well understood.

No single feature in the muscle biopsy is diagnostic of myotonic dystrophy. The most typical finding is type 1 fiber atrophy, as seen in 50% of cases. Ring fibers, sarcoplasmic mass, and central nuclei are classically described as common findings. Muscle fiber necrosis and increased endomysial connective tissue are uncommon in this disorder.

MAXIMS

1. Congenital (infantile) myotonic dystrophy occurs in infants of affected mothers. When this is suspected in floppy infants, it is essential to examine the mother.
2. Type 1 fiber atrophy is the most typical muscle biopsy finding in myotonic dystrophy.

REFERENCES

1. Hageman AT, Gabreels FJ, Liem KD, Renkawek K, Boon JM. Congenital myotonic dystrophy: a report on thirteen cases and a review of the literature. J Neurol Sci 1993;115:95–101.
2. Dubowitz V, Brooke MH. Muscle biopsy: a modern approach. Philadelphia: WB Saunders, 1973: 213–230.

CASE 5

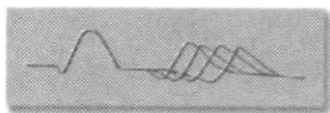

STRONG FAMILY HISTORY OF MUSCULAR DYSTROPHY AND HEART DISEASE

CASE PRESENTATION

A 40-year-old man (J.M.) with a strong family history of muscular dystrophy came to the MDA Clinic for a 1-year history of general fatigue. His two sisters, nephews, numerous cousins, and his grandmother and mother had muscular dystrophy. Several maternal uncles had suffered from heart attacks in their 40s. The patient had been very active, played high school football, and worked as a landscaper. For 2 years, he had been under the care of a cardiologist for mitral valve prolapse. He denied changes in his vision, swallowing function, or speech. With further questioning, the patient did report occasional difficulty opening bottles or jars. Neurological examination showed a thin, long face with mild facial diplegia, normal strength in all muscles except for myotonia in bilateral handgrips, and percussion myotonia of the thenar eminence.

His younger sister (C.B.) and nephew (C.M.) had been previously evaluated at the MDA Clinic. C.B. was a 39-year-old woman with a history of heart arrhythmias since 1978, requiring cardioversion. She reported some difficulty grasping objects due primarily to her inability to release them, which she claimed developed after a motor vehicle accident. She had two children: one had a heart problem and the other (C.M.) had a learning disability. Muscle strength was normal in all extremities except for mild weakness in the hands due to grasp myotonia.

C.M. was a 19-year-old man who complained of cramping in his legs. As a child, he had had trouble running and now experienced mild difficulty with tripping and getting out of bed. He was in a special class in high school and graduated at age 19. Abnormal neurological findings were thin face, nasal speech, percussion, and grasp myotonias.

CASE ANALYSIS

In view of its strong autosomal-dominant inheritance pattern, myotonic dystrophy was a definite possibility. Among the various muscular dystrophies, myotonic dystrophy is one of two that is inherited by autosomal-dominant pattern. The other is facioscapulohumeral muscular dystrophy. What was striking in these three patients was the apparent lack of two of the cardinal features of myotonic dystrophy: frontal balding and distal muscle atrophy or weakness. Clearly, the presence of percussion and grasp myotonia, subtle facial features of myotonic dystrophy in males, and cardiomyopathy in two members were indicative of myotonic dystrophy.

PLAN OF TESTING

1. Needle EMG: To confirm the diagnosis of myotonic disorder.
2. Trinucleotide CTG test: To further confirm the diagnosis of myotonic dystrophy in view of the mild clinical features.
3. CPK: As a routine test for myopathy.
4. EKG in J.M.: To see whether there is any cardiac dysrhythmia.

ELECTROPHYSIOLOGICAL TESTS AND FINDINGS

Needle EMG (Table 12.5)

1. Myotonic potentials in most muscles tested in all three patients (Fig. 12.10).
2. Fibrillations and PSWs in two tested muscles in J.M.

TABLE 12.5. Needle EMG Data in Case 5

				Spontaneous Potentials				Motor Unit Potential				Interference	
Muscle	**Root**	**Nerve**	**Insertion Activity**	**Fib**	**PSW**	**Fasc**	**Myotonic Potential**	**Amplitude (K)**	**Duration (ms)**	**Polyphasic Potential**	**SASD MUP**	**Pattern**	**Mean Amplitude (K)**
MJ													
Rt APB	C8, T1	Median	+	+	±	–	+ + +	0.5–2	6–12	N	–	RIP	2
Ant tibial	L3,4	Peroneal	+	+	+	–	+ + +	0.5–4	6–14	N	–	FIP	3
CB													
Rt deltoid	C5,6	Axillary	+	–	–	–	+	1–4	9–15	N	–	FIP	3
Biceps	C6,7	Musc cut	+	–	+	–	+	1–2	8–15	N	–	FIP	2
Triceps	C7	Radial	+	–	–	–	+	1–3	8–15	N	–	FIP	3
APB	C8, T1	Median	+	–	–	–	+ +	1–3	8–15	N	–	RIP	2
MC													
Rt deltoids	C5,6	Axillary	N	–	–	–	–	0.5–2	6–10	+	–	FIP	2
EDC	C6,7	Radial	+	–	–	–	+ +	0.5–2	3–8	+	+	FIP	2
APB	C8, T1	Median	+	–	–	–	+ + +	0.6–1.5	6–12	N	–	FIP	2.5
Ant tibial	L4,5	Peroneal	+	–	–	–	+	0.6–2	4–10	+	+	FIP	1.5

EDC, extensor carpi communis.

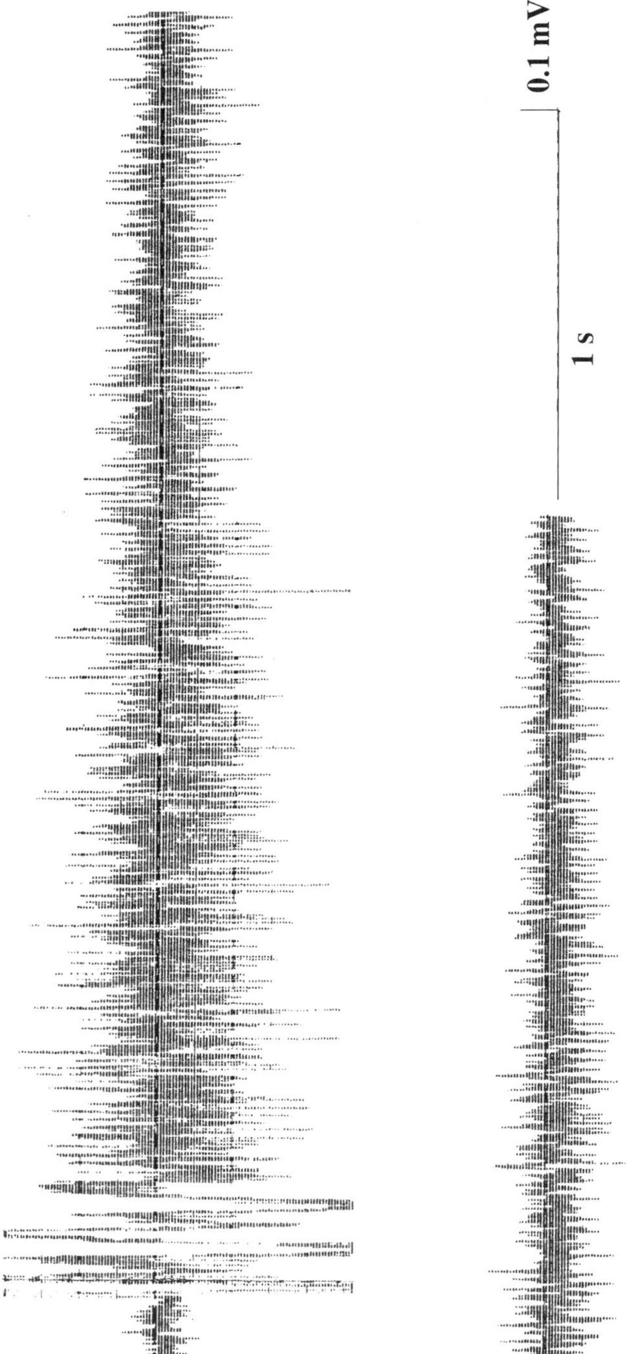

FIGURE 12.10. Continuous recording of myotonic potentials showing waxing and waning of frequency, amplitude, and shape.

3. Normal MUPs in all tested muscles in J.M. and C.B.
4. Some SASD MUPs in the extensor digitorum communis and anterior tibialis muscles in M.C.

ELECTROPHYSIOLOGICAL INTERPRETATION

Myotonic disorder in J.M. and C.B. and myotonic myopathy typical of myotonic dystrophy in M.C.

OTHER TEST FINDINGS

Trinucleotide CTG test detected an expansion greater than 50 repeats.

FINAL DIAGNOSIS

Myotonic dystrophy

TREATMENT AND FOLLOW-UP

CPK values were all normal in three of the members. EKG in J.M. was normal. For muscle cramps, quinine sulfate was effective in J.M. and Valium in C.M. Their course was stable over the next 5 years of the follow-up period.

COMMENTS

Despite a strong known family history, none of these three patients thought they were affected by myotonic dystrophy because of minimal clinical symptoms. They did not have the classic features of myotonic dystrophy that clinch the diagnosis easily. In fact, the resident physician presented the proband as a case of facioscapulohumeral muscular dystrophy in view of his facial weakness and strong family history.

In 1992, three groups simultaneously discovered in leukocyte DNA from myotonic dystrophy patients abnormal expansion of the unstable trinucleotide repeat CTG located on the untranslated 3′ end on chromosome 19. This segment codes for a protein kinase. Normal individuals have approximately 5 to 27 copies of this repeated DNA segment, whereas myotonic dystrophy patients have a CTG repeat greater than 50 copies. Patients with mild myotonic dystrophy have 50 to 70 copies, whereas those that are severely affected may have up to several thousand copies of the unstable fragment. The repeat generally expands from generation to generation correlating with worsening severity. This is more likely to occur when the mother is the affected parent. It appears that the ovum is able to support continued expansion of the unstable repeat throughout meiosis, whereas the sperm is not. Thus, infants with congenital myotonic dystrophy have the largest repeats and on average their mothers have larger repeats than mothers of infants without congenital myotonic dystrophy.

As a result of the discovery of the dystrophica myotonia (DM) gene, specific DNA diagnostic tests are now available to determine whether one has myotonic dystrophy or not in at-risk individuals. DNA testing can now play a critical role in establishing the prenatal diagnosis of myotonic dystrophy, and it can be used to predict the likelihood of whether a pregnant myotonic dystrophy woman will have a baby with the severe congenital form of myotonic dystrophy. Using cultured amniocytes or chorionic villus samples, one study found that the analysis of CTG repeat size was accurate in excluding or identifying the presence of myotonic dystrophy in the fetus and in predicting the severity of symptoms.

MAXIMS

1. Myotonic dystrophy is one of three neuromuscular diseases with the abnormal trinucleotide repeat. Other diseases are Kennedy's disease (X-linked spinobulbar muscular atrophy) (CAG repeat) and spinocerebellar ataxia type 1 (CAG repeat).
2. In congenital myotonic dystrophy, CTG repeat is larger than in adult myotonic dystrophy.

REFERENCES

1. Ptacek LJ, Johnson KJ, Griggs RC. Genetics and physiology of the myotonic muscle disorders. N Engl Med 1993;328:482–489.

CASE 6

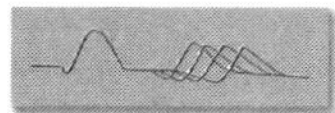

MUSCLE STIFFNESS SINCE EARLY CHILDHOOD

CASE PRESENTATION

A 20-year-old woman's development was normal in early childhood, but since the age of 5 or 6 she had complained of muscle stiffness that had been gradually getting worse. It is interesting that among five siblings, two brothers and three sisters, all the sisters had the same problem with stiffness of the muscles but none of the boys were affected. At this time, she had difficulty climbing stairs. Her stiffness was usually most prominent after prolonged rest and was improved by warm-up movements. Stress, nervousness, and cold weather seemed to aggravate it. Her mother noted that she had rather bulky muscles.

Abnormal neurological findings were bulky muscles, especially in biceps, quadriceps, and calf muscles; grasp myotonia; percussion myotonia in thenar and forearm extensor muscles; 5 – MRS strength in the neck flexor and extensor, deltoid, and iliopsoas muscles; and "stiff gait." There was no obvious speech difficulty, no myotonic eyelids, no bulbar abnormalities, or difficulty in knee bending.

CASE ANALYSIS

This patient had muscle stiffness since early childhood, "bulky muscles," a strong family history, and classic description of myotonia symptoms. There was no evidence of systemic manifestations or myopathy (muscle weakness or wasting) to suggest the possibility of myotonic dystrophy. Thus, findings are classic for myotonia congenita of Thomsen's disease.

PLAN OF TESTING

1. Needle EMG: To confirm myotonia and check for any EMG evidence of myopathy.
2. RNS test: To document PED and RNS features typical of myotonic disorder.
3. CPK

ELECTROPHYSIOLOGICAL TESTS AND FINDINGS

Needle EMG (Table 12.6)

1. Increased insertional activity in the right deltoid, anterior tibialis, and APB muscles.
2. PSW and fibrillations in the right deltoid.
3. Myotonic potentials in all tested muscles.
4. Difficulty of obtaining MUPs with minimal contracture because MUPs tended to disappear with minimal contraction. Those MUPs obtained were normal.

RNS Test Findings (Table 12.7)

1. Repetitive discharges in the CMAP (Fig. 12.11).
2. Normal CMAP amplitude at rest, but marked decrease in the CMAP amplitude after exercise (PED).
3. No decremental response at the low rate of stimulation.
4. Marked decremental response at the high rate of stimulation (Fig. 12.12).

ELECTROPHYSIOLOGICAL INTERPRETATION

Myotonic disorder compatible with myotonia congenita

FINAL DIAGNOSIS

Myotonia congenita of Thomsen's type

TREATMENT AND FOLLOW-UP

ECG was normal. Ophthalmological evaluation showed no cataracts. Mexiletine 750 mg/day relieved the patient's stiffness enough for her to take care of her daily activities without any trouble.

TABLE 12.6. Needle EMG Data in Case 6

				Spontaneous Potentials				Motor Unit Potential			Interference	
Muscle	**Root**	**Nerve**	**Insertion Activity**	**Fib**	**PSW**	**Fasc**	**Myotonic Potential**	**Amplitude (K)**	**Duration (ms)**	**Polyphasic Potential**	**Pattern**	**Mean Amplitude (K)**
Rt deltoid	C5,6	Axillary	+	+	+	–	+++	0.4–1	7–14	N	FIP	1
Ant tibial[a]	L3,4	Peroneal	+	–	–	–	+++	0.4–1	9–14	N	FIP	2
APB[b]	C8, T1	Median	+	+	–	–	+++	0.5–1.5	8–15	N	FIP	2

[a] MUPs disappear after exercise.

[b] Extremely difficult to obtain MUP on minimal contraction due to myotonic potentials.

TABLE 12.7. RNS Test Data in Case 6

	ADQ Muscle
CMAP (mV)	14.6
CMAP Ex (%)	−88
2 Hz (%)	0
3 Hz (%)	0
5 Hz (%)	0
50 Hz (%)	−58[a]
5 Hz PT 0 (%)	+5
5 Hz PT 4 m (%)	0

[a] Nonsmooth decrement. ADQ, abductor digiti quinti.

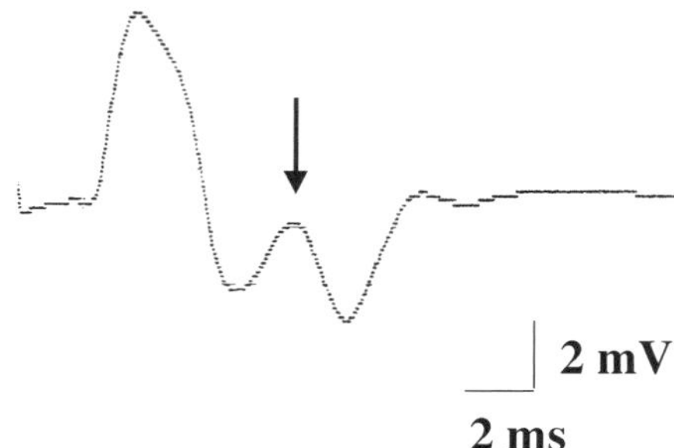

FIGURE 12.11. Repetitive discharge (*arrow*) of the CMAP in the median motor nerve conduction in myotonia congenita. This can be rarely observed in myotonic syndromes. The CMAP can be repetitive after two or three stimulations.

COMMENTS

Repetitive discharges in the CMAP are usually indicative of acetylcholine overactivity, as typically seen in anticholinesterase toxicity, organophosphate poisoning, and hyperirritable peripheral nerve disorder (neuromyotonia). This has also been reported in myotonic disorder and is due to hyperirritable muscle membrane in myotonic disorder.

Congenital myotonia is differentiated from myotonic dystrophy by the lack of muscle weakness and other system abnormalities. Thus, myotonia is the principal feature of myotonia congenita and the most disabling. This is in contrast to most patients with myotonic dystrophy, in whom myotonia is rarely disabling.

Myotonia congenita is classified into two forms depending on the basis of the inheritance pattern: autosomal-dominant Thomsen's disease and autosomal-recessive generalized myotonia (Becker's disease). In Thomsen's disease, described by Thomsen in 1876, myotonia is usually noted from infancy and generalized. There is no wasting or weakness of muscles. Instead, muscles are hypertrophied, giving sometimes a Herculean appearance. The disease is essentially nonprogressive.

Becker's disease, described in the 1960s and 1970s, is more common than Thomsen's disease. In certain cases, the clinical features are indistinguishable from those of Thomsen's disease. However, Becker found distinct overall differences between the two genetic varieties, although there is considerable overlap. Age of onset ranged from 4 to 12 years. In most patients, symptoms of myotonia began and were most severe in the legs. Muscle hypertrophy was common but usually spared the forearms, where mild atrophy was frequently evident. The disease tended to be progressive, and weakness was present to some degree in most patients.

Thomsen's and Becker's diseases are caused by at least seven different mutations in the ClCN1 (ClC-1) skeletal muscle chloride channel gene on chromosome 7q35.

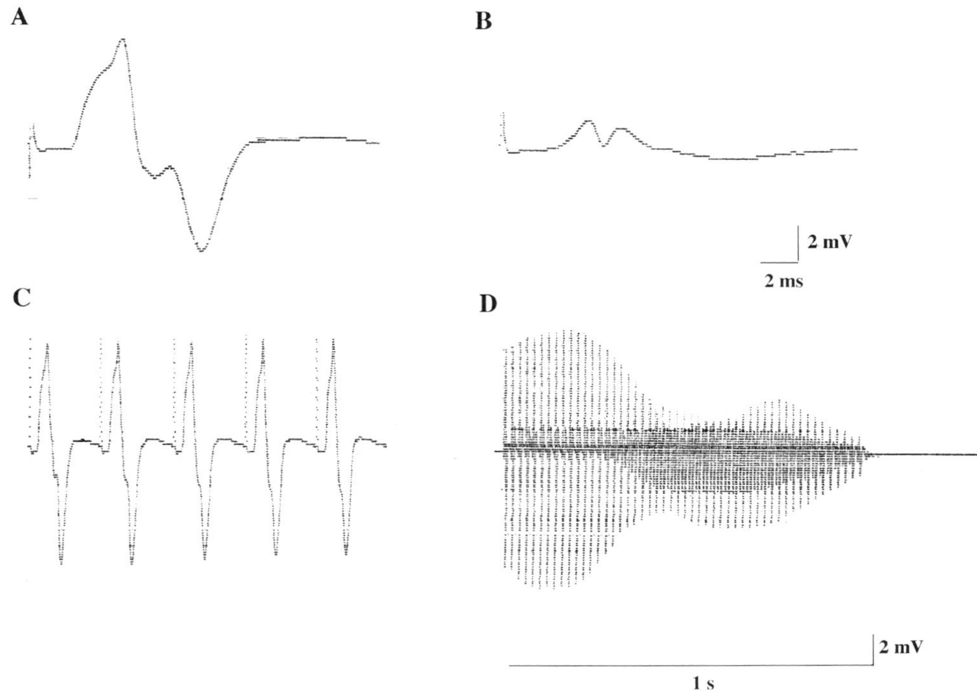

FIGURE 12.12. Repetitive nerve stimulation test in the ADQ muscles. **A.** The CMAP with a repetitive discharge at rest. **B.** Marked postexercise depression after 10 seconds of exercise. **C.** No decremental response at 5-Hz stimulation. **D.** Marked decremental response at 50-Hz stimulation. Notice the peculiar shape of decremental response that is different from the smooth decremental response in MG.

MAXIMS

1. The principal clinical feature of myotonia congenita is myotonia. Systemic abnormalities and obvious muscle atrophy or weakness are absent in myotonia congenita.
2. Thomsen's and Becker's diseases are chloride channel disorders.

REFERENCES

1. Streib EW. Differential diagnosis of myotonic syndromes. Muscle Nerve 1987;10:603–615.
2. Moxley R III. The myotonias: their diagnosis and treatment. Comp Ther 1996;22:8–21.

CASE 7

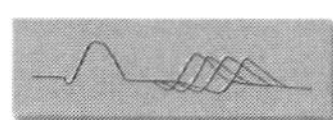

INCIDENTAL FINDINGS OF MYOTONIC POTENTIALS IN THE NEEDLE EMG

CASE PRESENTATION

A 32-year-old woman was referred to the EMG Laboratory for workup of left cervical radiculopathy. Three weeks previously, she had developed sudden sharp "neuralgic pain" in the left C3-4 distribution followed by numbness that lasted for 3 hours. This was soon followed by weakness in the left arm. The referring neurologist documented slight weakness in the left deltoid, supra- and infraspinatus muscles, and reduced pin-prick sensation over the left C2-4 dermatomes. Cervical spine x-ray showed spina bifida occulta at the C7-T1 spine. The patient had a history of migraine.

CASE ANALYSIS

The history and findings suggest two possibilities: high cervical radiculopathy and acute brachial plexus neuropathy (Parsonage-Turner syndrome; neuralgic amyotrophy). This patient was referred to the EMG Laboratory with a neurologist's impression of left acute brachial plexus neuropathy.

PLAN OF TESTING

1. NCS: To distinguish between cervical radiculopathy and brachial plexus neuropathy. Left median and ulnar motor and sensory nerve conductions, including left lateral antebrachial sensory nerve.
2. Needle EMG: In the left arm muscles and trapezius and cervical paraspinal muscles.

ELECTROPHYSIOLOGICAL TESTS AND FINDINGS

NCS Findings (Table 12.8)

1. Slow sensory NCV and low CNAP amplitude in the finger-wrist segments of the left median and ulnar nerves.
2. Slow mixed NCV and low CNAP amplitude in the elbow-axilla segment of the left median and ulnar nerves.
3. Slow sensory maximum NCV and low CNAP amplitude in the left lateral antebrachial nerve.
4. Normal motor NCS in the left median and ulnar nerves.

Needle EMG (Table 12.9)

1. Myotonic potentials, fibrillations, and PSW in all tested muscles, including the cervical paraspinal muscles (Fig. 12.13).
2. Increased polyphasic MUPs and RIP in the left deltoid, infra- and supraspinatus, and biceps muscles.

ELECTROPHYSIOLOGICAL INTERPRETATION

1. Widespread myotonic potentials indicative of myotonic disorder compatible with myotonia congenita.
2. Abnormal sensory and mixed nerve conductions in the left ulnar and median nerves and increased polyphasic MUPs and RIP in some tested muscles, which are compatible with acute left brachial plexus neuropathy.

FINAL DIAGNOSIS

1. Autosomal-recessive myotonia congenita (Becker type of myotonia congenita).
2. Acute left brachial plexus neuropathy (neuralgic amyotrophy).

TREATMENT AND FOLLOW-UP

With the first insertion of the EMG needle, prominent fibrillations and PSWs were noted. In addition, there was a classic "dive-bomber sound," indicating that fibrillations and PSWs were due to myotonic potentials. The patient was more thoroughly examined. The only abnormality detected was percussion and grasp myotonia. No weakness or atrophy of muscles was

TABLE 12.8. Nerve Conduction Data in Case 7

	Latent/NCV (ms/m/s)	Amplitude (mV/μV)	Shape
Left	**Median**	**Motor**	**Nerve**
TL	2.4	8.0	N
E-W	61.5	7.8	N
AX-E	68.6	7.5	N
F-wave	28.5		
	Ulnar	**Motor**	**Nerve**
TL	2.25	11.6	N
BE-W	65.6	9.0	N
AE-BE	60.0	9.2	N
AX-AE	70.8	8.5	N
F-wave	29.0		
	Median	**Sens/Mixed**	**Nerve**
F-W	38.5	6.0	N
W-E	52.1	12.2	N
E-AX	46.7	8.0	N
	Ulnar	**Sens/Mixed**	**Nerve**
F-W	33.3	7.5	N
W-E	51.9	11.0	N
E-AX	45.5	5.0	N
	Lateral antbebrachial	**Sens**	**Nerve**
E-Forearm	45.5	5.0	N

Height: 165 cm.

TL, terminal latency; W, wrist; E, elbow; BE, below elbow; AE, above elbow; AX, axilla; F, finger; N, normal.

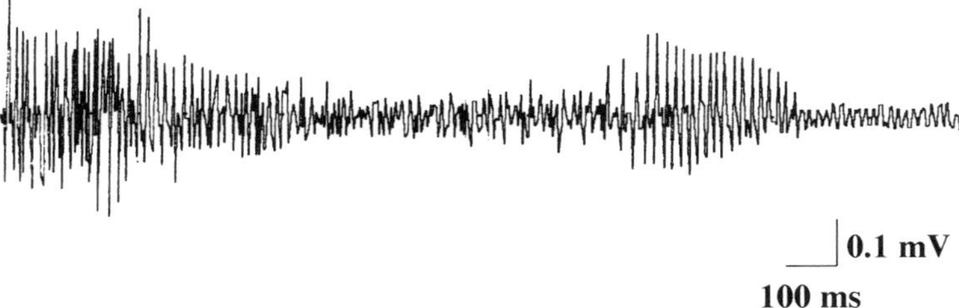

FIGURE 12.13. Myotonic potentials in Becker-type myotonia congenita.

noted, no sign of systemic manifestations. In retrospect, the patient admitted muscle cramps and stiffness all over the body since childhood. No family history of myotonia was obtained. In the ensuing 3 months, left arm weakness and sensory loss gradually improved completely, confirming the diagnosis of acute brachial plexus neuropathy. CT of the cervical cord was also normal. Since then, the patient's myotonia has been treated with 300 mg Dilantin/day with good results.

COMMENTS

In this case, myotonia congenita was not suspected until the classic "dive-bomber" sound was recognized as myotonia in the EMG laboratory during an unrelated workup. It is not unusual

TABLE 12.9. Needle EMG Data in Case 7

				Spontaneous Potentials				Motor Unit Potential			Interference	
Muscle	**Root**	**Nerve**	**Insertion Activity**	**Fib**	**PSW**	**Fasc**	**Myotonic Potential**	**Amplitude (K)**	**Duration (ms)**	**Polyphasic Potential**	**Pattern**	**Mean Amplitude (K)**
Lt C5-8 paraspinal	C5-8		+	+++	+++	−	+++					
Trapezius	C2-4	Accessory	+	++	++	−	+++	0.5–1.5	5–10	N	FIP	1
Supraspinatus	C5	Suprascapular	+	++	++	−	+++	0.5–1.7	6–12	+	RIP	1.5
Infraspinatus	C5	Suprascapular	+	+	+	−	+++	0.4–1.2	6–10	+	RIP	1
Deltoid	C5,6	Axillary	+	+	+	−	+++	0.5–2.0	7–15	+	RIP	2
Biceps	C5,6	Axillary	+	+	+	−	+++	0.3–2.5	6–15	+	RIP	2
Triceps	C7	Radial	+	+	+	−	+++	0.4–1.7	6–12	N	FIP	1.5
OP	C8, T1	Median	+	++	++	−	+++	0.5–1.5	6–10	N	FIP	1
Rt OP	C8, T1	Median	+	+++	+++	−	+++	0.4–1.8	6–12	N	FIP	1.5

OP, opponens pollicus.

that mild cases of myotonia congenita go unrecognized, as noted in this patient. In view of the sporadic nature of the disease, this case is an example of the autosomal-recessive form of myotonia congenita (Becker's disease).

Fibrillations and PSWs are invariably observed in myotonic muscles. Thus, in patients with myotonic disorder, denervation process can not be identified by fibrillations or PSWs and normal MUP, but it should be identified on the basis of the HALD MUPs.

There are many drugs effective for relief of myotonia. In this case, phenytoin was effective in relieving myotonia. Historically, quinine and procainamide are the first two drugs used for this purpose and considered to be the most satisfactory treatment. They can be taken intermittently when symptoms are troublesome. In patients requiring chronic treatment for myotonia, phenytoin is the first agent of choice because of its relatively low incidence of side effects, but it is not always effective. In recent years, mexiletine and tocainide were found to be the most potent antimyotonic agents. The antimyotonic efficacy of mexiletine and tocainide is explained by their fast-blocking effect on voltage-dependent sodium channels in the muscle membrane. They have been reported to be effective in myotonia congenita and paramyotonia congenita and have the added benefit of preventing weakness in paramyotonia. Thus, these agents can be tried if phenytoin is not effective. The benefits of myotonia control with pharmacological agents must be weighed against the risk of therapy in the individual patient. Because of the risks of hematologic problems, we do not recommend tocanide for the treatment of myotonia. In patients with cardiac conduction defects, as often seen in myotonic dystrophy, phenytoin is theoretically preferable because it speeds conduction through the atrioventricular node. Acetazolamide, the commonly used drug for periodic paralysis, was found to be effective in paramyotonia congenita with potassium-sensitive periodic paralysis, but it was most dramatic in alleviating myotonia in acetazolamide-responsive myotonia and more effective than other antimyotonic agents in this condition. There are a few agents that aggravate myotonia: anticholinesterase agents and potassium.

MAXIMS

1. Fibrillations and PSWs are invariably present in myotonic muscles.
2. Antimyotonic drugs are most effective in treating myotonia in myotonia congenita syndromes and less effective in myotonic dystrophy.

REFERENCES

1. Kwiecinski H, Ryniewicz B, Ostrzycki A. Treatment of myotonia with antiarrhythmic drugs. Acta Neurol Scand 1992;86:371–375.
2. Streib EW. Successful treatment with tocainide of recessive generalized congenital myotonia. Ann Neurol 1986;19:501–504.

CASE 8

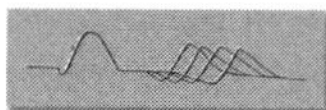

MUSCLE STIFFNESS AND WEAKNESS INDUCED BY COLD

CASE PRESENTATION

A 17-year-old boy noted painless spasms in his hands when exposed to cold since the age of 1.5 years. These episodes usually were not precipitated by cold immersion of the hands, but by chilling of the entire body. At times, swallowing ice cubes induced a choking sensation and difficulty speaking because of dysarthria. He also had intermittent stiffness and paralysis since 12 years of age, when he first noted symptoms of weakness in his legs; while attempting to get up from a desk at the end of a period at school, he was unable to move his legs. This lasted 1 to 2 hours and passed spontaneously. At 15, he had the worst attack. He went to bed with a high fever and awakened the following morning unable to move any muscles except his eyes, neck, and bulbar muscles. He was able to breathe and speak normally, however. During these episodes, observers noted that the involved muscles were firm and tense and that his skin was generally cool. Since then, the patient had many minor episodes of stiffness and weakness in his lower legs. These occurred often while resting after periods of exercise and occasionally were related to missing a meal. When he experienced an aura before a spell, he could avoid some episodes by moving around. His mother and a half-sister from a different father had similar problems.

Abnormal neurological examination showed somewhat hypertrophied gastrocnemius; mild weakness in neck flexor, deltoid, and hand muscles; percussion myotonia in the tongue and thenar muscles; and paradoxical myotonia in the eyelids.

CASE ANALYSIS

This patient had autosomal-dominant neuromuscular disease characterized by two major problems: spasms of the hands and bulbar muscles induced by cold and episodic attacks of weakness or paralysis of the limb muscles sparing bulbar and respiratory muscles. Cold-induced spasms are typical of paramyotonia. The clinical description of these episodic attacks of weakness is typical of periodic paralysis. Neurological examination clearly showed that this patient had myotonia, pseudohypertrophy of the gastrocnemius muscles, and mild proximal myopathy, confirming the diagnosis of myotonic myopathy. The constellation of findings clearly suggested paramyotonia congenita together with potassium-sensitive (hyperkalemic) periodic paralysis.

PLAN OF TESTING

1. Needle EMG: To document myotonic potentials.
2. CPK
3. Provocative tests for periodic paralysis: To decide whether periodic paralysis was hypokalemic or potassium-sensitive periodic paralysis.

ELECTROPHYSIOLOGICAL TESTS AND FINDINGS

Needle EMG (Table 12.10)

1. Myotonic discharges and normal MUP in all tested muscles (Fig. 12.14).
2. After cooling with ice, myotonic discharges were less prominent and fewer MUPs were recruited.

ELECTROPHYSIOLOGICAL INTERPRETATION

Myotonic disorder compatible with paramyotonia congenita.

OTHER TEST FINDINGS

CPK was normal. No paresis occurred with oral K loading test (serum K 7.5 mEq/dL) or glucose-insulin infusion test (serum K 3.2 mEq/dL versus pretest K 4.3). Vigorous exercise test induced a brief period of stiffness and weakness in the lower legs (serum K 4.1 mEq/dL). Cold-exposure test in a walk-in refrigerator for 15 minutes induced marked cramping in the hands, some stiffness in the face, thick speech, and marked myotonic eyelids. Marked spasms in the hands lasted 4 to 5 hours (serum K 3.8 mEq/dL). One hour after a low Na diet and

TABLE 12.10. Needle EMG Data in Case 8

				Spontaneous Potentials				Motor Unit Potential			Interference	
Muscle	**Root**	**Nerve**	**Insertion Activity**	**Fib**	**PSW**	**Fasc**	**Myotonic Potential**	**Amplitude (K)**	**Duration (ms)**	**Polyphasic Potential**	**Pattern**	**Mean Amplitude (K)**
Rt APB[a]	C8, T1	Median	+	+	++	−	++	0.5–2.0	6–14	N	RIP	2
Deltoid	C5,6	Axillary	+	−	++++	−	++	0.3–1.5	5–12	N	RIP	1
Vast lat	L3,4	Femoral	+	−	+++	−	++	0.7–1.8	6–10	N	RIP	1

[a] With ice cooling to 22 C, myotonic potentials became less prominent and a fewer MUPs were recruited.

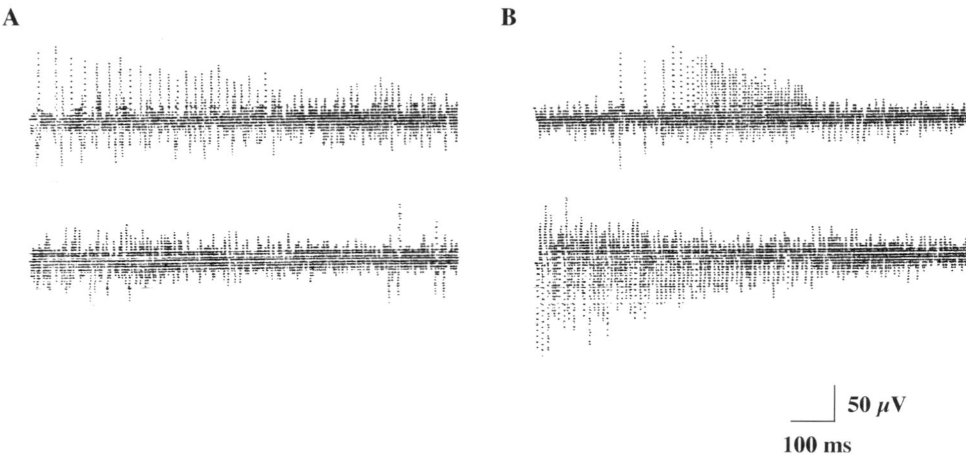

FIGURE 12.14. Myotonic potentials in the deltoid muscle at room temperature in paramyotonia congenita. **A.** Continuous recordings of myotonic potentials. **B.** Two separate recordings of myotonic potentials.

12 g of oral KCl, the patient developed attacks of weakness of the legs, neck, and lower jaw (K was 5.2 mEq/dL).

FINAL DIAGNOSIS

Paramyotonia congenita and potassium-sensitive periodic paralysis

TREATMENT AND FOLLOW-UP

This patient is now a 42-year-old man who is fully employed. He has been taking dilantin and acetazolamide 500 mg/day. A cholesterol-rich diet such as spaghetti and potatoes led to improvement in his overall condition. A bowl of cereal loaded with sugar between 10:00 PM and midnight each evening ensures improved motor ability the following day. Neurological examination showed myotonia of the eyelids with paradoxical myotonia. Neck extensors and flexors were 5 in strength; deltoids 5; biceps 4+; triceps 5−; wrist extensors, flexors, and handgrip 5; iliopsoas 4+. Further study showed that two of his three daughters had the same problem.

COMMENTS

The salient features of paramyotonia congenita are prolonged muscle stiffness and weakness induced by cold; episodic flaccid weakness, usually related to cold; myotonic eyelid; and paradoxical myotonia. Facial, hand, tongue, and pharyngeal muscles are most sensitive to this reaction. Myotonia is typically diminished with repeated exercise. If myotonia worsens with repeated activity, it is termed paradoxical myotonia. This is particularly well observed in eyelid closure in paramyotonia congenita. Grasp and percussion myotonia may be seen as unrelated to cold. Muscle hypertrophy is usual. In addition to the cold/exercise-induced localized muscle paralysis, some patients have independent generalized attacks of paralysis that is usually potassium-sensitive. Paramyotonia congenita is rare and manifests itself in early childhood and is nonprogressive. It is autosomal-dominantly inherited with a high penetrance of the gene. Potassium-sensitive paralysis does not occur in all families but in fact is rare. This syndrome is now well recognized as a sodium-channel disorder—sodium channel gene on chromosome 17. An elevated serum K level during a paralytic attack is diagnostic of hyperkalemic periodic paralysis, but serum levels need not be elevated during repeated attacks in the same patient. A diagnosis of hyperkalemic periodic paralysis can also be confirmed with a positive K challenge.

TABLE 12.11. Needle EMG Findings in Paramyotonia Congenita and Myotonia Congenita

	Paramyotonia Congenita	Myotonia Congenita
At rest[a]	No clear difference in myotonic discharges and MUPs between two	
Ice-water cooling[a]		
Myotonic discharges	Disappear	Increase
MUP recruitment:	MUP: dropout and finally electrically silent	Normal
Postexercise fibrillations[b,c]	(+)	(−)
RNS test with cooling[c]		
Amplitude of the CMAP	Significant fall	Minimal change
2-Hz stimulation	Decremental response is induced or worsened	No change

[a] Nielson (1982).

[b] Needle EMG immediately after an exercise to the degree of exhaustion.

[c] Subramony (1983).

Needle EMG in paramyotonia congenita shows a characteristic myotonic discharge with normal MUP at room temperature. With cooling, myotonic discharges gradually disappear and MUPs drop out, finally reaching electrical silence as noted in this case. With cooling, there is a significant decline in the CMAP amplitude, and 2-Hz stimulation induces or worsens decremental response in the RNS test. These are distinctly different from those found in myotonia congenita and thus can be used for confirmation of paramyotonia (Table 12.11).

In addition to paramyotonia congenita, two more rare sodium-channel myotonic disorders have been described: myotonia fluctuans and acetazolamide-responsive myotonia. Myotonia fluctuans, which was first described in 1990, follows an autosomal-dominant mode of transmission. In contrast to classic myotonia congenita and paramyotonia congenita, the myotonia fluctuates to an unusual degree and does not worsen with cold but increases markedly with potassium loading. Needle EMG shows a characteristic exercise-induced delayed-onset myotonia; relaxation of muscle is normal immediately after exercise, but within a few minutes a minor stimulus may provoke severe myotonia.

Acetazolamide-responsive myotonia, first described in 1987, is also inherited in an autosomal-dominant manner. This is characterized by painful muscle stiffness that is provoked by fasting and oral potassium (some patients require a banana-free diet) and relieved by carbohydrate-containing foods. Myotonia is dramatically relieved by acetazolamide and exacerbated by cold. Cold never produces weakness or paralysis. Needle EMG shows classic myotonic potentials with normal MUPs.

MAXIMS

1. Paradoxical myotonia is one of the characteristic features of paramyotonia congenita and myotonia becomes worse with warm-up exercises.
2. In paramyotonia congenita, myotonic discharges diminish and MUPs dropout with cooling, finally reaching electrical silence.

REFERENCES

1. Nielsen V, Friis M, Johnson T. Electromyographic distinction between paramyotonia congenita and myotonia congenita. Neurology 1982;32:826–832.
2. Subramony SH, Malhotra CP, Mishra SK. Distinguishing pramyotonia congenita and myotonia congenita by electromyography. Muscle Nerve 1983;6:374–379.

CASE 9

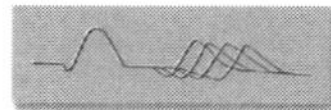

PROXIMAL MUSCLE WEAKNESS, ELEVATED CPK, AND MYOTONIA

CASE PRESENTATION

A 35-year-old man was referred to the UAB Clinic to rule out familial myopathy. He had noticed a gradual bilateral hand weakness over the preceding 2 years. He worked as a chef in a restaurant and had noticed increasing difficulty in using his hands to cook and carry things at work. He also has noticed difficulty climbing stairs for approximately 1 year, which was gradually worsening. He stated that the difficulty stemmed from both weakness and a feeling of stiffness. He reported severe nocturnal cramps in the calf muscles, which were relieved by mild narcotics. He stated that the problems were worse at the end of the day and complained of generalized fatigue. He denied any dysphagia but had some mild dysarthria from time to time. Many members of his family were affected with a similar muscle disease. Examination by the referring neurologist showed increased bulk in the trapezius and upper shoulder girdle muscles, 5 − MRC strength in neck flexors and shoulder girdle muscles, 4 − MRC strength in iliopsoas and quadriceps. The patient had difficulty doing knee bends. No myotonic facial features, frontal balding, or atrophy of muscles was observed. CPK was 737 units. Our evaluation showed additional findings of eyelid, grasp, and percussion myotonia.

CASE ANALYSIS

This patient developed subacute hand weakness and proximal leg weakness. The referring neurologist rightfully suspected the possibility of muscular dystrophy in view of the autosomal-dominant inheritance, proximal weakness, and elevated CPK. Myotonic dystrophy was not suspected because of the lack of classic "myotonic face" and distal muscle weakness. However, the absence of obvious atrophy is unusual for muscular dystrophy. Our findings of eyelid, grasp, and percussion myotonia clinched the diagnosis of proximal myotonic myopathy.

PLAN OF TESTING

1. Needle EMG: To document myotonia and myopathy.
2. Short-exercise test: To document PED, a typical finding for myotonia.
3. Repetitive nerve stimulation: To clarify further the nature of myotonia in proximal myotonic myopathy (PROMM).
4. Muscle biopsy: To delineate further the muscle histology in PROMM.
5. CTG triplet repeat test for DM.

ELECTROPHYSIOLOGICAL TESTS AND FINDINGS

Needle EMG (Table 12.12)

1. Increased insertional activity and myotonic potentials in the APB and vastus lateralis muscles.
2. Fibrillations in the vastus lateralis muscles.
3. Significant decrease in the mean duration of MUPs in the vastus lateralis muscle (Fig. 12.15).

RNS Test Findings (Table 12.13)

1. Fluctuating incremental and decremental responses at 50-Hz stimulation (Fig. 12.16).
2. Repetitive CMAP at the end of HRS.
3. Discrepancy between the amplitude and area change in the CMAPs at HRS.

Short-Exercise Test

1. Significant decrement of CMAP amplitude after 10 seconds of exercise and subsequent recovery of CMAP amplitude after 2 minutes in the left APB muscle (Fig. 12.17).

ELECTROPHYSIOLOGICAL INTERPRETATION

Myotonic myopathy typical of PROMM.

TABLE 12.12. Needle EMG Data in Case 9

				Spontaneous Potentials				Motor Unit Potential			Interference	
Muscle	**Root**	**Nerve**	**Insertion Activity**	**Fib**	**PSW**	**Fasc**	**Myotonic Potential**	**Amplitude (K)**	**Duration (ms)**	**Polyphasic Potential**	**Pattern**	**Mean Amplitude (K)**
Lt APB	C8, T1	Median	+	–	–	–	++	1–3	5–10	N	FIP	2
Lt vast lat	L3,4	Femoral	+	+	–	–	+++	1.6	7.8[a]	27%	FIP	1

[a] Normal duration: 12.2 ms.

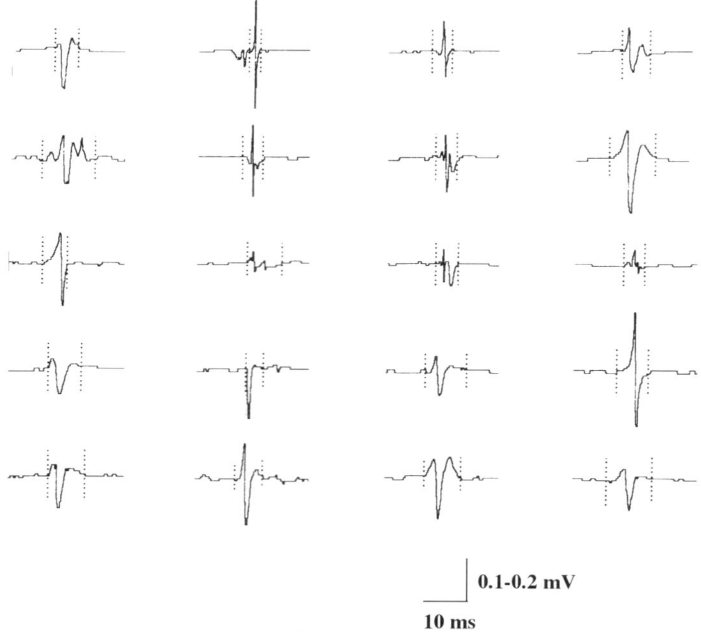

FIGURE 12.15. Twenty MUPs in the vastus lateralis muscle in PROMM.

TABLE 12.13. RNS Test Data in Case 9

	ADQ Muscle
CMAP (mV)	15
CMAP Ex (%)	−88
2 Hz (%)	−3
3 Hz (%)	−2
5 Hz (%)	−2
10 Hz (%)	−23
20 Hz (%)	−15
50/s (%)	−67

Ex, after 30 s exercise.

OTHER TEST FINDINGS

Normal number of CTG repeats (no expansion of CTG repeats). Normal muscle biopsy.

FINAL DIAGNOSIS

PROMM

TREATMENT AND FOLLOW-UP

With mexiletine 750 mg/day, there was improvement in myotonia and strength in the shoulder girdle muscles returned to normal. We were not able to control his muscle pain with nonsteroidal anti-inflammatory agents but were able to relieve pain with mild narcotics.

COMMENTS

Our case represents an example of PROMM. In 1994, a new autosomal-dominant inherited disease of PROMM was described. Patients often have findings suggestive of myotonic dystrophy, but unlike in myotonic dystrophy, they have proximal myopathy and do not have abnormal expansion of the CTG repeat in the DM gene on chromosome 19. The core clinical features of PROMM are muscle stiffness, myotonia, weakness, muscle pain, and cataracts.

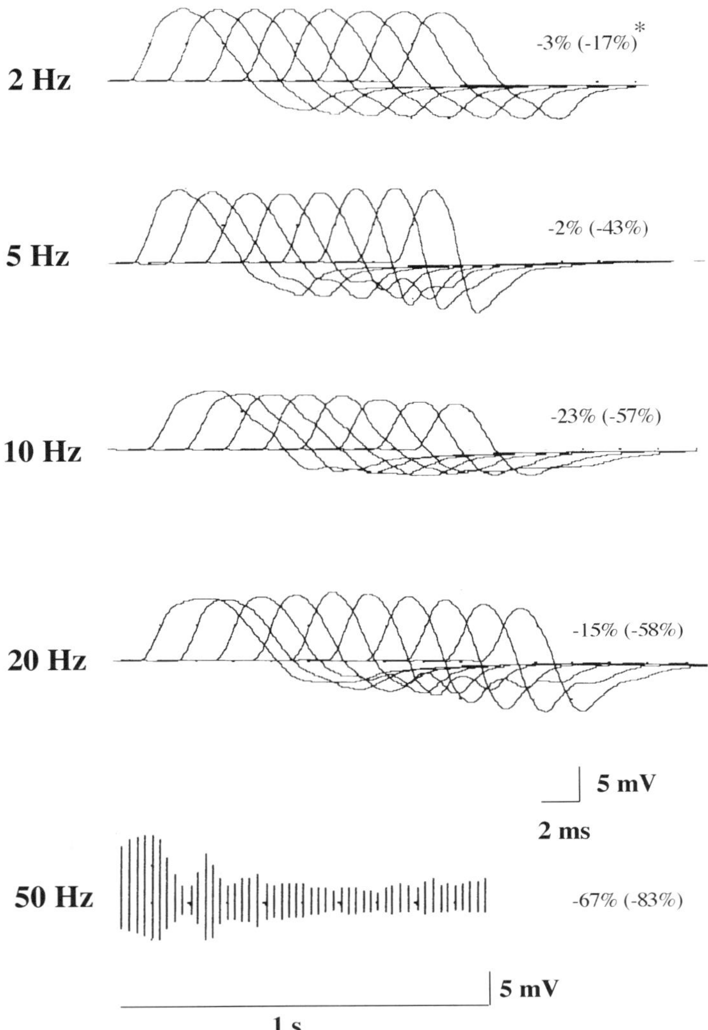

FIGURE 12.16. RNS test in PROMM, showing many findings typical of myotonic muscle membranes: repetitive discharges in some responses at 5- and 20-Hz stimulations and marked discrepancy in the decrement (*) between the negative-peak amplitude and negative-peak area (% in parenthesis). Notice also marked change in the duration at high rate of stimulation and fluctuating decrement at 50-Hz stimulation.

Initial symptoms usually develop between 20 and 60 years of age. The most striking difference from myotonic dystrophy is proximal muscle weakness, especially in the legs. Muscle pain is a rather prominent finding in this disorder and is most apparent at rest. Cataracts in PROMM are indistinguishable from those in myotonic dystrophy, being posterior capsular, iridescent, multicolored opacities. None of these patients had distal weakness or wasting of muscles in the arms and legs or in the face. Testicular atrophy and cardiac arrhythmias, two common features in cases of DM, were present in a small number of patients with PROMM. The clinical course was mild, showing only slow progression. Elevated CPK was reported in 50% of cases. Muscle biopsy showed a nonspecific mild myopathy.

In myotonic dystrophy, the RNS test shows a decremental response in 60 to 100% of cases

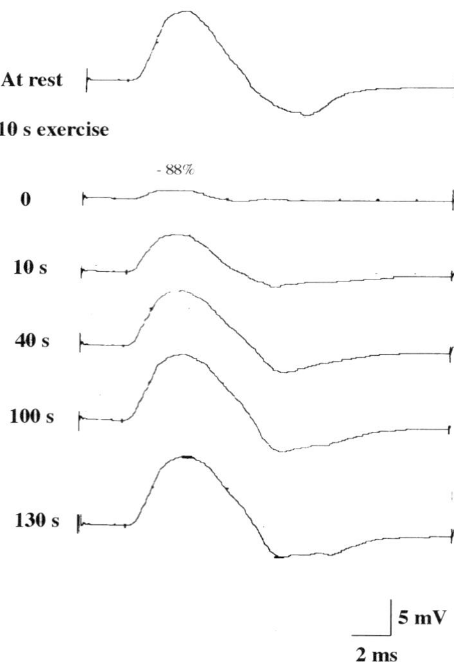

FIGURE 12.17. Postexercise depression in the short-exercise test in PROMM. There is an 88% decrease in the CMAP amplitude immediately after 10 seconds of exercise.

and HRS causes an earlier and more marked decremental response than the low rate of stimulation. Decremental response occurs in all forms of myotonic disorder but is most prominent in myotonia congenita. Decremental response is more prominent when the test is performed after rest (more than 5 min) than when done immediately after prolonged stimulation or activity. As discussed above, PED or post-tetanic depression is one of the typical findings of myotonic disorder.

There are certain qualitative differences between the response on the RNS test in MG and in myotonic disorder. In MG, the decremental response is more prominent at 2 to 5 Hz, stimulation decline of the CMAP is maximal in the first five responses, and the decremental response becomes more prominent after exercise and local warming. On the other hand, in myotonic disorder, decremental response usually occurs after prolonged stimulation and is more prominent at HRS, decline of the CMAP progresses beyond the fifth response, and decremental response becomes more prominent in the rested or cold muscles. Decremental response in myotonia is due to altered function in the muscle fibers, as has been clearly shown by documenting decremental response when the muscle itself is stimulated.

MAXIMS

1. PROMM is an autosomal-dominant inherited disease characterized by myotonia, predominant proximal muscle weakness, and normal CTG repeat.
2. The RNS test is commonly abnormal in myotonic disorders, especially at the HRS.

REFERENCES

1. Moxley R III. Proximal myotonic myopathy: mini-review of a recently delineated clinical disorder. Neuromusc Dis 1996;6:87–93.
2. Oh SJ. Electromyography. Neuromuscular transmission studies. Baltimore, MD: Williams & Wilkins, 1988:171–173.

CHAPTER 13

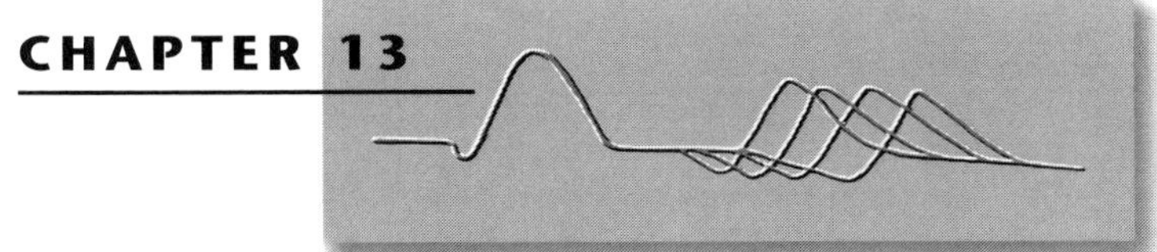

Myasthenia Gravis and Related Diseases

Myasthenia, defined as exertional weakness or easy fatigability, is a typical clinical feature of the neuromuscular transmission (NMT) disorders. It is characterized by weakness that is fluctuating in nature, worsens with repeated exercise, and improves with rest. Classically, myasthenic symptoms are least prominent early in the morning after waking from a restful night and most prominent late in the afternoon or early in the evening after a full day's work. Depending on the involved muscles, myasthenic symptoms vary from diplopia to walking difficulty. However, the most serious myasthenic symptom is respiratory failure, the major cause of death in patients with NMT disorders.

There are four major NMT disorders: myasthenia gravis, Lambert-Eaton myasthenic syndrome (LEMS), botulism, and congenital myasthenic syndrome (CMS).

MYASTHENIA GRAVIS

Myasthenia gravis (MG) is due to an antibody-induced postsynaptic defect of the neuromuscular junction, producing exertional weakness or easy fatigability and, commonly, oculobulbar palsy. Electronmicroscopic studies show simplification of the postsynaptic fold at the neuromuscular junction, which is induced by the acetylcholine receptor (AChR) antibody.

There is considerable evidence indicative of an autoimmune mechanism in the pathogenesis of MG. The strongest evidence is seen in experimental autoimmune myasthenia gravis. Within 2 weeks after injection of AChR antigen purified from electric eels, animals develop weakness that is reversed by edrophonium. Their electrophysiological and pharmacological responses are identical to those in human MG. The thymus seems to be the major organ initiating AChR antibody formation in MG, which eventually damages the postsynaptic fold.

MG is suspected in the presence of classic exertional weakness and oculobulbar symptoms. In 90% of MG patients, oculobulbar dysfunction is present. Commonly, such patients complain of diplopia, swallowing or speech difficulty, and proximal muscle weakness. Rarely, respiratory difficulty is the initial symptom. Exertional weakness should be documented on examination by the repetitive exercise test.

The diagnosis of MG is easily confirmed by the intravenous edrophonium test, a short-acting anticholinesterase (anti-ChE). Dramatic improvement is noted within 1 minute of injection. This test is invariably positive in MG.

The serum AChR antibody has become the more specific test for MG, although it is positive in only 85% of cases. Thus far, false-positive responses have not been reported in disease. However, the titer is not correlated with disease severity.

Other helpful diagnostic tests include the repetitive nerve stimulation (RNS) test (Jolly test) and the single-fiber electromyography (SFEMG). The RNS test is positive in 75% of cases. The SFEMG, which tests the microphysiological state of end plates, shows "abnormal jitter" in 95% of cases.

There are two main modes of treatment in MG: symptomatic treatment and immunotherapy. The mainstay of symptomatic treatment is anti-ChE, which is effective in almost all cases. The least success is noted in ocular MG. Mestinon (pyridostigmine) is the most commonly used drug because of the 6 to 8-hour duration of the drug effect.

Because MG is an autoimmune disease, it is natural to treat this disorder with various immunotherapies, including thymectomy, steroid therapy, immunosuppressives, and plasmapheresis.

Thymectomy is indicated in cases in which generalized MG is not satisfactorily controlled with anti-ChE alone. Thymectomy induces long-term improvement and remission. About 50% of patients who will be in remission achieve remission in the first 3 years after thymectomy and 100% do within 10 years. Thymectomy produces a stable remission by eliminating thymic centers. The effects are delayed because of the long life span of the existing pool of small immunocompetent lymphocytes.

Long-term steroid therapy is known to be effective in 75% of MG cases that are not responsive to anti-ChE. Improvement is also remarkable in ocular MG. Steroid treatment is different from thymectomy in that improvement occurs within a few days or weeks of treatment. Transient worsening may occur in the first weeks of steroid therapy.

Immunosuppressive agents, azathioprine, or cyclophosphamide are also used in MG cases resistant to anti-ChE and steroid treatment. In European centers, azathioprine is preferred to steroids. The effectiveness of these agents is usually seen after 6 weeks of treatment.

Plasmapheresis is most effective in improving the worsening symptoms during a myasthenic crisis. This therapy induces a rapid reduction of the AChR antibody and produces improvement within a few days. However, to maintain long-term improvement, the patient should be maintained on steroid or immunosuppressives.

Crisis in MG is defined as an acute progressive respiratory failure due to weakness in the bulbar or respiratory muscles. This is associated with a high mortality rate (7%). Crisis is due to three different causes: myasthenic crisis due to worsening of MG, cholinergic crisis from overmedication of anti-ChE, and drug insensitivity crisis. Myasthenic crisis is often precipitated by a mild "infection." The most important step in the management of crisis in MG patients is to maintain adequate respiration, either by endotracheal tubing or tracheostomy.

LAMBERT-EATON MYASTHENIC SYNDROME (OR EATON-LAMBERT SYNDROME)

LEMS is a myasthenic syndrome often associated with bronchogenic carcinoma. Clinically, exertional weakness and leg weakness are the cardinal symptoms. The NMT in LEMS is blocked due to a decrease in the release of acetylcholine from the nerve terminal. This syndrome is now proven to be autoimmune mediated. It is reproducible in animals passively injected with serum IgG from patients with this syndrome. Many of these patients are known to have other autoimmune diseases or antibodies against other tissues. Some patients respond to steroid or plasmapheresis. A recent study showed that antibody against the voltage-gated calcium channel (VGCC) is positive in 52 to 90% of cases.

The clinical, electrophysiological, and pharmacological differences between MG and LEMS are given in Table 13.1. Diagnosis of LEMS is confirmed by the RNS test. Three characteristics are noted: low CMAP amplitude, a decremental response at the low rate of stimulation, and an incremental response at the high rate of stimulation.

In the treatment of LEMS, guanidine HCl or aminopyridine, which increases the release of acetylcholine at the nerve endings, is the drug of choice. In patients with small cell lung cancer (SCLC), treatment of the tumor induces remission of this syndrome. Corticosteroids, immunosuppressives, and plasmapheresis are the next treatments of choice when guanidine or aminopyridine is not effective.

There are certain drugs that aggravate MG and LEMS: antiarrhythmic drugs (quinidine and procainamide, etc.), antibiotics (neomycin, kanamycin, gentamycin), muscle relaxants (curare, pavulone, succinylcholine), and magnesium preparations.

BOTULISM

Botulism is a neuromuscular disorder caused by the toxin of *Clostridium botulinum*. The basic defect and electrophysiological findings are similar to those in LEMS. The clinical symptoms simulate acute Guillain-Barré syndrome of descending type. Dysautonomia (fixed pupils, ileus, and urinary retention) and areflexia are two important features in botulism, in addition to muscle weakness. Diagnosis of botulism is made by the detection of botulinum toxin in the serum.

TABLE 13.1. Differences Between MG and LEMS

	MG	LEMS
Sex	F:M 2:1	Almost all men
Presenting signs	Weakness of ocular, bulbar, and facial muscles	Weakness of proximal leg muscles
Exertion	Exertional weakness	Transient improvement after brief exercise followed by weakness
Reflexes	Normal	Reduced or absent
Tumor	Thymoma in 16% of cases	SCLC in 75% of cases
Basic defect	Postsynaptic defect	Presynaptic defect
RNS test		
CMAP at rest	Normal	Low
After exercise	No change	Marked increase
Low rate stimulation	Decremental response	Decremental response
High rate stimulation	Normal or decrement	Incremental response
Antibodies	AChR antibody (+) in 85%	VGCC antibody (+) in 90%
Drugs	Anticholinesterases	Guanidine, aminopyridine
Immunotherapies	Steroids, immunosuppressives, plasmapheresis, and IVIG in both	
Thymectomy	Effective	Not indicated

Historically, foodborne botulism, caused primarily by faulty home-canned or preserved vegetables, has been the classic form of botulism. However, in recent years, infant botulism has become the most common form of botulism in the United States. Infant botulism presents itself as acute "floppy infant syndrome." Diagnosis is suggested by the RNS test and confirmed by the detection of clostridium in the stool. Wound botulism has been known to occur predominantly among intravenous drug users in recent years.

CONGENITAL MYASTHENIC SYNDROMES

CMS refers to a heterogeneous group of presynaptic or postsynaptic NMT disorders characterized by myasthenic symptoms since infancy, exertional weakness, negative AChR antibody, and decremental response on the RNS test. A positive family history and responsiveness to anti-ChE medications are present in many, but not all, CMS. Unfortunately, the detailed nature of this defect can be studied by only a few medical centers in the world, and thus a referral to such a center is recommended if CMS is suspected.

CASE 1

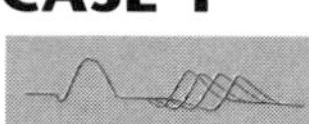

DROOPING OF EYELID FOR 20 YEARS AND LOW MONOTONOUS SPEECH

CASE PRESENTATION

A 73-year-old man with a history of high blood pressure controlled by medication reported drooping of the left eyelid for approximately 20 years. This problem became worse about 4 years ago and was associated with double vision on vertical gaze. His symptoms became worse as the day progressed. He denied any muscle weakness, chewing or swallowing difficulties, breathing problems, tiredness, or unusual fatigue, but he noticed slurring of his speech. A tensilon (edrophonium) test was performed in the past with no improvement in his ptosis or double vision. AChR antibody was reported to be negative. A CT of the head was normal according to the patient. He also reported a resting tremor in the right hand but denied any slowing of movement. Neurological examination showed moderate left ptosis that was fatigable, mild left superior rectus paresis, resting tremor in the right hand, masked face, and low monotonous speech without any pitch. There was no rigidity or bradykinesia.

CASE ANALYSIS

This patient had mild left ptosis for 20 years. Onset of double vision in recent years prompted him to seek medical attention. Worsening of symptoms late in the day and fatigable ptosis were strongly suggestive of MG. However, two important tests for MG were negative: tensilon test and AChR antibody. His speech was not of nasal phonation as is typical of MG but was a typical parkinsonian dysarthria (low monotonous and pitchless speech). Further confirmation of the diagnosis of MG was necessary. In addition, the patient had parkinsonism characterized by masked face and resting tremor.

PLAN OF TESTING

1. RNS test: To confirm the diagnosis of MG.
2. SFEMG: To corroborate the NMT defect.
3. Prostigmine test: To confirm the diagnosis of MG by testing responsiveness of ophthalmoparesis to anti-ChE medication.

ELECTROPHYSIOLOGICAL TESTS AND FINDINGS

RNS Test Findings (Table 13.2)

1. Normal RNS test in the ADQ, FCU, and trapezius muscles.
2. Significant decremental response in the orbicularis oculi muscle (Fig. 13.1).

SFEMG (Table 13.2). Normal fiber density and mildly prolonged MCD.

TABLE 13.2. NMT Study Data in Case 1

RNS Test Data				
	ADQ	**FCU**	**OO**	**Trapezius**
CMAP (mV)	13.5	1.8	2.4	7.5
CMAP Ex (%)	7.4	5.8		
2 Hz (%)	3.7	−2.8	−15	9.6
3 Hz (%)	1.8	0	−26	−6.2
5 Hz (%)	12.9	2.9	−24	−5.1
50 Hz (%)	−17	2.7		
5 Hz PT 0 (%)	3.7	−5.4		
5 Hz PT 4 (%)	9.5	0		

SFEMG Data	
	EDC
Fiber density	1.36
# of Pot pairs	10
Mean MCD (μs)	43
Normal MCD (μs)	40.4
No. PP with MCD >53 μs (%)	0
No. PP with blocking (%)	20

ADQ, abductor digiti quinti; FCU, flexor carpi ulnaris; OO, orbicularis oculi; EDC, extensor digitorum communis; CMAP, compound muscle action potential, CMAP Ex, CMAP after 30-second exercise; MCD, mean consecutive difference; PP, potential pair; PT 0, posttetanic response immediately after 50 Hz stimulation; PT4, posttetanic response 4 minutes after 50 Hz stimulation; −, decrement.

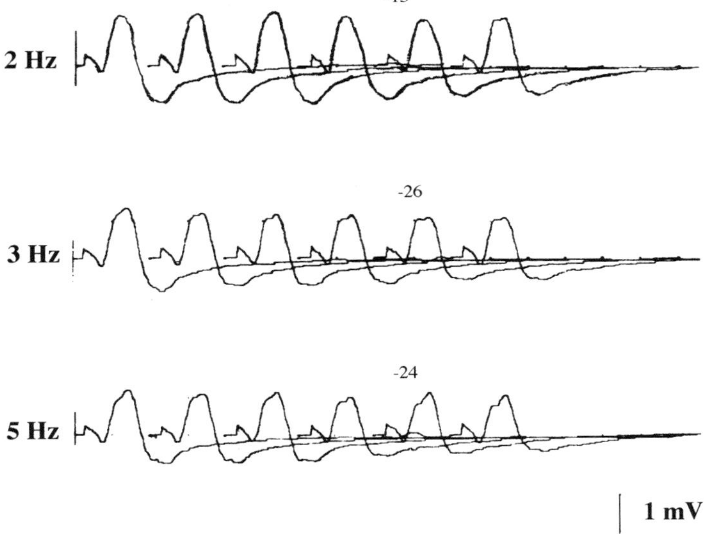

FIGURE 13.1. Decremental responses in the RNS test in the orbicularis oculi muscle. Numbers above the tracings represent decremental or incremental responses. 2 Hz, 3 Hz, and 5 Hz represent 2-Hz, 3-Hz, and 5-Hz stimulation.

ELECTROPHYSIOLOGICAL INTERPRETATION

Postsynaptic NMT defect typical of MG in the RNS test in the orbicularis oculi muscle and SFEMG.

OTHER TEST FINDINGS

Prostigmine test (2.0 mg prostigmine intramuscular injection after 0.4 mg atropine intramuscular injection 15 minutes before) showed improvement of left ptosis and superior rectus paresis.

FINAL DIAGNOSIS

Ocular MG and parkinsonism

TREATMENT AND FOLLOW-UP

The patient's speech and facial expression were dramatically improved with three tablets of carbidopa-levodopa 25/100 a day. Pyridostigmine was tried for 1 month without any definite improvement. After discussing the pros and cons of steroid treatment with the patient, we decided to follow him without steroid treatment. Within a year, his ocular MG was in remission.

COMMENTS

Ocular MG is quite different from generalized MG in several aspects. It is definitely benign in that if ocular MG does not progress to generalized MG within 4 years, it remains ocular with no increase in mortality. Diagnosis of ocular MG can be challenging in view of the often negative tensilon test, the nonresponsiveness to pyridostigmine medications, and the low diagnostic sensitivity of the routine RNS test. The prostigmine test, a forerunner of the tensilon test, is extremely helpful in this regard, because it is usually positive even in ocular MG. This is most likely due to the fact that with the prostigmine test, there is more time for an objective evaluation of response. Prostigmine (1.0 to 2.5 mg) is given intramuscularly after intramuscular atropine (0.4 to 0.6 mg) injection. The patient is then evaluated 30 minutes after prostigmine injection. Usually, the prostigmine effect lasts 3 to 4 hours, thus allowing plenty of time for adequate evaluation of response.

The routine distal RNS test is less sensitive in ocular MG. A previous study showed that it is positive in only 13 to 19% of patients with ocular MG. However, our latest study showed positive results in about 30% of cases. Even with the RNS test in the deltoid, biceps, and trapezius muscles, there is no higher diagnostic yield. However, a combined test on the orbicularis oculi and a distal muscle showed a significantly higher diagnostic yield (63%) in ocular MG compared with the distal muscle test alone. The AChR antibody is positive in 70% of cases of ocular MG. SFEMG is positive in 80% of cases, if testing of the frontalis or orbicularis oculi muscle is included. Thus, considering everything, the AChR antibody is the most helpful diagnostic test for ocular MG. In many patients with ocular MG, pyridostigmine is not effective in relieving the troublesome symptoms as noted in this case. Steroid is effective in ocular MG and in generalized MG.

MAXIMS

1. In ocular MG, the tensilon test is often negative and pyridostigmine is often not effective for treatment.
2. In ocular MG, the RNS test in the orbicularis oculi muscle is the test of choice if the routine RNS in the distal muscle is normal.

REFERENCES

1. Schwab RS, Viets HR. The prostigmine test in myasthenia gravis. Third report. N Engl J Med 1938; 219:226–228.
2. Sommer N, Melms A, Weller M, Dichgans J. Ocular myasthenia gravis. A critical review of clinical and pathophysiological aspects. Doc Ophthalmol 1993;84:309–333.

CASE 2

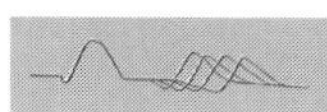

TRANSIENT ATTACKS OF DIFFICULTY CHEWING, SWALLOWING, AND SPEAKING

CASE PRESENTATION

In 2 months, a 75-year-old man with history of hypertension and hypothyroidism had visited the emergency room twice for possible stroke because of episodic attacks of difficulty chewing, swallowing, and speaking lasting 5 to 10 minutes while eating a steak. He denied vertigo, perioral paresthesia, unsteadiness, or weakness of arms or legs. In the preceding 4 months, he had similar but milder attacks provoked only by eating and chewing. Neurological evaluation in the emergency room documented only double vision on left lateral gaze at the first visit and normal findings at the second visit. No obvious ophthalmoplegia was noted. Other neurological findings were normal. No bruit was heard over the supraclavicular areas. MRI of the head revealed white matter ischemic changes. Aspirin was prescribed for possible basilar-vertebral insufficiency. The patient was sent to us for further evaluation. Neurological examination was again unremarkable.

CASE ANALYSIS

This patient had episodic transient attacks of "bulbar palsy" with no obvious neurological deficit at the time of examination. Thus, it was natural to suspect "basilar vertebral insufficiency," especially in a patient with hypertension. Considering multiple lower cranial nerve involvement, it was extremely unusual that other symptoms typical of basilar-vertebral symptoms were lacking. On the other hand, there were two important pieces of information to suggest MG: the episodic attacks were provoked only by repetitive movement of the bulbar muscles, and they rapidly resolved with rest. In fact, a detailed history revealed that 10 years previously, the patient had been evaluated for possible ocular MG because of episodic double vision but was told that he did not have MG after tests were performed.

PLAN OF TESTING

1. RNS test: To confirm the diagnosis of MG.
2. AChR antibody: To confirm the diagnosis of MG.
3. SFEMG test: To corroborate the diagnosis of MG

ELECTROPHYSIOLOGICAL TESTS AND FINDINGS

The first RNS test (Table 13.3; Fig. 13.2)

1. Normal findings in the ADQ, FCU, and trapezius muscles.
2. Decremental response in the orbicularis oculi muscle.

The First SFEMG (Table 13.3)

1. Normal fiber density for his age.
2. Increased mean MCD value.
3. Increased number of SFPP with MCD greater than 53 μs or with blocking.

ELECTROPHYSIOLOGICAL INTERPRETATION

Postsynaptic NMT defect typical of MG on the RNS test in the orbicularis oculi muscle and the SFEMG.

OTHER TEST FINDINGS

AChR antibody was positive.

FINAL DIAGNOSIS

Oculobulbar MG

TREATMENT AND FOLLOW-UP

The tensilon test was not possible because of the lack of objective neurological deficits at the time of evaluation. RNS test confirmed the diagnosis of MG on the day of evaluation. Mestinon

TABLE 13.3. NMT Study Data in Case 2

	RNS Test Data								SFEMG Data		
	First Test				Second Test[a]				EDC		
	ADQ	FCU	OO	Trapezius	ADQ	FCU	OO	Trapezius		First Test	Second Test
CMAP (mV)	7.6	10.1	2.6	13	10.4	8.4	3.3	11	Fiber density	1.55	1.93
CMAP Ex (%)	−5	2			0.9	−7.1			No. Pot pairs	17	16
2 Hz (%)	−3	2	−11	−4	0.9	−2.4	−16.6	−9.2	Mean MCD (μs)	97	73
3 Hz (%)	−5	1	−11	−3	1.9	−2.4	−19.4	−11.2	Normal MCD (μs)	40.4	40.4
5 Hz (%)	−3	1	−11	−1	5.8	1.1	−21.0	−15.3	No. PP with MCD >53 μs (%)	75	63
50 Hz (%)	0	5			−8.6	−5.3			No. PP with blocking (%)	47	19
5 Hz PT 0 (%)	−1	1			4.8	2.4					
5 Hz PT 4 (%)	−1	8			6.9	−1.1					

[a] Sixteen-month interval between the first and second tests.

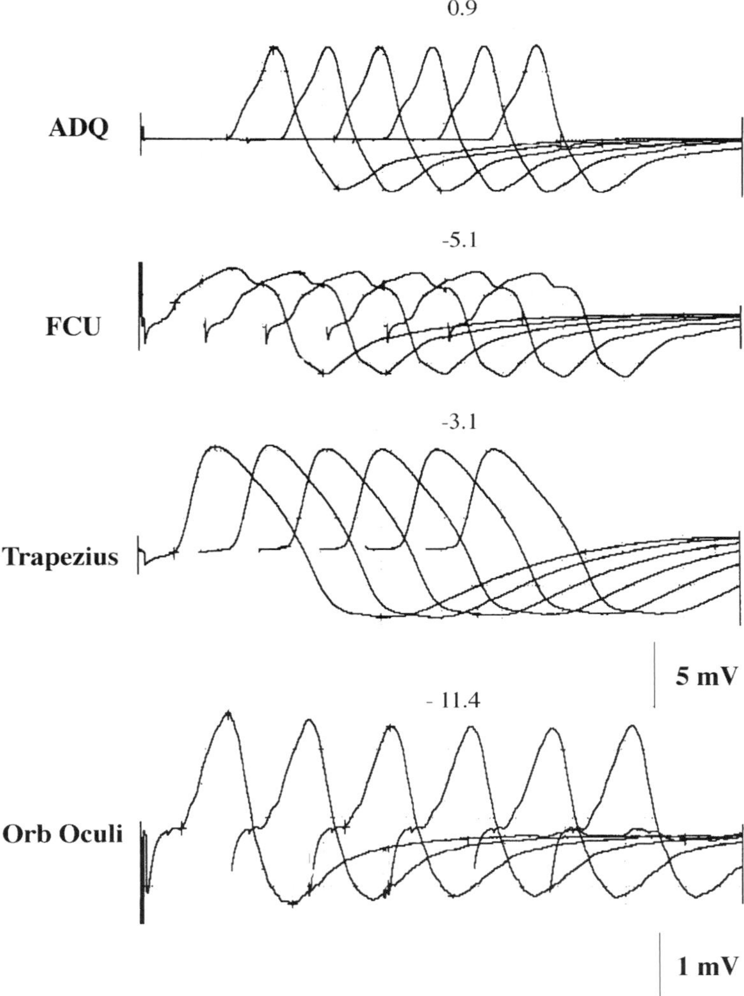

FIGURE 13.2. RNS responses at 3-Hz stimulation in the various muscles. Decremental response in the orbicularis (*Orb*) oculi muscle but normal response in the ADQ, FCU, and trapezius muscles.

(90 mg/day) dramatically abolished the episodic attacks of speech, swallowing, and chewing difficulty. However, because of severe diarrhea unrelieved by glycopyrrolate (Robinul, Robins Co.), the patient was not able to take pyridostigmine continuously. Fourteen months after the first evaluation, he developed severe bulbar palsy with swallowing, chewing, and speaking difficulty. A second RNS test showed electrophysiological worsening (Table 13.3; Fig. 13.3). Initially, this patient was treated with plasma exchange followed by a high dose of prednisone (60 mg/day). In 2 months, he became symptom free with prednisone 60 mg/day and pyridostigmine 90 mg/day.

COMMENTS

The RNS test is the time-honored test for the NMT disorders and offers the advantages of relative simplicity and rapid results. Although certain patterns on the RNS test are indicative of MG, it is less specific than the AChR antibody assay. The distinct advantages of the RNS test over the AChR antibody assay are that this test can provide a rapid and objective diagnosis of MG and can be used serially for evaluation of severity of disease, as noted in this case.

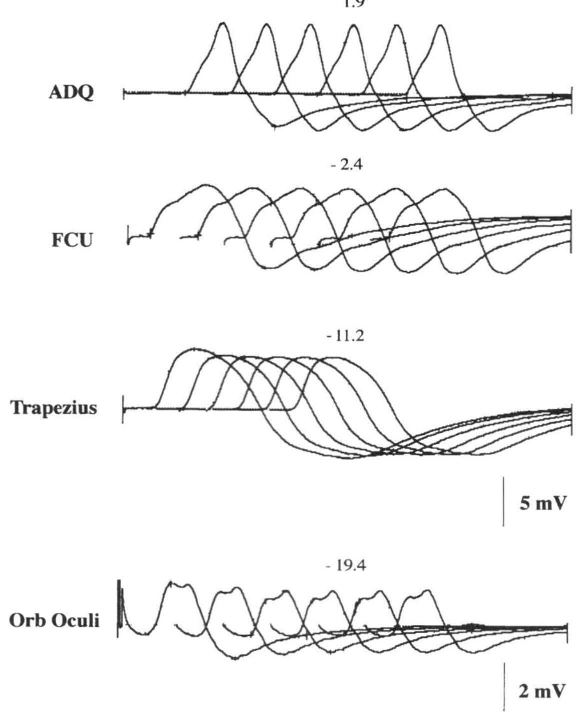

FIGURE 13.3. RNS responses at 3-Hz stimulation in the various muscles. Worsening of decremental response in the orbicularis (*Orb*) oculi and trapezius muscles.

The RNS test should preferably be performed before any anti-ChE inhibitor medication is administered, because it is well known that the anti-ChE inhibitor can normalize the RNS abnormality in mild cases of MG. In patients who are taking anti-ChE inhibitors, the drugs should be withdrawn, if possible, at least 12 hours before the test. The diagnostic sensitivity of the RNS test for MG has been found to be about 55% in distal muscles and about 70% in proximal muscles. Because of its technical reliability, the RNS test on the distal hand muscles (ADQ and FCU muscles in our laboratory) remains the most commonly used test and the first test of choice in our laboratory. When the distal muscles are normal, then the RNS test in the proximal muscles (orbicularis oculi and trapezius muscle in our laboratory) is recommended. This strategy increases the diagnostic sensitivity in MG by 15%. The test on the orbicularis oculi or the trapezius muscle is technically reliable as long as the stimulus is barely supramaximal and the rate of stimulation is less than 5 Hz.

The most common type of RNS abnormalities are those typical of postsynaptic NMT blocks: normal CMAP amplitude, normal or minimal PEF, decremental response at LRS, normal or decremental response at HRS, and PTF followed by PTE. Among these, the decremental response at LRS is the most common and characteristic RNS finding in MG. In many laboratories, HRS is not performed as a routine test because it is painful. We use HRS routinely for the RNS test and have found an increased diagnostic yield of 5% in MG. This test further ensures that LEMS has been ruled out completely. Abnormal decremental response at HRS was observed in 22% of cases in our series and in 47% in that of Slomic and coworkers. More typically in MG, postexercise or posttetanic responses are better reflected in the decremental response than in the CMAP amplitude. In our series, PTF was observed in 40% of cases and PTE in 17% of cases. In 5% of our series, PTE was the only abnormality on the RNS test.

MAXIMS

1. The RNS abnormalities in MG are characterized by the classic triad: normal CMAP amplitude, decremental response at LRS, and normal or decremental response at HRS. Decremental response at LRS is the most common abnormality in MG.
2. The proximal RNS test should be performed when the distal RNS test is normal in patients suspected of having MG, because it significantly increases the diagnostic sensitivity.

REFERENCES

1. Oh SJ. Electromyography. Neuromuscular transmission studies. Baltimore: Williams & Wilkins, 1988.
2. Keesey JC. Electrodiagnostic approach to defects of neuromuscular transmission. Muscle Nerve 1989; 12:613–626.

CASE 3

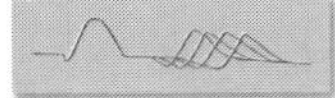

MG DURING PREGNANCY

CASE PRESENTATION

A 24-year-old woman who was in the 21st week of pregnancy had begun to notice episodic weakness in her legs 6 months previously. During these episodes, she would become profoundly weak in her legs with occasional sudden falls. These problems became progressively worse and included weakness in her upper extremities and some difficulty with slurred speech. She finally had to quit her job as a cashier in a department store. Three months later, the diagnosis of MG was made on the basis of a high AChR antibody (184 nmol/L versus normal 0.02) and abnormal decremental response on the Jolly test performed by a neurologist. Previous workups had included a normal CPK, thyroid function test, B_{12} and folate, sedimentation rate, antinuclear antibody, and rheumatoid factor. CT examination of the chest was negative. The patient was begun on pyridostigmine (180 mg/day) with some improvement in her weakness. She remained weak and had episodic dysphagia and shortness of breath. She denied any frank diplopia.

Abnormal neurological findings included diplopia on extreme gaze to the right and upward, moderate facial weakness and MRC strength of 4 in bilateral deltoid and iliopsoas muscles.

CASE ANALYSIS

This patient had fluctuating weakness and oculobulbar symptoms characteristic of MG. Diagnosis of MG was confirmed by AChR antibody and abnormal decremental response. She was referred to UAB for a special program for pregnant patients with MG. It is important to assess the severity of MG and achieve a steady stable status of MG within the shortest possible time.

PLAN OF TESTING

1. RNS test: To assess the degree of MG.
2. SFEMG: To corroborate the diagnosis of MG.

ELECTROPHYSIOLOGICAL TESTS AND FINDINGS

RNS Test Findings (Fig. 13.4; Table 13.4)

1. Normal CMAP amplitude.
2. Decremental response at LRS.
3. Normal response at HRS.
4. Posttetanic facilitation and exhaustion phenomena.

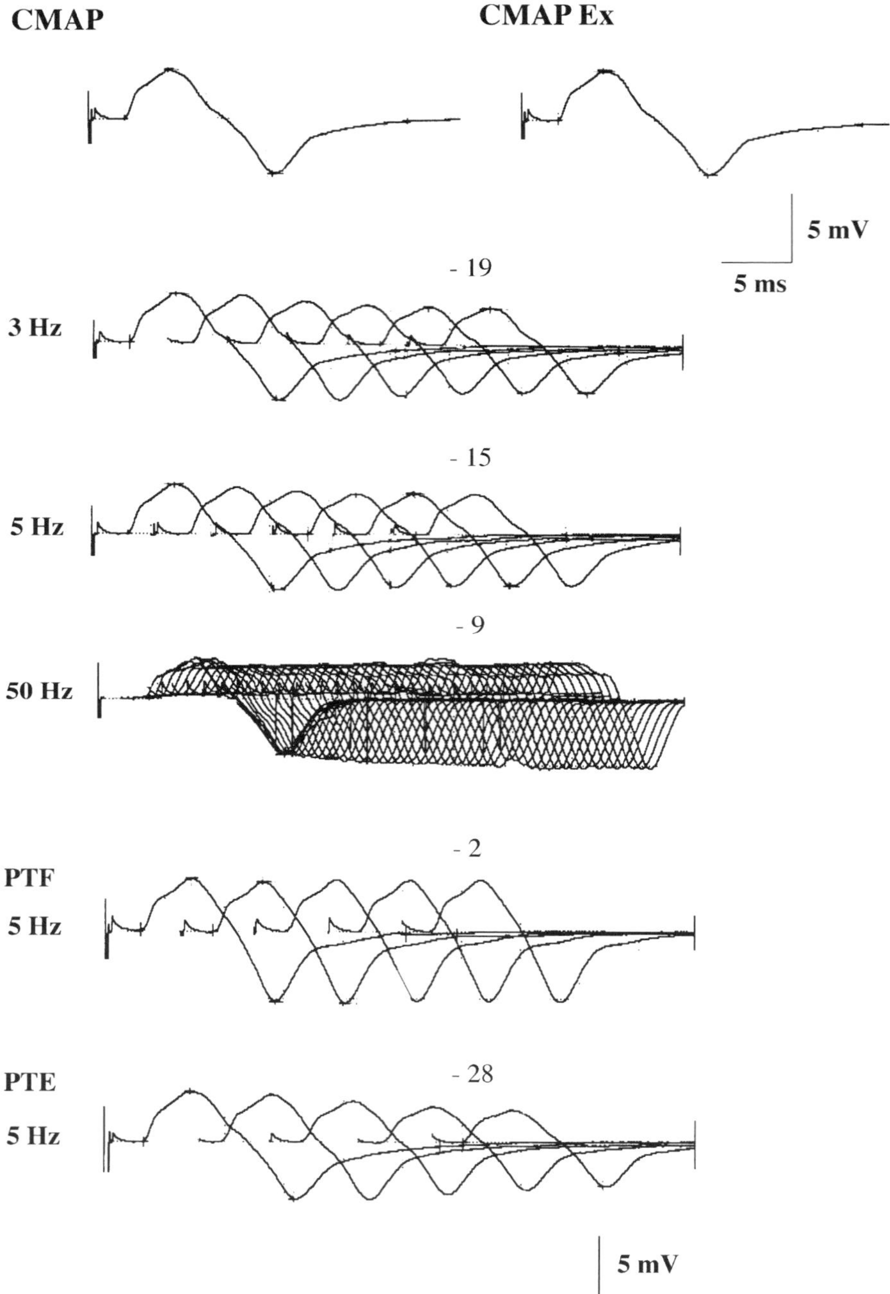

FIGURE 13.4. RNS response in the FCU muscle. RNS pattern typical of mild MG: normal CMAP, decremental responses at LRS, normal response at HRS, posttetanic facilitation (*PTF*), and posttetanic exhaustion (*PTE*) phenomena. PTE, 5-Hz stimulation immediately after the tetanic (50-Hz) stimulation. PTE, 5-Hz stimulation 4 minutes after the tetanic stimulation.

TABLE 13.4. NMT Study Data in Case 3

RNS Test Data			SFEMG Data	
	ADQ	FCU		EDC
CMAP (mV)	16.6	7.8	Fiber density	1.55
CMAP Ex (%)	12	0	No. Pot pairs	20
2 Hz (%)	−20	−12.6	Mean MCD (μs)	83
3 Hz (%)	−27.3	−18.7	Normal MCD (μs)	40.4
5 Hz (%)	−24.7	−15.1	No. PP with MCD >53 μs (%)	72.7
50 Hz (%)	−10	4.0	No. PP with blocking (%)	18.1
5 Hz PT 0 (%)	−5.5	−2.1		
5 Hz PT 4 (%)	−33.7	−28.3		

SFEMG (Table 13.4)
1. Normal fiber density.
2. Prolonged mean MCD.
3. Increased number of SFPP > 53 μs and with blocking.

ELECTROPHYSIOLOGICAL INTERPRETATION

Postsynaptic NMT defect typical of mild MG.

FINAL DIAGNOSIS

Mild generalized MG

TREATMENT AND FOLLOW-UP

Pyridostigmine was increased to 480 mg/day. The patient was put on prednisone 30 mg/day. Monthly evaluations showed gradual improvement in her MG and symptom-free status in 3 months. We were able to sustain her stable status until a healthy baby was delivered without any complications. No postpartum exacerbation of MG occurred.

COMMENTS

The effect of pregnancy on MG is variable: some patients worsen, some improve, and some are unchanged. In general, MG becomes worse in the first trimester and better in the last two trimesters. Many patients have worsening of MG in the postpartum period. To achieve a steady stable course of MG during pregnancy and the partum period, steroid is the drug of choice, because it can bring about a stable or improved status within a few weeks and does not have any major side effects on the baby. Following this regimen, we were able to achieve a steady stable condition without any major worsening of MG or any complications during delivery of the baby. Azathioprine and cyclophosphamide, two common immunosuppressives for MG, are known to be tetratogenic.

Depending on the severity of MG, there are two distinct responses on the RNS tests: in mild MG, an abnormal decremental response at LRS, normal response at HRS, and prominent PTF and PTE phenomena; and in severe MG, an abnormal decremental response at LRS and at HRS with less common PTF and rare PTE phenomena. In mild MG, the normal mechanism of increase in ACh release during HRS can compensate for the minimally diminished safety factor, producing a normal response at HRS and subsequent PTF and PTE. In severe MG, however, the neuromuscular block is so severe that the normal mechanism of increased ACh release during HRS cannot compensate for the markedly diminished safety factor, thus producing a decremental response at HRS, less common PTF, and subsequent lack of PTE.

MAXIMS

1. The effect of pregnancy on MG is variable. In general, MG is worse in the first trimester, better during the last two trimesters, and worse in the postpartum period. To achieve a stable MG status in the shortest time during pregnancy, steroid is the drug of choice.
2. The RNS test in mild MG is characterized by an abnormal decremental response at LRS, normal response at HRS, and prominent PTF and PTE.

REFERENCES

1. Burke ME. Myasthenia gravis and pregnancy. J Perinat Neonatal Nurs 1993;7:11–21.
2. Floyd RC, Roberts WE. Autoimmune diseases in pregnancy. Obstet Gynecol Clin North Am 1992; 19:719–32.

CASE 4

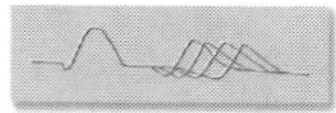

SUSPECTED PROGRESSIVE EXTERNAL OPHTHALMOPLEGIA WITH NORMAL MUSCLE BIOPSY

CASE PRESENTATION

A 23-year-old left-handed man developed drooping of the right eye and double vision a year ago. These symptoms would come and go throughout the day but were particularly worse at night. He later developed drooping of his left eye and nasal speech, which became worse after prolonged talking. He also noted increased fatigue at the end of the day. Two months ago, he developed difficulty climbing stairs and difficulty with his handwriting. In recent days, he had fallen about once a day and his eye movements were completely gone. Workup to date by the neuroopthalmologist included a tensilon test, which showed transient improvement of ptosis, a normal AChR antibody, and normal brain MRI. The patient was put on a short course of pyridostigmin (Mestinon, ICN Pharmaceutical) (four tablets a day) without any obvious improvement. At that point, the referring neuroophthalmologist suspected mitochondrial myopathy with progressive external ophthalmoplegia. However, a muscle biopsy was reported to be normal without any "ragged-red fibers." A second opinion, including another muscle biopsy, was requested.

Examination showed moderately severe bilateral ptosis with exertional worsening, almost total ophthalmoplegia with only minimal down-gaze movement, and normal pupillary light response. Despite bilateral facial weakness, no bulbar abnormality was noted. Muscle strength was 5 − in the deltoids, 4 + in biceps, 4 + in triceps, 4 in iliopsoas, and 4 + in anterior tibialis and quadriceps muscles. Exertional weakness (gradual worsening of strength on repeated or sustained muscle contraction) was present in these muscles. He was unable to rise from a squatting position or do deep knee bends. He had some difficulty with heel and toe walking. Reflexes and sensory function were normal.

CASE ANALYSIS

This patient had all the elements of a classic history of MG except for a lack of obvious improvement with pyridostigmine and a negative AChR antibody. His oculofacial weakness, proximal muscle weakness, and exertional weakness were almost diagnostic of MG. Even though this patient had a negative AChR antibody and poor response to a small dose of pyridostigmine, the diagnosis of MG needed to be pursued further. Performance of a muscle biopsy for mitochondrial myopathy (chronic external ophthalmoplegia) was premature.

PLAN OF TESTING

1. RNS test: To confirm MG.
2. SFEMG: To corroborate NMT disorder.
3. Repeat tensilon test: To confirm MG.

TABLE 13.5. NMT Study Data in Case 4

RNS Test Data					SFEMG Data	
			OO			
	ADQ	FCU	Before Ice Pack	After Ice Pack		EDC
CMAP (mV)	15.1	4.8	1.0	1.3	Fiber density	1.3
CMAP Ex (%)	15.1	−1.6			No. Pot pairs	12
2 Hz (%)	−37.1	−79.1	−59.8	−37	Mean MCD (μs)	85
3 Hz (%)	−37.1	−81.9	−75	−47	Normal MCD (μs)	40.4
5 Hz (%)	−32.9	−77.7	−73.7		No. PP with MCD >53 μs (%)	75
50 Hz (%)	−39.5	−55.8			No. PP with blocking (%)	16
5 Hz PT 0 (%)	−5.9	−33.5				
5 Hz PT 4 (%)	−31	−87.4				

ELECTROPHYSIOLOGICAL TESTS AND FINDINGS

Repetitive Nerve Stimulation Test (Table 13.5; Fig. 13.5)
1. Normal CMAP amplitude in the ADQ and FCU muscles.
2. Decremental responses at LRS and HRS in the ADQ and FCU muscles.
3. PTF phenomenon.
4. Improvement of decremental responses in the orbicular oculi after ice-pack testing.

SFEMG (Table 13.5)
1. Normal fiber density.
2. Marked increased mean MCD.
3. Increased number of SFPP with blocking and MCD > 53 μs.

ELECTROPHYSIOLOGICAL INTERPRETATION

Postsynaptic NMT defect typical of severe MG.

OTHER TEST FINDINGS

1. The tensilon test showed marked improvement in the palpebral fissure from 0.6 to 2 cm and in MRC strength in the deltoid from 5− to 5 and in the iliopsoas muscle from 4 to 5. Placebo injection did not show any improvement.
2. Ice-pack test on the right eye showed marked widening of the palpebral fissure from 0.6 to 1.3 cm.

FINAL DIAGNOSIS

Generalized MG, severe

TREATMENT AND FOLLOW-UP

Under the diagnosis of MG, this patient was treated with Mestinon (420 mg/day) and a high dose of prednisone (60 mg/day), which brought gradual improvement in muscle strength. One year later, he was free of myasthenic symptoms on prednisone 20 mg every other day and Mestinon 360 mg/day. CT of the mediastinum and thyroid function studies were normal.

COMMENTS

The tensilon test is still the most helpful, simple, and rapid test for diagnosis of MG. In 95% of MG patients, it is positive. To perform an adequate tensilon test, placebo injection and objective measurement of two or three clinical parameters are crucial (Table 13.6). Placebo

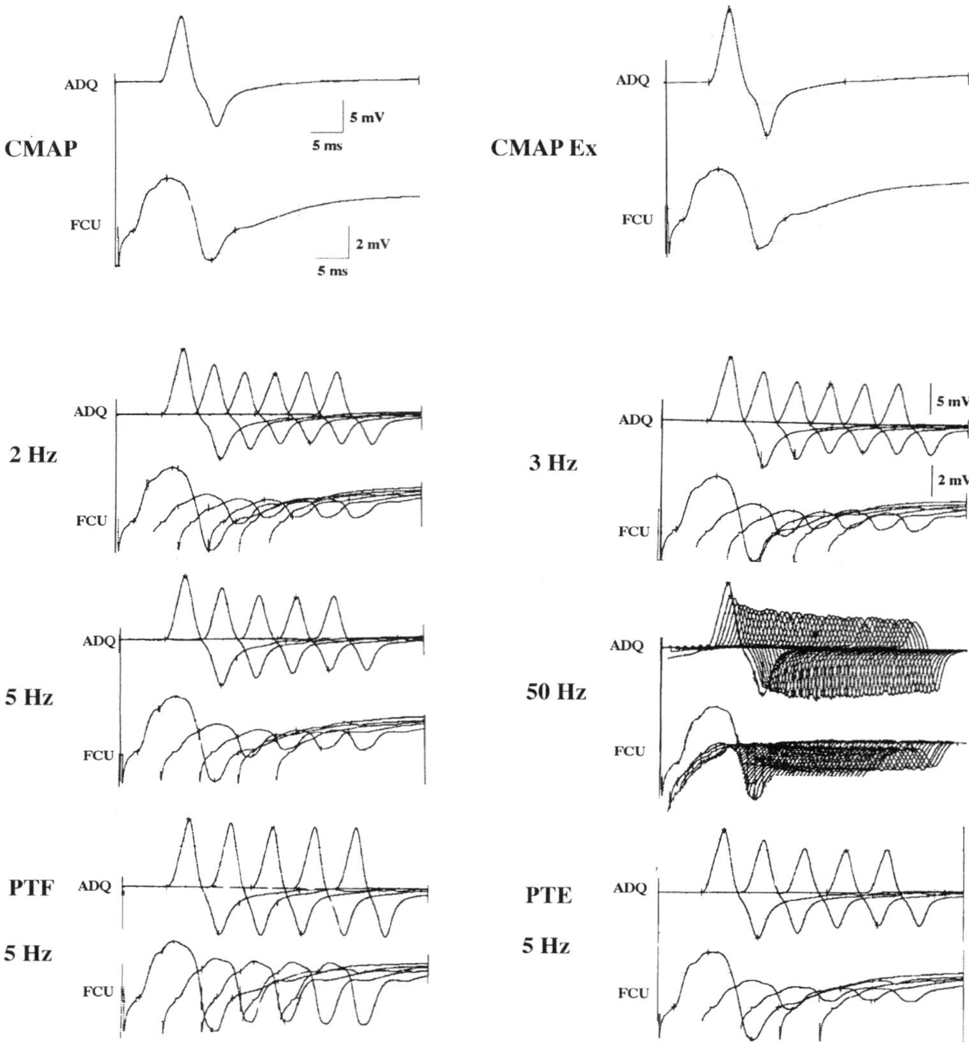

FIGURE 13.5. RNS responses in the ADQ and FCU muscles. RNS pattern typical of severe MG: normal CMAP amplitude, decremental responses at LRS and HRS. *PTF*, posttetanic facilitation; *PTE*, posttetanic exhaustion.

injection has been helpful in sorting out many pseudo-MG patients in whom both the tensilon test and placebo test were positive. A positive tensilon test has also been reported in other diseases. Understandably, it is positive in penicillamine-induced MG and in MG unmasked or precipitated by drugs. The tensilon test was positive in 89% of overlap MG/LEMS cases, in 37% of patients with LEMS and in 27% of those with botulism. Among the congenital myasthenic syndromes, patients with end-plate AChR deficiency and familial infantile myasthenia showed a positive test. False-positive tensilon tests have been reported in a single case of Guillain-Barré syndrome, three cases of amyotrophic lateral sclerosis, one case of brainstem glioma, and eight cases of parasellar tumor and aneurysm. Thus, an unequivocally positive edrophonium test alone is not necessarily diagnostic of MG. The diagnosis of MG should be based on the clinical features together with edrophonium responsiveness and other laboratory findings. A false-negative tensilon test may be seen in ocular MG, especially when ophthal-

TABLE 13.6. Single-Blind Tensilon (Edrophonium Chloride) Test[a]

Preparation materials

One tensilon (edrophonium chloride) 10-mg ampule
One butterfly IV connector
One 1-mL syringe with placebo (saline)
One 1-mL syringe with tensilon
One atropine 0.4-mg ampule ready in case needed[b]

Procedures

1. Explain procedure and reason for the test. Emphasize that two drugs are used for testing that may have side reactions. Do not go into the details of side reactions, so that the patient may notice which is genuine medication.
2. Choose two or three objective measurements (e.g., palpebral fissure opening measurement, MRC strength of deltoids or iliopsoas muscles, FVC, etc.).
3. Place a butterfly IV connector and be sure to have free flow of fluid.
4. Inject 0.2 mL of placebo first and observe whether there is any side reaction. Also check heart beat by the radial pulse.
5. If no side reaction is observed, inject the remaining 0.8 mL of placebo and wait 1 minute. While waiting 1 minute, check the radial pulse for irregularity or slow pulses.
6. Check objective measurements for any improvement.
7. Then, inject 0.2 mL of tensilon first and observe whether there is any side reaction. Again check heart beat.
8. If no side reaction is observed, inject the remaining 0.8 mL tensilon and wait 1 minute. Again, check the radial pulse and any side reactions.
9. Check objective measurements for any improvement.
10. Write down the accurate measurements in the chart and decide whether the test was positive or negative. Do not just write down "positive" or "negative" test.[c]

[a] Ideally speaking, the tensilon test should be "double-blind." However, sometimes the IV tensilon effect lasts longer than 5 minutes (supposedly the duration of effect of tensilon). If that occurs, there will be a continued improvement even with placebo. Thus, it is impossible to have a "double-blind" test.

[b] Cardiac complication is extremely rare. When this occurs, atropine should be given intravenously.

[c] Physicians who review the record later would like to know exactly what is measured and how good responses are.

moplegia is severe, as noted in this case, or when ophthalmoplegia is too minimal for objective measurement. In this case, the prostigmine test is often positive, as discussed in case 1. In recent years, a simple and inexpensive ice-pack test (application of ice over the eyes for 3 to 4 minutes) was found to be positive for ocular MG. This test was investigated in patients with MG, normal individuals, and a few cases of third nerve palsy and was positive only for MG.

This patient's RNS response is typical of severe MG: abnormal decremental response at LRS and at HRS with less common PTF and rare PTE.

MAXIMS

1. An adequate tensilon test should include a placebo injection and objective measurement of two or three clinical parameters.
2. A positive tensilon test is not necessarily diagnostic of MG.

REFERENCES

1. Oh SJ, Cho HK. Edrophonium responsiveness not necessarily diagnostic of myasthenia gravis. Muscle Nerve 1990:13:187–191.
2. Osserman KE, Genkins G. Clinical reappraisal of the use of edrophonium (tensilon) chloride tests in myasthenia gravis and significance of clinical classification. Ann NY Acad Sci 1965;135:312–326.

CASE 5

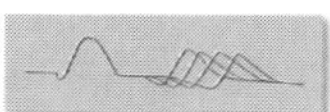

RECURRENT BULBAR PALSY DUE TO PYRIDOSTIGMINE?

CASE PRESENTATION

A 20-year-old woman had had a confirmed diagnosis of severe generalized MG in 1988, after a 6-month history of progressive bulbar palsy and generalized weakness. For the next 2 years, her course of MG was unstable even after treatment with pyridostigmine, prednisone (up to 80 mg/day), thymectomy, azathioprine (200 mg/day), and several plasma exchanges for repeated myasthenic crises. As side effects of these immunotherapies, she developed diabetes mellitus, a Cushingoid appearance, septicemia due to infection associated with vascular and Hickman catheters, and a right atrial thrombus. In early 1990, her MG was finally stabilized on 200 mg azathioprine daily, 30 mg of prednisone, and 180 mg of Mestinon. In April and May 1990, she was admitted to UAB twice for bulbar palsy after discontinuation of Mestinon. She was convinced that pyridostigmine was responsible for her bulbar palsy because this drug made her "sick at the stomach," short of breath, caused too much secretion in the mouth, and made talking difficult. On admission, abnormal neurological findings were mild bilateral ptosis and facial diplegia, nasal speech, and inability to clear oral secretion due to swallowing difficulty. FVC was 1400 to 1700 mL. No other neurological abnormality was noted.

CASE ANALYSIS

It seemed obvious to the clinician that this patient's bulbar palsy was due to myasthenic weakness that could be treated with pyridostigmine, avoiding costly admission. However, the patient was adamant that her bulbar palsy was due to pyridostigmine. Thus, it was the clinician's job to convince her that she needed pyridostigmine.

PLAN OF TESTING

1. RNS test: To confirm the diagnosis of MG in 1988, to assess the severity of MG in 1990, and to rule out pyridostigmine toxicity.
2. Special RNS test: To convince the patient objectively whether her bulbar palsy was due to too little pyridostigmine. This should be done with an edrophonium test 1 hour after her last dose of pyridostigmine.

ELECTROPHYSIOLOGICAL TESTS AND FINDINGS

RNS Test Findings (Table 13.7)

1. 1988 test:
   a. Normal CMAP amplitude, marked decremental responses at LRS and HRS, PTF and PTE in the ADQ and FCU muscles.

TABLE 13.7. RNS Test Data in Case 5

	7/7/88			5/20/90			
	ADQ	**FCU**	**OO**	**ADQ**	**FCU**	**OO Before Edrophonium**	**OO with Edrophonium**
CMAP (mV)	13.5	10	2.05	19.5	12.2	2.4	3.0
CMAP Ex (%)	18.5	−10		2.6	0		
2 Hz (%)	−11.7	−15.6	−38.0	−4.8	10	−9.0	−2.0
3 Hz (%)	−17.1	−27.5	−53.8	−4.8	−4.8	−18.0	0
5 Hz (%)	−14.1	−27.5	−52.9	−5.0	10	−19.0	13
50 Hz (%)	−22.5	−32.5		−20	20		
5 Hz PT 0 (%)	−3.2	−9		0	0		
5 Hz PT 4 (%)	−19.1	−40		−5.3	0		

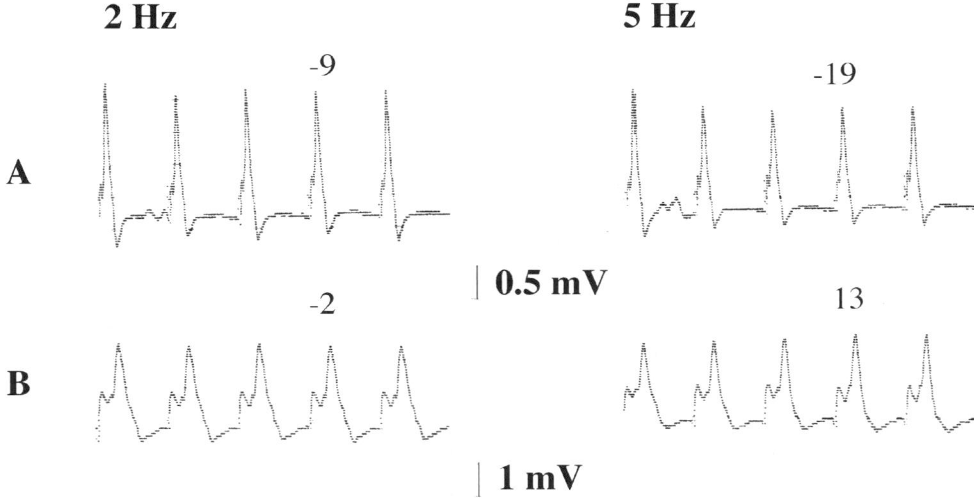

FIGURE 13.6. Definite improvement in the RNS test in the orbicularis oculi muscle after edrophonium test. **A.** Before edrophonium injection. **B.** After edrophonium injection.

   b. Normal CMAP amplitude and marked decremental response at LRS in the orbicularis oculi muscle.
2. 1990 routine test: Normal CMAP amplitude and no decremental response at LRS or HRS in ADQ and FCU muscles.
3. 1990 special test on the orbicularis oculi muscle (Table 13.7; Fig. 13.6):
   a. Normal CMAP amplitude and abnormal decremental response at LRS before edrophonium test.
   b. Increase in the CMAP amplitude and no decremental response at LRS after edrophonium test.

ELECTROPHYSIOLOGICAL INTERPRETATION

1. 1988 test: Postsynaptic transmission defect typical of severe MG.
2. 1990 test: No electrophysiological evidence of pyridostigmine toxicity. Compared with the 1988 test, there was a definite improvement.
3. RNS test in the orbicularis oculi muscle:
   a. Before edrophonium: Postsynaptic transmission defect typical of MG.
   b. With edrophonium: Normal response and definite improvement with edrophonium.

FINAL DIAGNOSIS

Bulbar MG improved by edrophonium treatment

TREATMENT AND FOLLOW-UP

On the first admission, a routine RNS test ruled out pyridostigmine overtoxicity, and for 2 days the patient was observed without any pyridostigmine. Her bulbar symptoms worsened. When Mestinon was restarted, she complained of nausea, abdominal cramps, and diarrhea, which were not controllable with atropine. Thus, two 10-mg tablets of ambostigmine were given without any muscarinic effect but with much improvement of bulbar symptoms. After discharge from the hospital, she was not able to continue ambostigmine. Thus, 30 mg of pyridostigmine was restarted. Her bulbar symptoms recurred and she was admitted again to UAB. An edrophonium test that showed definite improvement on the RNS test in the orbicularis oris muscle convinced her that she needed pyridostigmine. With Mestinon Timespan (90 mg twice a day), her bulbar palsy was improved without any muscarinic effect.

COMMENTS

Even in the era of the AChR antibody assay, the RNS test has its place in the diagnosis and management of MG (see Table 4.6). It is obvious that the RNS test is indicated for objective confirmation of disease in seronegative MG. Our study showed a statistically significant difference between seronegative and seropositive groups in the overall abnormality rate of the RNS test: 65.8% in seronegative and 83.3% in seropositive groups. Decremental responses at LRS in the ADQ and FCU muscle were worse in the seropositive group, indicating that seronegative MG is milder. When rapid and objective diagnosis of MG is needed, the RNS study is the test of choice because the result is immediately available. Results of the AChR antibody test may require a few days to a few weeks. The RNS test can also be used for objective measurement of the severity of MG because there is a good correlation between electrophysiological and clinical assessment of disease severity of MG.

When an objective titration of anti-ChE is needed, as in our case, the RNS test is most helpful in resolving the issue. Tensilon (edrophonium) improves the RNS abnormalities in roughly 87% of cases. After edrophonium injection, there is usually improvement in decremental response at LRS and an increase in the CMAP amplitude as noted in our case. Electrophysiological improvement became maximal within 2 to 3 minutes after edrophonium injection. This is in contrast to clinical improvement, which is maximal within 1 minute after edrophonium injection.

The most common side effects of anti-ChE are muscarinic effects: abdominal cramps, nausea, and diarrhea. These are not dose related and do not necessarily reflect anti-ChE toxicity. These side effects can easily be relieved by Atropine or Robinul (glycopyrrolate). Atropine or Robinul do not mask anti-ChE toxicity. Thus, it is important to use Atropine or Robinul liberally to reduce the uncomfortable muscarinic effects as much and as early as possible. This is because the anti-ChE is a most effective symptomatic drug of choice. Among the various anti-ChE agents, Mytelase (ambostigmine) has the fewest muscarinic effects, followed by Mestinon Timespan (long-acting pyridostigmine).

MAXIMS

1. Muscarinic effects of pyridostigmine are not necessarily indicative of pyridostigmine toxicity.
2. After edrophonium injection, an increase in the CMAP amplitude and improvement in decremental response are the usual findings on the RNS test in MG.

REFERENCES

1. Oh SJ. Electrophysiological characteristics in seronegative myasthenia gravis. Ann NY Acad 1993; 681:584–587.
2. Horowitz SH, Genkins G, Kornfeld, Papatestas AE. Electrophysiologic diagnosis of myasthenia gravis and the regional curare test. Neurology 1976;26:410–417.

CASE 6

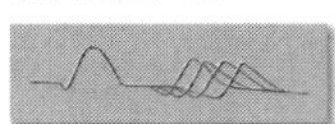

"SHAKING ARMS" IN THE RECOVERY ROOM IN A PATIENT WITH RHEUMATOID ARTHRITIS

CASE PRESENTATION

A 57-year-old woman with rheumatoid arthritis underwent general anesthesia including succinylcholine during corrective surgery for a deformed foot. On awakening, she was noted to have "shaking arms" and severe right ptosis. A neurological consultation for "convulsion" was requested. Examination in the recovery room by the chief neurology resident showed an alert woman with marked right fatigable ptosis, vertical diplopia without any obvious ophthalmoplegia, nasal speech, and 3 MRC strength in deltoid muscles.

CASE ANALYSIS

Neurological examination showed oculobulbar palsy and proximal muscle weakness with fatigable ptosis. An astute chief resident ruled out convulsion and recognized the patient's problem right away upon reviewing the history and performing a simple tensilon test, which showed marked improvement in right ptosis and resolution of diplopia. For her rheumatoid arthritis, she had been on penicillamine for 2 years. In retrospect, she recalled a 2-month history of diplopia, easy fatigability, and drooping of the right eyelid. She had penicillamine-induced MG unmasked by muscle paralyzing agents.

PLAN OF TESTING

1. RNS test: Portable test to confirm the diagnosis of MG.
2. SFEMG: To corroborate the diagnosis of MG.
3. AChR antibody: To confirm penicillamine-induced MG. This test must be positive.

ELECTROPHYSIOLOGICAL TESTS AND FINDINGS

RNS Test Findings (Table 13.8; Fig. 13.7)

1. Normal response in ADQ, FCU, orbicularis oris, and trapezius muscle.
2. Severe decremental response in deltoid muscle.

SFEMG

1. Normal fiber density.
2. Mildly prolonged mean MCD.

ELECTROPHYSIOLOGICAL INTERPRETATION

Postsynaptic NMT defect typical of MG on the RNS test in the deltoid and on the SFEMG in the EDC muscle.

TABLE 13.8. NMT Study Data in Case 6

RNS Test Data						SFEMG Data	
	ADQ	FCU	OO	Trapezius	Deltoid		EDC
CMAP (mV)	10.4	4.0	2.7	10	14.0	Fiber density	1.6
CMAP Ex (%)	17.4					No. Pot pairs	12
2/s (%)	0	0	0	0	−38	Mean MCD (μs)	43
3/s (%)	0	−3.7	13.7	1.9	−38	Normal MCD (μs)	40.4
5/s (%)	0	3.8	0	15.7	−40	No. PP with MCD >53 μs (%)	8.3
50/s (%)	8.7	40				No. PP with blocking (%)	0
5/s PT 0 (%)	0	1.9					
5/s PT 4 m (%)	7.0	0					

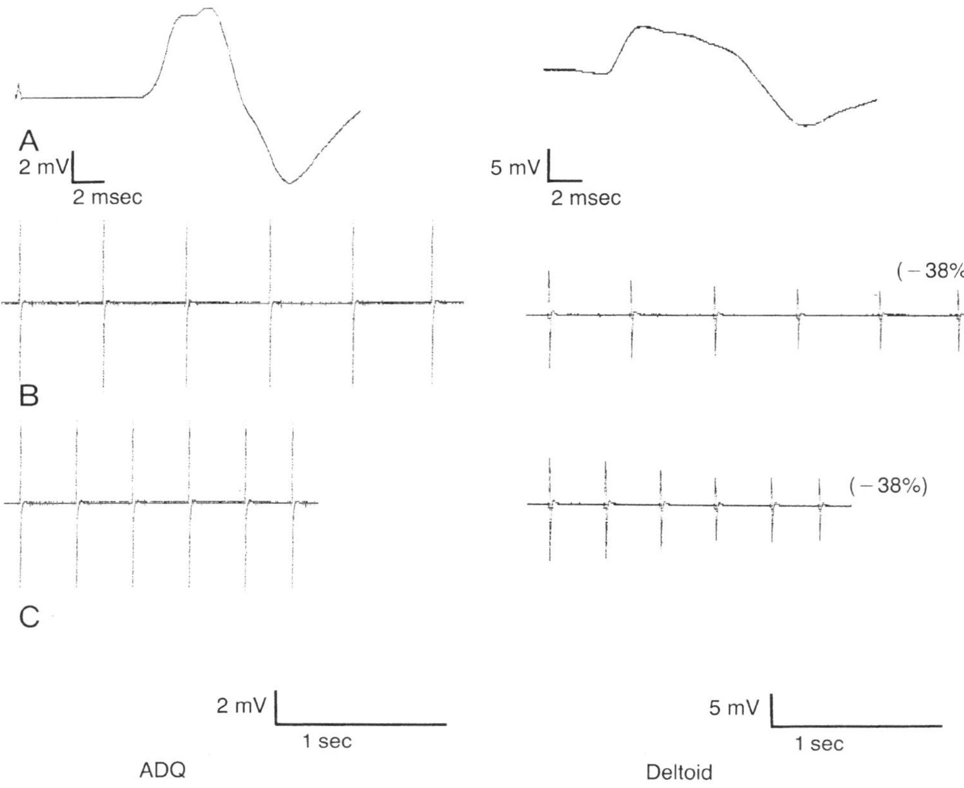

FIGURE 13.7. Normal RNS responses in ADQ and decremental responses in deltoid. **A.** CMAPs at rest. **B.** Responses at 2-Hz stimulation. **C.** Responses at 3-Hz stimulation. Normal responses were also found in ADQ, FCU, and orbicularis oculi muscles in this patient.

FINAL DIAGNOSIS

Penicillamine-induced MG

TREATMENT AND FOLLOW-UP

AChR antibody was positive. In view of the confirmation of penicillamine-induced MG, penicillamine was discontinued and no anti-ChE medication was prescribed. Examination 1 month later showed only mild right ptosis with fatigable weakness. Within 4 months, all her symptoms disappeared.

COMMENTS

Autoimmune MG has been known to occur in a few patients undergoing long-term penicillamine treatment for rheumatoid arthritis, scleroderma, or Wilson's disease. This syndrome is indistinguishable clinically, electrophysiologically, pharmacologically, and immunologically from classic MG except by its high remission rate after discontinuation of penicillamine and positive AChR antibody. Symptoms usually disappear within 8 months after penicillamine withdrawal, as noted in this case. Anti-ChE medications were effective in relieving symptoms. Edrophonium and neostigmine tests were positive. The RNS test and SFEMG showed findings identical to those seen in classic MG.

It has been well-known that certain drugs or agents can aggravate MG or LEMS. Penicillamine is contraindicated because it is known to produce MG, as is seen in this case. Any neuromuscular blockade (depolarizing or nondepolarizing agents) should be avoided because

TABLE 13.9. Drug Alert Lists for MG or LEMS Patients

Drug that is absolutely contraindicated
  D-Penicillamine[a]
Drugs that unmask or aggravate myasthenic symptoms definitely
  All neuromuscular blocking agents: competitive blocking agents (e.g., pancuronium, tubocurarine) and depolarizing agents (e.g., succinylcholine)
Drugs that unmask or aggravate myasthenic symptoms in most patients
  Antibiotics, particularly aminoglycosides[b]
    Neomycin, streptomycin, kanamycin, gentamycin, polymyxin, colistin, erythromycin, lincomycin, ampicillin, tobramycin, clindamycin, oxy- and rolie-tetracycline, bacitracin, cephalexin
  Cardiovascular drugs
    Quinidine, quinine, procainamide, trimethaphan; beta-blockers (e.g., propranolol, nodolol, practolol); calcium channel blockers (e.g., verapamil)
  Eye drops: timolol and betalol (beta-blockers)
  Magnesium salts
Drugs that unmask or aggravate myasthenic symptoms in some patients
  Anticonvulsants (e.g., phenytoin, trimethadione, ethsuccinamide)
  Antipsychotics (e.g., lithium salts, chloropromazine, phenelzine)
Diagnostic agents
  Iodinated contrast media

[a] Long-term D-penicillamine treatment can produce AChR antibody positive MG.

they definitely aggravate MG or LEMS (Table 13.9). They can bring out symptoms of MG or LEMS for the first time, aggravate existing symptoms, and produce prolonged paralysis or respiratory failure. Many aminoglycosides and antiarrhythmic agents are also well known to aggravate symptoms of MG or LEMS. Thus, these drugs should be avoided if there is any alternative. In this case, penicillamine-induced MG was unmasked by curare and succinylcholine. Because of these effects, systemic curarization was used as a diagnostic test for MG in the past and regional or systemic curarization was used as activation for the RNS test. Regional and systemic curarization were known to increase the diagnostic yield in generalized and ocular MG. However, these tests are no longer used because better diagnostic test, such as the SFEMG or AChR antibody test, are available and the possibility of respiratory failure exists.

The RNS test on the deltoid muscle is technically most difficult. It is extremely hard to keep the stimulating electrodes firmly in place during stimulation. Stimulation at 2 Hz produces the most technically satisfactory responses. If the test shows abnormalities, it must be repeated to check whether the results are reproducible. In recent studies, the axillary RNS test showed a higher diagnostic sensitivity for MG than the accessory RNS test. Nevertheless, we prefer the accessory and facial RNS tests as the second-line tests because of greater patient tolerance and technical dependability.

MAXIMS

1. Long-term penicillamine treatment can induce seropositive MG in a few patients.
2. MG can be unmasked or aggravated by neuromuscular blocking agents. Thus, such drugs should be avoided in MG and LEMS patients.
3. The RNS test on the deltoid muscle is technically difficult. If the test is abnormal, the test should be repeated to see whether the result is reproducible.

REFERENCES

1. Fawcell PRW, McLachlan SM, Nicholson LVB, Mataglia FL. D-Penicillamine myasthenia gravis: immunological and electrophysiological studies. Muscle Nerve 1982;5:328–334.
2. Howard JF. Adverse drug effects on NMT. Semin Neurol 1990;16:89–102.

CASE 7

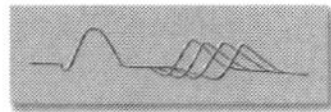

MG OR CHRONIC FATIGUE SYNDROME

CASE PRESENTATION

A 44-year-old man had a flu-like illness with adenopathy 1.5 years ago. Since then, he had general weakness, easy fatigability, difficulty walking, and occasional double vision and droopy eyelids. His weakness and walking difficulty worsened as the day went by, and especially in the evening, his double vision and droopy eyelids became prominent and he had trouble climbing the stairs to go to bed. Abnormal neurological findings were mild left ptosis, 5− MRC strength, which was fatigable to 4, in proximal muscles of the upper and lower extremities.

CASE ANALYSIS

The history of a flu-like illness and subsequent generalized weakness and fatigue were strongly suggestive of chronic fatigue syndrome. His occasional double vision, droopy eyelids, and good history of exertional weakness also suggested the possibility of MG. Fatigable weakness of the proximal muscles is strong objective evidence of MG.

PLAN OF TESTING

1. Needle EMG: To check for any varying amplitude of MUP or myopathic pattern.
2. RNS test: To determine whether there is a genuine decremental response.
3. SFEMG: To confirm the diagnosis of MG when the RNS test is normal and AChR antibody is negative.
4. Other tests: Tensilon test and AChR antibody.

ELECTROPHYSIOLOGICAL TESTS AND FINDINGS

Needle EMG
1. No varying amplitude of MUP is noted.
2. SASD MUPs in some spots in the iliopsoas muscle.

RNS Test Findings (Table 13.10). Normal test in the ADQ, FCU, orbicularis oculi, and trapezius muscles.

SFEMG (Table 13.10; Fig 13.8)
1. Normal fiber density.
2. Increased mean MCDs.
3. Increased number of SFPP with more than 53 μs and blocking.

ELECTROPHYSIOLOGICAL INTERPRETATION

Abnormal jitter compatible with MG.

TABLE 13.10. NMT Study Data in Case 7

RNS Test Data					SFEMG Data	
	ADQ	FCU	OO	Trapezius		EDC
CMAP (mV)	7.2	2.8	4.5	14.8	Fiber density	1.25
CMAP Ex (%)	10.4	15.2			No. Pot pairs	10
2 Hz (%)	−6.6	1.5	0.9	1.3	Mean MCD (μs)	99
3 Hz (%)	0	−4.1	−0.8	1.3	Normal MCD (μs)	40.4
5 Hz (%)	0	−0.5	2.6	−1.9	No. PP with MCD >53 μs (%)	40
50 Hz (%)	−10.1	5.0			No. PP with blocking (%)	40
5 Hz PT 0 (%)	2.2	8.7				
5 Hz PT 4 m (%)	4.5	−9.4				

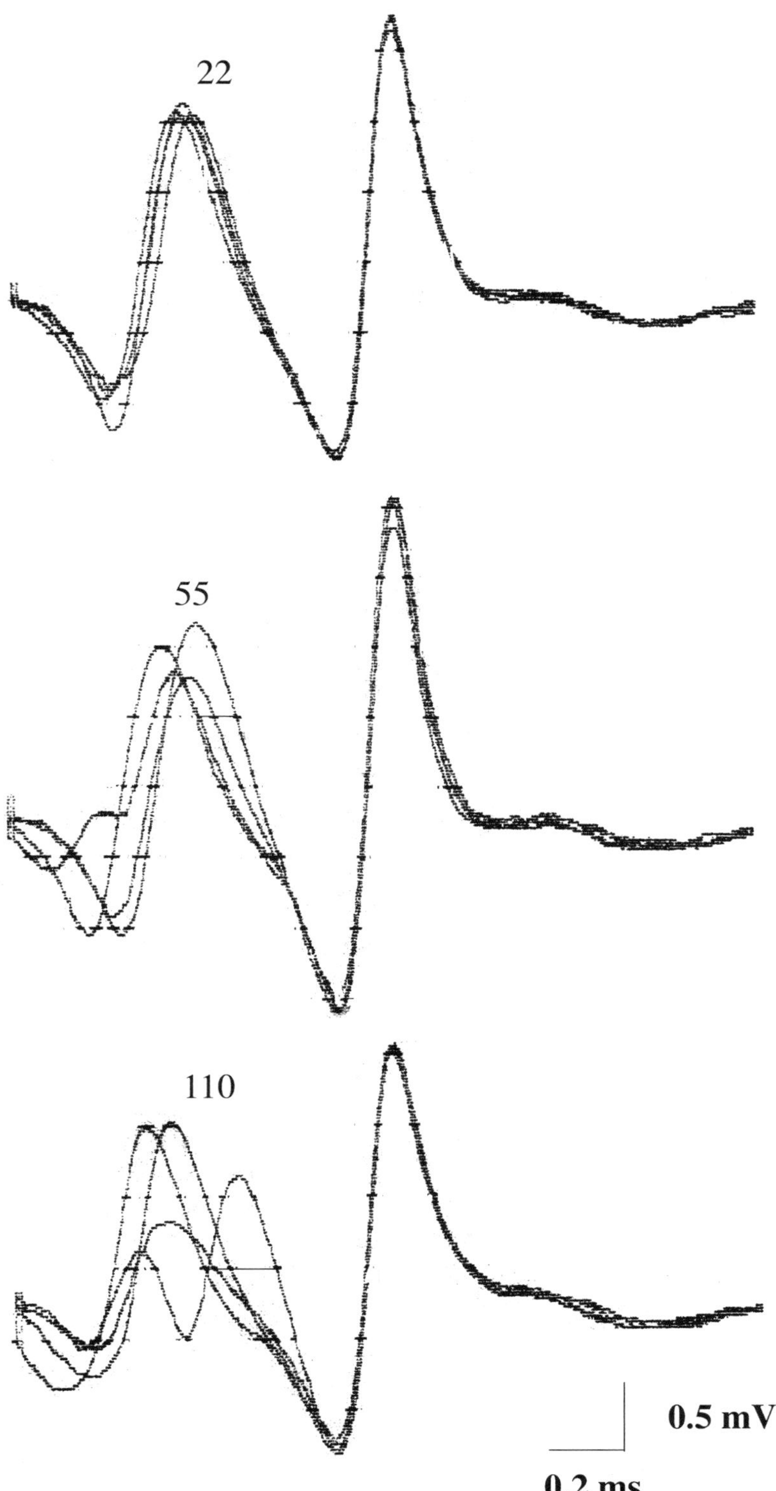

FIGURE 13.8. Normal jitter to markedly abnormal jitter in one SFPP in SFEMG in the EDC muscle.

FINAL DIAGNOSIS

Mild seronegative generalized MG

TREATMENT AND FOLLOW-UP

The tensilon test was positive. However, AChR binding, modulating, and blocking antibody tests were all normal. The definite SFEMG abnormality ruled out chronic fatigue syndrome and supported the clinical impression of MG. The patient was treated with pyridostigimine 240 mg/day with almost complete relief of his symptoms, as would be expected in MG.

COMMENTS

Often, it is difficult to differentiate MG from chronic fatigue syndrome or a neurotic reaction. Complaints of patients with chronic fatigue syndrome or neurotic reaction are usually characterized by constant generalized fatigue from morning to evening, other psychosomatic complaints, and a lack of any definite oculobulbar dysfunction such as double vision, ptosis, and chewing or speech difficulty. They cannot describe difficulty with any specific task and often report, "I feel tired all the time and cannot do anything," as if describing a lack of energy rather than easy fatigability. On examination, such patients may show a generalized "give-in weakness." The tensilon test is typically positive to placebo injection. All laboratory studies including the SFEMG are normal. Some of these patients will respond to Mestinon and are able to consume an excessive amount of Mestinon.

The SFEMG is the single most sensitive clinical test for MG, being positive in 77 to 100% of MG cases. The test is so sensitive that Stålberg and Trontelj concluded that the diagnosis of MG can be abandoned if abnormal jitter is not present in a weak muscle. However, this test has a drawback in that it requires fairly elaborate equipment and extensive training for the electromyographer, as well as patient cooperation. For this reason, this test is performed in only a limited number of EMG laboratories. Another drawback has been the nonspecificity of the SFEMG for MG, because similar abnormalities may be observed in many neuromuscular diseases.

The classic SFEMG pattern in MG is characterized by a definite increase in jitter with or without neuromuscular blocking and normal fiber density. The jitter abnormality usually increases with a higher discharge rate in MG. For obvious reasons, the SFEMG is most useful in seronegative MG cases in which the RNS test was negative and is thus the "must test" in 9% of MG cases. In mild generalized and ocular MG, in which the RNS test and AChR antibody are often normal, this test can be the crucial means of confirming the diagnosis of MG. Comparing all three diagnostic tests, the AChR antibody is the most specific and is positive in about 85% of cases. The RNS test has a relative specificity for MG and is positive in about 75% of cases. In none of our MG patients were all three tests found to be negative. Thus, MG can be confidently ruled out if all three tests are negative.

One advantage of the SFEMG is that its diagnostic sensitivity is not affected by ongoing treatment with anti-ChE drugs. It has been well demonstrated that anti-ChE drugs can modify the result of the RNS test and that a 12-hour anti-ChE-off period is essential in obtaining an accurate response to the test in mild MG. An earlier study showed that the SFEMG was abnormal in all studied MG patients, regardless of the anti-ChE status. Even though a few exceptions to this rule have been reported, these are extremely rare. Thus, the SFEMG can be performed in MG patients on anti-ChE drugs without loss of diagnostic sensitivity.

MAXIMS

1. The SFEMG is most useful and the "must test" in seronegative MG cases with normal RNS tests.
2. The diagnosis of MG is not tenable if the SFEMG is normal in clinically weak muscles.

REFERENCES

1. Oh SJ, Kim DE, Kuruoglu R, Bradley RJ, Dwyer D. Diagnostic sensitivity of the laboratory tests in myasthenia gravis. Muscle Nerve 1992;15:720–724.
2. Sanders DB, Stålberg E. SFEMG. AAEM Monograph #25. Single Fiber Electromyography 1996;19: 1069–1083.

CASE 8

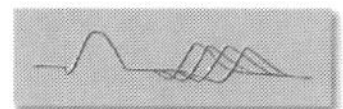

THYMECTOMY IN AN MG PATIENT WITH AREFLEXIA

CASE PRESENTATION

A 53-year-old woman was admitted to the UAB Hospital for thymectomy for MG. Seven months before admission, she experienced easy fatigability and double vision. She had left ptosis that was improved dramatically with edrophonium, and thus her internist made a diagnosis of MG. Pyridostigmine was given with initial improvement. Serum AChR antibody was negative. Rheumatology profile and thyroid studies were also normal. Mediastinal CT did not show any evidence of thymoma. Because of subsequent development of dysphagia, double vision, and increasing leg weakness, a daily 60-mg dose of prednisone was added with some initial improvement, which was not sustained. Thus, thymectomy was recommended and the patient was admitted. Neurological examination showed fatigable left ptosis, 3 MRC strength in the shoulder and pelvic girdle muscles, and areflexia. There was a transient improvement of strength in the proximal muscles after brief exercise. Knee and ankle reflexes were also elicitable immediately after a short period of strenuous exercise.

CASE ANALYSIS

Initially, the diagnosis of MG was correctly made on the basis of oculobulbar symptoms and a positive edrophonium test, which are typical findings in MG (see Table 13.1). Basic workup for MG, including the mediastinal CT, were normal. In view of the patient's resistance to prednisone therapy, thymectomy was rightfully recommended. Areflexia is not typical of MG. Careful examination showed clinical findings typical of LEMS. A transient improvement of muscle strength and muscle stretch reflexes after brief exercise is pathognomonic of LEMS.

PLAN OF TESTING

1. NCS: To rule out demyelinating peripheral neuropathy, which can explain diffuse areflexia and proximal weakness.
2. RNS test: To confirm the diagnosis of LEMS.
3. H-reflex and T-reflex test: To document a transient improvement of muscle stretch reflexes after brief exercise.
4. SFEMG: To corroborate the diagnosis of LEMS.

ELECTROPHYSIOLOGICAL TESTS AND FINDINGS

RNS Test Findings (Table 13.11; Fig. 13.9)

1. Low CMAP amplitude in the ADQ and FCU muscles.
2. PEF > 100%.
3. Abnormal decremental responses at the low rate of stimulation.

TABLE 13.11. NMT Study Data in Case 8

RNS Test Data			SFEMG Data	
	ADQ	FCU		EDC
CMAP (mV)	1.25	0.9	Fiber density	1.8
CMAP Ex (%)	540	420	No. Pot pairs	12
2 Hz (%)	−15	−26	Mean MCD	141
3 Hz (%)	−25	−21	Normal MCD	40.4
5 Hz (%)	−11	−16	No. PP with MCD >53 μs (%)	100
50 Hz (%)	325	350	No. PP with blocking (%)	76
5 Hz PT 0 (%)	0	5		
5 Hz PT 4 (%)	9	7		

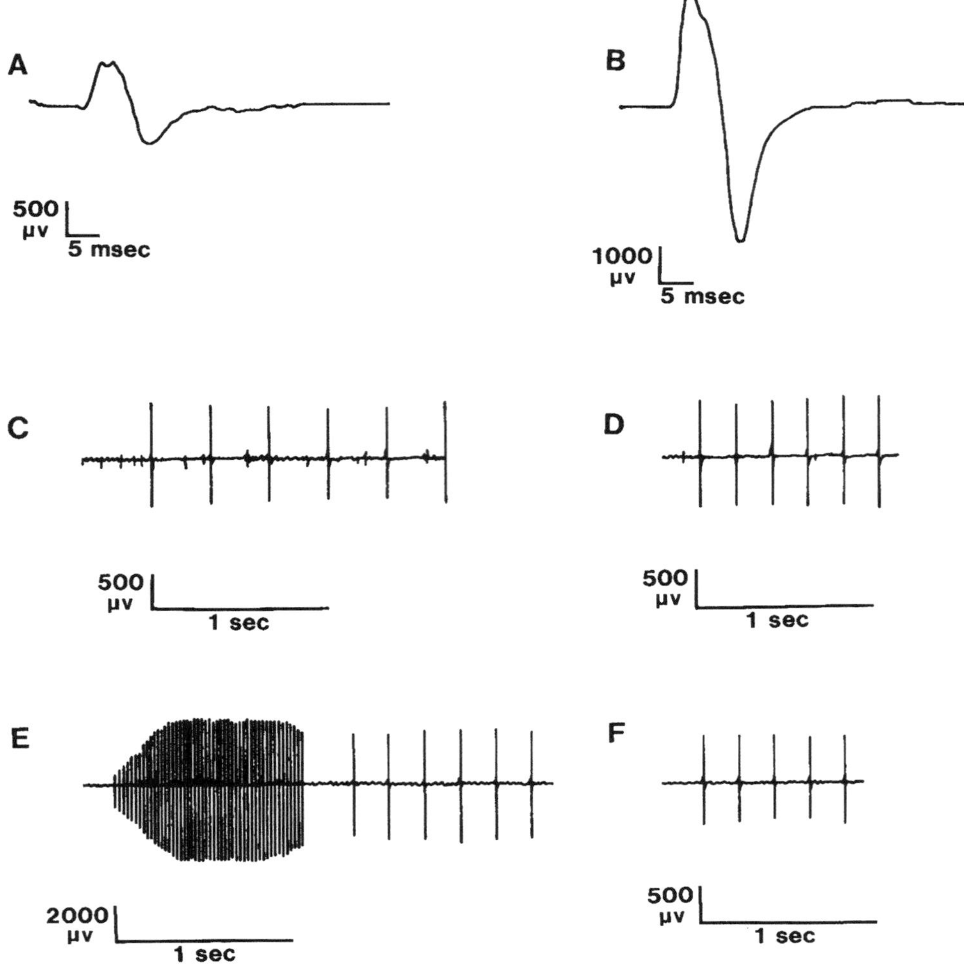

FIGURE 13.9. RNS pattern typical of LEMS. **A.** Low CMAP amplitude. **B.** Marked facilitation (540%) after 30 seconds of exercise. **C.** Twenty-five percent decrement at 3-Hz stimulation. **D.** Eleven percent decrement at 5-Hz stimulation. **E.** Marked facilitation (325% incremental response) at 50-Hz stimulation and normal response at 5-Hz stimulation immediately after tetanic stimulation. **F.** Nine percent decrement at 5-Hz stimulation 4 minutes after tetanic stimulation.

4. Marked incremental response (>100%) at the high rate of stimulation.
5. PTF but no PTE.

SFEMG

1. Increased mean MCD.
2. Increased number of potential pairs > 54 μs.
3. Increased number of SFPP with blocking.

H- and T-Reflexes

1. Marked increase in the H-reflex amplitude after exercise (Fig. 13.10).
2. Absent T-reflex before exercise and elicitation of ankle T-reflex after exercise.

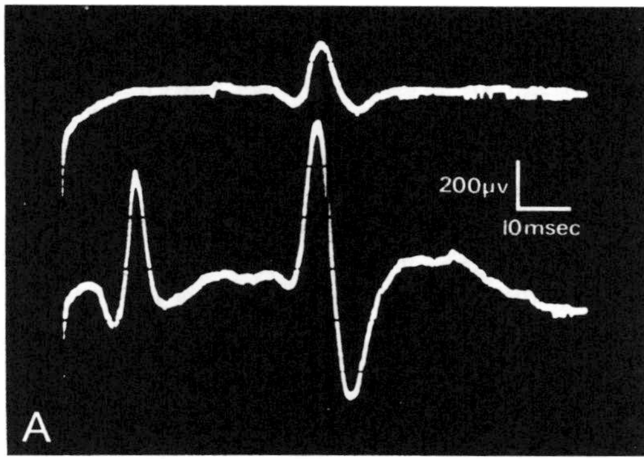

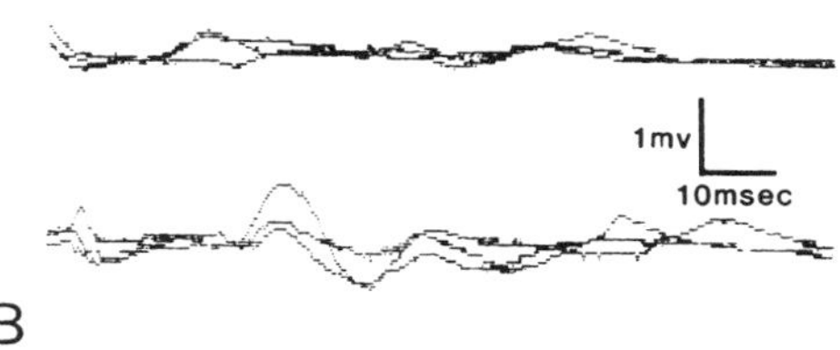

FIGURE 13.10. H-reflex (**A**) and T-reflex (**B**) improvement after exercise in LEMS. The first line represents the response before exercise and the second line, after exercise. Marked increase of the H-reflex amplitude and elicitation of the M-response after exercise. T-reflex was elicited after exercise. (Reprinted with permission from Joy JL, Baysal A, Oh SJ. Reflex improvement after exercise in the Eaton-Lambert syndrome. Muscle Nerve 1987;10:672.)

NCS Findings. In motor NCS, an extremely low CMAP amplitude in all tested nerves. Normal sensory and mixed NCS.

ELECTROPHYSIOLOGICAL INTERPRETATION

Presynaptic NMT defect typical of LEMS.

OTHER TEST FINDINGS

Initial cancer workup including CT chest and bronchial washing was negative.

FINAL DIAGNOSIS

LEMS

TREATMENT AND FOLLOW-UP

Thymectomy was not performed. However, 3 months later, a right hilar mass was found on the chest x-ray, and the diagnosis of small-cell lung cancer was confirmed histologically. The SCLC was treated with radiation and chemotherapy. LEMS was treated with 1500 mg guanidine hydrochloride and 300 mg pyridostigmine daily. In 2 months, the patient had mild weakness. For 2 years, her carcinoma was in remission and she was asymptomatic with 625 mg guanidine and 300 mg pyridostigmine. Then, gradually her weakness recurred and became worse even with additional prednisone and azathioprine therapy. Recurrence of the tumor was found 8 months after the return of weakness. The patient subsequently died.

COMMENTS

The classic triad of LEMS was observed on the RNS test in this case: low CMAP amplitude that increased after exercise (>100% increase), decremental response at the low rate of stimulation, and incremental response (>100%) at the high rate of stimulation. H-reflex and T-reflex testing with exercise showed the classic findings of LEMS (Fig. 13.10). Thus, the RNS data and the H-reflex and T-reflex data are pathognomonic of LEMS.

LEMS was first described in 1956 in association with small-cell carcinoma of the lung by Lambert and Eaton. Thus, it is called either "Lambert-Eaton myasthenic syndrome" or "Eaton-Lambert syndrome." Twelve years after the first description of LEMS, Elmqvist and Lambert pinpointed the basic mechanism of this disorder as a presynaptic defect of ACh release by means of an elegant MEPP study with intercostal nerve-muscle preparation. A recent study showed that this presynaptic defect of ACh release is induced by the voltage-gated calcium channel antibody.

The clinical diagnosis of LEMS is almost always elusive, as noted in this case. According to our experience, LEMS can mimic MG, myopathy, motor neuropathy, conversion reaction, or lumbar radiculopathy. Clinical suspicion is the key for the diagnosis of LEMS. The most common symptoms are easy fatigability and leg weakness. The classic clinical triad of LEMS includes proximal leg weakness, hyporeflexia or areflexia, and easy fatigability. A transient improvement in muscle strength and muscle stretch reflexes immediately after brief exercise is classically observed in LEMS. These findings, if observed, are pathognomonic of LEMS. This facilitation is most easily detected in moderately affected muscles, often the deltoid or iliopsoas muscles. This is the clinical counterpart of postexercise facilitation on the RNS test. Unfortunately, these are not common observations, noted in only one of three cases, according to our experience. Thus, when LEMS is suspected, these simple bedside tests are extremely helpful for confirmation of the disease. In this connection, in LEMS patients, it is important to assess the muscle strength on the first effort made by the patient after rest, before facilitation has increased the force of the contraction. Normally, the nerve action potential increases the calcium influx at the presynaptic membrane, which then stimulates release of ACh. In LEMS, antibody attacks at the nerve terminal produce morphologic disruption of active zones with reduction in the number of active zone particles and thereby impair the stimulus-induced calcium influx. This results in deficient quantal release of ACh and muscle weakness. With brief exercise and tetanic nerve stimulation, more calcium is available at the presynaptic membrane that increases ACh release, subsequently improving NMT. This is an explanation for postexercise improvement of muscle strength or reflexes.

Although there are overlap symptoms as noted in this case, distinct differences exist between MG and LEMS (see Table 13.1). MG is common in females under 40 and in males over 40 years of age. In contrast, LEMS is more common in people over 40 years of age. In the past, this disease was seen predominantly in males, with a 5:1 male-to-female ratio, but recent studies have shown a male-to-female ratio of 2:1, indicating that more female patients have been identified in recent years. In both diseases, easy fatigability is one of the major symptoms. In LEMS, the most common symptoms are proximal leg weakness and hyporeflexia or areflexia; oculobulbar weakness, the most common symptom in MG, is rare. Dysautonomic symptoms such as dryness of the mouth and impotence are also common in LEMS. The most crucial findings indicative of LEMS are a transient improvement of muscle strength and reflexes after brief exercise. These are not observed in MG or in any other disease. The tensilon response is also different in LEMS and MG. The tensilon test is positive in 90 to 95% of patients with MG and in 37% of those with LEMS. Usually in MG, the tensilon response is unequivocal, but in LEMS, the response is mildly positive, thus requiring more careful objective evaluation in these patients. In MG, association with thymoma is well known, being observed in 16% of cases, whereas SCLC is closely associated with LEMS. Although earlier studies showed SCLC in 75% of LEMS cases, O'Neil's report showed that this association is 50%. This difference is attributable to our increased capability in recent years to find more patients with noncarcinomatous LEMS. According to our experience, females have a smaller chance of having SCLC than do males.

Three groups of patients deserve diagnostic consideration of and testing for LEMS: any patient with proximal leg weakness and hyporeflexes or areflexia, any MG patients who are not responding well to conventional MG treatment modes, and any patients with unexplainable low CMAPs in the motor nerve conduction study.

MAXIMS

1. The classic clinical triad of LEMS is proximal leg weakness, hyporeflexia or areflexia, and easy fatigability.
2. Transient improvement of muscle strength and reflexes after brief exercise in the bedside examination is pathognomonic of LEMS.

REFERENCES

1. O'Neill J, Murry M, Newsom-Davis J. The Lambert-Eaton myasthenic syndrome. Brain 1988;111: 577–596.
2. McEvoy KM. Diagnosis and treatment of Lambert-Eaton myasthenic syndrome. Neurol Clin North Am 1994;12:387–399.

CASE 9

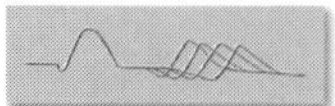

SJÖGREN'S SYNDROME AND WALKING DIFFICULTY FOR 3 YEARS

CASE PRESENTATION

A 56-year-old man was well until 3 years ago when while bird hunting, he noticed difficulty keeping up with his hunting partners because of weakness in both legs. This weakness gradually worsened to the point that he had considerable difficulty walking long distances, was quite slow, and tended to trip and fall. He had difficulty getting up from a sitting position and climbing stairs. Because of easy fatigability, he felt physically unable to keep up with the demands of his work. This symptom was helped by a small dose of pyridostigmine prescribed experimentally by a neurologist who suspected the possibility of MG. The patient also had carried a diagnosis of Sjögren's syndrome for 3 years because of dry mouth, dry eyes, and decreased sweating over the palms. Neurological examination showed moderate weakness in the proximal muscles of the legs and arms. Biceps, triceps, and patellar reflexes were diminished and ankle jerks were absent. He had difficulty doing knee bends. Sensory examination was normal. There was no fasciculation or atrophy of muscle. There was no improvement of muscle strength or reflexes with brief exercise. Serum AChR antibody, CPK, thyroid, and rheumatology profiles were normal.

CASE ANALYSIS

Initially, polymyositis was suspected because of the patient's history of Sjögren's syndrome and proximal leg weakness. Normal serum CPK was extremely unusual for polymyositis. The patient was referred to the EMG laboratory to rule out myopathy and MG. In retrospect, this patient had symptoms typical of LEMS: fatigability, proximal muscle weakness, and dysautonomia (dry mouth and eyes). Dysautonomia in this patient was not due to Sjögren's syndrome but to LEMS. This patient had the clinical triad of LEMS, proximal leg weakness, areflexia, and easy fatigability, but did not have pathognomonic findings of LEMS.

PLAN OF TESTING

1. Needle EMG: To confirm or document myopathy in the proximal muscles.
2. NCS study: To rule out neuropathy such as CIDP and diabetic neuropathy as responsible for his proximal muscle weakness.
3. RNS test: To confirm LEMS.
4. SFEMG: To corroborate LEMS.

ELECTROPHYSIOLOGICAL TESTS AND FINDINGS

Needle EMG (Fig. 13.11)

1. No fibrillation or positive sharp wave (PSW).
2. Significantly short mean duration (5.8 ms versus normal 9.4 ms), normal mean amplitude (0.28 mV), and increased polyphasic MUPs (29%) in deltoid muscle.

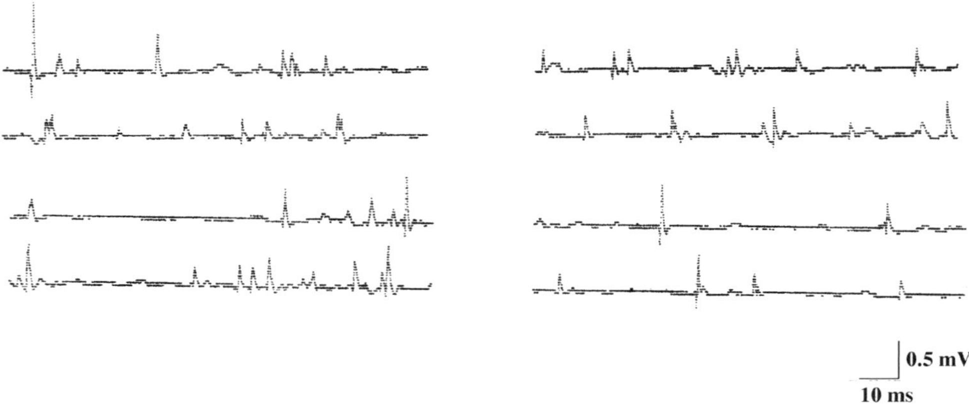

FIGURE 13.11. Many SASD MUPs in LEMS.

TABLE 13.12. NMT Study Data in Case 9

RNS Test Data			SFEMG Data	
	ADQ	**FCU**		**EDC**
CMAP (mV)	0.45	1.2	Fiber density	1.8
CMAP Ex (%)	133	142	No. Pot pairs	9
2 Hz (%)	−53	−33	Mean MCD (μs)	114
3 Hz (%)	−43	−31	Normal MCD (μs)	40.4
5 Hz (%)	−52	−25.6	No. PP with MCD >53 μs (%)	100
50 Hz (%)	233	163	No. PP with blocking (%)	100
5 Hz PT 0 (%)	−29	−29.3		
amplitude (%)[a]	122	167		
5 Hz PT 4 (%)	−29	−29.3		
amplitude (%)[a]	94	67		

[a] By the amplitude of first CMAP.

NCS Findings. Normal sensory and motor NCS in median, ulnar, peroneal, posterior tibial, and sural nerves except low CMAPs (2 mV in median; 0.42 mV in ulnar; 0.4 mV in peroneal; and 2 mV in posterior tibial nerves).

RNS Test Findings (Table 13.12; Fig. 13.12)

1. Low CMAP with abnormal incremental response after exercise.
2. Abnormal decremental response at LRS.
3. Abnormal incremental response at HRS.
4. PTF by amplitude in ADQ and FCU muscles and by decremental response in ADQ muscle.
5. Absence of PTE either by decrement or amplitude.

SFEMG. Marked increase in mean MCD with many SFPP with blocking and >53 μs MCD.

ELECTROPHYSIOLOGICAL INTERPRETATION

Presynaptic NMT disorder typical of LEMS.

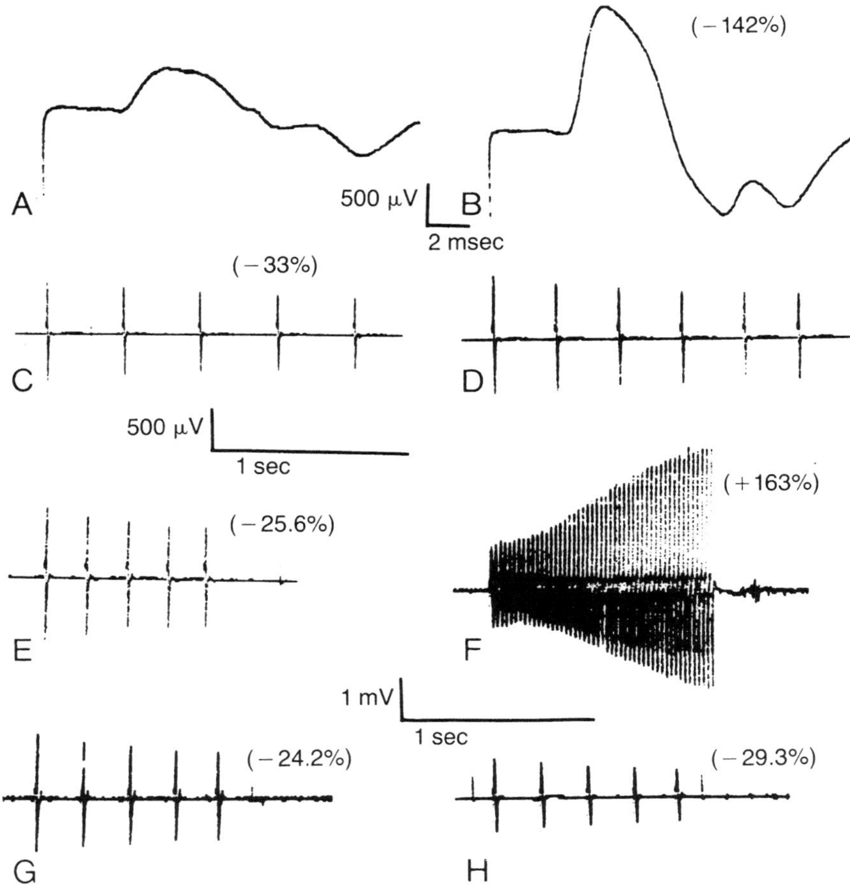

FIGURE 13.12. The classic RNS pattern in the FCU muscle in LEMS. **A.** Low CMAP at rest. **B.** CMAP after exercise. Postexercise facilitation is obvious. **C.** Decremental response at 2-Hz stimulation. **D.** Decremental response at 3-Hz stimulation. **E, G, H.** Decremental responses before, immediately after, and 4 minutes after 50-Hz stimulation. **F.** Note the marked incremental response at 50-Hz stimulation.

OTHER TEST FINDINGS

The workup for lung cancer was unrevealing.

FINAL DIAGNOSIS

LEMS

TREATMENT AND FOLLOW-UP

The patient was treated with guanidine HCl (750 to 2500 mg/day) with improvement of muscle strength to normal and increased moisture in mouth and palm. He was able to play golf, which he had not been able to do before guanidine. Because of the strong association with SCLC, he was checked semiannually with a chest x-ray. Two years after the diagnosis of LEMS, chest x-ray showed a deviation of the trachea to the right and a small mass in the left cervical area that turned out to be a thyroid medullary carcinoma. This was treated by radical neck surgery. Postoperatively, his improved muscle strength was maintained with guanidine 1000 mg/day for many years. No major side reaction was noted.

COMMENTS

LEMS is a pivotal example of a paraneoplastic neurological syndrome. From the first description of LEMS, its association with SCLC has been well known. As noted previously, an earlier study showed that 75% of LEMS patients had SCLC, whereas a more recent study showed this association in only 50% of cases, suggesting a trend toward a lower tumor frequency in recent years. Certainly, a smoking history is a risk factor for LEMS because it is a risk factor for SCLC. It is estimated that LEMS occurs in about 3% of patients with SCLC. Although other tumors have been reported to be associated with LEMS, most cancer-associated LEMS is due to SCLC. A recent study suggested that lymphoproliferative disorders may constitute another risk group for LEMS.

LEMS is a disease of the elderly, with the most common age of onset of symptoms being about 60 years of age. Paraneoplastic LEMS typically develops in the middle aged to elderly and was originally seen more commonly in men. More recent studies show less male predominance. Our latest series showed a 1:1 ratio. Paraneoplastic LEMS was clearly more common in males, whereas autoimmune LEMS was more frequent in females. In subjects younger than 30 years of age, the chance of cancer association is small. Usually, the discovery of LEMS precedes that of cancer by several months to years. In all cases, cancer develops within 4 years after diagnosis of LEMS. Thus, it is important to do a workup for occult cancer, especially SCLC, at the time of diagnosis of LEMS and serially thereafter, as noted in our case. There are no clinical and electrophysiological differences that separate paraneoplastic LEMS from autoimmune LEMS. According to our experience, cancer is less likely associated with LEMS if the patient is a young female and if cancer is not found within 4 years after the diagnosis of LEMS is made.

Unlike other paraneoplastic neurological syndromes that are usually resistant to any therapy, LEMS is known to be consistently responsive to immunotherapy or anticancer therapy. Thus, treatment of cancer is of paramount importance in paraneoplastic LEMS. Successful cancer treatment may result in remission or otherwise usually in improvement. Other treatments for noncancer-associated LEMS are also effective for paraneoplastic LEMS. The clinical improvement is usually associated with an improvement in the RNS test and SFEMG. It has been well known that recurrence of cancer may be heralded by reemergence or worsening of LEMS. Thus, it is important to treat paraneoplastic LEMS aggressively with anticancer therapy as well as other therapies for LEMS.

The needle EMG finding in LEMS is characterized by absence of fibrillation and PSW, SASD MUPs, and a varying amplitude of MUPs. Usually, the needle EMG abnormalities in LEMS are much more conspicuous than those in MG. The most striking abnormality in MUPs is a markedly varying amplitude from moment to moment, the most characteristic EMG feature of the NMT disorders. At the onset of contraction, the MUPs are small and variable in amplitude. However, there is frequently a gradual increase in MUP amplitude as contraction continues. This is due to facilitation of NMT with continued activity and is comparable with postexercise facilitation and an incremental response at HRS. Lambert and associates stated that this increase is observed when care is taken to observe MUPs during initiation of a contraction after several minutes of rest. It is the single most important EMG finding in differentiation of LEMS from MG. The only problem with this is that, in practice, it is not easy to document this phenomenon. SASD MUPs, the most classic EMG pattern in myopathy, are another frequent finding. A significant decrease of the mean MUP duration has been observed in LEMS.

MAXIMS

1. A diligent search for cancer is mandatory once the diagnosis of LEMS is made because of the close association of LEMS and SCLC. Cancer is usually found within 4 years of the diagnosis of LEMS. LEMS improves with successful anticancer therapy alone.
2. The most striking needle EMG abnormality in LEMS is a markedly varying amplitude from moment to moment, the most characteristic EMG feature of the NMT disorders.

REFERENCES

1. Chalk CH, Murray NM, Newsom-Davis J, O'Neill JH, Spiro SG. Response of the Lambert-Eaton myasthenic syndrome to treatment of associated small-cell lung carcinoma. Neurology 1990;40: 1552–1556.
2. Lambert E, Rooke E. Myasthenic state and lung cancer. In: Brain L, Norris F Jr, eds. The remote effects of cancer on the nervous system. New York: Grune & Stratton, 1965:67–80.

CASE 10

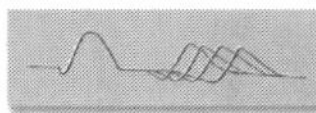

IS IT LEMS OR MG IN A PATIENT WITH SCLC

CASE PRESENTATION

A 55-year-old man with a confirmed diagnosis of SCLC for 6 months complained of progressive easy fatigability and weakness of the arms and legs. Neurological examination showed MRC strength of 3 in the proximal muscles, 5− in the distal muscles of arms and legs, mildly decreased triceps and biceps reflexes, absent ankle reflexes, and normal knee reflexes. We were able to obtain a trace of reflex in the ankle jerk after brief exercise. However, there was exertional weakness in muscle strength in the proximal muscles. CPK was normal. The patient denied any dysautonomic or oculobulbar symptoms.

CASE ANALYSIS

Because this patient had a confirmed diagnosis of SCLC, the clinician suspected the possibility of LEMS and polymyositis. In view of the normal CPK, polymyositis was less likely. This patient had the clinical triad of LEMS: proximal muscle weakness, decreased reflexes, and easy fatigability. Clearly, there was a postexercise facilitation in the reflex that was pathognomonic of LEMS, but there was exertional weakness instead of postexercise facilitation of muscle strength.

PLAN OF TESTING

1. NCS: To rule out any paraneoplastic peripheral neuropathy.
2. Needle EMG: To confirm myopathy and NMT disorder.
3. RNS test: To confirm the diagnosis of LEMS.

ELECTROPHYSIOLOGICAL TESTS AND FINDINGS

NCS Findings. Normal sensory and motor NCS except for low CMAP amplitudes in the right median, ulnar, peroneal, and posterior tibial nerves.

Needle EMG. No abnormal spontaneous potentials but many SASD MUPs in the right deltoid muscle.

Routine RNS Test Findings (Fig. 13.13; Table 13.13)

1. Low CMAP in ADQ and FCU muscles and no PEF.
2. Marked decremental response at LRS and at HRS for 1 second.
3. PTF by decremental response but not by amplitude.

Long HRS Test. Marked incremental response (>100%) in ADQ and minimal incremental response in FCU at HRS in a 10-second test.

ELECTROPHYSIOLOGICAL INTERPRETATION

Postsynaptic NMT disorder typical of LEMS.

FINAL DIAGNOSIS

LEMS

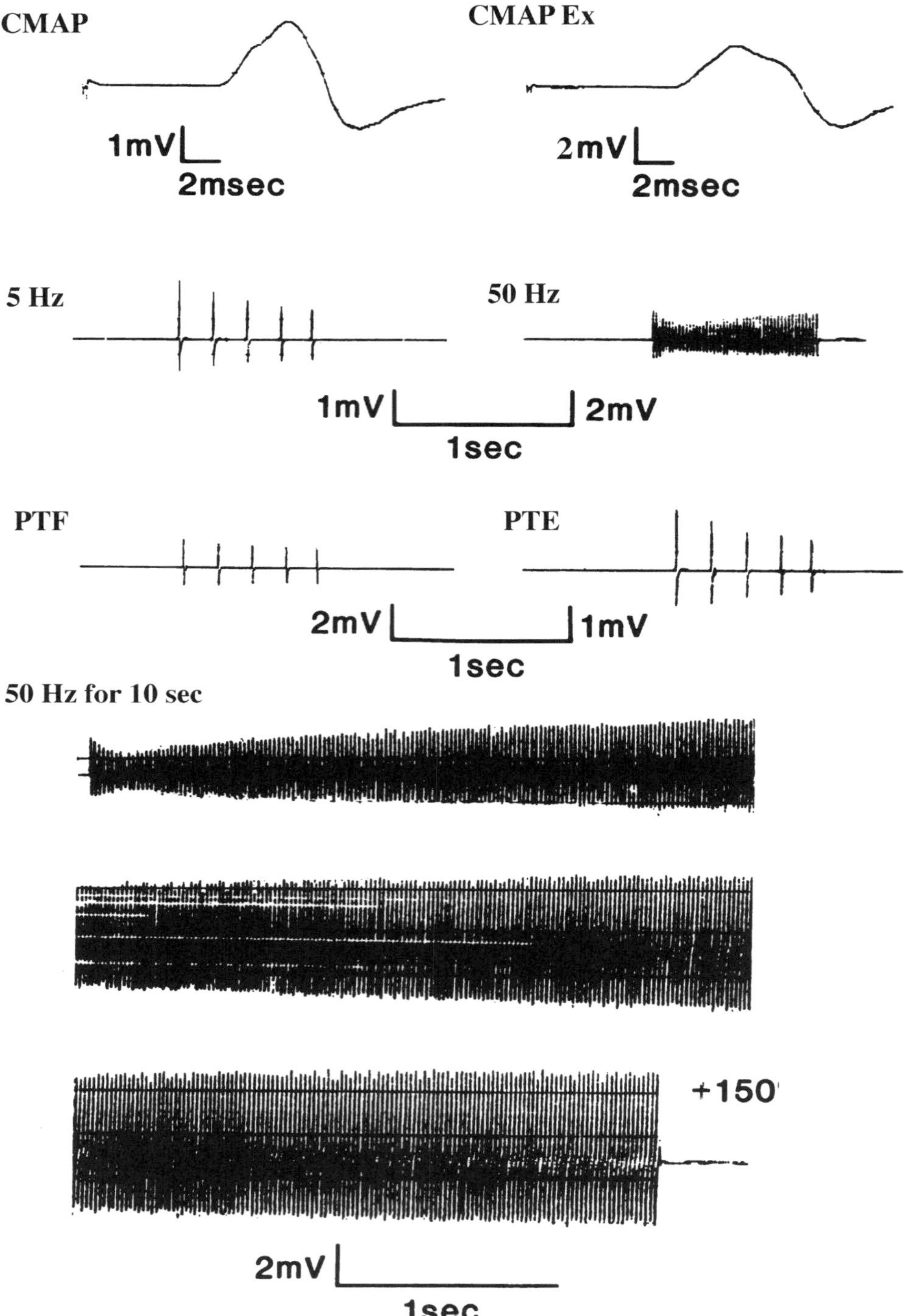

FIGURE 13.13. Type III pattern in LEMS showing low CMAP amplitude, decremental response at LRS, and initial decremental response at HRS. Significant incremental response is achieved at 50-Hz stimulation for 10 seconds. *PTF*, posttetanic facilitation; *PTE*, posttetanic exhaustion. (Reprinted with permission from Oh SJ. Diverse electrophysiological spectrum of the Lambert-Eaton myasthenic syndrome. Muscle Nerve 1989;12:468.)

TABLE 13.13. RNS Test Data in Case 10

	ADQ	FCU
CMAP (mV)	2.8	2.1
CMAP Ex (%)	44	23.3
2 Hz (%)	−43	−52
3 Hz (%)	−51	−51.7
5 Hz (%)	−48	−57.4
50 Hz (%)		
1 s	−50	−37.5
5 s	90	44
10 s	150	100
5 Hz PT 0 (%)	−29	−39.4
amplitude (%)	0	−9.5
5 Hz PT 4 (%)	−46	−55.0
amplitude (%)	0	−4.8

TREATMENT AND FOLLOW-UP

The routine RNS test did not confirm LEMS; there was no postexercise facilitation or incremental response at HRS. In fact, the test showed a severe MG pattern with low CMAP. At this point, we decided to prolong HRS for 5 seconds. The test showed a clear incremental response, which was still not enough to be indicative of LEMS. Thus, we extended HRS to 10 seconds. With a 10-second stimulation, we were able to document a 150% incremental response in the ADQ muscle, which was abnormal enough to be indicative of LEMS.

COMMENTS

The RNS test is still the gold standard for diagnosis of LEMS. Thus, without the typical RNS abnormalities, one cannot make a diagnosis of LEMS. The RNS test is always abnormal in LEMS. The classic triad of the RNS test in LEMS is a low CMAP amplitude, a decremental response at LRS, and an incremental response at HRS (posttetanic facilitation), which are typical of a presynaptic neuromuscular block. Posttetanic facilitation can be replaced by an increase of CMAP after exercise (postexercise facilitation) when it is present. Among this triad, low CMAP amplitude and posttetanic facilitation (>100% incremental response at HRS) or postexercise facilitation (100% increase of CMAP after exercise) are the two required diagnostic criteria for LEMS.

Low CMAP is seen in all cases of LEMS by definition. If the first test shows a low normal value, the diagnosis may have to be deferred until a low CMAP is achieved. One of the most dramatic RNS abnormalities in LEMS is PEF: an increase of the CMAP amplitude after brief exercise for 10 or 30 seconds. In LEMS, the CMAP increases by 120 to 1800%. This is beyond the values observed in normal or MG patients. Thus, a more than 100% increase of CMAP amplitude after exercise is typical of LEMS. Unfortunately, postexercise facilitation is not observed in all cases of LEMS. In our series, it was lacking in 25% of cases because of the patient's lack of cooperation or severe weakness of the hand muscles. Thus, it is important to remember that the absence of postexercise facilitation does not rule out LEMS. However, because this test is simple and relatively painless and is abnormal in most LEMS patients, this procedure should be used in all suspected cases. The decremental response at LRS is present in most cases but is not required for diagnosis of LEMS. The most dramatic RNS abnormality in LEMS is posttetanic facilitation, which by definition is seen in all cases of LEMS. The incremental response at HRS ranges from 100 to 4000%. In most cases, an incremental response was clearly documented with 50-Hz stimulation for 1 second. In a few cases, prolonged HRS for up to 10 seconds was needed to document a significant incremental response (>100%). Thus, it is important to remember that a lack of posttetanic facilitation with 50-Hz stimulation for 1 second does not rule out LEMS.

As noted in our patient, the RNS test in LEMS can mimic the "MG pattern": decremental response at LRS and normal or decremental response at HRS. This is seen in mild cases and some severe cases. In mild cases, low normal CMAP amplitude, decremental response at LRS, and normal response at HRS (type 1 pattern) are observed. In severe cases, low CMAP amplitude, decremental response at LRS, and initial decremental response at HRS (type 3 pattern) are observed. The type 2 pattern is the classic triad. These three patterns represent different degrees of blocking in LEMS, from the mildest in type 1 to the most severe in type 3. Because types 1 and 3 can be misinterpreted as the MG pattern, they must be recognized in LEMS, and an incremental response must be documented by prolonged stimulation, as in our case. If we had not prolonged the HRS stimulation up to 10 seconds in this patient, we would not have been able to confirm the diagnosis of LEMS. Thus, prolonged stimulation is essential. The initial decremental response at HRS can be explained by an extremely severe presynaptic block of ACh release. The physiological ACh increase at HRS is the basis for postexercise and HRS facilitation in LEMS. If the presynaptic block is severe enough that this mechanism cannot compensate for the depletion of immediately available ACh, an initial decrement will occur, and there may be a delay in increment. This is what happens with the type 3 pattern, in which prolonged stimulation at HRS is required to induce an incremental response.

MAXIMS

1. The classic RNS triad in LEMS is a low CMAP amplitude, a decremental response at LRS, and an incremental response at HRS (posttetanic facilitation). A low CMAP amplitude and posttetanic facilitation are the two most important diagnostic criteria for LEMS.
2. In LEMS, the RNS pattern may mimic MG, and a prolonged stimulation at HRS is essential in documenting an incremental response, making it possible to reach the diagnosis of LEMS in these cases.

REFERENCES

1. Oh SJ. Diverse electrophysiological spectrum of the Lambert-Eaton myasthenic syndrome. Muscle Nerve 1989;12:464–469.
2. Lambert EH, Rooke ED, Eaton LM. Myasthenic syndrome occasionally associated with bronchial neoplasm: Neurophysiological studies. In Viets HR (ed): Myasthenia Gravis. Springfield, IL, Charles C Thomas 1961;:pp 362–410.

CASE 11

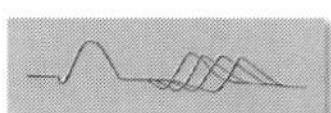

GUILLAIN-BARRÉ SYNDROME OR MG?

CASE PRESENTATION

A 36-year-old woman noticed weakness of the legs beginning 3 months previously. She had the greatest difficulty getting up from a chair. There was no history of diplopia or bulbar symptoms. She tired easily but felt better in the evening than in the morning, which was her worst time. The first neurologist who evaluated her within a month of onset of symptoms told her that she probably had Guillain-Barré syndrome and would improve. Because of continued weakness, she saw a second neurologist, who performed a tensilon test that was minimally positive. She was begun on Mestinon, which had been increased to as high as 120 mg every 3 hours. She noted a definite improvement of strength around the second hour after Mestinon intake but developed difficulty with nausea and vomiting, which were controlled with atropine. She had normal thyroid and rheumatoid profiles, a negative AChR antibody, and normal CPK. In the past, she had a benign breast cyst removed in 1981 and a "frozen shoulder" 6 months ago. She had never smoked.

Abnormal neurological findings were MRC strength of 4 in the iliopsoas and 5 − in the deltoid muscles, and 1 + symmetrical reflexes with reinforcement. There was no fatigability or facilitation, and no change in reflexes after brief exercise. Her gait was waddling, and she was not able to do knee bends.

CASE ANALYSIS

This patient had subacute proximal muscle weakness, easy tiredness, and decreased reflexes. Differential diagnoses included CIDP, polymyositis, limb-girdle MG, and LEMS. CIDP should be ruled out by the NCS. Polymyositis was less likely in view of the normal CPK level. The absence of oculobulbar symptoms made MG less likely. However, the patient's minimal but definite therapeutic responsiveness to pyridostigmine suggested the possibility of limb-girdle MG. The constellation of clinical symptoms and findings suggested the possibility of LEMS, but the pathognomonic findings, facilitation of muscle strength, and reflexes after brief exercise were not documented.

PLAN OF TESTING

1. NCS: To rule out chronic demyelinating neuropathy.
2. RNS test: To rule out or confirm the diagnosis of MG or LEMS.
3. SFEMG: To corroborate the diagnosis of LEMS.
4. Voltage-gated calcium channel antibody.
5. Parietal cell antibody.

ELECTROPHYSIOLOGICAL TESTS AND FINDINGS

NCS Findings. Normal motor and sensory NCS.

The First RNS Test Findings (Table 13.14; Fig 13.14)

1. Normal CMAP amplitude in the ADQ and low CMAP amplitude in the FCU muscles.
2. PEF (>100%) in the ADQ muscle.
3. Decremental response at LRS in the ADQ and FCU muscles.
4. Normal response at HRS on routine 1-second stimulation.
5. Incremental response at HRS for 4 seconds in the ADQ muscle.
6. PTF.

The Second RNS Test (Table 13.14)

1. Low CMAP amplitude in the ADQ and FCU muscles.
2. PEF in the ADQ muscle.
3. Decremental response at LRS in the ADQ and FCU muscles.
4. Incremental response at HRS in the ADQ muscle.
5. PTF.

TABLE 13.14. NMT Study Data in Case 11[a]

	First RNS Test		Second RNS Test		SFEMG Data	
	ADQ	FCU	ADQ	FCU		EDC
CMAP (mV)	6.0	1.8	4.5	2.1	Fiber density	1.4
CMAP Ex (%)	+150	+61	+140	+61.9	No. Pot pairs	20
2 Hz (%)	−27.0	−22.0	−31.0	−25	Mean MCD	78
3 Hz (%)	−20.0	−25.0	−33.0	−29.6	Normal MCD	43
5 Hz (%)	−30.0	−28.0	−24.0	−15.9	No. PP with MCD >53 μs	5 (25%)
50 Hz (%)	+64/+193[b]	+50	+111	− +72.9	No. PP with blocking	2 (10%)
5 Hz PT 0 (%)	−24.0	−24.0	−17.0	−16.6		
5 Hz PT 4 m (%)	−28.0	−28.0	−21.0	−26.0		

[a] Interval between first and second test was 13 days.

[b] Increment in 1 second/increment in 4 second-stimulation.

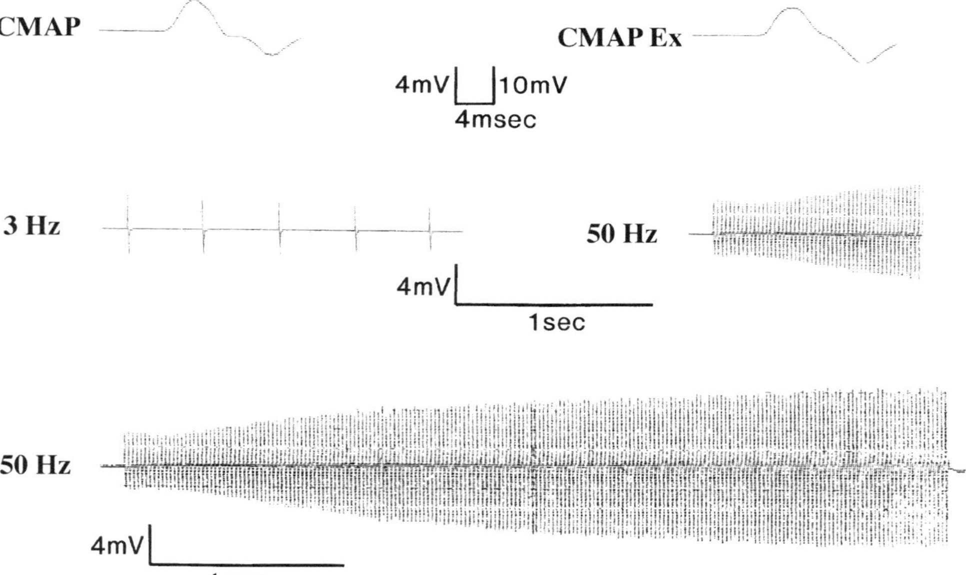

FIGURE 13.14. Type I pattern in LEMS showing normal CMAP amplitude, decremental response at low rate of stimulation, and relatively normal response at high rate of stimulation. There was an incremental response after exercise (CMAP Ex) and 50 Hz stimulation for 4 seconds.

SFEMG (Table 13.14)

1. Normal fiber density.
2. Prolonged MCD.
3. Increased number of MCD >53 μs.

ELECTROPHYSIOLOGICAL INTERPRETATION

The first RNS test was compatible with a presynaptic NMT disorder and the second was indicative of a presynaptic NMT disorder typical of LEMS.

OTHER TEST FINDINGS

1. Anti-parietal cell antibody 1:320 (<1:10).
2. Vitamin B_{12} 173.
3. Hemoglobin 11.5 g%.
4. Schilling test 16.5% (<0.10%).

FINAL DIAGNOSIS

LEMS

TREATMENT AND FOLLOW-UP

The initial workup for cancer was negative. The patient was initially treated with plasma exchange followed by prednisone, pyridostigmine, and guanidine hydrochloride. Gradually her condition improved. Within 1.5 years, she became symptom free and her strength was normal even with complete discontinuation of prednisone. Seven years later, she remains symptom free with 500 mg of guanidine and 360 mg of pyridostigmine. She also receives monthly vitamin B_{12} shots. So far there has not been any sign of cancer.

COMMENTS

Guanidine and aminopyridine, which are known to increase the release of ACh at the presynaptic membrane by blocking potassium channels, are the symptomatic drugs of choice. This is in good contrast to pyridostigmine, which is effective for symptomatic treatment of MG. However, pyridostigmine has been found to be effective in LEMS if used together with guanidine and aminopyridine. Aminopyridine is the drug of choice when available, because guanidine is known to be associated with bone-marrow suppression as a short-term side-reaction and renal dysfunction as a long-term side-reaction. The most serious side reaction with aminopyridine is seizure, which was reported in three cases. In countries where aminopyridine is not available (including the United States), low-dose (<1000 mg/day) guanidine combined with a liberal dose of pyridostigmine is recommended because we found this combination effective and relatively safe. If symptomatic treatment is not satisfactory, then immunotherapies (steroid, azathioprine, plasma exchange, and IVIG treatment) must be added. Immunotherapies are effective in LEMS but less dramatic and slower to act than in MG.

Over the years, an autoimmune pathogenesis of LEMS has been suggested. This is based on a strong association with organ-specific autoimmune disorders as noted previously (antibodies to striate muscle, thyroid organ, or gastric parietal cells in 45% of LEMS cases), the effectiveness of immunotherapies, passive transfer of the syndrome to mice with purified IgG from LEMS patients, and VGCC antibody. Among these, the most compelling evidence for the autoimmune pathogenesis of LEMS is the detection of VGCC antibodies in the serum of LEMS patients. However, the sensitivity and specificity of the VGCC antibody test vary depending on the type of antibody and the specific testing laboratory. The N-type antibody was positive in 41 to 91% of LEMS patients and false positive in 9% of controls and in 67% of RA/SLE (rheumatoid arthritis/systemic lupus erythematosus) patients. It was positive in patients both with and without cancer. The P-type antibody was positive in 85% of LEMS patients in Newsom-Davis' laboratory and rather specific, because it was not positive in other neurological diseases or MG. However, at the Mayo Clinic Laboratory, the P/Q-type antibody was positive in 95% of LEMS patients, but it was also positive in 54% of patients with paraneoplastic neurological syndromes, 24% of patients with cancer, and in 23% of patients with ALS.

MAXIMS

1. Aminopyridine is the drug of choice for symptomatic treatment of LEMS, if it is available. Low-dose guanidine together with pyridostigmine is also safe and effective.
2. The sensitivity and specificity of the VGCC antibody test for the diagnosis of LEMS vary depending on the type of antibody and the testing laboratory. Because of this, the VGCC antibody can not be used as a gold standard for the diagnosis of LEMS.

REFERENCES

1. Sanders DB. Lambert-Eaton myasthenic syndrome: pathogenesis and treatment. Semin Neurol 1994; 14:111–117.
2. Motomura M, Johnston I, Lang B, Vincent A. An improved diagnostic assay for Lambert-Eaton myasthenic syndrome. J Neurol Neurosurg Psychiatry 1995;58:85–87.

CASE 12

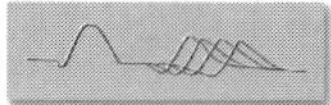

MG OR LEMS?

CASE PRESENTATION

A 26-year-old woman with pernicious anemia and migraine headache had intermittent leg weakness and diplopia 8 months before our initial evaluation. AChR antibody was positive. Her right ptosis and proximal leg weakness were reversed by edrophonium. CT revealed no thymoma. Muscle biopsy of the quadriceps showed type II fiber predominance and atrophy. The patient was treated with pyridostigmine and later with prednisone (60 mg daily) with no improvement. In the 4th month of disease, the RNS test showed a typical MG pattern, and the SFEMG showed increased jitter and blocking (Table 13.15). Another AChR antibody was positive. After plasmapheresis, substernal total thymectomy was performed at another university hospital. Postoperatively, the patient's symptoms improved, and she was discharged on no medications. Two months after thymectomy, because of leg weakness and extreme fatigue, she was placed back on a small dose of prednisone and pyridostigmine without any benefit. Initial examination at UAB 4 months after thymectomy showed right ptosis, mild weakness of hip flexors and gluteal muscles, waddling gait, difficulty doing knee bends, absent muscle stretch reflexes, and slightly diminished vibration perception on the toes. No exertional fatigue was documented in the hip flexor evaluation. There were no complaints of dry mouth, slurring of speech, or swallowing difficulty.

CASE ANALYSIS

This patient had a classic history of MG: ocular symptoms, proximal muscle weakness, positive AChR antibody, positive tensilon test, and the MG pattern on RNS testing. Absent muscle stretch reflexes were thought to be due to pernicious anemia. Thus, thymectomy was performed. Usually, after thymectomy there is a "honeymoon period" of improved status lasting a few months. In this case, it lasted 4 months. Even with reintroduction of pyridostigmine and prednisone, there was no satisfactory improvement. Thus, there was a need for reevaluation of her MG.

PLAN OF TESTING

1. NCS: To assess the degree of B_{12} deficiency neuropathy.
2. RNS test: To assess the severity of MG.
3. SFEMG: To corroborate the diagnosis of MG.

ELECTROPHYSIOLOGICAL TESTS AND FINDINGS

NCS Findings

1. Except for low CMAPs, motor conduction was normal in median, ulnar, peroneal, and posterior tibial nerves.
2. Sensory and mixed NCS in ulnar and median nerves were normal.
3. Mild slowing of NCV in sural nerves (33 to 35 m/s) with normal CNAP amplitude.

RNS Test Findings (Table 13.15; Fig. 13.15)

1. Low CMAP amplitude.
2. Abnormal PEF (>100%).
3. Significant decremental response at low rate of stimulation.
4. Significant incremental response (>100%) at high rate of stimulation.

SFEMG (Table 13.15; Fig. 13.16):

1. Because of frequent blocking, only one single-fiber potential pair was obtained: abnormal MCD (314 μs) with 14% blocking.
2. An inverse relationship between MCD and the discharge rate of single-fiber potential pairs in the SFEMG after improvement.

ELECTROPHYSIOLOGICAL INTERPRETATION

LEMS. SFEMG findings typical of presynaptic NMT disorder.

TABLE 13.15. NMT Study Data in Case 12

	RNS Test Data		SFEMG Data	
	Pre-UAB Test ADQ	**UAB Test ADQ**		**EDC**
CMAP (mV)	10	4.8	Fiber density	1.5
CMAP Ex (%)	16	151	No. Pot pairs	19
2 Hz (%)		−30.7	Mean MCD (μs)	152
3 Hz (%)	−15	−32.0	Normal MCD (μs)	40.4
5 Hz (%)		−33.4	No. PP with MCD >53 μs (%)	100
50 Hz (%)		150	No. PP with blocking (%)	47
3 Hz PT 0 (%)		−32.8		
3 Hz PT 4 (%)		−33.2		

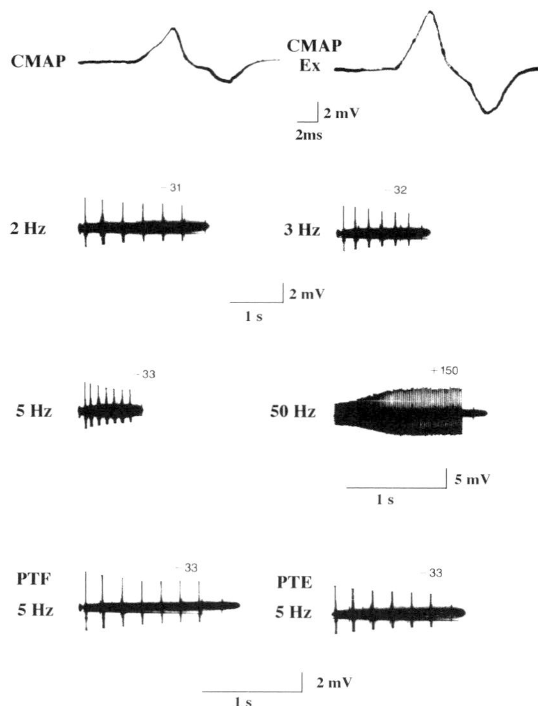

FIGURE 13.15. RNS responses in overlap MG/LEMS syndrome. Classical presynaptic RNS pattern (low CMAP amplitude, marked increment in the CMAP after exercise, decremental responses at LRS and marked incremental response at HRS) is typical of overlap MG/LEMS syndrome. *PTF*, posttetanic facilitation; *PTE*, posttetanic exhaustion.

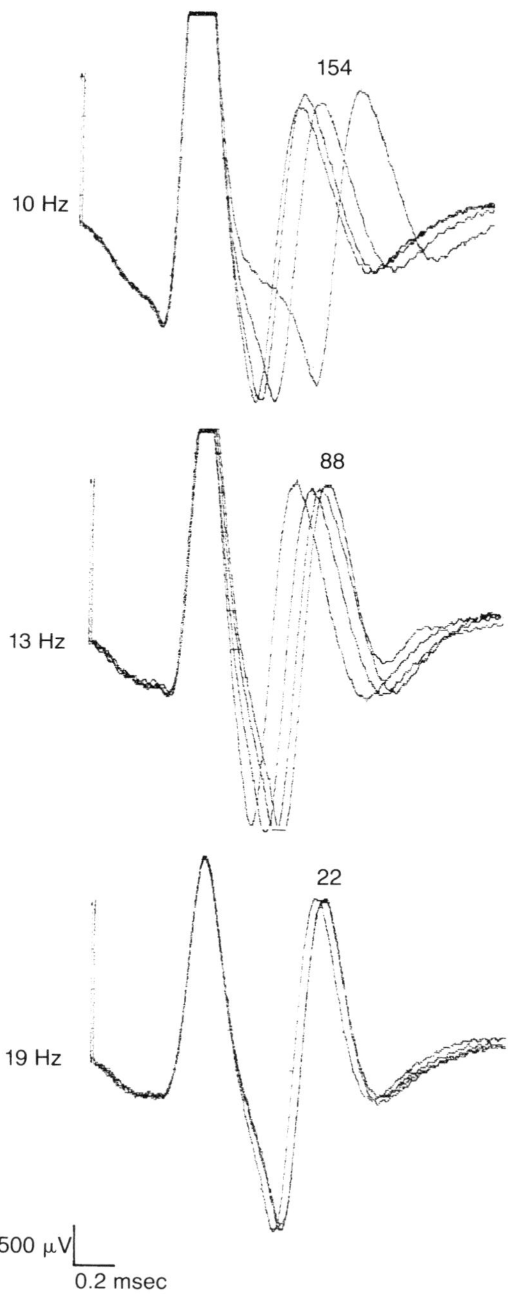

FIGURE 13.16. Decreasing mean consecutive difference values with increasing discharge rates from 10 to 19 Hz.

OTHER TEST FINDINGS

Thyroid function was normal. Schilling test was positive. Her HLA type was B8. AChR antibody was again positive. No cancer was found.

FINAL DIAGNOSIS

Overlap MG/LEMS syndrome

TREATMENT AND FOLLOW-UP

The RNS test showed a pattern consistent with LEMS (Table 13.1). With pyridostigmine (~300 mg/day) together with guanidine (1000 mg/day), there was clinical and electrophysiologic improvement within 3 days. Thereafter, with guanidine (325 mg/day) and pyridostigmine (300 mg/day), her leg weakness gradually improved. Since then, the patient's condition has been stable, mostly with pyridostigmine alone and occasionally with a supplement of guanidine. A few episodes of exacerbation of her symptoms were controlled with IVIG treatment. Voltage-gated calcium-channel antibody was positive.

COMMENTS

The term "overlap MG/LEMS syndrome" is used to refer to a combined syndrome of MG and LEMS in a single patient. A review of the literature revealed a dozen cases of overlap MG/LEMS syndrome based on the strict diagnostic criteria of MG and LEMS. The clinical features of these cases are best explained as a combination of MG and LEMS. Oculobulbar symptoms and a positive edrophonium test, two classic features of MG, were common. Areflexia, a typical feature of LEMS, was also common. In these cases, there was definite clinical improvement with anticholinesterase, as well as with guanidine and 3,4-diaminopyridine. In all cases except one patient with SCLC, cancer was not found. AChR antibody and voltage-gated calcium channel antibodies were found to be positive in all tested cases.

The RNS test showed findings typical of classic LEMS: a low CMAP amplitude, postexercise facilitation, decremental response at LRS, incremental response at HRS, and posttetanic facilitation. PTE was less common. The present case showed a typical MG pattern in an earlier study and a typical LEMS pattern in a subsequent study. The needle EMG showed SASD MUPs, typical of myopathy. The SFEMG showed abnormal jitter in all tested cases. In our case, SFEMG showed findings typical of a presynaptic NMT block: abnormal jitter, frequent blocking, and MCD improvement at the higher discharge rate.

MAXIMS

1. MG can coexist with LEMS in the same individual.
2. The classic LEMS triad in RNS test in seropositive MG patient is diagnostic of overlap MG/LEMS syndrome.

REFERENCES

1. Newsom-Davis J, Vincent A, Ferguson L, Modi G, Mills K. Immunological evidence for the coexistence of the Lambert-Eaton myasthenic syndrome and myasthenia gravis in two patients. J Neurol Neurosurg Psychiatry 1991;54:452–453.
2. Oh SJ, Dwyer DS, Bradley RJ. Overlap myasthenic syndrome: combined myasthenia gravis and Eaton-Lambert syndrome. Neurology 1987;37:1411–1414.

CASE 13

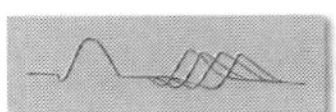

SERONEGATIVE "MG" WITH A POSITIVE FAMILY HISTORY

CASE PRESENTATION

An 8-year-old boy (Z.A.) had fatigue and substantial weakness of the eyes and limbs since birth. There was no medical problem at the time of his birth, and his developmental milestones were normal except that he had been a "lazy" boy. At the time of initial examination, his main complaint was constant fatigue, which was worse in the evening. He became choked easily when he ate but did not complain of double vision or speech problems. Abnormal neurological findings included moderate ptosis in both eyes, mild ophthalmoparesis in all directions, moderate facial weakness, prominent nasal voice, MRC strength of 3 in neck flexors, 4 in all extremity muscles except hand grips and quadriceps, which were 3, and 2 in iliopsoas and deltoid muscles. Exertional fatigability was easily demonstrable in all muscles. Reflexes were normal. He was not able to get up by himself from the floor.

A 4-year-old brother (J.A.) had similar problems, fatigue, nasal phonation, and ophthalmoplegia, again since birth. Examination showed moderate bilateral ptosis, mild facial weakness, moderate ophthalmoplegia, nasal phonation, and 4 MRC strength in deltoid and iliopsoas muscles. Clearcut exertional fatigability was noted.

CASE ANALYSIS

The history and findings were strongly diagnostic of MG. However, the fact that the patients had symptoms of MG since birth and a positive family history, which are extremely unusual for acquired autoimmune MG but are strongly supportive of CMS. To confirm the diagnosis of CMS, a negative AChR antibody and decremental response at LRS are required. Moreover, it is important to demonstrate the effectiveness of anti-ChE inhibitors in CMS because anti-ChE is the sole effective medication for many forms of CMS.

PLAN OF TESTING

1. RNS test: To confirm the diagnosis of CMS.
2. AChR antibody test: To rule out seropositive acquired MG.
3. Tensilon test: To confirm the diagnosis of some form of CMS and test the effectiveness of the anti-ChE as a therapeutic agent.

ELECTROPHYSIOLOGICAL TESTS AND FINDINGS

RNS Test on Z.A. (Table 3.16; Fig. 13.17)

1. Normal CMAP amplitude in the ADQ, FCU, and orbicularis oculi muscles.
2. Decremental response at LRS in all muscles.
3. Decremental response at HRS in the FCU muscle.
4. PTF but not PTE in the ADQ and FCU muscles.

RNS Test on J.A. (Table 13.16; Fig. 13.18)

1. Normal CMAP amplitude in the ADQ muscle.
2. Decremental response at 5-Hz stimulation.

ELECTROPHYSIOLOGICAL INTERPRETATION

Postsynaptic neuromuscular transmission disorder typical of postsynaptic CMS.

OTHER TEST FINDINGS

Tensilon test was positive. Binding, modulating, and blocking AChR antibodies were negative. Thyroid and rheumatology profiles were also normal.

FINAL DIAGNOSIS

Postsynaptic anti-ChE responsive CMS

TABLE 13.16. RNS Test Data in Case 13

	Z.A.[a]			J.A.[b]	
	ADQ	FCU	OO		ADQ
CMAP (mV)	10	20	1.0	CMAP (mV)	12.2
CMAP Ex (%)	−12.5	12.5		3 Hz at rest	3.0%
2 Hz (%)	−13.6	−16.3	−60.3	3 Hz 30 s PE	11.0%
3 Hz (%)	−14.3	−25.6	−50.0	3 Hz 1 m PE	1.0%
5 Hz (%)	−23.8	−40.5	−36.8	3 Hz 3 m PE	−8.0%
50 Hz (%)	−13.8	−59.5		3 Hz 4 m PE	−12.0%
5 Hz PT 0 (%)	0	−9.5		3 Hz 5 m PE	−8.0%
5 Hz PT 4 (%)	−9.1	−31.0			

[a] Oh's method.

[b] Lambert's method: PE, after 10 s exercise.

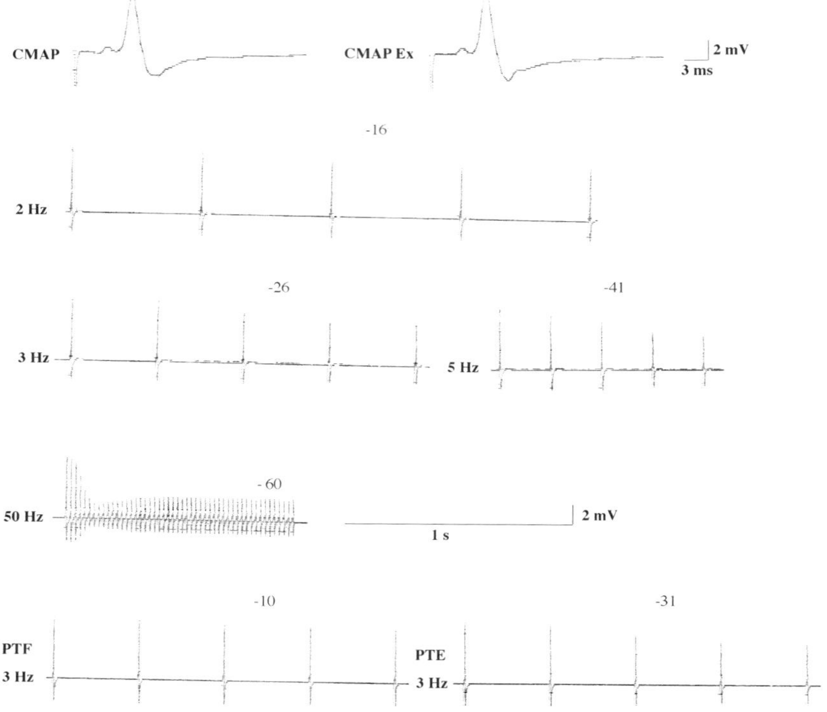

FIGURE 13.17. RNS responses in the FCU muscle following Oh's method. Decremental responses at LRS and HRS, posttetanic facilitation (*PTF*), and posttetanic exhaustion (*PTE*) are present.

TREATMENT AND FOLLOW-UP

With Mestinon 60 mg alternating with 90 mg every 3 hours and with Timespan 180 mg at night, Z.A. is doing relatively well. No major side reaction has been noted with Mestinon. He feels much stronger but becomes tired about 5 o'clock in the evening. Certainly, he is making better grades in school. Mestinon was also effective in J.A., but its benefit was not as dramatic as in Z.A.

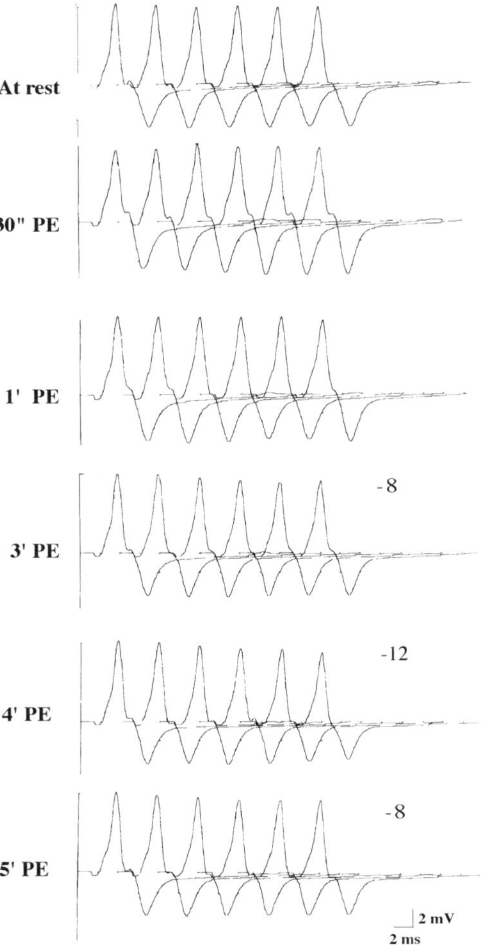

FIGURE 13.18. Postexercise exhaustion (*PE*) in 3-Hz RNS response in the ADQ muscle following Lambert's method. Before exercise, there was no decremental response.

COMMENTS

The clinical features, positive Tensilon test, and RNS findings in these patients are not different from seronegative acquired MG. The main differences from acquired seronegative MG are the long-standing myasthenic history since childhood and positive family history. Considering the autosomal-recessive family history, prominent ophthalmoparesis, good response to anti-ChE, and postsynaptic RNS test, these patients most likely had a form of AChR deficiency. Familial infantile myasthenia (CMS attributed to a defect of ACh resynthesis or mobilization) is another possibility. This is less likely because of the lack of history of feeding difficulties and respiratory crises in infancy and prominent eye involvement in our cases. In familial infantile myasthenia, the symptoms can be episodic, with severe weakness and respiratory insufficiency appearing with fever, excitement, or without known cause. A decremental response at HRS is not easily demonstrable in this disorder.

CMSs are genetically determined disorders in which the safety margin of NMT is affected by one or more pathologic mechanisms. The various forms of CMS have been described by Engel in the past decade and new syndromes are added almost every year. These disorders are present at birth by definition, but some patients are not evaluated until later in childhood or adult life because the symptoms are mild or not recognized. A positive family history is consistent with the diagnosis of CMS, but a negative family history does not exclude autosomal-recessive inheritance. Most cases of CMS are inherited by an autosomal-recessive pattern except one. The classic slow-channel syndrome has an autosomal-dominant inheritance. On examination, the most important clue to a NMT disorder is increasing weakness on sustained exertion (myasthenic weakness). There are some findings suggestive of the specific forms of CMS: scoliosis and delayed pupillary light reflex in acetylcholine esterase (AChE) deficiency, selective severe weakness of cervical muscles and of wrist and finger extensor muscles in end-plate AChE deficiency and slow-channel syndrome, lack of ocular muscle involvement in AChE deficiency, slow-channel syndrome, or familial limb-girdle myasthenia, and hyporeflexia in congenital LEMS. A positive tensilon test is consistent with the diagnosis of CMS, but a negative test does not rule out CMS, because this test is negative in patients with end-plate AChE deficiency and in familial infantile myasthenia between attacks of weakness. The diagnosis must be supported by a decremental response at LRS in at least one muscle or by abnormal jitter and blocking on SFEMG, according to Engel. The decremental response may be absent in familial infantile myasthenia between attacks; here, a decremental response can be elicited by prolonged 10-Hz stimulation or by exercise for several minutes before 2-Hz stimulation. Repetitive discharge is typically observed in two forms: end-plate AChE deficiency and slow-channel syndrome. The LEMS pattern was reported in congenital LEMS. In all CMS, the AChR antibody was negative. Responsiveness to anti-ChE is present in many CMS, but not in end-plate AChE deficiency and slow-channel syndrome.

Thus, the clinical history and examination, tensilon response, and RNS test findings can provide sufficient information for a specific diagnosis of CMS in some cases, but detailed microphysiological, ultrastructural, and histochemical studies are required for accurate diagnosis and classification. These latter studies can only be performed in a few centers in the world.

In practice, the best diagnostic criteria of CMS are myasthenic symptoms since birth, demonstrable exertional weakness, negative AChR antibody, and decremental response at LRS. Other features are variable.

MAXIMS

1. Diagnosis of CMS can be made on basis of myasthenic symptoms since birth, exertional weakness on examination, negative AChR antibody, and decremental response at LRS. However, the specific form of CMS should be made by detailed microphysiological, ultrastructural, and histochemical studies.
2. Clinical and RNS findings in AChR deficiency CMS syndromes are not different from those of seronegative MG patients except for the history of myasthenic symptoms since birth.

REFERENCES

1. Engel AG. The investigation of congenital myasthenic syndrome. Ann NY Acad Sci 1993;681:425–434.

CASE 14

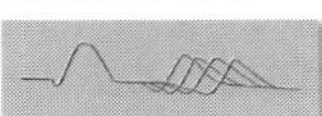

SLOWLY PROGRESSIVE WEAKNESS OF THE RIGHT HAND WITH FAMILY HISTORY

CASE PRESENTATION

A 54-year-old woman had slowly progressive weakness of the right hand for 10 years. She experienced leg cramps and easy fatigability since childhood and heavy feelings in her legs on and off since 17 years of age. During two pregnancies in her 20s, she had "falling episodes," which resolved spontaneously after delivery. These falling episodes were characterized by difficulty getting up from a chair or climbing stairs and inability to lift her arms above her shoulders to comb her hair or put dishes on the shelves. About 20 years ago, she had another episode of weakness: she could not get up from a chair or walk for long periods of time. This episode had been dramatically improved with quinine. Since then, she continued to take quinine, which had improved her leg cramps and "heaviness."

The patient's father was known to have short periods of weakness in his forearms, which was thought to be due to lead poisoning. Her uncle had distal arm weakness, predominantly involving the extensor surface of the forearms, which had been evaluated by three neurological institutes without a definite diagnosis. At one neurological institute, MG was suspected in her uncle on the basis of a positive curare test. Mestinon was effective for the first 2 weeks of treatment but was ineffective thereafter.

On examination, the patient had atrophy of the right thenar, first dorsal interosseous, and possibly the medial aspect of the flexor surface of the right forearm and mild weakness in the right abductor pollicis breves muscle and opponens pollicis, interosseous, and finger-extensor muscles. No exertional weakness was observed. Reflexes and sensory examination were normal.

CASE ANALYSIS

This patient was originally referred to us with the tentative diagnosis of right median and ulnar neuropathy. Clinical examination showed involvement of the finger extensor muscles that were innervated by the radial nerve. The initial working diagnoses included benign focal amyotrophy, right C7-8 radiculopathy, and multifocal motor neuropathy. A tentative diagnosis of multifocal motor neuropathy was entertained on the basis of "dispersion of CMAPs" and prolonged terminal latencies in the radial, median, and ulnar nerves until we examined her uncle, who showed a similar clinical presentation and a more dramatic history of remission and relapse of weakness of the arms and head and a possible diagnosis of MG. His RNS test showed repetitive discharge and a marked decremental response at low and high rates of stimulation.

PLAN OF TESTING

1. NCS in both arms and one leg to document or rule out "demyelinating neuropathy," including the proximal segments to document any conduction block.
2. Needle EMG to document any chronic denervation process in the right C7-8 innervated muscles.
3. RNS test to document the repetitive discharge and decremental response at low and high rates of stimulation. This was performed after the patient's uncle was examined.
4. SFEMG: To corroborate the NMT disorder.
5. Muscle biopsy: To rule out AChE deficiency syndrome.
6. AChR antibody and CPK: To rule out acquired MG and myopathy.

ELECTROPHYSIOLOGICAL TESTS AND FINDINGS

NCS Findings

1. NCS showed mildly prolonged terminal latencies in median nerve.
2. CMAPs showed repetitive discharge in all CMAPs.
3. No other motor or sensory nerve conduction abnormalities. No conduction block. Normal F-wave latency.

Needle EMG

1. No evidence of chronic or active denervation in the right cervical paraspinal, deltoid, biceps, triceps, FDI, APB, or ADQ muscles.

TABLE 13.17. NMT Study Data in Case 14

RNS Test Data			SFEMG Data	
	ADQ	FCU		EDC
CMAP (mV)	8.5[a]	9.5[a]	Fiber density	1.30
CMAP Ex (%)	9.0	−13.6	No. Pot pairs	11
2/s (%)	−13.6	−20.0	Mean MCD (μs)	93
3/s (%)	−13.6	−30.0	Normal MCD (μs)	40.4
5/s (%)	−12.2	−29.0	No. PP with MCD >53 μs (%)	73
50/s (%)	−24[b]	−24.0[b]	No. PP with blocking (%)	46
5/s PT 0 (%)	3.4	20.0		
5/s PT 4 (%)	−10.6	−33.0		

[a] Repetitive discharge.
[b] Second or third response showed the most prominent decrement.

2. Needle EMG in the right extensor digitorum communis muscles showed "short-duration MUPs."

RNS Test Findings (Table 13.17; Fig. 13.19)
1. Repetitive discharges in the CMAPs in the ADQ and FCU muscles.
2. Marked decremental response at the low rate of stimulation.
3. Minimal decremental response ("dip phenomenon") at the high rate of stimulation.
4. PTF and exhaustion phenomena.

SFEMG (Table 13.17). Normal fiber density and markedly abnormal jitter.

ELECTROPHYSIOLOGICAL INTERPRETATION

ACh overactivity pattern typical of slow-channel syndrome or acetylcholinesterase deficiency. No definite evidence of multifocal motor neuropathy.

OTHER TEST FINDINGS

All blood tests including GM and MAG antibody were normal.

FINAL DIAGNOSIS

"Slow-channel syndrome" as CMS.

TREATMENT AND FOLLOW-UP

A detailed family history showed that this patient's disease was inherited by an autosomal-dominant inheritance pattern. Muscle biopsy of her uncle showed myopathy with a few "rimmed vacuoles." Acetylcholinesterase activity was normal. Thus, an alternative diagnosis of "slow channel syndrome" was made. Quinine sulfate and ephedrine sulfate relieved her cramps and "heavy feelings" in the legs. She believed that her son had problems similar to hers.

COMMENTS

Quinine sulfate, which is known to stabilize muscle membrane irritability, was effective for this patient. This is understandable because repetitive discharge represents a hyperirritable muscle membrane state that should be stabilized by quinine. Mestinon should worsen symptoms of this myasthenic syndrome. The cardinal clues for diagnosis of slow-channel syndrome in this patient were a positive family history, lingering neurological problems since childhood, forearm or finger extensor weakness, and repetitive discharge in the CMAPs. Repetitive discharge in the CMAPs was originally interpreted as "dispersion phenomenon." Usually, repetitive discharge follows the main component of the response as an "after-discharge," as

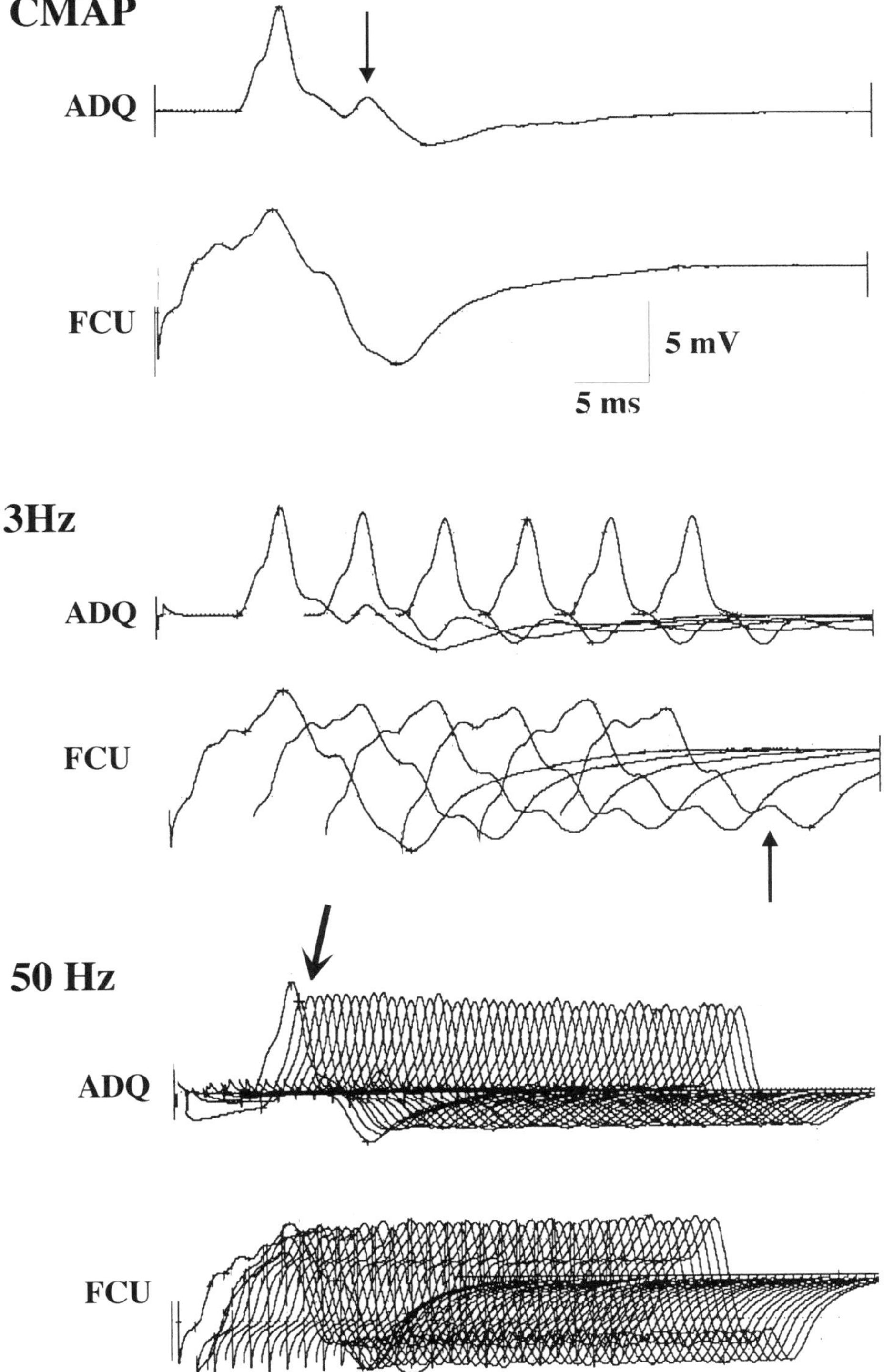

FIGURE 13.19. RNS responses in the ADQ and FCU muscles. Repetitive discharge (*thin arrow*) in the CMAP. Decremental response at LRS. Dip phenomenon (*thick arrow*) at HRS.

noted in our case. Abnormal temporal dispersion is characterized by CMAPs of many phases and long duration. Once the repetitive discharge was recognized, in the presence of a decremental response on the RNS test, we were able to narrow the diagnostic possibilities to two congenital myasthenic syndromes: slow-channel syndrome and acetylcholinesterase deficiency syndrome. The latter was ruled out by the demonstration of acetylcholinesterase in the muscle biopsy. Acquired NMT disorders characterized by repetitive discharge are organophosphate intoxication and anti-ChE toxicity. RNS features in this case were almost identical to those seen in organophosphate intoxication and anticholinesterase toxicity: repetitive discharge and "dip phenomenon."

Slow-channel syndrome is characterized by autosomal dominant inheritance pattern; onset of symptoms in infancy or later life; selective involvement of cervical, scapular, and finger extensor muscles; ophthalmoparesis; variable involvement of other muscles; and repetitive discharge and decremental response on the RNS test. Microphysiological studies show prolonged duration of the end-plate potential due to a prolonged open time of the AChR ion channel, the basic defect in this order. This is the only congenital myasthenic syndrome so far reported that has an autosomal dominant pattern. The most characteristic clinical feature of this syndrome is prominent involvement of neck, wrist, and finger extensor muscles. It is noteworthy that the patient's father was thought to have lead neuropathy that is characterized by wrist-drop. Muscle weakness may be asymmetric, as noted in our case. The most characteristic RNS finding in this disorder is the repetitive discharge of CMAP. This repetitive discharge is not different from that observed in AChE deficiency. LRS produces a 5 to 50% decremental response. In our case, there was a dip phenomenon that is classically observed in ACh overactivity. Harper reported that administration of anti-ChE has no effect on the decrement of the main CMAP wave but causes an increase in the amplitude of the number of repetitive CMAPs. In contrast, the repetitive CMAPs observed in congenital AChE deficiency are unchanged by anti-ChE. The needle EMG in slow-channel syndrome shows SASD MUPs of varying amplitude. In view of the RNS pattern typical of ACh overactivity, physiologically, slow-channel syndrome represents ACh overactivity and a hyperirritable membrane state. Thus, any drugs that reduce the hyperirritable membrane state will be of benefit. Quinine sulfate and quinidine sulfate are two such drugs. In 1997, Engel et al. reported clinical and electrophysiological improvement with quinidine sulfate in this syndrome.

MAXIMS

1. Repetitive discharge in the CMAP in CMS are indicative of either classic slow-channel syndrome or acetylcholinesterase deficiency syndrome.
2. The repetitive discharge follows the main component of the response as "after-discharge." Dispersion phenomenon (abnormal temporal dispersion) is characterized by abnormal CMAPs with multiple phases and prolonged duration.

REFERENCES

1. Engle AG, Lambert EH, Mulder DM, et al. A newly recognized congenital myasthenic syndrome attributed to a prolonged open time of the acetylcholine-induced ion channel. Ann Neurol 1982;11: 553–569.

CASE 15

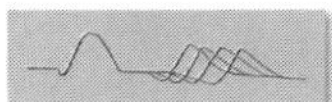

ACUTE OCULOBULBAR-RESPIRATORY PARALYSIS

CASE PRESENTATION

A 54-year-old man began to vomit one day in February 1974 and on the following day developed dysarthria, diplopia, and dysphagia, which were soon followed by shortness of breath and difficulty walking. Because of progression of these symptoms, he was admitted 3 days later to a local hospital. Within 2 days, he was transferred to the UAB Hospital because of progressive respiratory distress. By the time of transfer, he also had urinary retention. The patient was alert but mute because of bulbar paralysis. His blood pressure was 105/70 mm Hg. Respirations were shallow at 40/min. Except for absence of bowel sounds, no abnormalities were found at the time of physical examination. Neurological examination showed complete ophthalmoplegia, midsized pupils without any light response, mild bilateral ptosis, bilateral facial weakness, dysarthria, absent gag reflex, hyperactive patellar (3 +) and absent ankle reflexes, bilateral Babinski signs, and 3 MRC strength of deltoid muscles and hip flexors. No sensory or cerebellar abnormalities were noted. Soon after initial examination, respiratory arrest developed. This was treated by endotracheal intubation and mechanical ventilation. The patient was unconscious for about 15 hours after this episode. Injection of 10 mg edrophonium chloride intravenously did not affect the ophthalmoplegia. Spinal fluid examinations disclosed no abnormalities.

CASE ANALYSIS

This patient presented a diagnostic challenge to the neurology housestaff and faculty. The working diagnosis of the housestaff physician was brainstem infarction in view of the bulbar palsy, hyperactive knee jerk, and Babinski sign. The neurology attending thought that normal consciousness with this degree of bulbar palsy was incompatible with brainstem infarction. Three other possibilities to be considered in acute bulbar palsy were MG, the descending form of the Guillain-Barré syndrome, and botulism. A negative endrophonium test and pupillary involvement ruled out MG. Pupillary involvement can be seen in Guillain-Barré syndrome and botulism. Guillain-Barré syndrome was less likely in view of the normal spinal fluid evaluation. Botulism was clinically suspected. A careful history was taken with regard to the possibility of toxin exposure. The patient had eaten home-preserved tomatoes 5 hours before onset of vomiting.

PLAN OF TESTING

1. NCS: To rule out Guillain-Barré syndrome.
2. RNS: To rule out MG and confirm botulism.
3. Needle EMG: To corroborate the diagnosis of botulism.
4. Send the serum and stool for botulinum toxin test to the Centers for Disease Control and Prevention, Atlanta.

ELECTROPHYSIOLOGICAL TESTS AND FINDINGS

NCS Findings

1. Normal sensory, mixed, and motor NCS except for prolonged H-reflex (43 ms) and low CMAP amplitudes.

Needle EMG Findings on the 5th Day of Admission

1. No fibrillation or PSW in any tested muscles.
2. In the deltoid muscle, mean duration was 7.3 ms and mean amplitude, 832 μV. In the anterior tibialis, mean duration was 11.0 ms and mean amplitude, 1150 μV.

RNS Test Findings (Table 13.18; Fig. 13.20)

1. Low CMAP amplitude.
2. Decremental response at LRS and no decremental response at HRS.
3. PTF by amplitude (58%) as well as decrement.
4. No PTE.

TABLE 13.18. RNS Test Data in Case 15

	ADQ[a]
CMAP (mV)	1.95
2 Hz (%)	−22.0
5 Hz (%)	−21.0
50 Hz (%)	25.0
5 Hz PT 0 (%)	−9.0
amplitude (%)	55.9
5 Hz PT 4 (%)	−11.0
amplitude (%)	14.9

[a] Second hospital day.

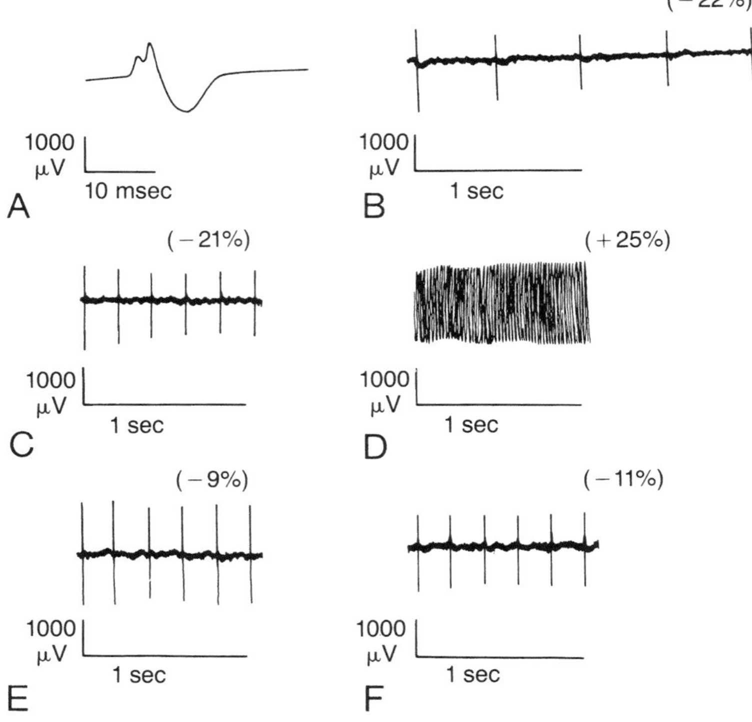

FIGURE 13.20. RNS responses in severe botulism. **A.** CMAP at rest. **B.** Two-Hz stimulation. **C, E, F.** Responses at 5-Hz stimulation before, immediately after, and 4 minutes after 50-Hz stimulation. **D.** Notice the absence of any substantial incremental response in **D.** (Reprinted with permission from Oh SJ. Botulism: electrophysiological studies. Ann Neurol 1977;1:482.)

ELECTROPHYSIOLOGICAL INTERPRETATION

Atypical presynaptic NMT block compatible with botulism.

OTHER TEST FINDINGS

Botulinum toxin was found in the serum and in the home-preserved tomatoes by means of the mouse neutralizing test performed by the CDC.

FINAL DIAGNOSIS

Foodborne botulism

TREATMENT AND FOLLOW-UP

The RNS test on the second day of hospitalization showed findings consistent with botulism. Thus, the serum and stool were sent to the CDC for confirmation of botulinum toxin. A tracheostomy was performed on the third hospital day. The patient was treated with three vials of trivalent botulism antitoxin (type A, 22,500 units; type B, 16,500; type E, 25,500) on the fourth hospital day. The diagnosis of botulism type B was confirmed in pretreatment sera and stools with the use of the mouse neutralizing test at the Laboratory of the National Communicable Disease Center in Atlanta. X-ray films of the cervical spine showed moderate spondylosis. Hyperactive knee jerks and bilaterally positive Babinski signs were unchanged even after recovery from botulism and were most likely due to preexisting cervical spondylotic myelopathy. During hospitalization, guanidine was tried twice with clinical and electrophysiological improvement. The patient was completely recovered in a month. The RNS test on the thirty-seventh hospital day was normal.

COMMENTS

Botulism is an uncommon, but often fatal, NMT disease caused by a potent neurotoxin produced by *Clostridium botulinum*. Three distinct clinical syndromes have been described: foodborne botulism, wound botulism, and infant botulism. Foodborne botulism, the best-known form, is due to ingestion of preformed toxin in improperly preserved foods. Vegetables are the most commonly implicated foods. Wound botulism, the least common form, results from wounds infected with *C. botulinum* in which the toxin is produced in vivo. In infant botulism, the most recently recognized and now most common form, the toxin is produced in vivo in the gut of the infant after ingestion of the *C. botulinum* organism.

Botulinum toxins interfere with the release of ACh at the cholinergic transmission sites of the peripheral nervous system. As a rule, neuromuscular block is the most prominent of these symptoms, producing paralysis of the extraocular, bulbar, and limb muscles. Because of the involvement of the parasympathetic system, autonomic dysfunction is common but less prominent and includes pupillary abnormality, paralytic ileus, urinary retention, diminution of secretions, and orthostatic hypotension. The hallmark of botulism is an acute, descending, symmetrical motor paralysis first affecting muscles supplied by the cranial nerves. In addition to motor weakness, areflexia and dysautonomia (fixed pupils, ileus, and urinary retention) are prominent findings. MG is differentiated from botulism by preserved reflexes, normal pupillary response, and positive tensilon test. The descending form of Guillain-Barré syndrome, which is more common than botulism, can mimic botulism, producing areflexia and dysautonomia. High spinal fluid protein and nerve conduction abnormalities are the key findings for Guillain-Barré syndrome.

The most effective way to confirm a diagnosis of botulism is to demonstrate botulinum toxin in the serum or botulinum toxin and *C. botulinum* organisms in the feces or wound. Electrophysiological studies are extremely helpful in the diagnosis of botulism. Because the RNS test provides the only relatively specific responses in botulism, this test has been found to be the most convincing objective evidence of botulism until microbiological confirmation is achieved. The most characteristic RNS abnormalities are those of presynaptic NMT blocks: low CMAP, postexercise increase of CMAP, decremental response at LRS, and incremental response at HRS. Depending on the severity of disease, these parameters may vary, being normal in mild cases. However, among the most consistent abnormalities in the RNS test is the incremental response at HRS. In some cases, a longer (>1 second) tetanic stimulation is required to document an incremental response. Other unique features of the RNS test in botulism are minimal but persisting posttetanic facilitation and lack of PTE. Two types of responses on the RNS test have been observed depending on the degree of severity. In the mild form (respiratory failure not present), the RNS abnormalities are characterized by a normal CMAP amplitude, a normal response at LRS, and a significant incremental response at HRS. In the severe form (respiratory failure present), the RNS abnormalities are characterized by a low CMAP amplitude, a normal or decremental response at LRS, and an insignificant incremental response at HRS. In severe case, prolonged HRS may be needed to document an incremental response.

MAXIMS

1. The descending form of motor paralysis, areflexia, and dysautonomia comprise the classic constellation of botulism. More commonly, this constellation is seen in the descending form of Guillain-Barré syndrome.
2. The most characteristic RNS abnormalities in botulism are those of presynaptic NMT blocks: low CMAP, postexercise increase of CMAP, a normal or decremental response at LRS, and an incremental response at HRS. Among these, the incremental response at HRS is the most consistent.

REFERENCE

1. Oh SJ. Botulism: electrophysiological studies. Ann Neurol 1977;1:481–485.

CHAPTER 14

Hyperexcitable Peripheral Nerve Disorders (Neuromyotonia)

Hyperexcitable peripheral nerve disorders are characterized by sustained muscle activity due to hyperexcitability in the distal motor axons. *Neuromyotonic discharges are the electrophysiological hallmark of these disorders.* However, myokymic discharges and fasciculations are also the electrophysiological expressions of hyperexcitable peripheral nerve. In recent years, there has been a tendency to label hyperexcitable peripheral nerve disorders loosely as "neuromyotonia."

Hyperexcitability of the distal nerves is classically documented by pharmacological tests; sustained muscle activity persists during sleep, under general anesthesia, and after epidural spinal block but is abolished by regional curare administration. Depending on the site of the "excitable" generator and peripheral nerve block, continuous muscle activity persists or is blocked by peripheral nerve block.

Hyperexcitable peripheral nerve disorders can be associated with peripheral neuropathy. In these cases, there is usually clinical evidence of peripheral neuropathy in addition to sustained muscle activity. Nerve conduction is abnormal in these cases, most of which are due to demyelinating neuropathies.

There are three well-known hyperexcitable peripheral nerve disorders without clinically obvious peripheral neuropathy: Isaacs' syndrome, myokymia-cramp syndrome, and cramp-fasciculation syndrome. Isaacs' syndrome is characterized by stiffness, continuous muscle contraction, clinical improvement after phenytoin or carbamazepine therapy, and continuous motor unit activity on needle electromyography (EMG). On the other hand, myokymia-cramp syndrome and cramp-fasciculation syndrome are characterized by cramp, myokymia, or fasciculation and clinical improvement with phenytoin or carbamazepine therapy. *The diagnosis of myokymia-cramp syndrome or cramp-fasciculation syndrome is made depending on whether myokymic discharges or fasciculations are seen in the needle EMG.* We believe that these three clinical syndromes represent the spectrum of hyperexcitable peripheral nerve disorders and are caused by differences in the degree of hyperexcitability: continuous muscle fiber activity in Isaacs' syndrome as the most extreme, myokymia-cramp syndrome as an intermediate, and cramp-fasciculation syndrome as the mildest form.

In this chapter, hemifacial spasm and stiff-man syndrome (SMS) are included. Hemifacial spasm is a type of facial dystonia clinically characterized by paroxysmal bursts of involuntary tonic or clonic activity occurring in muscles innervated by the facial nerve. It is thought to be due to the ectopic excitation and ephatic transmission of proximal facial nerves, thus representing a hyperexcitable peripheral nerve disorder.

SMS is not caused by hyperexcitable peripheral nerve disorder but by motor neuronal hyperexcitability, producing persistent painful axial and proximal limb-muscle rigidity and spasms that are exacerbated by sensory or motor stimuli and abolished by sleep and general anesthesia. SMS is included here because of its clinical similarities to hyperexcitable peripheral nerve disorders. The differences between SMS and Isaacs' syndrome are listed in Table 14.1.

TABLE 14.1. Differential Diagnostic Features of Stiff-Man Syndrome and Isaacs' Syndrome

	Stiff-Man Syndrome	**Isaacs' Syndrome**
Involuntary continuous muscle activity	+ +	+ +
Painful	+ +	+ +
Predominant location	Trunk, axial	Limb
Induced by tactile or emotional stimuli or volitional movements	+ +	−
Hyperhidrosis	±	+ +
Continuous muscle activity abolished by		
General anesthesia	+ +	−
Epidural spinal block	+ +	−
Sleep	+ +	−
Peripheral nerve block	+ +	± [a]
Curare or pancuronium	+ +	+ +
Pharmacological response		
Anticonvulsants (phenytoin or carbamazepine)	−	+ +
GABAergic agents (valium and baclofen)	+ +	−
Neurophysiological responses		
Neuronal hyperexcitability	+ +	−
Repetitive discharge	−	±

[a] Depending on the site of hyperexcitability generator and location of block. If the generator is proximal and the block is distal to it, the continuous activity will be abolished. If the reverse is true, then the continuous activity will not be abolished.

CASE 1

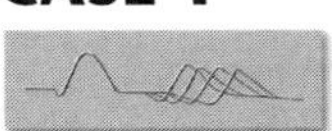

PROGRESSIVE MUSCLE WEAKNESS, MUSCLE SPASMS, AND MYOKYMIA IN THE ARMS FOR 9 MONTHS

CASE PRESENTATION

A 45-year-old man was evaluated for a 9-month history of progressive weakness, muscle spasms, and stiffness in the arms, gradually spreading from his hands up to his shoulders. He complained of spasms and twitching of his arm muscles at rest or at night while sleeping. When he attempted to raise his arms to perform any task, he noted spasms in the arms. In the past, he had been treated with penicillin for asymptomatic neurosyphilis and positive VDRL. There was no family history of neuromuscular disease.

Neurological examination revealed constant, coarse, undulating muscle movements (myokymia) involving the proximal muscles of the arms. On the MRC scale, right and left deltoids and right wrist extensor and flexor muscles were graded 2 and bilateral biceps, hand grip and left wrist extensor and flexor muscles were grade 3. Muscle strength in the trapezius, triceps, and leg muscles was normal. There was no muscle atrophy. Relaxation of the right biceps was difficult because of continuous muscle contraction, necessitating mechanical extension of the right arm. There were spontaneous spasms of both trapezius muscles but no percussion or grasp myotonia. Sensory examination was intact to pinprick, light touch, vibration, and proprioception. Tendon reflexes were diffusely absent bilaterally. There was no evidence of hyperhydrosis. Routine laboratory studies revealed only an elevated CPK of 617 IU/L (normal up to 275 IU/L). Serum and cerebrospinal fluid VDRL was negative. CSF was normal with no cells and 43 mg/dL of protein.

CASE ANALYSIS

This patient had a subacute motor syndrome characterized by continuous muscle contraction (myokymia) in the proximal muscles of the arms, preventing normal relaxation of muscles, weakness of some arm muscles, and diffuse areflexia. Considering the continuous muscle contraction, Isaacs' syndrome, SMS, and myokymia-cramp syndrome were the diagnostic possibilities. SMS usually involves truncal muscles; myokymia-cramp syndrome is generally less severe. Possible causes for the continuous muscle contraction should include multifocal motor neuropathy, cervical polyradiculopathy, and adult-onset spinal muscular atrophy. EMG and NCS were the crucial tests in identifying the nature of the continuous muscle contraction in the lower motor neuron axis.

PLAN OF TESTING

1. Needle EMG: To document whether clinical myokymia represents continuous muscle fiber activity or electrophysiological myokymia and to document the nature of the disease.
2. Nerve conduction study: To see whether peripheral neuropathy is the cause for clinical myokymia.
3. Pharmacological test: To differentiate between Isaacs' syndrome and SMS.

ELECTROPHYSIOLOGICAL TESTS AND FINDINGS

NCS Findings (Table 14.2)

1. No sensory CNAP in median, ulnar, and sural nerves.
2. Abnormal mixed nerve conduction in ulnar and median nerves, either by absent CNAP, slow NCV, or low CNAP amplitude.
3. Prolonged terminal latency, abnormal temporal dispersion, conduction block, and mildly slow motor NCV in ulnar nerve.
4. Prolonged terminal latency, low CMAP amplitude, and conduction block in median nerve.
5. Prolonged terminal latency, low CMAP amplitude, slow motor NCV but with abnormal temporal dispersion in peroneal and posterior tibial nerves (Fig. 14.1).
6. No repetitive discharges after the motor response.

Needle EMG (Table 14.3)

1. In most tested muscles in the arms and some muscles in the legs, motor unit potentials (MUPs) were increased in amplitude and duration with a reduced recruitment pattern and rare fibrillation potentials or positive sharp waves were identified.

TABLE 14.2. Nerve Conduction Data in Case 1

	Latent/NCV (ms/m/s)	Amplitude (mV/μV)	Shape		Latent/NCV (ms/m/s)	Amplitude (mV/μV)	Shape
	Median	**Motor**	**Nerve**		**Peroneal**	**Motor**	**Nerve**
TL	3.9	2.2		TL	6.5	2	
E-W	NP		CB	FH-A	36.2	1.33	D
AX-E	NP			PF-FH	70.4	1.30	D
	Ulnar	**Motor**	**Nerve**		**Post-Tibial**	**Motor**	**Nerve**
TL	3.1	6		TL	6.5	1	
BE-W	43.9	1.8	D/CB	PF-A	36.2	0.65	D
AE-BE	41.2	1.2	D				
AX-AE	NP		CB				
	Median	**Sens/Mixed**	**Nerve**		**Sural**	**Sens/Mixed**	**Nerve**
F-W	NP			MC-A	NP		
W-E	42.8	3					
E-AX	48.3	15					
	Ulnar	**Sens/Mixed**	**Nerve**		**Superficial Peroneal**	**Sens/Mixed**	**Nerve**
F-W	NP			MC-A			
W-E	NP						
E-AX	37.7	20					

Height: 170 cm.
TL, terminal latency; E, elbow; W, wrist; AX, axilla; BE, below elbow; AE, above elbow; F, finger; FH, fibular head; A, ankle; PF, popliteal fossa; MC, midcalf; CB, conduction block; D, dispersion; NP, no potential.

2. In muscles in which clinical myokymia was prominent, there was a state of constant dysrhythmic discharges of MUPs at rest with bursts of rapid-firing MUPs.
3. Electrical stimulation of the median nerve at the wrist produced high-frequency discharges of MUPs followed by a gradual decrease in amplitude and frequency that lasted more than 2 seconds (Fig. 14.2). This pattern differed from that of true myotonia, in which there is a waxing and waning discharge of muscle fibers, and also from that of bizarre high-frequency potentials, which show abrupt onset and termination. Somewhat less dramatic MUP discharges were noted with percussion of the median nerve at the wrist.

ELECTROPHYSIOLOGICAL INTERPRETATION

Demyelinating neuropathy and neuromyotonia (continuous muscle fiber activity).

PHARMACOLOGICAL STUDIES

1. The right median nerve was blocked at the wrist by a local injection of 2% lidocaine. Continuous muscle activity in the right APB muscle was attenuated but not abolished (Fig. 14.3). After administration of 0.2 mg of D-tubocurarine locally, it disappeared totally.
2. Continuous muscle fiber activity was not affected during spinal anesthesia in the left gastrocnemius muscle (Fig. 14.3).

FINAL DIAGNOSIS

Isaacs' syndrome due to chronic inflammatory demyelinating neuropathy

TREATMENT AND FOLLOW-UP

The patient was treated with phenytoin 300 mg/day and gradually had subjective improvement of muscle spasms, twitching, and weakness. The weakness never completely resolved, but the patient improved enough that in 3 months he was able to work as a shipping clerk

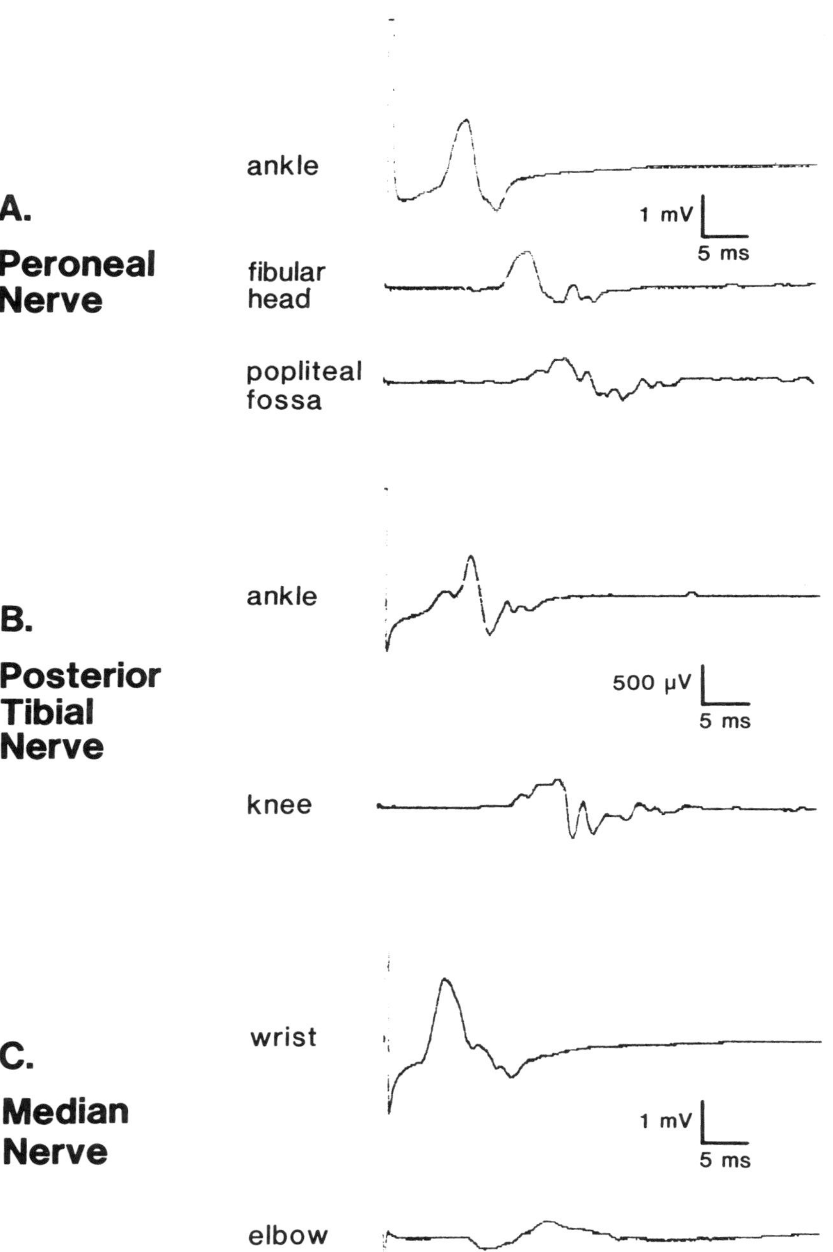

FIGURE 14.1. Nerve conduction studies. **A** and **B** demonstrate increased temporal dispersion and reduced amplitude of the CMAP in the peroneal and the posterior tibial nerves. **C** shows conduction block in the median nerve at the forearm segment. (Reprinted with permission from Odabasi Z, Joy JL, Claussen GC, et al. Isaacs' syndrome associated with chronic inflammatory demyelinating polyneuropathy. Muscle Nerve 1996;19:213.)

TABLE 14.3. Needle EMG Data in Case 1

				Spontaneous Potentials				Motor Unit Potential				Interference	
Muscle	**Root**	**Nerve**	**Insertion Activity**	**Fib**	**PSW**	**CMFA**	**Myokymia Fasc**	**Amplitude (K)**	**Duration (ms)**	**Polyphasic Potential**	**HA MUP**	**Pattern**	**Mean Amplitude (K)**
Rt C5-C8 paraspinal	C5–8		N	–	–	–	–						
Deltoid	C5,6	Axillary	+	–	+	++	+	1.88	12.8	4%	–	FIP	2
Biceps	C5,6	Musc cut	+	–	–	++	++	1–7	7–16	N	+	RIP	5
Trapezius	C3,4	Sp acces	+	–	–	++	++	1–3	8–16	N	–	RIP	2.5
Left deltoid	C5,6	Axillary	+	–	–	++	+	1–4	6–15	N	–	RIP	3
EDC	C7	Radial	N	–	–	+	–	0.8–4	6–12	N	–	RIP	3
FDI	C8,T1	Ulnar	N	–	–	+	–	1–3	6–13	++	–	DA	2
OP	C8,T1	Median	+	–	–	+++	+	1–4	7–14	N	–	RIP	3
Rt vast lat	L3,4	Fem	N	–	–	–	–	0.7–2.5	8–16	N	–	RIP	2.5
Ant tibial	L4,5	Peroneal	+	–	–	–++	–+	1–6	8–16	N	+	RIP	2.5
Right gastroc	S1,2	Post tibial	+	–	–	+++	+	1–3	8–16	N	–	RIP	3

Fib, fibrillations; PSW, positive sharp wave; CMFA, continuous muscle fiber activity; Fasc, fasciculations; HA MUP, high-amplitude MUP; N, normal; –, absent; +, present or increased; FIP, full interference pattern; RIP, reduced interference pattern; EDC, extensor digitorum communis; FDI, first dorsal interosseous; DA, discrete activity; OP, opponens pollicis.

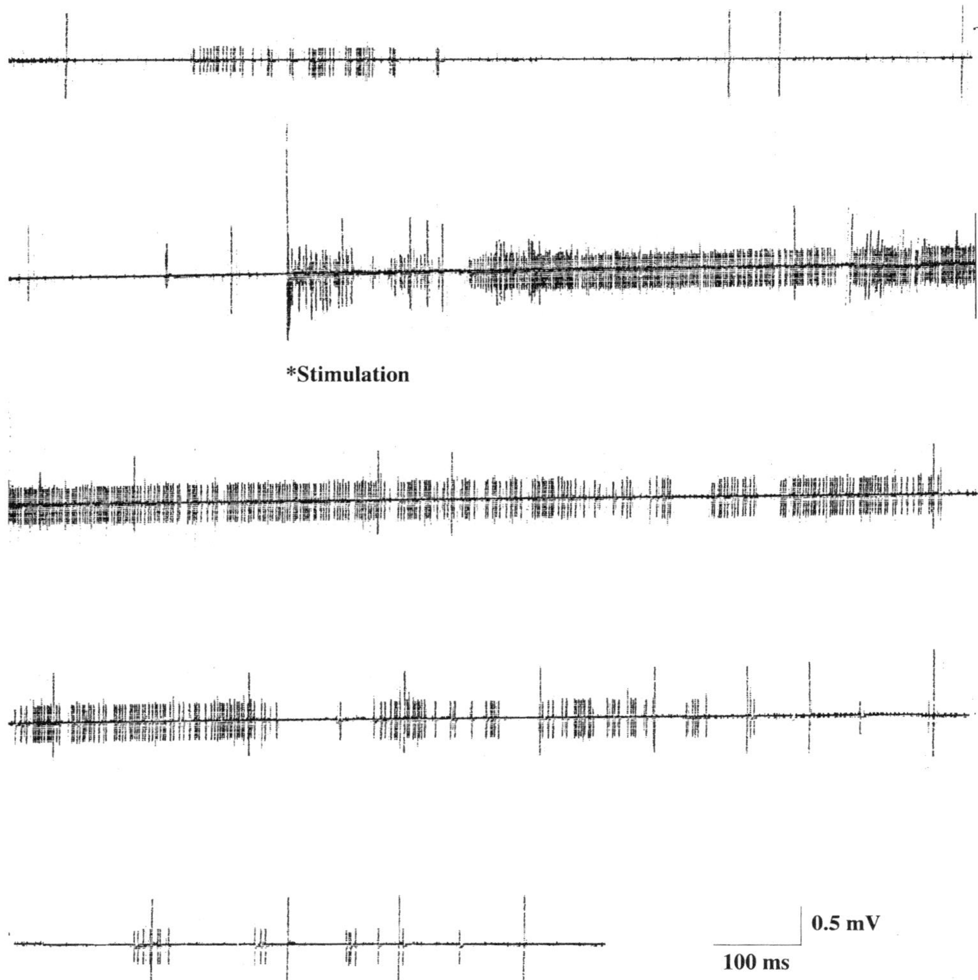

FIGURE 14.2. Continuous muscle fiber activity (MUP discharge) from APB muscle before and after a single electrical stimulation (*) of median nerve at the wrist. Continuous muscle fiber activity lasted for 2 seconds after the electrical stimulation.

and stopped taking phenytoin. A year later there had been a recurrence of symptoms with additional moderate weakness of the legs. The patient underwent a sural nerve biopsy, which was indicative of inflammatory demyelinating neuropathy. He was started on prednisone and phenytoin with subsequent improvement over several months. Since then, there have been three relapses of Isaacs' syndrome and neuropathy that were treated successfully with phenytoin, prednisone, and azathioprine.

COMMENTS

Isaacs' syndrome (neuromyotonia) is characterized by involuntary sustained muscle contraction that persists during sleep and general or spinal anesthesia. The electrophysiological hallmark of this syndrome is neuromyotonia: continuous muscle fiber activity at rest. The abnormal EMG activity of this syndrome is believed to arise in peripheral nerve axons because it persists in sleep and after generalized or spinal anesthesia (Table 14.1). Conflicting results from many reported peripheral nerve block studies suggest that multiple trigger zones might

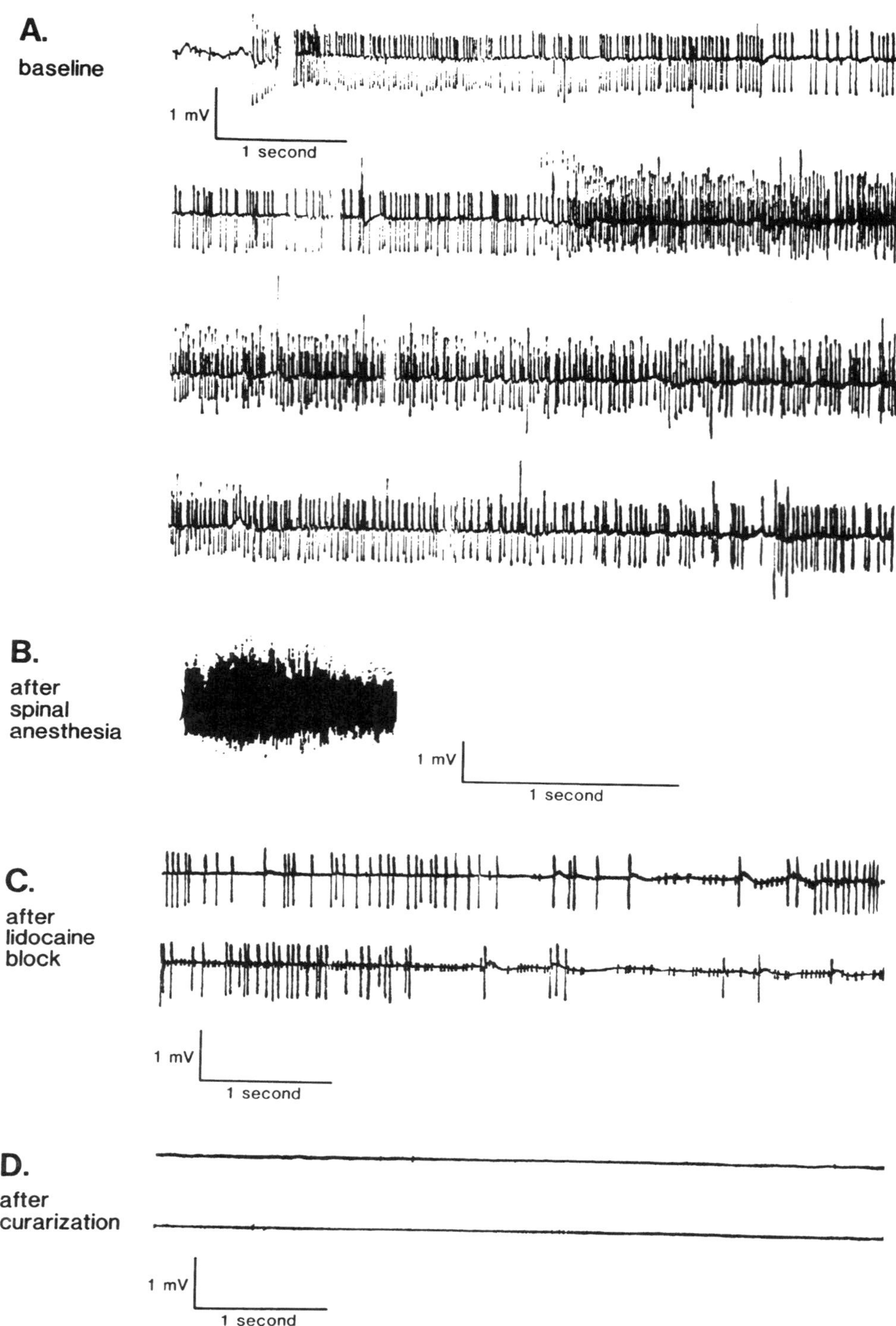

FIGURE 14.3. Spontaneous activity recorded from the muscles with a concentric needle. **A.** From APB muscle at rest. **B.** No change from gastrocnemius muscle during spinal anesthesia. **C.** Marked improvement from APB muscle after lidocaine block at the wrist. **D.** Abolition of spontaneous activity from APB muscle after regional curarization. (Reprinted with permission from Odabasi Z, Joy JL, Claussen GC, et al. Isaacs' syndrome associated with chronic inflammatory demyelinating polyneuropathy. Muscle Nerve 1996;19:213.)

be present anywhere in the axon from the anterior horn cell down to the nerve terminal. In our case, the spontaneous activity arose from multiple demyelinated areas along the nerve proximal and distal to the wrist. To confirm the diagnosis of Isaacs' syndrome, it is important to document peripheral hyperexcitability; high-frequency discharges of MUPs with electrical and percussion stimulation of the median nerve in our case.

Terms used to describe this syndrome include continuous muscle fiber activity, Isaacs-Merten syndrome, neuromyotonia, pseudomyotonia, neurotonia, myokymia with delayed muscle relaxation, and idiopathic generalized myokymia. Involuntary muscle contraction persisting during sleep is a constant feature of this syndrome and presents as undulation of the overlying skin (myokymia). Associated phenomena may include absent tendon reflexes, muscle hypertrophy, action or percussion myotonia, excessive sweating, and elevated CPK. The syndrome can occur without an associated peripheral neuropathy, may be inherited or sporadic, and can also occur in association with polyneuropathy or malignancies (thymoma or small cell lung carcinoma) as a paraneoplastic syndrome.

Needle EMG of the involved muscles demonstrates four main abnormalities, alone or in combination: neuromyotonic discharge (continuous muscle fiber activity); myokymic discharges; doublets, triplet, and multiplets; and fasciculations.

Nerve conduction studies may vary depending on whether there is an associated peripheral neuropathy. In patients with peripheral neuropathy, the results depend on whether it is axonal or demyelinating neuropathy. More often, this is seen in demyelinating neuropathy, as in our case. In some cases, repetitive discharges (electrophysiological hallmark of peripheral nerve hyperexcitability) were documented. In cramp-fasiculation syndrome, repetitive after discharges were documented after the RNS test but not after a single stimulation according to Tahmous et al.

Phenytoin or carbamazepine is the drug of choice for relieving continuous muscle fiber activity in Isaacs' syndrome. This effect is most likely the result of the reduced flux of sodium ions during action potentials. Recently, Isaacs' syndrome has been thought to be an autoimmune entity, and immunotherapy has been tried with some success. A recent study found voltage-gated potassium channel autoantibodies in 12 of 12 neuromyotonia patients, establishing neuromyotonia as a new antibody-mediated channelopathy.

MAXIMS

1. The electrophysiological hallmark of Isaacs' syndrome is neuromyotonia (continuous muscle fiber activity) at rest that is present during sleep and under general or spinal anesthesia.
2. Phenytoin or carbamazepine is the drug of choice in Isaacs' syndrome.

REFERENCES

1. Odabasi Z, Joy JL, Claussen GC, Herrera GA, Oh SJ. Isaacs' syndrome associated with chronic inflammatory demyelinating polyneuropathy. Muscle Nerve 1996;19:210–215.
2. Hart IK, Waters C, Vincent A, et al. Autoantibodies detected to expressed K+ channels are implicated in neuromyotonia. Ann Neurol 1997;41:238–246.

CASE 2

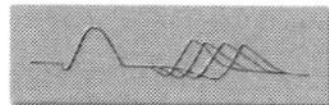

PAINFUL MUSCLE CRAMPS FOR 7 WEEKS

CASE PRESENTATION

A 13-year-old white male had pain in his back and thighs for 7 weeks and muscle twitching in the calves for 3 weeks, which progressed to involvement of his thighs and lower back. These painful cramps awakened him at night and were so disabling that he was not able to attend school. Studies, including MRI of the spinal cord and bone scan, were all normal. He had no significant past medical history or family history. Therapy with phenytoin by the referring pediatric neurologist had been ineffective.

General physical examination was normal. Neurological examination revealed full motor strength throughout without evidence of atrophy. Continuous visible myokymia was noted in the calves and posterior thighs and minimally in the deltoid muscles bilaterally. Muscle stretch reflexes were normal and symmetrical with the exception of bilateral ankle clonus. Plantar response was flexor. There was no other neurological abnormality.

Abnormal laboratory tests included a white blood cell count of 2700/mm^3 with a normal differential count and slightly elevated SGOT and GGT. CPK was normal. CSF was normal in protein and 0 in white cells.

CASE ANALYSIS

This patient had a subacute course of painful cramp characterized by continuous myokymia in the legs and otherwise normal neurological findings. Pain was due to the continuous contraction of muscle (myokymia). In this case, there was not any finding clearly localizing the site of lesion. Thus, it was important to identify the source of myokymia: anterior horn cells or peripheral nerve.

PLAN OF TESTING

1. Needle EMG in the deltoid, hamstring, gastrocnemius, and anterior tibialis muscles to document myokymic discharge and denervation process.
2. NCS for peripheral neuropathy workups to document peripheral neuropathy, especially demyelinating neuropathy, or hyperexcitability of peripheral nerve. Hyperexcitability of peripheral nerve can be documented by the repetitive discharge of CMAPs or multiple discharges of CMAPs with single stimulation of nerve.
3. RNS in the peroneal nerve to document the repetitive afterdischarge after the repetitive nerve stimulation.
4. H-reflex and T-reflex study to document the repetitive discharge. Late wave or reflex study is known to show the repetitive discharge more clearly.
5. Once hyperexcitable peripheral nerve is identified, the pharmacological test is needed to localize the source of myokymia.

ELECTROPHYSIOLOGICAL TESTS AND FINDINGS

NCS Findings (Table 14.4)

1. A barely noticeable repetitive discharge in the CMAPs in the peroneal and posterior tibial nerves with higher sensitivity (Fig. 14.4*A*).
2. Definite repetitive discharge in the CMAPs with higher sensitivity (Fig. 14.4*B*).
3. More prominent repetitive discharges in the H- and T-reflexes (Fig. 14.4, *C* and *D*).
4. Otherwise, normal motor NCS in the peroneal and posterior tibial nerves.
5. Normal sural NCS.
6. Normal motor, sensory, and mixed NCS in the ulnar and median nerves.

Needle EMG (Table 14.5)

1. Normal needle EMG findings in the arm muscles.
2. Myokymic discharges and fasciculations in the vastus lateralis, gastrocnemius, and anteror tibialis muscles (Fig. 14.5).

TABLE 14.4. Nerve Conduction Data in Case 2

	Latent/NCV (ms/m/s)	**Amplitude (mV/μV)**	**Shape**		**Latent/NCV (ms/m/s)**	**Amplitude (mV/μV)**	**Shape**
Right	**Peroneal**	**Motor**	**Nerve**	**Left**	**Peroneal**	**Motor**	**Nerve**
TL	4.8	6	RD		4.8	6	RD
FH-A	46.5	6			47.2	5.5	
PF-FH	58.8	6			52.5		
F-wave	48.0		RD		46.0		RD
	Posterior Tibial	**Motor**	**Nerve**		**Posterior Tibial**	**Motor**	**Nerve**
TL	4.5	14	RD		4.4	15	RD
PF-A	50.0	13			55.4	15	
F-wave	46.0				46.0		
H-reflex	27		RD				
	Sural	**Sensory**	**Nerve**		**Sural**	**Sensory**	**Nerve**
MC-A	42.4	25			44.4	30	
	Ankle	**T-Reflex**					
	30.0	3					

Height, 170.2 cm. RD, repetitive discharge.

3. Myokymia in the gastrocnemius muscle persisted even after complete sciatic nerve block with 2% lidocaine but was abolished with local 2% lidocaine infiltration in the periphery of exposed muscle during biopsy of the gastrocnemius muscle (Fig. 14.5).

RNS Test Findings. Normal response. No afterdischarge after 2 to 5-Hz stimulation. In the cramp-fasciculation syndrome, the afterdischarge occurs after repetitive stimulation but not after a single stimulation.

ELECTROPHYSIOLOGICAL INTERPRETATION

Myokymic discharges and hyperexcitable peripheral nerve disorder typical of myokymia-cramp syndrome.

FINAL DIAGNOSIS

Myokymia-cramp syndrome

TREATMENT AND FOLLOW-UP

Because of leucopenia and abnormal liver function due to phenytoin, carbamazepine was not tried. Instead, the patient was treated with quinine sulfate. He slept comfortably the first night of therapy, and myokymia and cramps gradually resolved over 2 months with two tablets of quinine sulfate 520 mg/day. Repeat nerve conduction studies 2 months later were normal without evidence of repetitive discharges.

COMMENTS

Our patients had a benign disorder clinically characterized by myokymia and cramps and electrophysiologically by myokymic potentials and repetitive discharge in the CMAPs. Their clinical features best fit myokymia-cramp syndrome, a rare disorder described by Denny-Brown and Foley in 1948. These patients presented clinically with cramps and myokymia and had normal routine nerve conduction studies with myokymic discharges noted in the needle EMG. Most responded well to treatment with either phenytoin or carbamezepine.

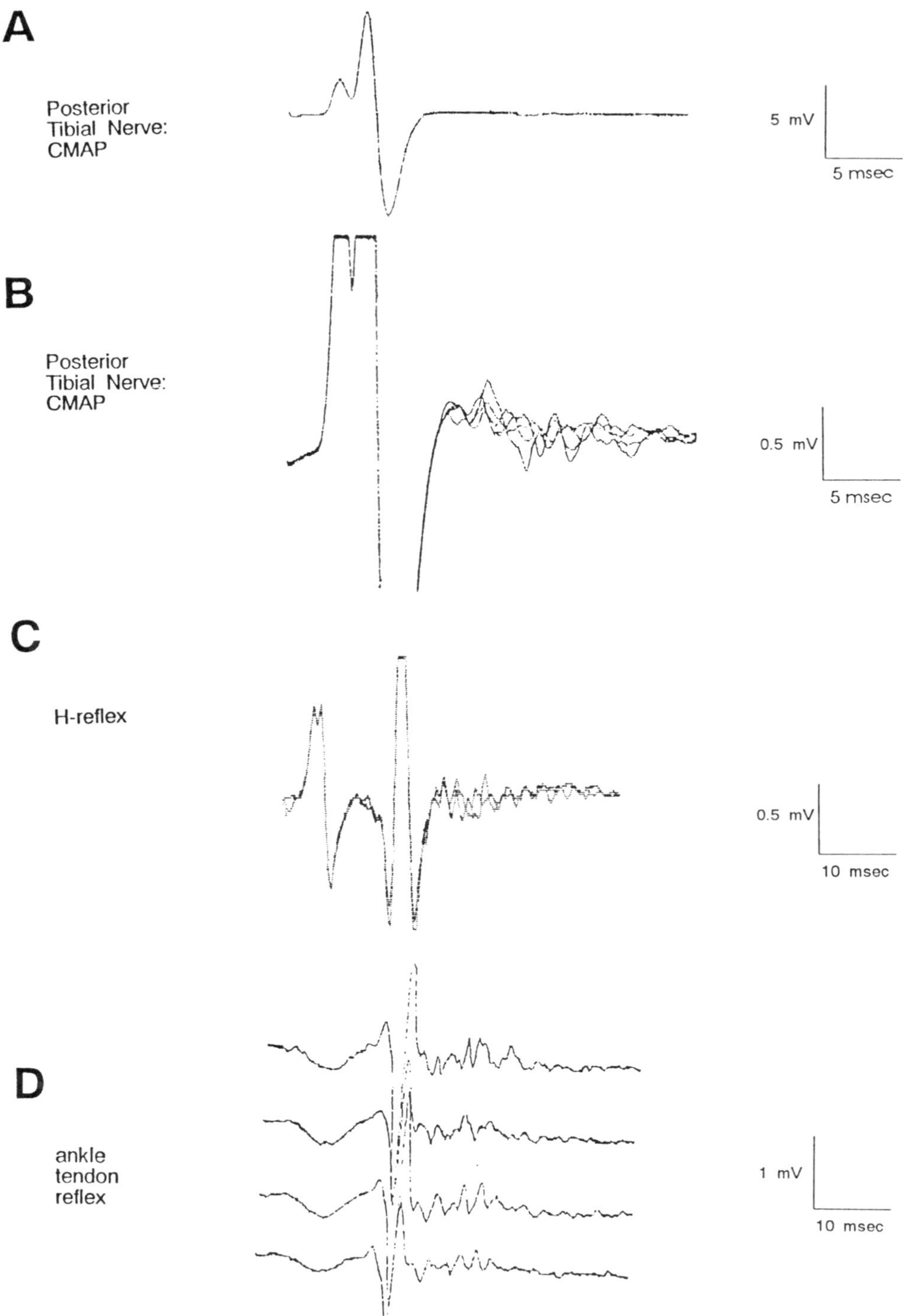

FIGURE 14.4. Repetitive discharges. RDs are absent with 5 mV sensitivity (**A**) but suggestive with 0.5 mV sensitivity (**B**). However, RDs are obvious in the H- (**C**) and ankle-tendon (**D**) reflexes. (Reprinted with permission from Smith KK, et al. Myokymia-cramp syndrome: evidence of hyperexcitable peripheral nerve. Muscle Nerve 1994;17:1066.)

TABLE 14.5. Needle EMG Data in Case 2

				Spontaneous Potentials				Motor Unit Potential				Interference	
Muscle	Root	Nerve	Insertion Activity	Fib	PSW	Fasc	Myokymia	Amplitude (K)	Duration (ms)	Polyphasic Potential	HA MUP	Pattern	Mean Amplitude (K)
Rt ant tibial	L4,5	Peroneal	N	–	–	–	+ + +	0.5–2	10–16	N	–	RIP	2
Vast lat	L3,4	Femoral	N	–	–	–	+ + +	0.5–1.5	10–16	N	–	RIP	1
Gastroc	S1,2	Post tib	N	–	–	–	+ + +	0.5–2	6–12	N	–	RIP	1.5
Biceps fem longus	S1,2	Sciatic	N	–	±	–	+ + +	0.5–2.5	7–12	N	–	RIP	1.5

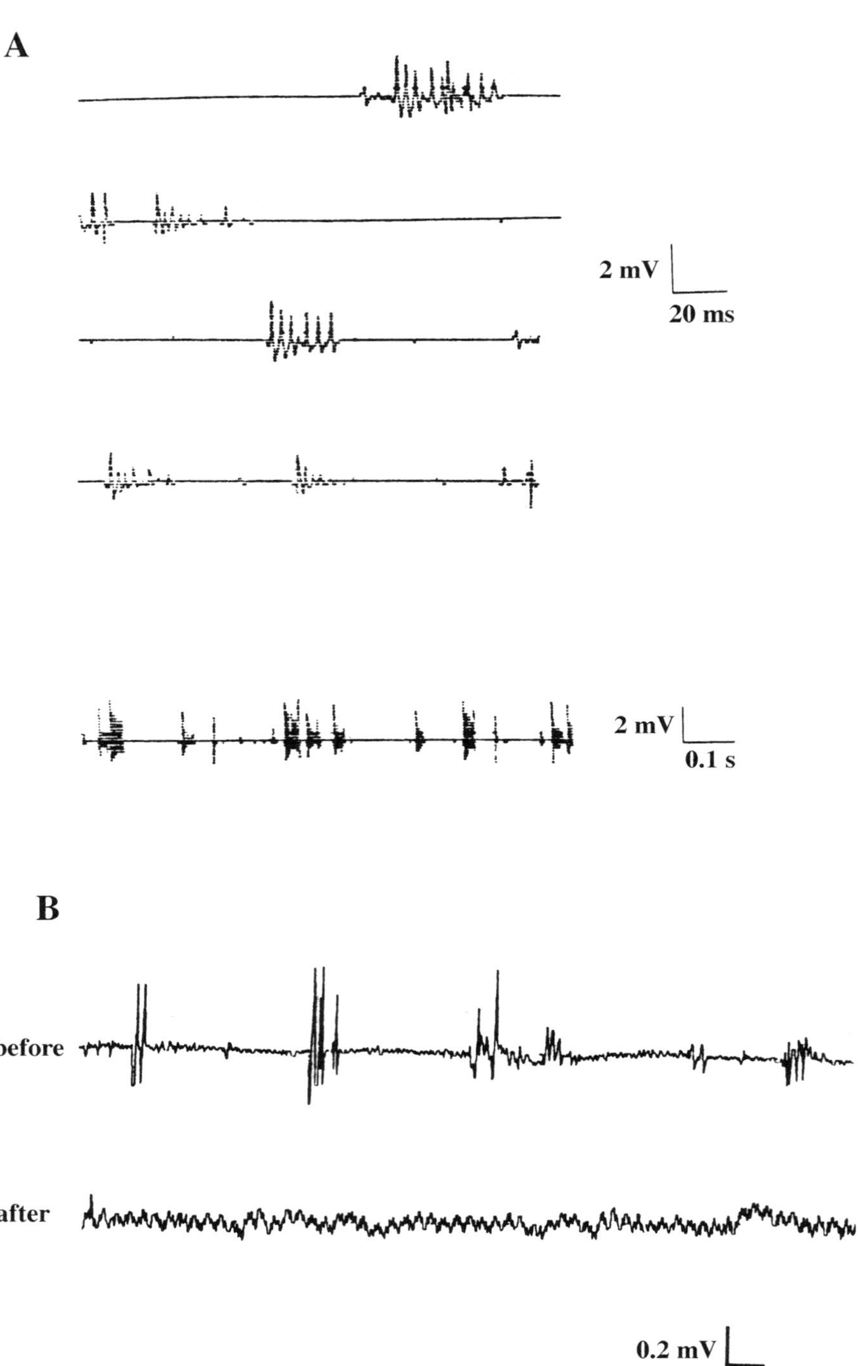

FIGURE 14.5. A. Myokymic discharges from the gastrocnemius muscle. **B.** Myokymic discharges before and after terminal axon block. Myokymic discharges are abolished after terminal axonal block with lidocaine.

Quinine sulfate was effective in our cases, but this is rare. This syndrome is characterized by painful cramps, clinical and electrophysiological myokymia, and no other major neurological deficits. The consensus is that this syndrome is due to an abnormal excitability of the peripheral nerves, especially in the distal portion of nerves as observed in our case: repetitive discharge and abolishment of myokymic discharge with axonal block. Thus, we believe that myokymia-cramp syndrome is an intermediate form of hyperexcitable peripheral nerve disorder with Isaacs' syndrome as the most severe form and cramp-fasciculation syndrome as the mildest form. There are clinical and needle EMG differences among these three syndromes: continuous muscle contraction and continuous muscle fiber activity in Isaacs' syndrome, clinical and EMG myokymia in myokymia-cramp syndrome, and clinical and EMG fasciculations in cramp-fasciculation syndrome.

Repetitive discharges in the CMAP are seen in a handful of neuromuscular diseases: anticholinesterase toxicity such as myasthenia gravis overtreated with anticholinesterase or organophosphate poisoning; congenital myasthenic syndromes; end-plate acetylcholinesterase deficiency and slow channel-syndrome; MG treated with germine acetate; and some cases of neuromyotonia as seen in myokymia-cramp syndrome. The common pathway for all these disorders is too much acetylcholine at the neuromuscular junction. Thus, repetitive discharge in the CMAP is physiologically indicative of too much acetylcholine.

MAXIMS

1. Repetitive discharge in the CMAP is indicative of too much ACh, regardless of the cause.
2. Peripheral nerve hyperexcitability can be detected with the motor nerve conduction study by documenting repetitive discharge in the CMAP.

REFERENCES

1. Auger RG. AAEM Minimonograph #44. Diseases associated with excess motor unit activity. Muscle Nerve 1994;17:1250–1263.
2. Gutmann L. AAEM Minimonograph #37. Facial and limb myokymia. Muscle Nerve 1991;14:1043–1049.

CASE 3

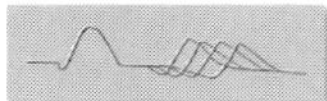

PAINFUL CRAMPS IN THE BACK AND LEGS FOR 3 MONTHS

CASE PRESENTATION

A 55-year-old man began to experience cramping pains in his back and legs in August 1993. He was initially treated for suspected tetanus, because he was employed as a roofer and had a history of cuts and nail-puncture wounds. He was then placed on valium and received four courses of antitetanus toxoid without much relief. In November 1993, his painful muscle contractions and spasms worsened, causing him to fall and strike his head. At that time, his neurological examination revealed diffuse hyperhidrosis and diffuse axial and lower limbs stiffness. Toes remained in fixed extension and pain was experienced when flexion of the ankles was attempted. Clinical myokymia was present in the calf muscles. Reflexes were brisk but symmetrical throughout with equivocal plantar responses. Coordination examination was consistent with his stiffness. He had difficulty lifting his legs off the floor due to movement-induced spasm. He refused to tandem walk or walk unassisted for fear of falling. The slightest attempt to elicit a jaw jerk produced painful opistotonus. This response was severe enough that it made it difficult for the patient to take medications because even bringing his hand to his mouth elicited this response. Auditory, emotional, and tactile stimuli also produced similar painful spasms.

CASE ANALYSIS

Painful spasms that prevent the patient from walking are typical of SMS. Painful opistotonus induced by jaw tapping (neuronal hyperexcitability) was the pivotal finding strongly suggestive of SMS in this case because such finding is observed in tetanus, tetany, and SMS. By exclusion, SMS was most likely the diagnosis.

PLAN OF TESTING

1. Anti-glutamic acid decarboxylase antibody.
2. Needle EMG: To document the continuous muscle fiber activity.
3. NCS: To document neuronal hyperexcitability and to exclude peripheral nerve hyperexcitability.

ELECTROPHYSIOLOGICAL TESTS AND FINDINGS

NCS Findings

1. Normal motor, sensory, and mixed nerve conduction.
2. No repetitive discharge in the CMAP.
3. Motor neuron excitability (Figs. 14.6 and 14.7): relatively high F-wave amplitude (1.2 mV) with F-wave/M-wave ratio of 0.15 (normal, <0.05); H-reflex amplitude (8-5 mV) with H-reflex/M-wave ratio of 0.38 to 0.62 (normal <0.38); T-reflex amplitude, 9 to 19 mV in the ankle T-reflex (normal, 8.8 mV) and 16 to 8.5 mV in the patellar T-reflex (normal, 3.9 mV).
4. Absent silent period in the masseter reflex testing.

Needle EMG (Table 14.6)

1. Continuous discharge of MUPs, supposedly at rest, in many leg muscles, some of which increased with effort and tapping of muscle (Fig. 14.8).
2. These continuous MUPs in the gastrocnemius muscles were abolished under general anesthesia (Fig. 14.9).

ELECTROPHYSIOLOGICAL INTERPRETATION

Involuntary MUP discharges that disappear with general anesthesia and motor neuron hyperexcitability typical of SMS.

FINAL DIAGNOSIS

SMS

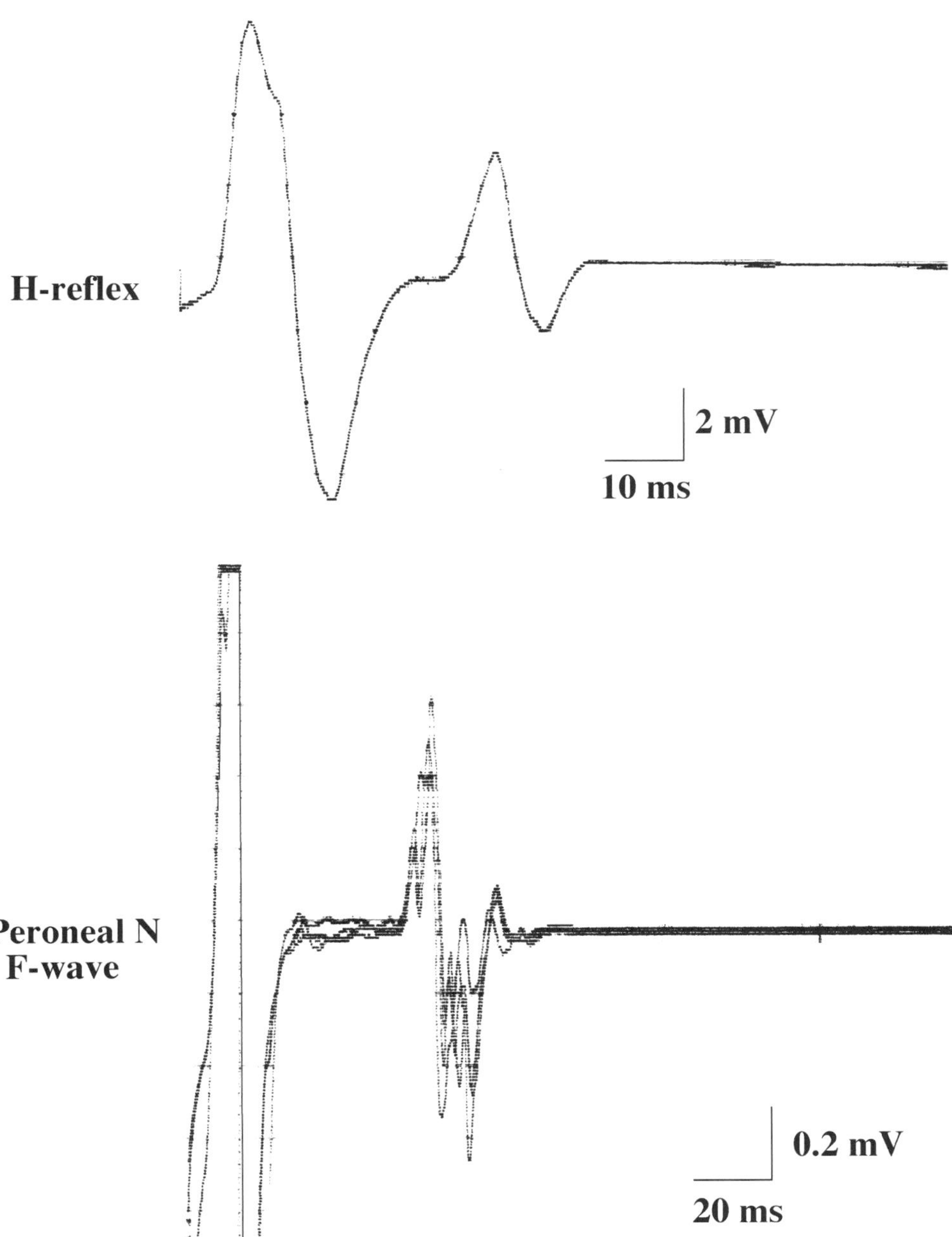

FIGURE 14.6. H-reflex from triceps surae and F-wave from peroneal nerve (*N*) with distal stimulation. Notice the high amplitude of H-reflex and F-wave, indicating neuronal hyperexcitability.

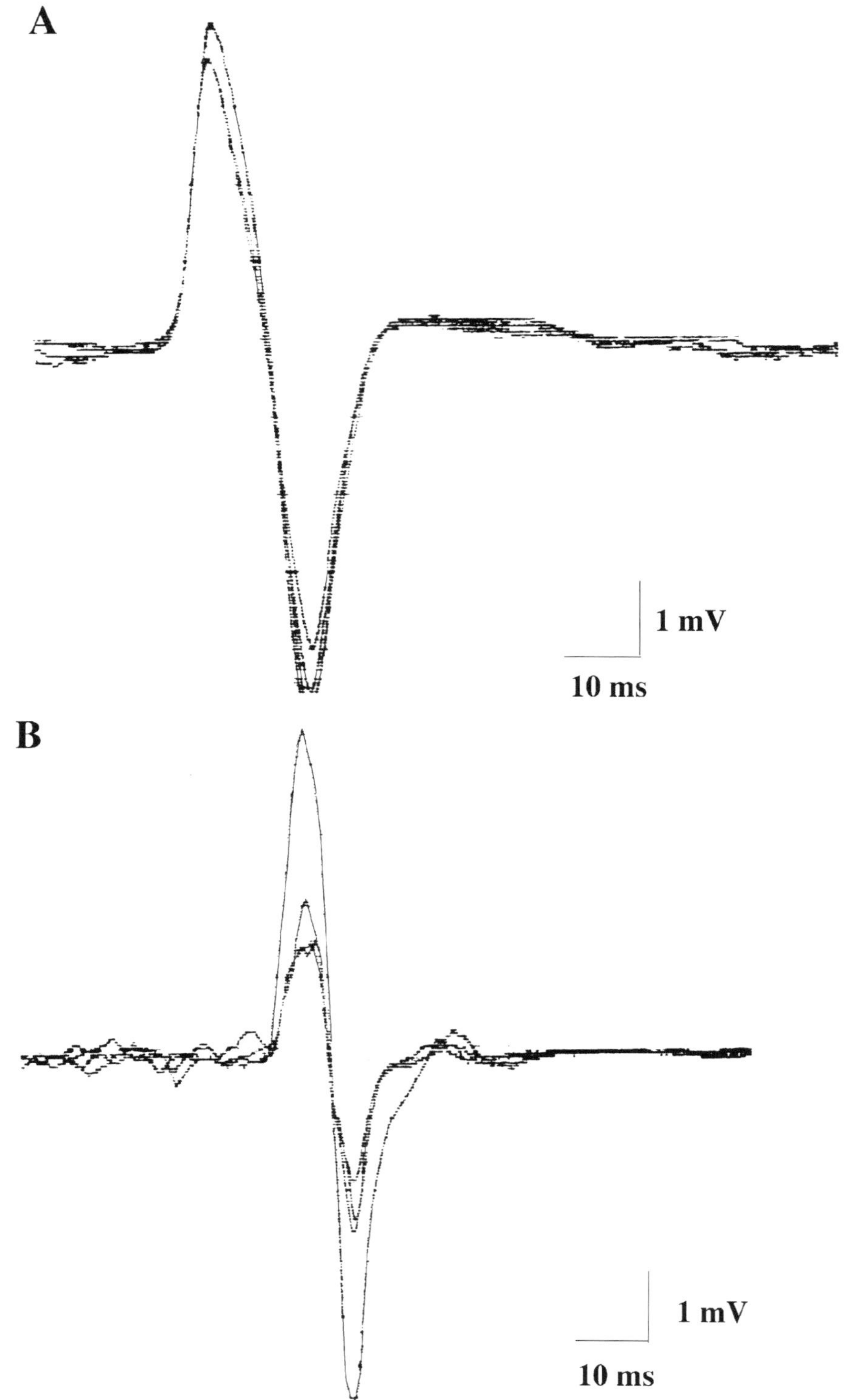

FIGURE 14.7. High amplitude of knee (**A**) and ankle (**B**) T-reflexes, indicating neuronal hyperexcitability.

TABLE 14.6. Needle EMG Data[a] in Case 3

				Spontaneous Potentials				Motor Unit Potential				Interference	
Muscle	**Root**	**Nerve**	**Insertion**	**Fib**	**PSW**	**Spontaneous MUP**	**Myotonia CRD**	**Amplitude (K)**	**Duration (ms)**	**Polyphasic Potential**	**HA MUP**	**Pattern**	**Mean Amplitude (K)**
Lt ant tibial	L4,5	Peroneal	N	–	–	+	–	0.5–3	6–12	N	–	RIP	1.5
Gastroc	S1,2	Post tibial	N	–	–	+	–	1–4	6–13	N	–	RIP	1.5
Rt ant tibial	L4,5	Peroneal	N	–	–	+	–	1–3	6–13	N	–	RIP	1.5
Gastroc	S1,2	Post tibial	N	–	–	+	–	1–4	6–13	N	–	RIP	2

[a] This needle EMG was difficult because of lack of good relaxation of muscle.
CRD, complex repetitive discharge.

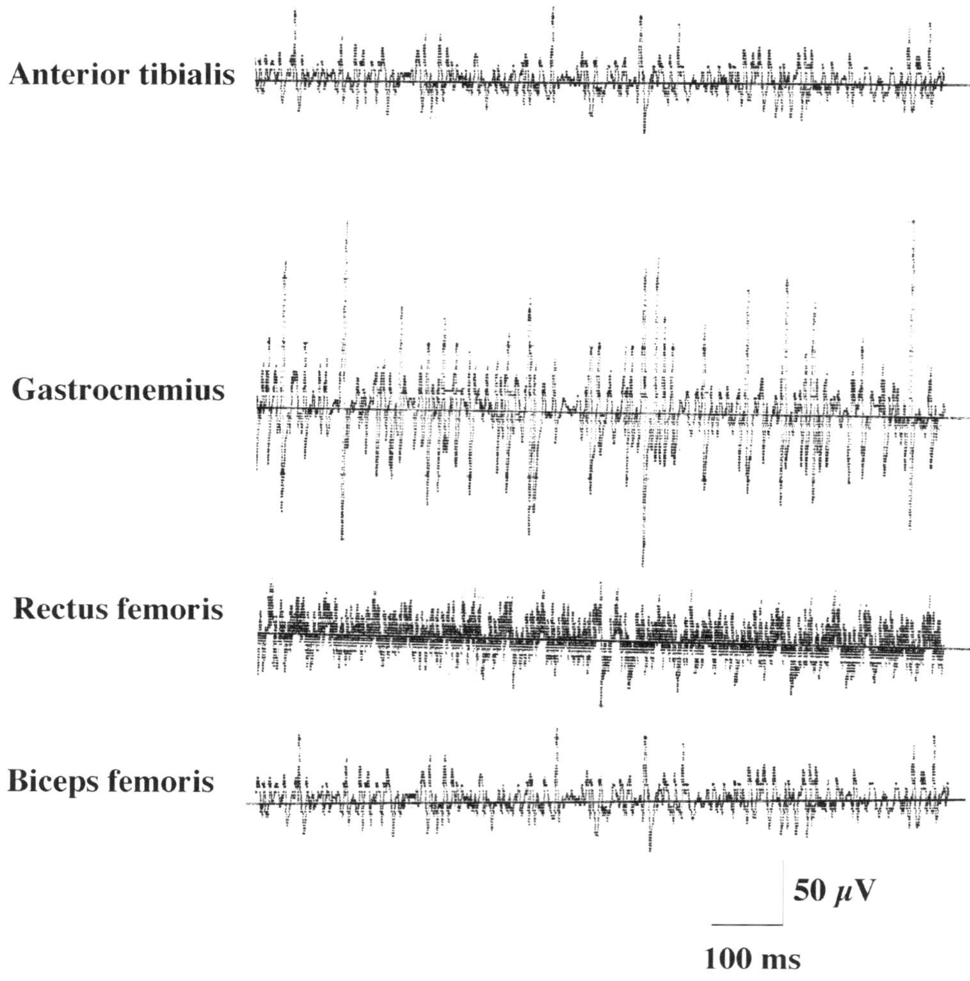

FIGURE 14.8. Spontaneous surface EMG activities from anterior tibialis, gastrocnemius, rectus femoris, and biceps femoris muscle on standing still. In normal individuals, there are no spontaneous surface EMG activities from these muscles on standing still in one place.

TREATMENT AND FOLLOW-UP

The patient was treated with valium 40 mg/day and baclofen 80 mg/day with moderate success. CSF was normal. Anti-MAG, anti-GM1, anti-GAD, and anti-Purkinje cell cytoplasmic antibodies were negative. CT of the chest showed a mass in the anterior mediastinum. Previous to thymectomy, the patient received five courses of intravenous IgG (400 mg/kg/day) without noticeable benefit, but after thymectomy he experienced profound clinical improvement. A few months later, ocular MG developed and lasted 2 months. ACh receptor antibody was negative. RNS tests in the ulnar, facial, and accessory nerves were all normal. Single-fiber EMG in the frontalis muscle (Table 14.7) was mildly abnormal, whereas one in the EDC was normal.

COMMENTS

Our case is unique in that this patient had SMS, MG, and thymoma. Such cases support the autoimmune basis of SMS. Paraneoplastic SMS has been reported with colon adenocarcinoma,

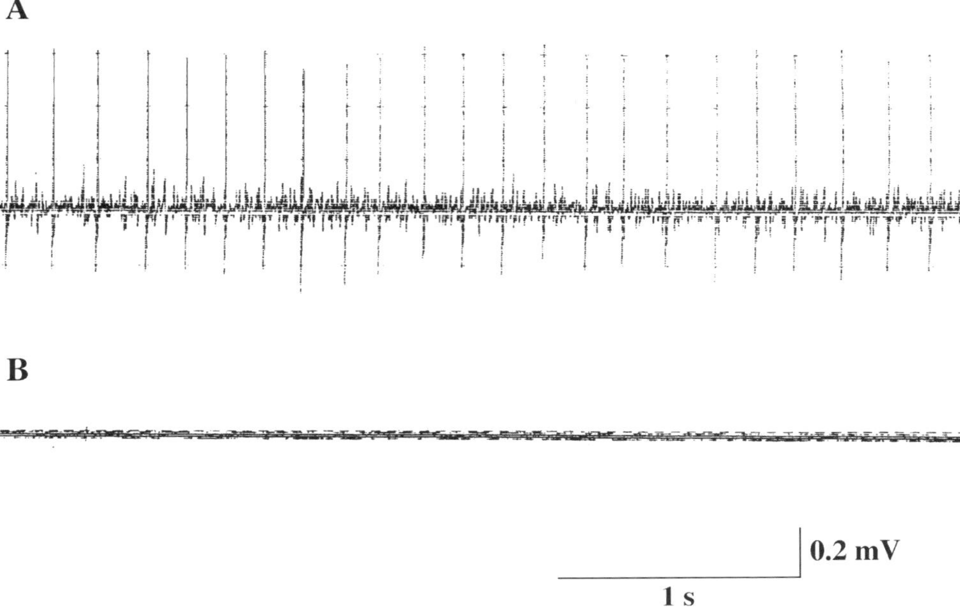

FIGURE 14.9. Needle EMG at rest in the left gastrocnemius muscle. (**A**) Spontaneous MUPs at rest. (**B**) Absence of spontaneous MUPs at rest during general anesthesia. (Reprinted with permission from Nicholas AP, et al. Stiff-person's syndrome associated with thymoma and subsequent myasthenia gravis. Muscle Nerve 1997;20:494.)

TABLE 14.7. Single-Fiber EMG Data in Case 3

	EDC	Frontalis
Fiber density	1.63	1.52
No. of pot pairs	16	17
Mean MCD	23	33
Normal MCD	40.4	30
No. of PP with MCD > ULN[a]	0	3 (17%)
No. of PP with blocking	0	0

[a] ULN: upper limit of normal; 53 μs for EDC and 45 μs for frontalis muscle.

breast adenocarcinoma, Hodgkin's lymphoma, vertebral plasmacytoma, small-cell carcinoma of the lung, and carcinoma of the pharynx. Unlike most SMS cases, paraneoplastic SMS has not been reported to have anti-GAD antibodies.

Piccolo reported a case of SMS and possible thymoma followed by sero-positive MG 6 years later. Six cases with thymoma and Isaacs' syndrome have been reported. In two cases, MG was additionally present. In Halbach's two cases without MG, ACh-receptor antibody was positive. In Isaac's syndrome, muscular hyperactivity was not abolished by general anesthesia.

SMS is a rare disorder first described by Moersch and Woltman in 1956 and characterized by persistent painful axial and proximal limb muscle rigidity and spasms that are exacerbated by sensory or motor stimuli and abolished by sleep and general anesthesia.

SMS typically presents with progressive severe muscle stiffness that fluctuates in intensity. Axial and proximal muscles are affected to a greater degree than distal muscles, and lower extremities are involved to a greater degree than upper extremities. Painful spasms occur spontaneously or are precipitated by sudden noises and other sudden stimuli. Often, walking becomes laborious and stiff. Unlike tetanus, the facial muscles are rarely involved and trismus does not occur. In some patients, hyperlordosis of the lumbar spine occurs. Considering the physiological and pharmacological similarities with tetanus, the most likely site of abnormality is at the inhibitory interneurons in the spinal cord, producing impairment of GABA-mediated central inhibition that subsequently causes motor neuronal hyperexcitability and sustained muscle contraction. GABAergic drugs such as valium, baclofen, and valproic acid are effective in relieving stiffness and spasms.

SMS is now considered to be an autoimmune disorder because anti-GAD antibody was found to be positive in two-thirds of patients, suggesting an impairment of GABAergic neurotransmission. Other organ-specific antibodies have also been reported in SMS. Treatment with immunotherapy (plasmapheresis, IVIG, or immunosuppressants) was successful in some cases. Recently, it has been recognized that SMS may occur as a paraneoplastic syndrome.

EMG recordings from stiff muscles show continuous discharge of MUPs resembling voluntary muscle contraction at rest. Classically, this activity is abolished by general anesthesia and sleep and exacerbated by external stimuli (auditory or tactile). This can best be achieved by the surface EMG recording from multiple muscles as in our case. We also found the motor neuron hyperexcitability test (H-reflex, T-reflex, and F-wave study) extremely helpful in diagnosis of SMS. We have found this phenomenon in all three cases of SMS in recent years.

MAXIMS

1. Continuous muscle activity that is abolished under general anesthesia is typical of SMS.
2. GABAergic medications such as diazepam, baclofen, and valproate are effective in relieving painful spasms in SMS.

REFERENCES

1. Grimaldi LME, Martino G, Braghi S, et al. Heterogeneity of autoantibodies in Stiff-Man syndrome. Ann Neurol 1993;34:57–64.
2. McEvory KM. Stiff-man syndrome. Semin Neurol 1991;11:197–205.

CASE 4

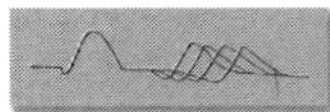

INVOLUNTARY CLONIC SPASMS OF FACIAL MUSCLES

CASE PRESENTATION

A 43-year-old woman was referred to Botox clinic for treatment of hemifacial spasm. She had involuntary clonic spasms of right facial muscles for 5 years, initially starting around the eye and now spreading to the mouth and platysma. It had affected her daily life and self-esteem. Neurological examination showed completely normal findings except for right hemifacial spasm.

CASE ANALYSIS

Diagnosis of HFS in this case was straightforward for the classic clonic muscle spasms involving the right facial muscles. Because Botox injection is extremely effective in HFS, we usually confirm the diagnosis of HFS by documenting synkinetic responses in the orbicularis oris muscles before Botox injection. Also, by means of the needle EMG study in the various involved facial muscles, we divided the total Botox units among the various involved muscles according to the severity of involuntary MUP discharges.

PLAN OF TESTING

1. Blink reflex with four-channel recording from the right and left orbicularis oculi and oris muscles.
2. Needle EMG in the clinically involved muscles to judge the most prominently involved muscles.

ELECTROPHYSIOLOGICAL TESTS AND FINDINGS

1. Blink reflex: Synkinetic responses in the right and left orbicularis oculi with the stimulation on the right supraorbital nerve. Synkinetic responses in the right and left orbicularis oculi with stimulation of the left supraorbital nerve (Fig. 14.10).
2. Needle EMG: Needle EMG showed the most prominent discharges from the right levator labii and outer orbicularis oculi muscles.

ELECTROPHYSIOLOGICAL INTERPRETATION

Synkinetic response in the right (affected) and left (unaffected) orbicularis oris muscles typical of HFS.

FINAL DIAGNOSIS

Right hemifacial spasm

TREATMENT AND FOLLOW-UP

A total of 30 Botox units was administered by EMG-guided injection to the right orbicularis oculi and oris, levator labii, and risorius muscles in a divided dose. This brought satisfactory relief of hemifacial spasm for 3 months. A repeat blink-reflex study a month later showed improvement by the reduction of synkinetic responses in the affected and unaffected sides. The patient needed injections of 30 to 40 Botox units every 3 to 5 months to sustain a satisfactory improved status.

COMMENTS

By simultaneously recording the responses of the orbicularis oculi and orbicularis oris muscles in the blink-reflex testing, the phenomenon of facial synkinesis can be assessed. In normal individuals, no response is elicited from the orbicularis oris muscle with supraorbital nerve stimulation unless an extremely strong stimulus is given. However, during the aberrant regeneration of the facial nerve after Bell's palsy or other facial nerve injury, a synkinetic response can be recorded in the orbicularis oris as well as other muscles innervated by the facial nerve on the involved side.

Rt (affected) stimulation

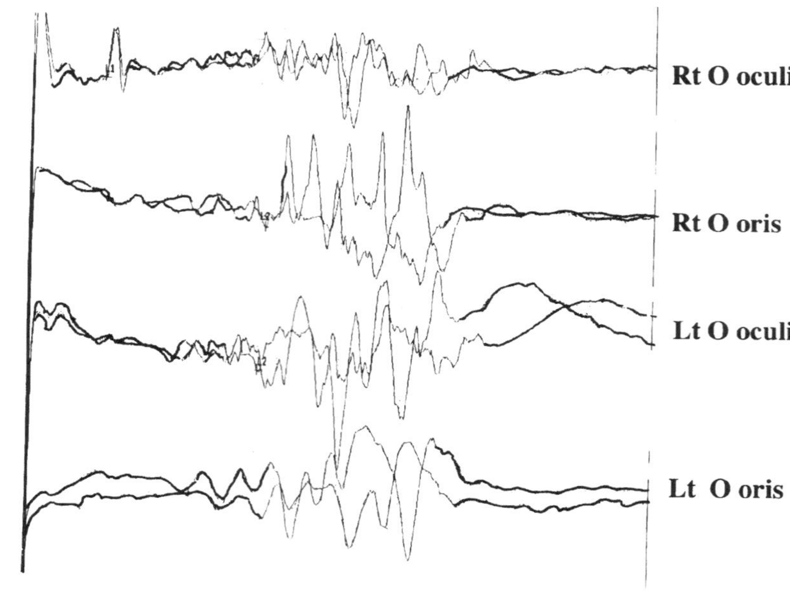

Lt (unaffected) stimulation

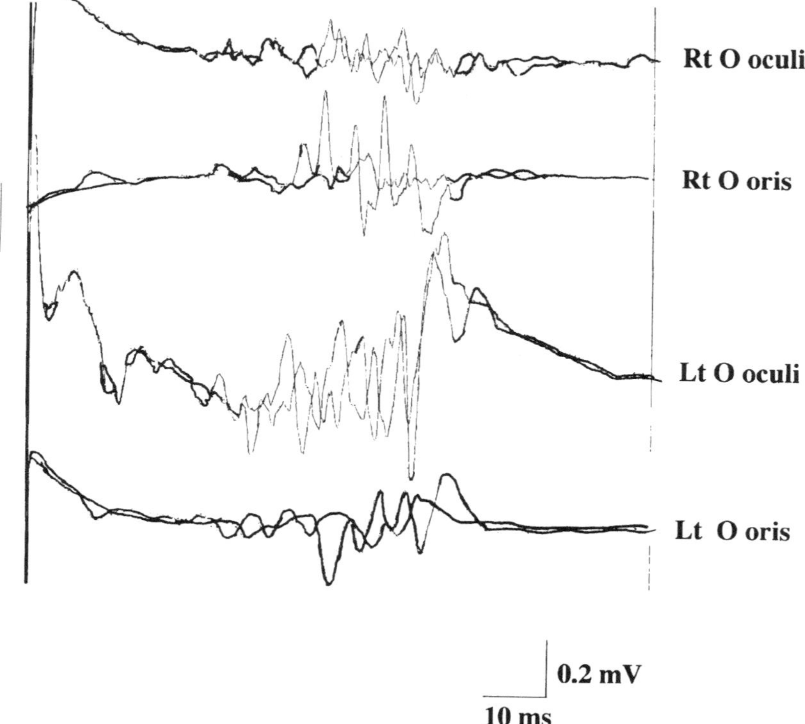

FIGURE 14.10. Synkinetic responses in the right (*Rt*) (affected) and left (*Lt*) (unaffected) orbicularis oris (*O oris*) muscles following the right and left supraorbital nerves. *O Oculi,* orbicularis oculi.

A similar phenomenon is observed in hemifacial spasm. This finding is useful in confirming the presence of hemifacial spasm in doubtful cases and in differentiating hemifacial spasm from other facial movement disorders, because this synkinetic response does not occur in the latter. A recent study from our laboratory showed that synkinetic response occurred also in the unaffected orbicularis oris muscles in two-thirds of patients. In the past decade, microsurgical decompression of the facial nerve has been performed in the cerebellopontine area in HFS. Several authors reported that the synkinetic response accompanying the blink reflex disappeared after surgery, rendering objective confirmation of the effectiveness of such surgery.

Drug therapy has been disappointing in HFS. Janetta has reported relief of the involuntary movements by exploring the facial nerve in the posterior fossa and then removing aberrant blood vessels that may compress the nerve. Since the introduction of Botox treatment, this has been extremely effective in relieving HFS and has become the preferred treatment for this disorder. As noted in our case, clinical and electrophysiological improvement was well documented. The most interesting finding is that the synkinetic response in the unaffected side was also improved by Botox on the affected side. This is more than would be expected from the remote effect of Botox injection.

MAXIMS

1. A synkinetic response in the orbicularis oris is the most typical electrophysiological finding in HFS and is useful in differentiating HFS from other facial movement disorders.
2. Botox treatment is the treatment of choice in HFS.

REFERENCES

1. Flanders M, Chin D, Boghem D: Botulinum toxin: preferred treatment for hemifacial spasms. Eur Neurol 1993;33:316–319.
2. Auger RC. Hemifacial spasm: clinical and electrophysiologic observations. Neurology 1979;29: 1261–1272.

CHAPTER 15

Pediatric Neuromuscular Diseases

In performing electrodiagnostic procedures in pediatric populations, there are four factors to be considered: the maturational factor, lack of cooperation, technical considerations, and special neuromuscular problems confined to children.

MATURATIONAL FACTORS

Age is an important variable in electrodiagnostic studies, especially in the nerve conduction. The nerve conduction velocities (NCVs) in motor, sensory, and mixed nerves are about 50% of the normal adult values in the full-term newborn, reaching about 75% of the adult value at 1 year of age and nearing 100% at 4 years of age. The motor, sensory, and mixed NCVs increase with age in a logarithmic function. Thus, it is imperative to compare the NCVs obtained in infants and babies with the normal values for that same age group. (Normal values for newborns and children are available in Chapter 8 in Oh SJ. Clinical EMG: nerve conduction studies. Baltimore: Williams & Wilkins, 1993.)

Age is the most important physiological factor for MUP parameters. The duration and amplitude of MUPs increase with age, although not as dramatically as the NCVs. In general, the duration and amplitude of normal MUPs in infants are substantially lower than those in the adults. Thus, it is important to compare the measured mean duration in a given individual with the age-matched duration in the quantitative analysis of MUPs. However, in routine practice, this factor is not that critical because the normal range of MUP duration is wide enough to include this factor. Because the duration of normal MUPs in children is shorter, the differentiation between the normal limit and subtle myopathy can be difficult. In fact, in David and Jones' study of floppy infant syndrome, neurogenic conditions were more easily recognized than myopathic ones. In children from birth to age 3 years, the normal MUP amplitude varied from 100 to 700 μV, and MUPs with an amplitude greater than 1000 μV were rare with a concentric needle. Considering this, it is reasonable to term MUPs > 4 mV amplitude with monopolar needle and >2 mV with concentric needle as HA MUPs in children under 3 years of age. In the routine repetitive nerve stimulation (RNS) test, age is not critical except for a lower CMAP amplitude in newborns and children than in adults.

LACK OF COOPERATION

The needle electromyography (EMG) has a definite limitation in the pediatric population because of poor cooperation from patients. Certainly, one cannot do a full battery of tests as in adult patients. It is difficult to obtain full relaxation of muscle to isolate fibrillation, positive sharp wave (PSW), or fasciculation. On the other hand, infants or younger children may not generate minimal contraction for MUP analysis. Thus, the examiner is often forced to draw a conclusion based on a limited amount of information. To obtain the maximum results with the limited cooperation of a child, the following strategies are used in our EMG laboratory.

1. To reduce fear and elicit the cooperation of a child, the presence of a parent in the examining room is usually helpful. We encourage the parent to participate by holding the child's hands or having the child sit on the parent's lap for the study. However, this has to be individualized because some parents cannot stand to watch their children having the electrodiagnostic test. Cooperation from the parent for the nerve conduction study (NCS) can be improved by allowing the parent to experience a brief electrical stimulus on the palm before beginning the study with the child.

2. In general, the NCS can be performed without difficulty in most pediatric patients. Thus, in the workup of suspected neuromuscular disorders in children, we recommend that the nerve conduction test be performed first. It often provides a definite diagnosis if the patient has peripheral neuropathy, and there is then no need for the more painful needle EMG study. Moreover, the nerve conduction test can be performed without much difficulty in infants and most older children. In small children who are not cooperative for the nerve conduction test, sedation is occasionally needed.

3. In general, the needle EMG in a limited number of muscles can be performed without too much difficulty in most older children once the procedure is explained. In younger children who have a fear of needles, we use Elma Cream (lidocaine and prilocaine) with the occlusive dressing for skin anesthesia over a predetermined site on the muscles 1 to 2 hours before needling to reduce the pain of needle insertion. This simple procedure has worked extremely well in our hands. For some young children who are not cooperative, premedication may be needed for sedation.

4. For premedication, chloral hydrate at a dose of 60 to 70 mg/kg body weight 20 to 40 minutes before EMG testing is recommended. This produces enough sedation for the motor and sensory NCS and evaluation of abnormal spontaneous potentials. However, too much sedation is a problem for MUP evaluation, which is critical for differentiation of myopathy from denervation. The child must be awake enough to produce MUPs. Clearly, the disadvantage of this approach is that it is more difficult to assess voluntary activity in muscles. The electromyographer may have to wait until the end of the study when the child is more aroused. This is the reason why children are not universally sedated for the EMG study.

5. In explaining the needle EMG study, it is better to explain that "a fine wire" will be inserted just under the skin into the muscle instead of "a needle." During the needle EMG procedure, it is helpful to distract the child's attention from the discomfort by allowing him or her to watch the responses on a video monitor and listen to the audio display. Often children are fascinated by the MUP activity that they can generate by voluntary movement.

6. To limit the discomfort of the needle EMG and maximize its value, the examiner must have a clear understanding of what to look for before insertion of the needle. He must attempt to solve the diagnostic problem with a needle EMG study in two muscles: one for proximal and the other for distal muscles. In most cases, two-muscle needle EMG studies have been sufficient to make the diagnosis according to my experience. If the limited study was not sufficient to make this determination, usually further studies were useless. In the workup of floppy infants, we prefer the anterior tibialis muscle for MUP evaluation and the quadriceps for resting abnormal potentials. An infant usually activates the anterior tibialis muscle better than the quadriceps when moving the leg voluntarily or in response to painful stimulation. The iliopsoas muscle below the inguinal ligament is good for activation of MUPs in the proximal muscles. At most, a three-muscle needle EMG study in children is the maximum in my experience.

TECHNICAL CONSIDERATIONS

Because of their small body size, special technical considerations have to be made for NCS in infants. For this, we recommended the following guidelines.

1. A pediatric simulator should be used because the distance between the active and reference electrodes is shorter.
2. As a reference recording electrode, a ring electrode can be used for fingers or toes.
3. The posterior tibial nerve should be tested first because it shows the most reliable and technically satisfactory response.
4. Often the response from the extensor digitorum brevis is difficult to record after stimulation of the peroneal nerve at the ankle in infants. This is again due to the proximity of the stimulating electrode to the recording electrode. In this situation, the latency from the knee may be the only objective finding in the peroneal nerve.
5. In motor conduction studies of the median and ulnar nerves, the NCV can be calculated over the elbow-axilla segment if the response with wrist stimulation is unrecordable.

6. Sensory nerve conduction is easier to study in the median and ulnar nerves. If there is difficulty in obtaining the CNAP from the wrist after stimulation at the fingers, the recording electrodes should be placed on the elbow. Usually, no difficulty is encountered when obtaining the sensory CNAP at the elbow.

FLOPPY INFANT SYNDROME

Floppy infant syndrome is a special neuromuscular problem confined to children. Generalized muscular hypotonia in infancy may be due to a variety of causes. Patients with this problem are diagnosed as having "floppy infant syndrome" until a definite diagnosis becomes clear. The causes for generalized muscular hypotonia range from cerebral palsy to myopathy. The most common cause of floppy infant syndrome is the atonic type of cerebral palsy.

From a practical point of view, the important distinction that should be made clinically is whether the floppy infant has underlying weakness with associated hypotonia or has reasonable muscle power despite marked hypotonia. This clinical observation will considerably narrow the diagnostic possibilities. Those infants with weakness are likely to have an underlying neuromuscular disorder, the most common being infantile spinal muscular atrophy. In those infants where the hypotonia is disproportionate to any apparent weakness, the underlying cause is likely to be outside the neuromuscular system; most common are disorders of the central nervous system (cerebral palsy), usually associated with intellectual retardation as well.

A definite diagnosis cannot be made on the clinical evaluation alone in most floppy infants. The most important diagnostic clue is obtained from a decent EMG study, and a muscle biopsy, with detailed histochemical and ancillary studies, is essential. The needle EMG can clearly differentiate spinal muscular atrophies from myopathies, and NCS clearly identify peripheral neuropathies. The muscle biopsy will confirm the diagnosis of myopathies and spinal muscular atrophy.

For the sake of prognosis, it is important to recognize many benign nonprogressive congenital myopathies, so that these patients can be supported aggressively. To diagnose these benign congenital myopathies, histochemical and often electron-microscopic evaluations are essential. These myopathies include nemaline myopathy, central core disease, fiber type disproportion syndrome, myotubular myopathy, and mitochondrial myopathy.

CASE 1

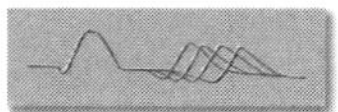

FLOPPY INFANT WITH RESPIRATORY FAILURE

CASE PRESENTATION

A 4-month-old infant had been a floppy infant since birth. During pregnancy, the mother noticed that the baby was not moving well in her womb. However, the child was delivered vaginally without any difficulty. Since then, the infant was quiet, with a weak cry and sucking reflex. It also failed to gain any weight and developed breathing difficulty in the preceding two months. There was no similar disease in two siblings.

Examination showed a quiet infant with a "frog-leg posture" and without any spontaneous movement of arms and legs. Its cry was weak and breathing was labored. Reflexes were absent. Tone was flaccid. No obvious fasciculation was observed in limb or tongue muscles.

CASE ANALYSIS

The history was indicative of rapidly progressing neuromuscular disease as a cause of floppy infant syndrome. Lack of fetal movement suggested onset of symptoms in utero. The classic frog-leg posture with labored breathing and absent reflexes was strongly suggestive of Werdnig-Hoffman disease.

PLAN OF TESTING

1. NCS: To rule out peripheral neuropathy.
2. Needle EMG: To identify denervation process and rule out myopathy.
3. Other tests: Muscle biopsy to confirm the presence of denervation process.

ELECTROPHYSIOLOGICAL TESTS AND FINDINGS

NCS Findings. Normal motor nerve conductions except for the decreased CMAP amplitudes in all of tested nerves (Figs. 15.1 and 15.2; Table 15.1).

Needle EMG (Table 15.2)

1. Fibrillations and PSW in the right anterior tibialis and vastus lateralis muscles.
2. Spontaneous MUP discharges in two muscles.
3. A few MUPs were generated in the tested muscles and MUPs were normal.

ELECTROPHYSIOLOGICAL INTERPRETATION

Denervation process and typical of infantile spinal muscular atrophy.

OTHER TEST FINDINGS

The muscle biopsy showed severe fascicular atrophy typical of infantile SMA.

FINAL DIAGNOSIS

WHD (infantile SMA)

TREATMENT AND FOLLOW-UP

The baby died 2 months after the diagnosis.

COMMENTS

The most common type of neuromuscular disease in floppy infant syndrome is infantile SMA. WHD is the most malignant form of SMA and is inherited by autosomal-recessive pattern. The infant becomes floppy in the first 6 months of life and grows relentlessly worse, usually dying before 18 months of age. In half the cases, poor fetal movement was observed by the mother, suggesting onset of symptoms in utero. Because of severe muscle weakness, the infant assumes a characteristic frog-leg posture, protuberant belly, diaphragmatic breathing, and jug-handle arms. DTRs are absent. Fasciculation is often seen in the tongue, but generalized fasciculation is not obvious due to prominent subcutaneous fat in the newborn infant. Recently, a very useful molecular diagnostic tool for SMA types I to III has been developed. It

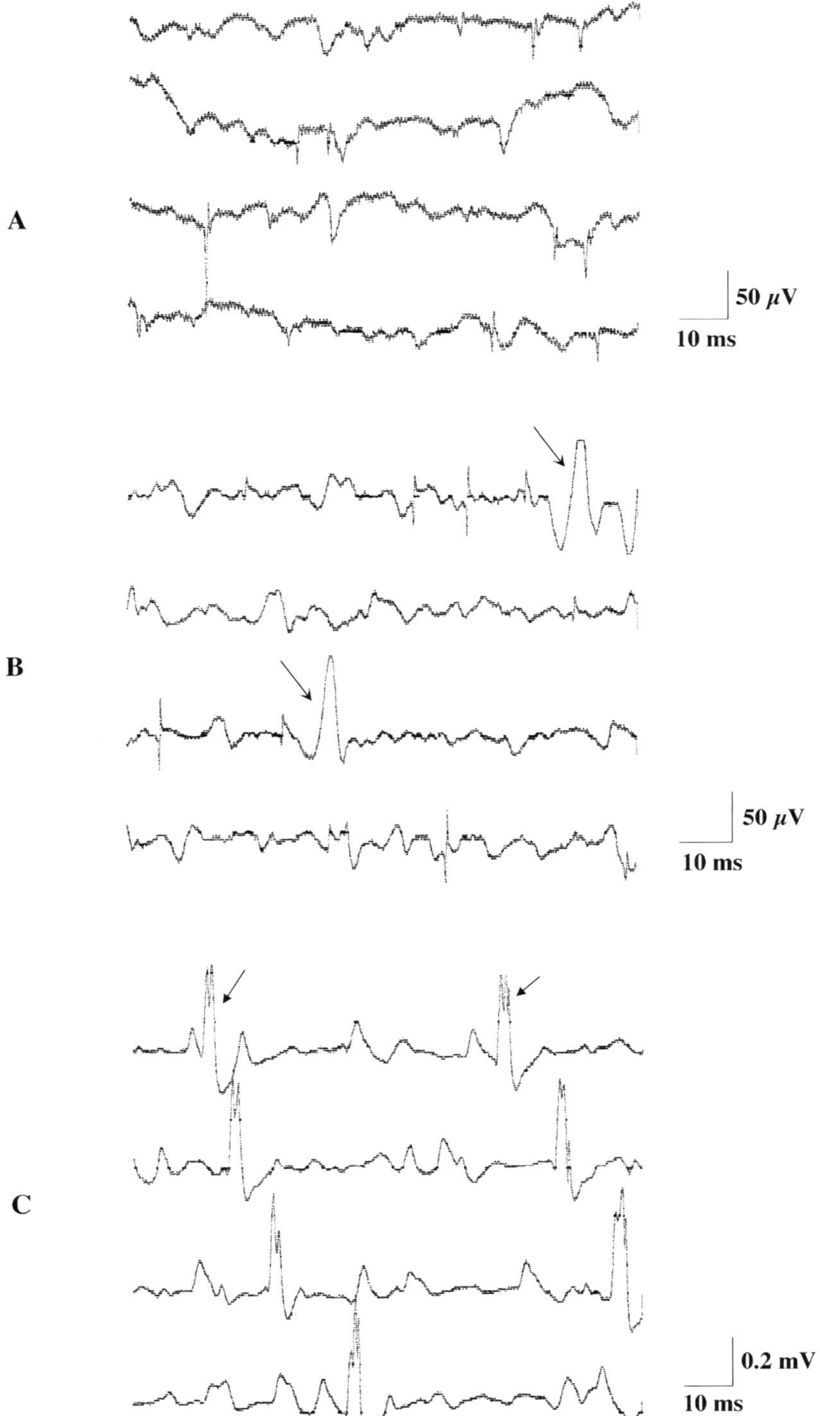

FIGURE 15.1. Abnormal spontaneous potentials. **A.** Fibrillations and PSWs. **B.** Fibrillations and fasciculations (*arrow*). **C.** Spontaneous MUP discharge (*arrow*). Notice a regular firing of spontaneous MUP discharge in contrast to an irregular firing of fasciculations.

TABLE 15.1. Nerve Conduction Data in Case 1

	Latency/NCV (ms/m/s)	Amplitude (mV/μV)		Latency/NCV (ms/m/s)	Amplitude (mV/μV)
	Median	**Motor N**		**Peroneal**	**Motor N**
TL	2.5	0.5	TL	4.1	0.1
E-W	25.5	0.4	FH-A	21.8	0.1
	Ulnar	**Motor N**		**Post-Tibial**	**Motor N**
TL	1.8	0.5	TL	4.5	0.2
BE-W	28.5	0.5	PF-A	18.7	0.15
	Median	**Sens N**		**Sural**	**Sens N**
F-E	33.3[a]	20	MC-A	[b]	
	Ulnar	**Sens N**		**Superficial Peroneal**	**Sens N**
F-E	36.8[a]	10	MC-A	44.4[a]	4

Height: 62 cm.

[a] Onset latency NCV.

[b] Technically difficult.

TL, terminal latency; E, elbow; W, wrist; FH, fibular head; A, ankle; BE, below elbow; PF, popliteal fossa; F, finger.

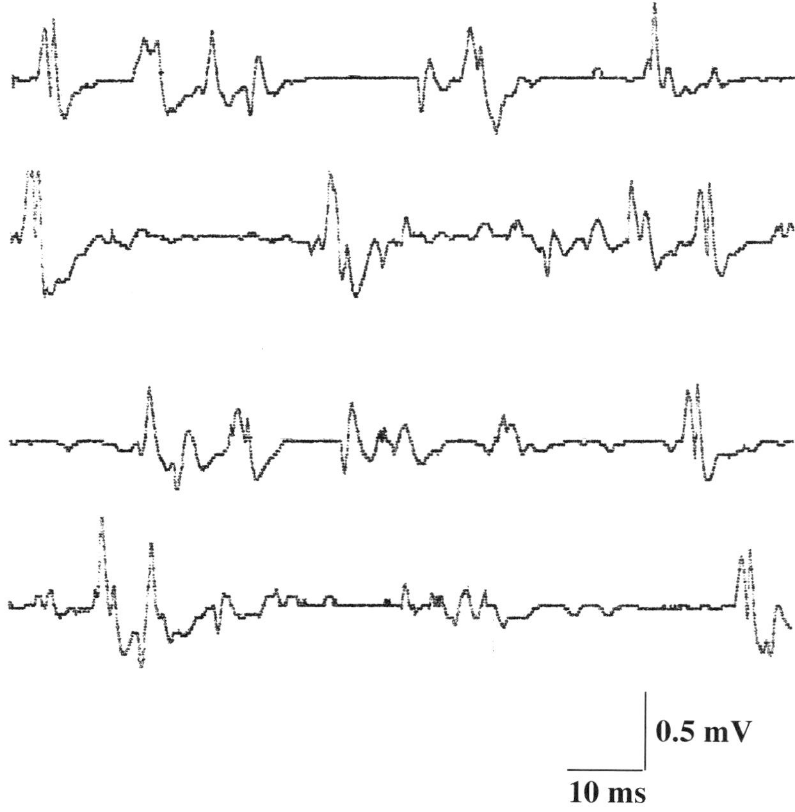

FIGURE 15.2. A few normal MUPs in the anterior tibialis muscle.

TABLE 15.2. Needle EMG Data in Case 1

				Spontaneous Potentials				Motor Unit Potential				Interference	
Muscle	**Root**	**Nerve**	**Insertion Activity**	**Fib**	**PSW**	**Fasc**	**Myotonia CRD**	**Amplitude (mV)**	**Duration (ms)**	**Polyphasic Potential**	**HA MUP**	**Pattern**	**Mean Amplitude (mV)**
Lt vast lat	L3,4	Femoral	+	+ + +	+ + +	+	–	No	MUP				
Gastroc	S1,2	Post tibial	+	+	+	+(1)	–	0.5–1.5	6–12	+	–	(3)	
Ant tibial	L4,5	Peroneal	+	+	–	+ +(2)	–	0.5–2	6–12	+	–	(3)	

1, A few spontaneous MUP discharges; 2, prominent spontaneous MUP discharges; 3, a reduced recruitment.
Fib, fibrillations; PSW, positive sharp wave; Fasc, fasciculations; CRD, complex repetitive discharge; HA MUP, high-amplitude MUP; +, present or increased; –, absent.

consists of a study of deletions in a gene called "survival motor neuron". Exon 7 has been shown to be deleted in 99% and exon 8 in 93% of individuals affected by SMA, independently of the severity of the disease. In WHD, prenatal carrier detection is extremely accurate and this technique should be applied in clinical practice.

The amplitude of the CMAPs in WHD is either normal or low. Low amplitude was reported in 73% of cases. The motor NCV is either normal or mildly slow, the latter finding being observed in 43% of Kunz's cases. Sensory nerve conduction is normal. Needle EMG is the most important diagnostic tool in making a definitive diagnosis of WHD. It shows the classic evidence of active denervation: widespread fibrillations and PSW with relatively normal MUPs. Fasciculations are rarely (7%) observed. This is in contrast to the SMA type III adult form of motor neuron disease. On the other hand, spontaneous MUP discharges, which were first described in this disorder by Buchthal, were found in two of three cases. Buththal thought that these spontaneous MUP discharges were specific to WHD, in which MUPs are usually normal in duration and amplitude. This is in contrast to other forms of childhood SMA in which HA or HALD MUPs are the classic finding. MUP recruitment is usually reported to be reduced and MUPs fire rapidly.

MAXIMS

1. Spontaneous MUP discharge is commonly observed in WHD and is typical of WHD.
2. Prenatal carrier detection is extremely accurate in WHD.

REFERENCES

1. Buchthal F, Olsen PZ. Electromyography and muscle biopsy in infantile spinal muscular atrophy. Brain 1970;93:15–30.
2. Hausmanowa-Petrusewicz I, Karwanska A. Electromyographic findings in different forms of infantile and juvenile proximal spinal muscular atrophy. Muscle Nerve 1986;9:37–46.

CASE 2

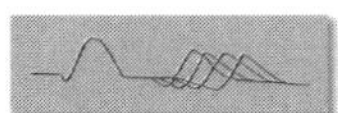

ACUTE FLOPPY INFANT SYNDROME IN A 17-DAY-OLD INFANT

CASE PRESENTATION

A 17-day-old infant had difficulty eating and breathing because of a 4-day history of severe weakness and poor formula intake. Up to that time, the infant was healthy. Examination showed normally reactive pupils, ptosis, weak cry, generalized weakness and hypotonia, and decreased stretch reflexes. In three separate double-blind trials documented with videotape, the infant's strength improved after 0.2 mg/kg intravenous edrophonium but did not respond to saline injection. Treatment with pyridostigmine was ineffective.

CASE ANALYSIS

In acute floppy infant syndrome in a previously healthy infant, three diagnostic possibilities have to be considered: infant botulism, myasthenia gravis, and Guillain-Barré syndrome. If pupillary response to light is sluggish or absent, MG is definitely ruled out. In this case, a positive edrophonium test was thought to be diagnostic of MG. Unfortunately, pyridostigmine treatment was ineffective. Thus, alternative diagnoses were sought. Decreased reflexes are unheard of in MG.

PLAN OF TESTING

1. NCS and cerebrospinal fluid test: To rule out GBS.
2. RNS test: To confirm the presence of a neuromuscular transmission block.
3. Edrophonium test.
4. Stool test for botulinum toxin and *Clostridium botulinum*.

ELECTROPHYSIOLOGICAL TESTS AND FINDINGS

NCS Findings

1. Normal motor NCS except a low CMAP amplitude in the median, ulnar, and posterior tibial nerves.
2. Normal sensory NCS in the median and ulnar nerves.

RNS Test Findings (see Fig. 4.12)

1. Low CMAP (1380 μV) in the ADQ muscle.
2. Eight percent decremental response at 2-Hz stimulation.
3. One hundred twenty-two percent incremental response at 50-Hz stimulation for 2 seconds.

ELECTROPHYSIOLOGICAL INTERPRETATION

Presynaptic neuromuscular transmission disorder typical of infant botulism. No electrophysiological evidence of demyelinating neuropathy.

OTHER TEST FINDINGS

CSF protein was normal.

FINAL DIAGNOSIS

Infant botulism

TREATMENT AND FOLLOW-UP

Stool culture revealed *C. botulinum* type A. The infant's strength gradually improved without treatment; 3 months later, he had only mild head lag.

COMMENTS

Infant botulism is the most common form of botulism in the United States. It is caused by the in vivo production of botulinum toxin from ingested *C. botulinum* organism. In adults, the ingested botulinum toxin, not the ingested botulinum organism, is the cause for botulism. It occurs exclusively in 1- to 20-week-old infants. Acute onset of floppy infant syndrome with ptosis, sometimes associated with enlarged sluggish pupils, decreased gag reflex, dysphagia, weak cry, and respiratory failure, are the classic features of infant botulism. It is relatively benign, and recovery is spontaneous without any botulinum antitoxin. Unlike the adult form of botulism, botulinum toxin is not detectable in the serum. A definite diagnosis can be made by detection of botulinum toxin or *C. botulinum* organism in the stool. The edrophonium test is usually positive in MG. However, it may be positive in other neuromuscular diseases. This test has been reported to be positive in 27% of adult cases of botulism. To our knowledge, this is the first patient with infant botulism to have a positive edrophonium test. A positive edrophonium test in a weak infant neither excludes infant botulism nor diagnosis congenital MG.

The RNS test should be performed in any previously healthy infant under 6 months of age who develops acute floppy infant syndrome with constipation and areflexia. The child is usually first suspected of having GBS. A high index of suspicion is the first step in the diagnosis of infant botulism.

In infant botulism, the classic RNS pattern of presynaptic block has been observed: low CMAP amplitude, decremental response at LRS, and incremental response at HRS. Compared with foodborne botulism, the typical pattern of presynaptic block was more often seen. In 25 cases of infant botulism, Cornblath found low CMAP in 100% of cases, decremental response in 56%, and incremental response at 20- to 50-Hz stimulation in 95% of cases. Cornblath used 20% increment at 20-Hz stimulation as the maximal normal value for infants. Considering normal adults that showed 43% increment at 50-Hz stimulation due to pseudofacilitation, a 20% increment criteria is too liberal. Many authorities believed that tetanic facilitation of greater than 100% should be used as a definite criterion for facilitation. In some patients with equivocal increment, a longer stimulation (sometimes up to 10 seconds) at 50-Hz stimulation is recommended to document facilitation. In severe cases, the presynaptic block is so severe that a longer stimulation is needed to bring out an incremental response.

The most consistent needle EMG finding in infant botulism is a classic myopathic pattern: SASD MUPs. This was observed in 90% of infants. Fibrillations and PSW were observed in 54% of cases.

MAXIMS

1. A positive edrophonium test is not always diagnostic of MG. This test can also be positive in botulism.
2. In infant botulism, RNS findings typical of presynaptic neuromuscular transmission block are the most convincing objective evidence of botulism until microbiological confirmation is obtained.

REFERENCES

1. Oh SJ, Cho HK. Edrophonium responsiveness not necessarily diagnostic of myasthenia gravis [see comments]. Muscle Nerve 1990;13:187–191.
2. Cornblath DR, Sladky JT, Sumner AJ. Clinical electrophysiology of infantile botulism. Muscle Nerve 1983;6:448–452.

CASE 3

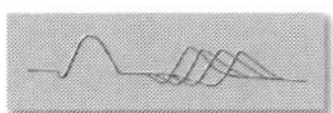

FLOPPY INFANT SYNDROME AND CARDIOMEGALY

CASE PRESENTATION

A 6-month-old infant was admitted for pneumonia. Chest x-ray revealed cardiomegaly and an echo study showed hypertrophic cardiomyopathy. CPK was 2043 units; SGOT, 363 units; SGPT, 198 units. The child was developmentally delayed and unable to sit up or roll over. On examination, he was alert, cooing, and smiling. Weight was 6.42 kg (<5th percentile), head circumference was 41 cm (<5th percentile), and height was 67.3 cm (25th percentile). Cranial nerves were normal. Tongue was not enlarged. Tone was decreased and there was diminished head control. Weakness was greater proximally than distally. No reflexes, clonus, or Babinski signs were observed. The child withdrew normally to pin-prick. Liver was not enlarged. Electrocardiogram showed large voltages, indicating biventricular hypertrophy.

CASE ANALYSIS

Delayed development and cardiomegaly were the reasons for ordering a neurological consultation. The pediatric neurologist was able to make a clinical diagnosis of Pompe's disease on the basis of the classic constellation of floppy infant syndrome, hypertrophic cardiomyopathy, and elevated CPK. It is possible that this patient developed pneumonia due to respiratory failure from this disease.

PLAN OF TESTING

1. NCS: To rule out hypomyelinative neuropathy as a cause for floppy infant syndrome.
2. Needle EMG: To detect genuine myotonic potentials and to confirm myopathy.
3. Muscle biopsy: To confirm acid maltase deficiency.

ELECTROPHYSIOLOGICAL TESTS AND FINDINGS

NCS Findings

1. Prolonged F-wave latency for age (19.2/18.0 ms) in the right median and ulnar nerves.
2. Otherwise, normal NCS in the right sural, posterior tibial, and peroneal nerves for age.

Needle EMG (Table 15.3)

1. Increased insertion activity, prominent fibrillation, PSW, and myotonic potentials in all tested muscles (Fig. 15.3).
2. Increased polyphasic MUPs, many short MUPs, and easily recruited full MUPs in all tested muscles (Fig. 15.4).

ELECTROPHYSIOLOGICAL INTERPRETATION

Active myotonic myopathy typical of acid maltase deficiency.

FINAL DIAGNOSIS

Pompe's disease (infantile form of acid-maltase deficiency)

TREATMENT AND FOLLOW-UP

As soon as the EMG needle was inserted into the muscle, myotonic potentials were detected easily in this patient. No clinical myotonia was observed. Muscle biopsy showed vacuolar myopathy with increased PAS-positive and acid-phosphatase activities. Biochemical analysis confirmed acid maltase deficiency.

COMMENTS

There are three types of acid maltase deficiency: the infantile form (Pompe's disease), the childhood form, and the adult form. The infantile form is characterized by a severe rapidly progressive myopathy producing hypotonia, generalized weakness, feeding difficulties, and respiratory insufficiency. Associated features include a dilated cardiomyopathy, hepatomeg-

TABLE 15.3. Needle EMG Data in Case 3

Muscle	Root	Nerve	Insertion Activity	Spontaneous Potentials				Motor Unit Potential				Interference	
				Fib	PSW	Fasc	Myotonic Potential	Amplitude (mV)	Duration (ms)	Polyphasic Potential	HA MUP	Pattern	Mean Amplitude (mV)
Rt ant tibial	L4,5	Peroneal	+	+++	+++	−	+++	0.3–2	3–10	++	−	[a]	
Quadriceps	L3,4	Femoral	+	+++	+++	−	+++	0.5–1.5	6–10	++	−	[a]	

[a] Early and excessive recruitment.

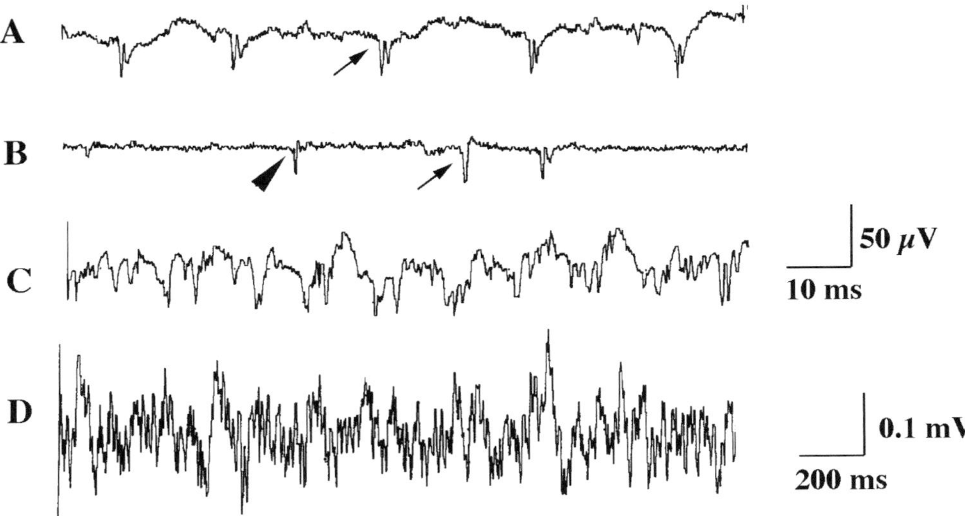

FIGURE 15.3. Abnormal spontaneous potentials. **A.** PSWs. **B.** Fibrillations (*thick arrow*) and PSW (*thin arrow*). **C** and **D.** Myotonic potentials characterized by waxing and waning of amplitude and frequency of potentials.

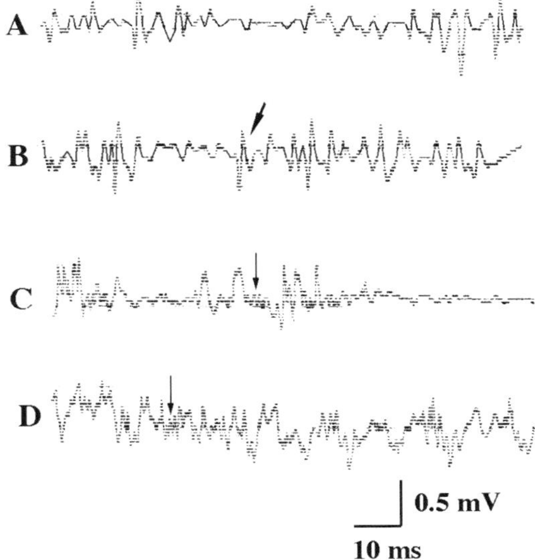

FIGURE 15.4. SASD MUPs. Because of early recruitment of MUPs, it is difficult to isolate an individual MUP clearly. **A** and **B.** Many simple SASD MUPs (*thick arrow*). **C** and **D.** Many polyphasic SASD MUPs (*thin arrow*).

aly, and enlargement of the tongue. Invariably, the patient dies before 2 years of age. In the childhood form, the patient has a delay in motor development, proximal myopathy with respiratory involvement, and variable organomegaly. He or she often dies before 19 years of age. In the adult form, the most characteristic presentation is respiratory failure in a patient with limb-girdle myopathy as noted in this patient. The disease is slowly progressive, but prognosis is much better than in other forms.

The most characteristic needle EMG finding in this disorder is prominent genuine myotonic potentials. Thus, prominent myotonic potentials in the needle EMG without clinical myotonia is indicative of acid maltase deficiency until proven otherwise. So far, this rule has not been broken in our laboratory. Additional evidence of active myopathy is invariably present in these disorders—fibrillation and PSW and SASD MUPs. In the childhood and adults forms, these EMG abnormalities may be confined to paraspinal and respiratory muscles.

MAXIMS

1. Myotonic potentials without clinical myotonia are pathognomonic of acid maltase deficiency until proven otherwise.
2. Floppy infant syndrome due to myopathy with cardiomyopathy is typical of Pompe's disease.

REFERENCES

1. Engel AG, Gomez MR, Seybold ME, Lambert EH. The spectrum and diagnosis of acid maltase deficiency. Neurology 1973;23:105–106.
2. Hogan G, Gutmann L, Schmidt R, et al. Pompe's disease. Neurology 1969;19:894–900.

CASE 4

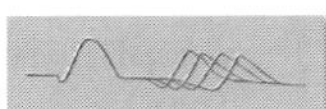

DELAYED WALKING AND HAND TREMORS IN A 27-MONTH-OLD INFANT

CASE PRESENTATION

A 27-month-old infant was referred to the pediatric neurologist for evaluation of delayed walking and hand tremors. Her birth was uneventful and her early development up to sitting at 6 months of age was normal. She crawled at 1 year and started to stand up without assistance at 18 months. Her mental development was normal. When she attempted to walk, she often began to shake in her arms and legs and fell down. Because of her hand shaking, she frequently spilled food or dropped objects. Family history was remarkable for a maternal second cousin with cerebral palsy and a maternal great-aunt who suffered from mental retardation. Abnormal neurological findings were increased tone in the legs, marked dysmetria in the upper and lower extremities, a very wide ataxic gait, absent DTRs, and upgoing toes. No telangiectasia was noted. Muscle strength was good. MRI of the brain was reported to be normal.

CASE ANALYSIS

The most salient feature in this patient was the combination of central nervous system and peripheral nerve involvement: ataxia, increased tone, Babinski signs with absent reflexes. Thus, obvious diagnostic possibilities at this age included metachromatic leukodystrophy, globoid leukodystrophy (Krabbe's disease), adrenoleukodystrophy, infantile axonal dystrophy, and ataxia telangiectasia. In view of the lack of telangiectasia, ataxic telangiectasia was most likely ruled out. Normal cognition and normal MRI of the brain were thought to rule our "leukodystrophy." NCS and EMG were included in the workup in view of the specific pattern of nerve conduction abnormalities seen in these conditions. After the NCS study, the pediatric neurologist ordered a nerve biopsy in desperation for a diagnosis.

PLAN OF TESTING

1. NCS: To identify any peripheral neuropathy or sensory neuropathy.
2. Needle EMG: To identify any denervation process.
3. Nerve biopsy.

ELECTROPHYSIOLOGICAL TESTS AND FINDINGS

NCS Findings (Table 15.4). Low CMAP amplitude and markedly slow NCV for her age. Some suggestion of uniform slowing.

Needle EMG. Normal in the anterior tibialis, quadriceps, and biceps muscles.

ELECTROPHYSIOLOGICAL INTERPRETATION

Demyelinating neuropathy.

OTHER TEST FINDINGS

Serum alpha-fetoprotein, pyruvate, and lactate were all normal. CPK was also normal. Nerve biopsy showed demyelinating neuropathy with metachromatic granules.

FINAL DIAGNOSIS

Metachromatic leukodystrophy due to arylsulfatase-A deficiency

TREATMENT AND FOLLOW-UP

Arylsulfatase-A level was 12% of normal.

COMMENTS

Disorders in early childhood with peripheral and central nervous system involvement can be divided into two main groups of neuropathy: demyelinating neuropathy and sensory neuronopathy. A sensory neuronopathy pattern is classically seen in Friedreich's ataxia, ataxia telangiectasia, and Bassen-Kornzweig's disease. Demyelinating neuropathy is classically seen in metachromatic leukodystrophy, adrenoleukodystrophy, Refsum's disease, and Krabbe's disease.

TABLE 15.4. Nerve Conduction Data in Case 4

	Latency/NCV (ms/m/s)	Amplitude (mV)		Latency/NCV (ms/m/s)	Amplitude (mV)
	Median	**Motor N**		**Peroneal**	**Motor N**
TL	10.1	0.83	TL	8.10	1.83
E-W	8.36	0.17	FH-A	8.83	0.48
AX-E	10.5	0.19	PF-FH	16.5	0.21
				Post Tibial	**Motor N**
			TL	8.22	0.14
			PF-A	9.72	0.12

The nerve biopsy was diagnostic of metachromatic leukodystrophy, even with normal MRI. In metachromatic leukodystrophy, the nerve biopsy is diagnostically specific by showing "metachromasia" in the frozen nerve biopsy specimen.

Melachromatic leukodystrophy is a rare demyelinating disorder of the central nervous system and peripheral nerves caused by a deficiency of arylsulfatase. Pathologically, this disorder is diagnosed by the presence of metachromatic granules in the CNS white matter and peripheral nerves. Among five different types, the late infantile form of metachromatic leukodystrophy is the most common, occurring between the ages of 1 and 4 years. Severe mental regression, ataxia, hypertonia, flaccid paraplegia with pyramidal signs, peripheral neuropathy, and optic atrophy are characteristic clinical features. Nerve conduction abnormalities in this disorder are characterized by a uniform demyelinating neuropathy pattern: marked motor NCV slowing (below 25 m/s) and absent sensory CNAPs. Thus, it is an example of Bolton's "high-low syndrome" (high stimulation threshold and low NCV). The same nerve conduction findings have been reported in juvenile cases. The needle EMG usually shows chronic denervation.

MAXIMS

1. In young children with CNS and peripheral nerve involvement, the NCS can narrow the diagnostic possibilities by differentiating the "demyelinating neuropathy group" from the "sensory neuronopathy group."
2. Uniform demyelinating neuropathy pattern is typical of metachromatic leukodystrophy.

REFERENCES

1. Cruz Martinez A, Ferrer MT, Fueyo E, Galdos L. Peripheral neuropathy detected on electrophysiological study as first manifestation of metachromatic leukodystrophy in infancy. J Neurol Neurosurg Psychiatry 1975;38:169–174.
2. Oh SJ. Clinical electromyography. Nerve conduction studies. Baltimore: Williams & Wilkins, 1993: 612–616.

CASE 5

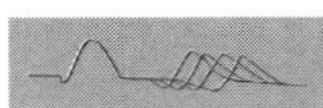

FAILURE TO THRIVE SINCE BIRTH IN A 3-YEAR-OLD GIRL WITH A HISTORY OF MUSCULAR DYSTROPHY

CASE PRESENTATION

A 3-year-old girl was the 6-pound, 8-oz product of a full-term pregnancy with little fetal movement noted in utero. She was delivered by cesarean section secondary to fetal distress, found to have decreased respiratory effort, and subsequently required intubation but was weaned to room air and was sent home. She continued to have poor feeding. At 2 months of age, she had been evaluated for failure to thrive. At that time, all metabolic profiles including thyroid study, sweat test, CPK, and amino acid screen were normal. TORCH workups were also nonproductive. Developmental milestones were somewhat delayed, with sitting at 9 months and walking at 18 months. She was toilet trained at 2 years and had good language development. At 11 months of age, neurological evaluation show marked hypotonia, "fish mouth" (tented upper lip), and areflexia. No tongue fasciculation, spasticity, or ataxia was noted. Family history was pertinent in that two first cousins of her mother had died with muscular dystrophy. Shortly before the present evaluation, the mother noticed some "worsening" in the child's condition. Neurological examination showed hypotonia, a positive Gower's sign, waddling gait, and areflexia. There was no pseudohypertrophy of calf muscles, fasciculation, or myotonia. She appeared to be normal mentally.

CASE ANALYSIS

This patient had a problem since birth, indicating the congenital nature of her hypotonia. However, she had slowly reached developmental milestones, ruling out WHD. Congenital muscular dystrophy, congenital myopathies, and congenital myotonic dystrophy were diagnostic possibilities. Fish mouth is due to weakness of facial and jaw muscles and is thought to be a characteristic facial feature of congenital myotonic dystrophy. No myotonia was detected. In congenital myotonic dystrophy, myotonia may not be present until 5 years of age. Needle EMG and muscle biopsy were critical in reaching a definite diagnosis in this patient.

PLAN OF TESTING

1. NCS: To rule out peripheral neuropathy as a cause of proximal girdle weakness.
2. Needle EMG: To rule out myotonic syndrome and identify a denervation process or myopathy as a cause of weakness.
3. Muscle biopsy: To confirm the type of congenital myopathy.

ELECTROPHYSIOLOGICAL TESTS AND FINDINGS

NCS Findings. Normal motor and sensory nerve conduction in right median, ulnar, peroneal, and posterior tibial nerves.

Needle EMG (Table 15.5; Fig. 15.5). Some SASD MUPs in the right anterior tibialis muscl No fibrillation, PSW, or myotonic potentials were identified.

ELECTROPHYSIOLOGICAL INTERPRETATION

Inactive myopathy compatible with benign congenital myopathy

OTHER FINDINGS

Muscle biopsy showed rod (nemalin) myopathy.

FINAL DIAGNOSIS

Rod (nemalin) myopathy

TREATMENT AND FOLLOW-UP

There has not been any progression in her myopathy.

COMMENTS

Congenital myopathies represent a heterogenous group of myopathies that are present at birth. Common congenital myopathies include nemalin myopathy, central core disease, myotubular (central nuclear) myopathy, and fiber type disproportion. They are characterized by a non- or slowly progressive course, frequent association with dysmorphic features, normal

TABLE 15.5. Needle EMG Data in Case 5

				Spontaneous Potentials				Motor Unit Potential			Interference	
Muscle	**Root**	**Nerve**	**Insertion Activity**	**Fib**	**PSW**	**Fasc**	**Myotonia CRD**	**Amplitude (mV)**	**Duration (ms)**	**Polyphasic Potential**	**Pattern**	**Mean Amplitude (mV)**
Ant tibial	L4,5	Peroneal	N	–	–	–	–	0.2–1	2–8	+	[a]	
Vast lat	L3,4	Femoral	N	–	–	–	–	0.3–1.5	2–10	+		

[a] Early recruitment.

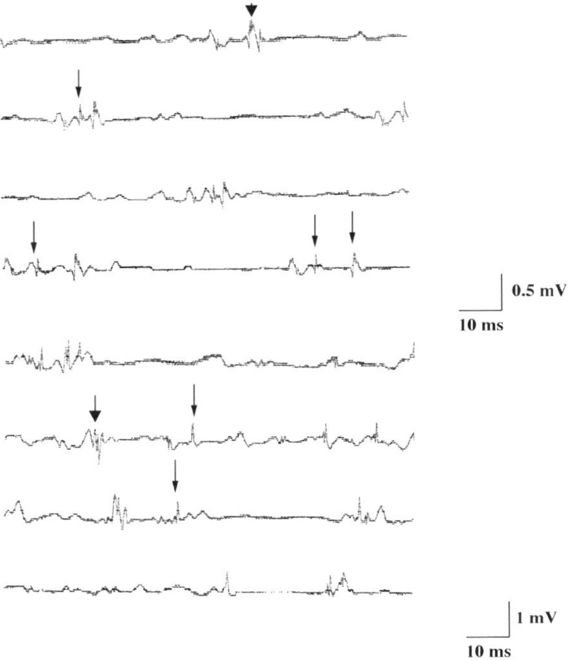

FIGURE 15.5. SASD MUPs. *Thin arrows* indicate simple SASD MUPs and *thick arrows*, polyphasic SASD MUPs.

CPK, and specific histological abnormalities in the muscle biopsy. Recognition of these entities is important in future planning for individual patients. Most present to the physician for diagnosis in late infancy and early childhood. Usually, these patients have a history of floppy infant syndrome, delayed motor milestones, or subtle signs of muscle weakness. Two of the most helpful clinical features are absent reflexes and dysmorphic or skeletal abnormalities, such as high palate, pectus excavatum, elongation of facies, and scoliosis, which are due to long-standing muscle weakness. On clinical evaluation, most patients have predominantly proximal muscle weakness. There are certain features that are rather specific for certain types of congenital myopathies: malignant hyperthermia for central core disease, and ptosis and ophthalmoplegia for myotubular myopathy. CPK is usually normal or mildly elevated in a few cases. However, CPK is valuable in differentiating congenital myopathies from muscular dystrophy because it is markedly elevated in the latter. The definite diagnosis of congenital myopathy rests unequivocally on the muscle biopsy, which shows specific diagnostic features. Type I fiber predominance is another common and typical finding in congenital myopathies.

The most helpful diagnostic tool in support of myopathy in congenital myopathies is a myopathic pattern on the needle EMG. Most articles we reviewed stated that the needle EMG is normal or shows the typical myopathic pattern of SASD MUPs, reflecting the general sentiment on the value of needle EMG in the study of congenital myopathies. According to the literature review, the needle EMG showed a myopathic pattern in 63% of cases, normal findings in 26%, and neurogenic EMG in 15%. In our experience, the needle EMG shows a classic myopathic pattern of SASD MUPs in 90% of cases, indicating a high diagnostic sensitivity in congenital myopathy, and is extremely helpful in differentiating myopathies from other disorders. The low sensitivity of the needle EMG in congenital myopathies is due to inexperience on the part of electromyographer in dealing with pediatric patients. Abnormal spontaneous potentials (fibrillation, PSW, and CRD) are reported in only 11% of cases in congenital myopathies. Although many review articles stated that fibrillation and PSW should suggest myotubular myopathy in the setting of congenital myopathy, these were observed in only 20% of cases, indicating that such a statement is unsubstantiated.

MAXIMS

1. CPK is usually normal in congenital myopathies.
2. Needle EMG shows a classic myopathic pattern of SASD MUPs in congenital myopathies.

REFERENCES

1. Bodensteiner JD. Congenital myopathies. Muscle Nerve 1994;17:131–144.
2. Dietzen CJ, D'Auria R, Fesenmeier J, Oh SJ. Electromyography in benign congenital myopathies. Muscle Nerve 1993;16:327–328.

CASE 6

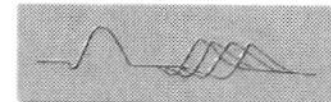

A 2-YEAR-OLD BOY WITH ENLARGED CALF MUSCLES

CASE PRESENTATION

A 5 year-old boy had progressive walking difficulty since beginning to walk at age 2. Until then, his motor and verbal developmental milestones had been normal. Neurological examination showed a boy with waddling gait, positive Gower's sign, prominent calf hypertrophy, 4 MRC strength in the iliopsoas, 4+ strength in the deltoid muscles, and absent reflexes. Family history was negative. His 7 year-old sister was healthy.

CASE ANALYSIS

This patient had a history and findings typical of Duchenne muscular dystrophy except for the negative family history.

PLAN OF TESTING

1. NCS: To rule out demyelinating neuropathy as a cause of proximal weakness.
2. Needle EMG: To document myopathy.
3. Other tests: CPK, DNA deletion test for DMD, and dystrophin assay of biopsied muscle.

ELECTROPHYSIOLOGICAL TESTS AND FINDINGS

NCS Findings. Normal motor and sensory NCS.

Needle EMG (Table 15.6; Fig. 15.6)

1. Fibrillation and PSW in the tested muscles.
2. Many simple or polyphasic SASD MUPs in the vastus lateralis and biceps muscles.

ELECTROPHYSIOLOGICAL INTERPRETATION

Active myopathy.

OTHER TEST FINDINGS

CPK was 50,000 units. Muscle biopsy from the vastus lateralis showed a marked increase in perimysial and endomysial connective tissue and several focal areas with many muscle fibers undergoing regeneration and phagocytosis typical of muscular dystrophy. DNA deletion test was negative for DMD. Dystrophin was absent in the biopsied muscle.

FINAL DIAGNOSIS

DMD

TABLE 15.6. Needle EMG Data in Case 6

				Spontaneous Potentials				Motor Unit Potential			Interference	
Muscle	**Root**	**Nerve**	**Insertion Activity**	**Fib**	**PSW**	**Fasc**	**Myotonia CRD**	**Amplitude (mV)**	**Duration (ms)**	**Polyphasic Potential**	**Pattern**	**Mean Amplitude (mV)**
Lt ant tibial	L4,5	Peroneal	+	+	+	–	–	0.1–0.3	2–5	+	[a]	
Vast lat	L3,4	Femoral	+	+	+	–	–	0.1–0.4	2–6	+		

[a] Early recruitment.

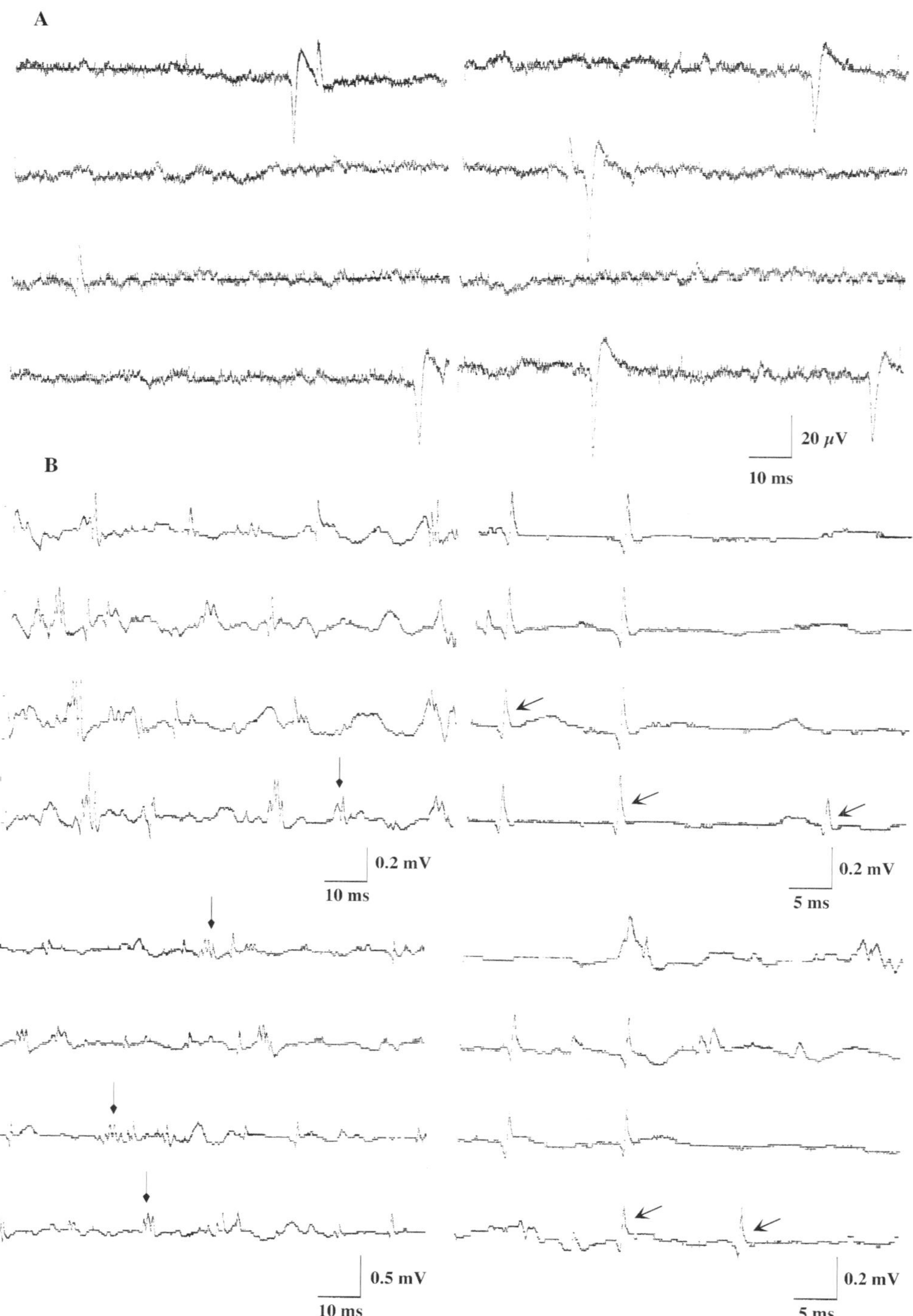

FIGURE 15.6. A. Fibrillations and PSWs. **B.** SASD MUPs. *Downward arrows* indicate a few polyphasic SASD MUPs. *Side-pointing arrows* indicate a few SASD MUPs with 2 ms duration.

TREATMENT AND FOLLOW-UP

The patient's myopathy progressed gradually even with a small daily dose of prednisone, and at 11 years of age he became wheelchair bound.

COMMENTS

DMD and Becker muscular dystrophy are sex-linked dystrophies characterized by progressive muscle weakness and pseudohypertrophy of calf muscles. Phenotypically, they are the same. However, Duchenne dystrophy is characterized by early onset between 2 and 3 years of age, rapid progression with loss of ambulation by 12 years of age, higher incidence of cardiomyopathy, and death in the late teens or early twenties. Becker dystrophy, on the other hand, has a similar presentation but a much milder clinical course in which the onset of symptoms is usually later, the muscle weakness is milder, and the disease progression is slower. Patients with BMD typically remain ambulatory beyond the age of 16 years of age and into adult life, thus allowing the clinical distinction from DMD patients. They usually survive beyond the age of 30. There is also an intermediate group of patients (with mild DMD or severe BMD) who become wheelchair dependent between the ages of 12 and 16.

Dystrophin is a subsarcolemmal protein that is deficient in DMD and BMD. Dystrophin testing, which measures the quantity and quality of dystrophin protein in the muscle tissue, is now available for the diagnosis of dystrophinopathies. In this regard, the Western immunoblot is the most sensitive and specific test for the diagnosis of DMD and BMD. The complete absence (<5% of normal) of dystrophin is very specific for the diagnosis of DMD, whereas the presence of an altered molecular weight form or reduced amount (5 to 25% of normal) of dystrophin is specific for BMD. Thus, the dystrophin test has become an important predictor of the severity of disease, distinguishing BMD from DMD. Other dystrophinopathies so far known include cardiomyopathy, isolated quadriceps myopathy, a syndrome with cramp and myoglobinuria, and subgroups of limb-girdle muscular dystrophy.

In approximately 65% of cases, a deletion in the dystrophin gene is the cause of DMD and BMD. Thus, the DNA deletion test in the blood can be used for diagnosis of DMD and BMD in the preclinical and the clinical stage. Because this test is noninvasive and highly accurate if positive, the DNA deletion test is the first laboratory test for diagnosis of DMD and BMD. Once a deletion is detected in an affected individual, this test can be used for carrier detection among family members and for prenatal diagnosis. One disadvantage is that this test cannot differentiate DMD from BMD. Carrier status is determined by gene dosage. If a deletion is not detected, the dystrophin test is the only way to confirm the diagnosis of DMD and BMD. If a deletion is not the basis of the mutation in the dystrophin gene causing BMD and DMD, linkage analysis using restriction fragment length polymorphisms may then be useful in identifying at-risk family members by detection of an abnormal gene.

CPK is the most important serum enzyme in the diagnosis of DMD. It is markedly elevated (>50 times of normal) in DMD, even in the preclinical stage. Griggs et al. stated that a CPK less than 10 times normal, at any age, is strong evidence against the diagnosis of Duchenne dystrophy. CPK gradually falls as the disease advances. The needle EMG shows typical features of myopathy: many simple and polyphasic SASD MUPs. Fibrillation and PSW may occur in early stages, but to a much lesser extent than in myositis or motor neuron disease.

MAXIMS

1. The most sensitive and specific diagnostic method for DMD is the dystrophin assay on the biopsied muscle. Dystrophin assay can differentiate DMD from BMD.
2. The DNA deletion test is diagnostic of DMD and BMD in 65% of cases. This can be used for prenatal diagnosis and carrier detection.

REFERENCES

1. Buchthal F, Rosenfalck P. Electrophysiological aspect of myopathy with particular reference to progressive muscular dystrophy. In: Bourne GH, Golarz MN, eds. Muscular dystrophy in man and animals. New York: Hafner, 1963:193–262.
2. Darras BT. Molecular genetics of Duchenne and Becker muscular dystrophy. J Pediatr 1990;117: 1–15.

CASE 7

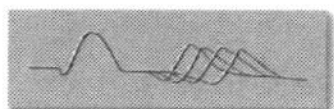

WEAKNESS IN THE LEGS AT 13 MONTHS OF AGE

CASE PRESENTATION

A 4-year-old boy was evaluated for progressive muscle weakness. He had a normal gestation, held his head up at 5 months, and rolled over at 6 months. He sat up at 9 months and crawled at 13 months. At 13 months, he was evaluated for weakness in the legs without any definite diagnosis and a follow-up evaluation was advised. He started walking at 18 months. At 4 years he returned for progressive muscle weakness. Over the past several months he had more difficulty walking; he could not get up from the floor to a standing position without help and had a positive Gower's sign. Family history was notable for similar disease in several relatives.

The boy was somewhat underdeveloped, with marked muscle atrophy in the hands and feet, only 2+ MRC muscle strength in proximal muscle groups and 1 to 2+ in the distal muscle groups. His DTRs were diminished. There was a fine tremor of fingers. His gait was obviously weak and knock-kneed. No fasciculations were noted.

CASE ANALYSIS

This patient was apparently normal until 6 months of age. Since then, there had been a delay in his developmental milestones and progressive muscle weakness. Examination showed diffuse weakness, more so distally with distal atrophy. Neurological findings were indicative of a neuromuscular disease, but there was no definite finding indicative of either myopathy or denervation process. Diminished reflexes did not help here because they are also diminished in many benign congenital myopathies. Thus, electrophysiological testing was crucial in identifying the disease process in this patient. In fact, the pediatric neurologist's impression was "familial myopathy" because of the strong family history.

PLAN OF TESTING

1. NCS: To rule out peripheral neuropathy as a cause of weakness.
2. Needle EMG: To identify myopathy or denervation process.
3. Other tests: CPK and muscle biopsy to confirm chronic denervation.

ELECTROPHYSIOLOGICAL TESTS AND FINDINGS

NCS Findings. Normal except for a low CMAP in the left peroneal nerve.

Needle EMG (Table 15.7; Figs. 15.7 and 15.8)

1. Many high-amplitude and long-duration MUPs in the left anterior tibialis muscle.
2. Spontaneous MUP discharges in the extensor digitorum communis muscles producing minipolymyoclonus.

ELECTROPHYSIOLOGICAL INTERPRETATION

Chronic denervation typical of type II SMA.

OTHER TEST FINDINGS

CPK, 200 U/L. Muscle biopsy showed chronic denervation typical of type II SMA.

FINAL DIAGNOSIS

Type II SMA

TREATMENT AND FOLLOW-UP

Gradually, the patient became weaker and died at 3 years of age.

COMMENTS

As in cases of floppy infant syndrome, the clinical findings alone are not enough to make a definite diagnosis in many early childhood neuromuscular diseases. In this case, the needle

TABLE 15.7. Needle EMG Data in Case 7

				Spontaneous Potentials				Motor Unit Potential				Interference	
Muscle	**Root**	**Nerve**	**Insertion Activity**	**Fib**	**PSW**	**Fasc**	**Myotonia CRD**	**Amplitude (mV)**	**Duration (ms)**	**Polyphasic Potential**	**HALD MUP**	**Pattern**	**Mean Amplitude (mV)**
Lt ant tibial	L4,5	Peroneal	N	–	–	–	–	2–6	10–20	N	+ + +	[a]	
Vast lat	L3,4	Femoral	N	–	–	–	–	1–5	10–25	N	+ + +	[a]	

[a] Difficult to judge because of lack of cooperation.

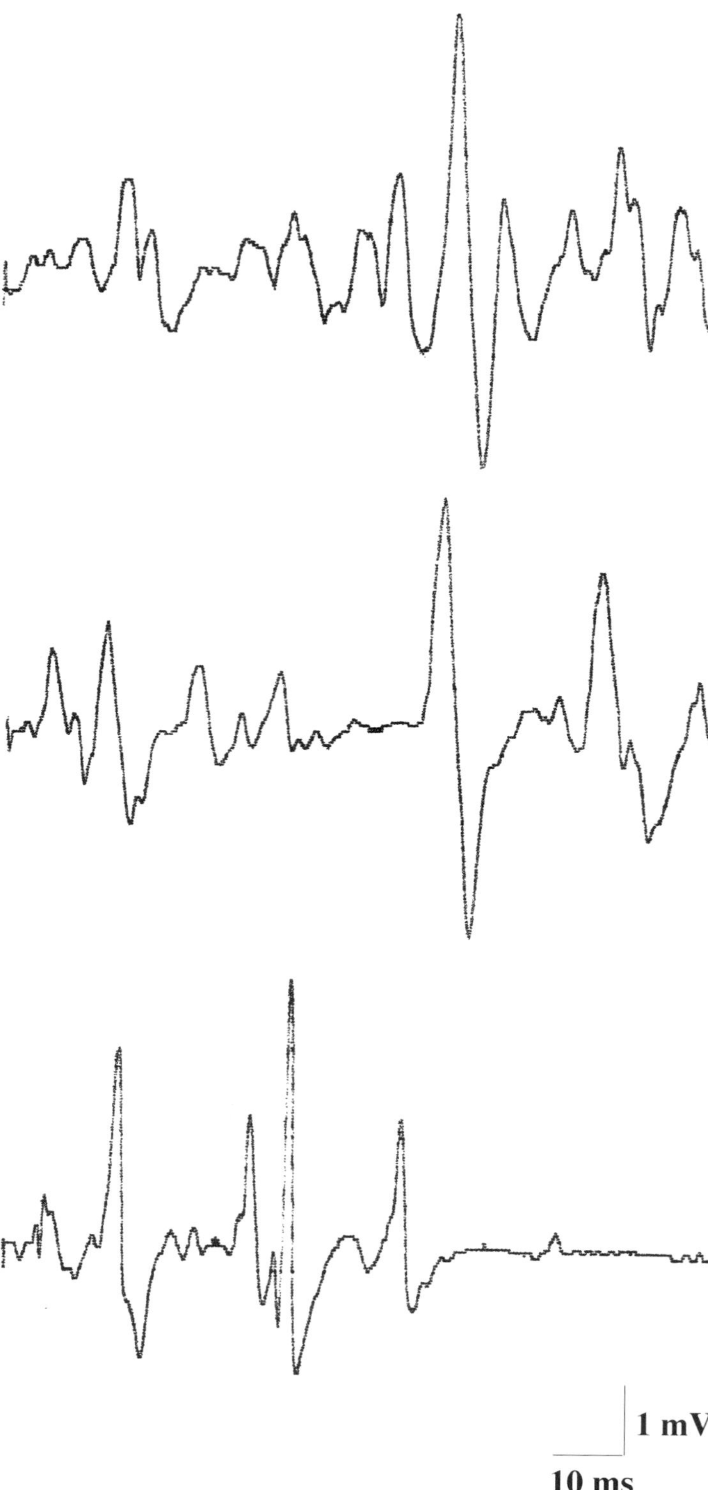

FIGURE 15.7. High-amplitude, long-duration MUPs.

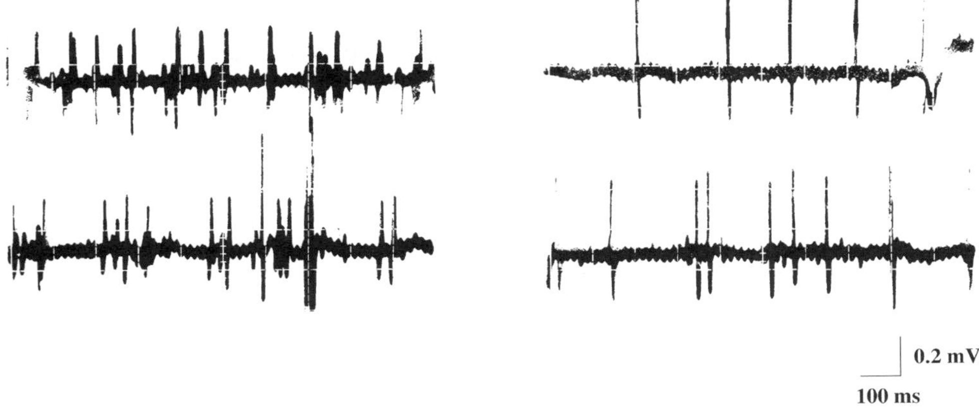

FIGURE 15.8. Continuous fasciculations in the extensor digitorum communis producing polyminimyoclonus.

EMG study was the crucial test indicative of SMA. This is a classic example of the usefulness of the needle EMG in childhood neuromuscular diseases.

SMA is a group of inherited disorders in which the primary defect is degeneration of the anterior horn cells of the spinal cord and often of the bulbar motor nuclei but with no evidence of peripheral nerve or long tract involvement. SMA can be divided into four main groups (see Table 10.2). Among these, WHD has the worst prognosis, with certain death before 18 months of age. It is now well accepted that there exists an intermediate type (SMA type II) between WHD and juvenile Kugelberg-Welander disease. Classically, type II SMA has an onset between 6 months and 2 years of age and autosomal-recessive inheritance. Weakness and wasting are generalized and do not show predominant distal or proximal involvement. Fasciculation and atrophy of the tongue may be present, but fasciculations are not seen in the limbs. However, tremor of the fingers (minipolymyoclonus) corresponding to the EMG findings of spontaneous MUP discharges is present in one-third of cases. Tendon reflexes are diminished or absent. The progression is very slow and the disease is more severe in males. Life expectancy is variable, with most patients living more than 2 years and some reaching adolescence.

MAXIMS

1. The needle EMG is the crucial test in establishing the diagnosis of SMA type II. It shows a chronic denervation pattern with HALD MUPs.
2. Minipolymyoclonus is due to spontaneous MUP discharges and is seen in one-third of patients with SMA type II.

REFERENCES

1. Campbell MJ, Liversedge LA. The motor neuron diseases (including spinal muscular atrophy). In: Walton J, ed. Disorders of voluntary muscle, 4th ed. Edinburgh and London: Churchill Livingstone, 1984:725–752.

CASE 8

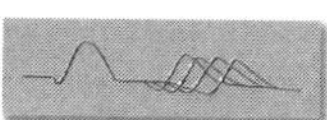

PROXIMAL MUSCLE WEAKNESS AND PSEUDOHYPERTROPHY IN THE CALF MUSCLES IN A 15-YEAR-OLD GIRL

CASE PRESENTATION

A 15-year-old girl was healthy as an infant. Except for frequent falls as a toddler and subtle difficulty getting up from the floor as a child, her childhood had been normal. In the past few years, she had noted more difficulty rising from a chair or after falling. Abnormal neurological findings were hypertrophy of calf muscles, mild atrophy in the deltoid and quadriceps, 4 MRC strength in the deltoids, 3 in right triceps, 2 in iliopsoas, 4− in quadriceps, 4 in hamstrings and anterior tibialis muscles, absent reflexes, waddling gait, and difficulty doing knee bends. The patient had a 28-year-old sister who had been in a wheelchair for the past 10 years due to "limb-girdle muscular dystrophy," which was diagnosed on the basis of clinical findings and elevated CPK.

CASE ANALYSIS

This patient has all the clinical features of myopathy together with hypertrophy of the calf muscles, strongly suggestive of limb-girdle muscular dystrophy. This was especially so in view of the positive family history of "limb-girdle muscular dystrophy" in her sister.

PLAN OF TESTING

1. NCS: To rule out peripheral neuropathy as a cause of weakness.
2. Needle EMG: To identify myopathy or denervation process.
3. Other tests: CPK and muscle biopsy to confirm chronic denervation.

ELECTROPHYSIOLOGICAL TESTS AND FINDINGS

NCS Findings. Normal motor and sensory NCS.

Needle EMG (Table 15.8; Fig. 15.9)

1. Rare fibrillations and PSWs in both tested muscles.
2. Many HALD MUPs in both tested muscles.
3. A few SASD MUPs in the vastus lateralis muscle.
4. Reduced interference pattern in both tested muscles.

ELECTROPHYSIOLOGICAL INTERPRETATION

Indicative of chronic denervation typical of type II SMA.

OTHER TEST FINDINGS

CPK, 350 U/L. Muscle biopsy showed chronic denervation process characterized by prominent fascicular atrophy, type I fiber grouping, minimal increase in the endomysial and perimysial space, and few small fibers undergoing phagocytosis.

FINAL DIAGNOSIS

KWD

TREATMENT AND FOLLOW-UP

The biggest surprise in this patient was the needle EMG findings, which were contrary to those expected in limb-girdle muscular dystrophy. Needle EMG findings were typical of KWD. The patient's sister was reexamined and found to have the same disease with more severe features. Her EMG also showed the same findings. Over a 15-year follow-up period, there has been extremely slow progression with a little more difficulty climbing stairs, weakness in the fingers and forearm muscles, and mild scoliosis. She has two healthy children.

COMMENTS

As noted in this patient, KWD (SMA type III, juvenile proximal SMA) simulates limb-girdle muscular dystrophy clinically because it produces a progressive proximal muscular weakness

TABLE 15.8. Needle EMG Data in Case 8

				Spontaneous Potentials				Motor Unit Potential				Interference	
Muscle	**Root**	**Nerve**	**Insertion Activity**	**Fib**	**PSW**	**Fasc**	**Myotonia CRD**	**Amplitude (mV)**	**Duration (ms)**	**Polyphasic Potential**	**HA MUP**	**Pattern**	**Mean Amplitude (mV)**
Lt deltoid	C5,6	Axillary	N	+	+	–	–	1–8 (4.1)[a]	7–20 (11.5)[a]	15%	+	RIP	7
Vast lat	L3,4	Femoral	N	+	+	–	–	1–10	2–25	N	+	RIP	6

[a] Mean amplitude and duration of 20 MUPs. Normal upper limit of MUP: 12.1 ms.

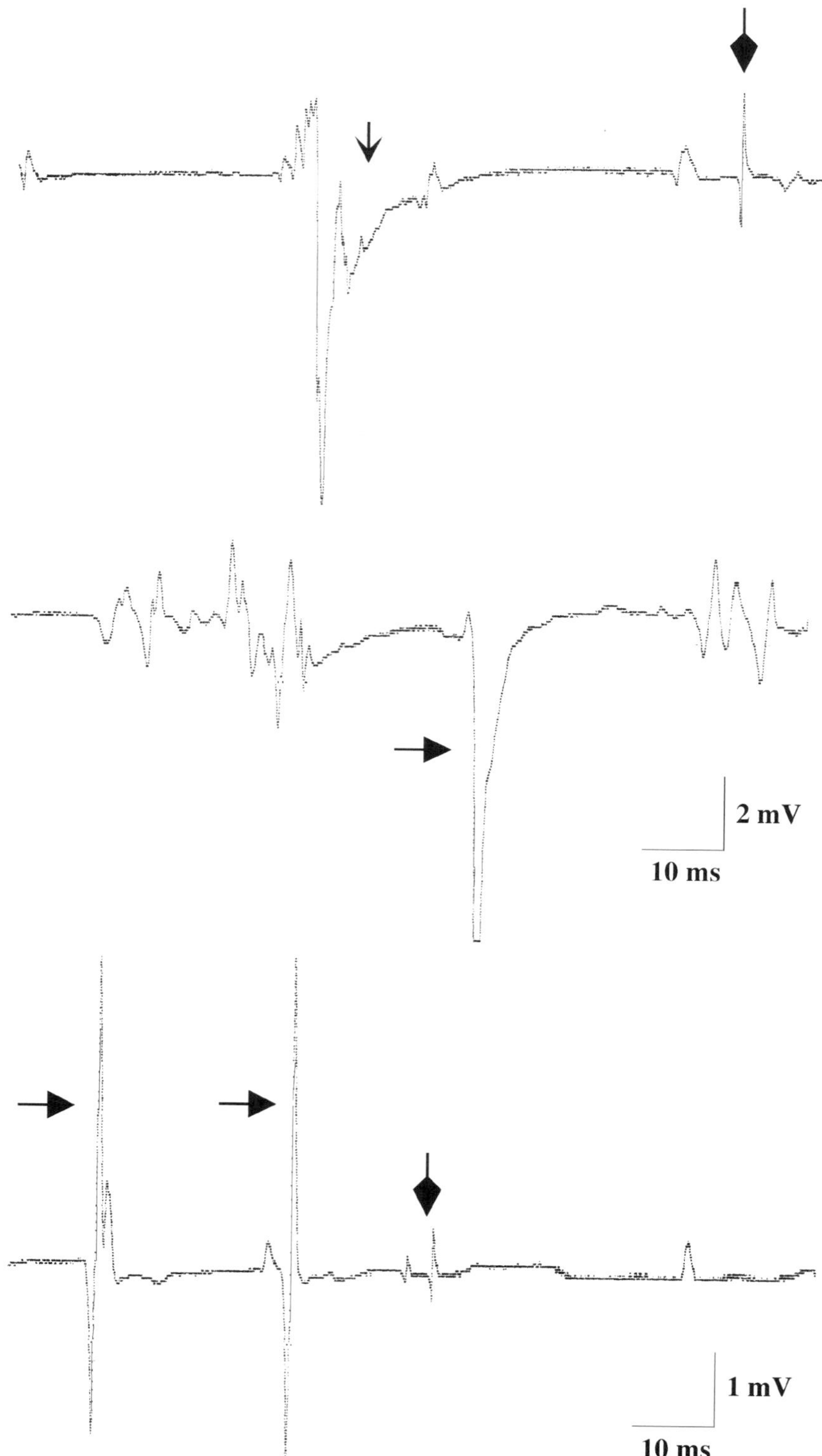

FIGURE 15.9. Various MUPs. ♦, SASD MUP; ➞, HA MUP; ↓, HALD MUPs.

in young adults. In fact, until an accurate needle EMG study is performed, limb-girdle myopathy is the clinician's diagnosis. This is rightfully so, because there is no clinical means of differentiating KWD from muscular dystrophy unless fasciculation is obviously observed. KWD, inherited in an autosomal-dominant or recessive fashion, is characterized by proximal muscle weakness and atrophy commencing in the lower extremities between 2 and 20 years of age. Family history is positive in two of three cases. Fasciculations are seen in the proximal muscles in one-half the cases. Muscle stretch reflexes are usually reduced or absent. The disease is slowly progressive, but many patients are capable of a normal life span. CPK is either normal or mildly elevated. The muscle biopsy typically shows chronic denervation process, and myopathic features may be present as a secondary feature, as noted in this patient.

The needle EMG is critical in reaching a definite diagnosis of KWD because it shows the typical findings of chronic denervation. Fibrillation and PSW have been observed in 20 to 60% of cases in different series. Fasciculation may be present. The most important EMG findings are the high-amplitude and long-duration MUPs with a reduced interference pattern. A few small-amplitude and short-duration MUPs may be present, reflecting secondary myopathic features as noted in this case.

MAXIMS

1. KWD simulates clinically limb-girdle muscular dystrophy. Thus, the most critical diagnostic test in KWD is the needle EMG. The most important needle EMG finding is the high-amplitude and long-duration MUPs.
2. Muscle fiber necrosis can be observed in chronic denervation as a secondary phenomenon. This is an explanation of the mild elevation of CPK and the few SASD MUPs in the chronic form of SMA.

REFERENCES

1. Kugelberg E, Welander L. Heredofamilial juvenile muscular atrophy simulating muscular dystrophy. Arch Neurol Psychiatry 1956;75:500–509.
2. Drachman DB, Murphy SR, Nigam P, Hills JR. Myopathic changes in chronically denervated muscles. Arch Neurol 1967;16:14–24.

CASE 9

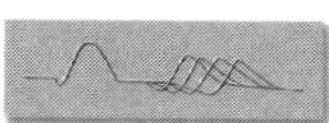

AN 8-YEAR-OLD GIRL WHO OVERCAME DIFFICULTY AS A FLOPPY BABY

CASE PRESENTATION

An 8-year-old girl had an uneventful gestation and birth but was noted to be a floppy baby. She had markedly delayed motor developmental milestones, walking at 21 months. She never really crawled but only scooted on the floor on her bottom. Her speech and intellectual development had been normal. She was an A/B student in the second grade. Over the years, she made some small developmental motor gains. She was able to walk alone and even jog somewhat but could still not climb stairs without a rail or get up from the floor without using the Gower's maneuver. The patient was an only child. Family history was negative. A previous needle EMG and muscle biopsy were reported to be normal. CPK was normal.

General examination was remarkable in that the girl was diffusely thin with a very long face, high arched palate, and prominent pectus excavatum. Abnormal neurological findings were bilateral facial diplegia; 4+ MRC strength in neck flexors and extensors; 3 in deltoid, biceps, and iliopsoas; 4 in wrist extensors and flexors, quadriceps, hamstrings, and anterior tibialis muscles; and 5− in hand grip and gastrocnemius muscles, diffuse areflexia, and scapular winging. She had a waddling gait and was unable to arise from a sitting position. Gower's sign was positive.

CASE ANALYSIS

Given the patient's history and physical examination, it was clear that she was suffering from a congenital myopathy. A fellow physician raised the possibility of nemalin myopathy on the basis of her facial features. Definite, although minimal, improvement over the years was suggestive of congenital fiber type disproportion. There is no single clinical finding that differentiates nemalin myopathy from CFTD. The needle EMG study confirms myopathy and the muscle biopsy confirms the definite diagnosis.

PLAN OF TESTING

1. NCS: To rule out neuropathy.
2. Needle EMG: To document myopathy.
3. Other tests: Review of previous muscle biopsy.

ELECTROPHYSIOLOGICAL TESTS AND FINDINGS

NCS Findings. Normal motor and sensory NCS

Needle EMG (Table 15.9; Fig. 15.10)

1. Many simple and polyphasic SASD MUPs.
2. Early recruitment of MUP and FIP.

ELECTROPHYSIOLOGICAL INTERPRETATION

Nonactive myopathy.

OTHER TEST FINDINGS

The muscle biopsy was reviewed. There was no histological feature of muscle fiber necrosis. Instead, it showed the classic findings of CFTD: type 1 fibers were smaller than type II fibers and comprised 90% of fibers.

FINAL DIAGNOSIS

CFTD

TREATMENT AND FOLLOW-UP

The patient's condition has been stable over the years.

TABLE 15.9. Needle EMG Data in Case 9

				Spontaneous Potentials				Motor Unit Potential				Interference	
Muscle	**Root**	**Nerve**	**Insertion Activity**	**Fib**	**PSW**	**Fasc**	**Myotonia CRD**	**Amplitude (mV)**	**Duration (ms)**	**Polyphasic Potential**	**HA MUP**	**Pattern**	**Mean Amplitude (mV)**
Lt deltoids	C5,6	Axillary	N	–	–	–	–	0.3–2	1.6–10	+ + +	–	FIP	1
Vast lat	L3,4	Femoral	N	–	–	–	–	0.3–1	2–12	+ + +	–	FIP	0.8

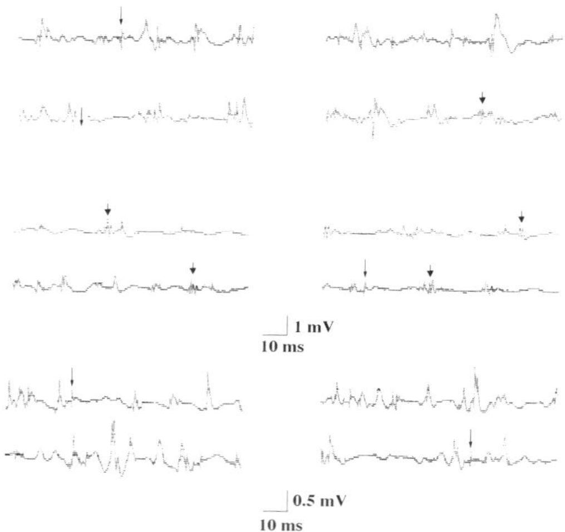

FIGURE 15.10. *Short arrows* indicate simple SASD MUPs and *long arrows*, polyphasic SASD MUPs.

COMMENTS

In 1973, Brooke introduced the term "CFTD" to describe 12 patients who fulfilled the criteria of having type 1 fibers with an average diameter 15% smaller than that of type 2 fibers. He stated that these patients had a favorable prognosis. Most patients present in infancy with hypotonia, delayed milestones, and generalized muscle weakness with prominent facial involvement. Dysmorphic features of the face and other skeletal deformities (high-arched palate, kyphoscoliosis, congenital hip dislocation, or club feet) as seen in our case are common. These children have normal intelligence. Most patients have a static course or show improvement. In the literature, the needle EMG showed a myopathic pattern in about 50% of cases. However, our study revealed a myopathic pattern (SASD MUPs) in all of eight patients. CPK was normal. Muscle biopsy showed two distinctive findings: smaller type 1 fibers than type 2 fibers and type 1 fiber predominance. Many children with this disorder have a favorable outcome. For this reason, aggressive supportive therapy should be provided.

MAXIMS

1. CFTD is indicative of a favorable prognosis. Thus, an aggressive supportive therapy should be provided to these patients.
2. Needle EMG shows myopathic pattern in most patients with CFTD.

REFERENCES

1. Brooke MH. Congenital fiber type disproportion. In: Kukulus BA, ed. Clinical studies in myology. Amsterdam: Excerpta Medica, 1973.

CASE 10

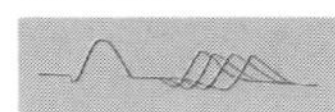

LIMB-GIRDLE MUSCULAR DYSTROPHY WITH LEUKOENCEPHALOPATHY ON THE MRI

This case is included here because this patient has a form of congenital muscular dystrophy.

CASE PRESENTATION

A 39-year-old man presented with a history of muscle weakness since approximately 2 years of age. Three muscle biopsies in childhood showed muscular dystrophy. He carried a diagnosis of limb-girdle muscular dystrophy, as did his sister. This disease had been very slowly progressive over his lifetime. He came to the clinic for migraine headaches, complaining of three to four migraines per week. He had tried many nonnarcotic medications for prophylaxis of his headaches without relief. He was currently taking mild narcotics. Abnormal findings were calf and deltoid enlargement due to hypertrophy; 4 MRC strength in the deltoid, biceps, triceps, iliopsoas, hamstrings, quadriceps, and anterior tibialis muscles; and trace DTRs. A previous MRI a year before because of migraine showed leukoencephalopathy.

CASE ANALYSIS

Compared with the classic limb-girdle muscular dystrophy, the patient had extremely early onset, slower progression, and no atrophy. Thus, benign congenital myopathy was a definite possibility, especially in view of his family history. Three muscle biopsies performed before the days of histochemistry were not helpful in identifying a definite pathological type of benign congenital myopathy. Because of leucoencephalopathy in the MRI of brain, we suspected that this patient had merosin-deficiency congenital muscular dystrophy.

PLAN OF TESTING

1. NCS: To rule out neuropathy.
2. Needle EMG: To document myopathy.
3. Other tests: CPK.

ELECTROPHYSIOLOGICAL TESTS AND FINDINGS

NCS Findings. Normal motor and sensory NCS.

Needle EMG (Table 15.10; Fig. 15.11)

1. Decreased insertional activity and many SASD MUPs in the deltoid muscle.
2. Decreased insertional activity, fibrillations and PSW, and many SASD MUPs in the biceps muscle.

ELECTROPHYSIOLOGICAL INTERPRETATION

Active myopathy.

OTHER TEST FINDINGS

Muscle biopsy showed many fibers with moth-eaten appearance, increased endomysial connective tissue, and a few muscle fibers undergoing granular change typical of chronic nonspecific myopathy. Merosin assay showed partial deficiency.

FINAL DIAGNOSIS

Merosin-deficiency (partial) congenital muscular dystrophy

TREATMENT AND FOLLOW-UP

His condition is stable. His migraine is controlled with narcotics and imitrex.

COMMENTS

Congenital muscular dystrophy is a heterogenous group of autosomal-recessive disorders that have nonspecific pathological features of a primary myopathy on muscle biopsy and are clinically characterized by the early onset of hypotonia, generalized weakness, muscle atrophy, and contractures. Congenital muscular dystrophy has recently been classified into four cate-

TABLE 15.10. Needle EMG Data in Case 10

				Spontaneous Potentials				Motor Unit Potential				Interference	
Muscle	**Root**	**Nerve**	**Insertion Activity**	**Fib**	**PSW**	**Fasc**	**Myotonia CRD**	**Amplitude (mV)**	**Duration (ms)**	**Polyphasic Potential**	**HA MUP**	**Pattern**	**Mean Amplitude (mV)**
Left deltoid	C5,6	Axillary	Decreased	–	–	–	–	0.2–2.7	2.8–6	+	–	FIP	3
Biceps	C6	Musc cut	Decreased	+	++	–	–	0.2–1	2–6	+	–	FIP	2

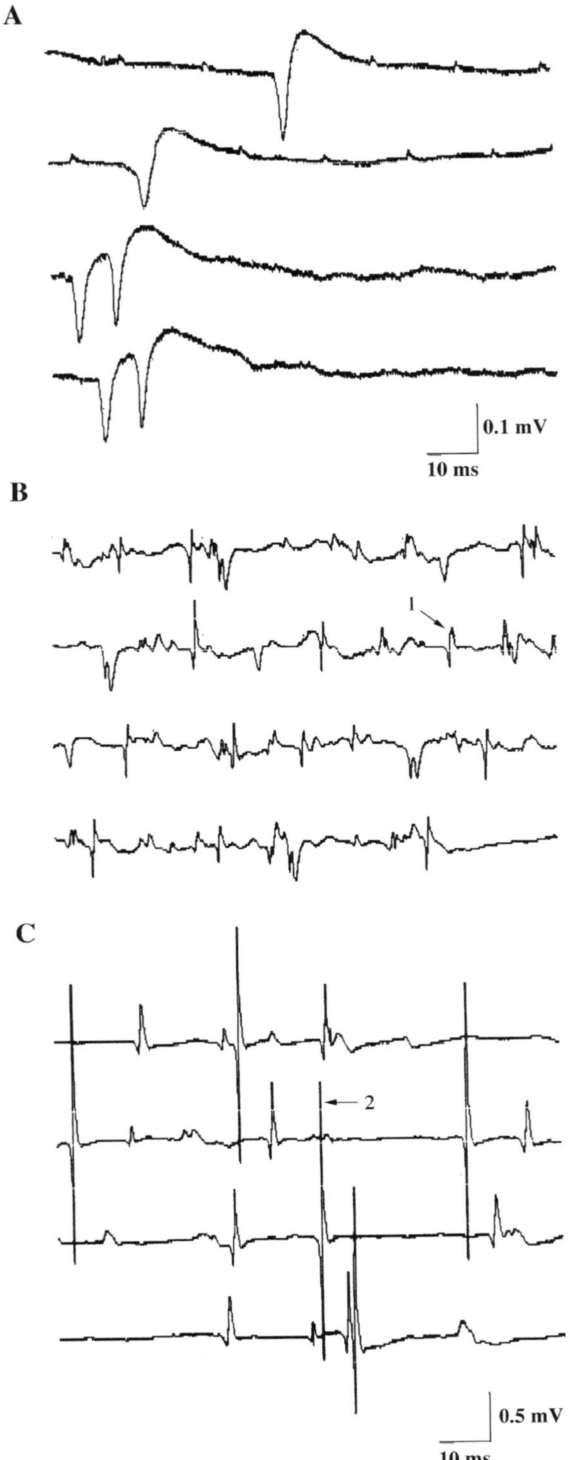

FIGURE 15.11. **A.** PSWs. **B.** SASD MUPs. *1*, MUP with 3.0-ms duration. **C.** Short-duration MUPs with normal amplitude. *2*, MUP with 4.4 ms and 3.0 mV.

gories: congenital muscular dystrophy I, the classic or "pure" congenital muscular dystrophy without severe impairment of intellectual development; congenital muscular dystrophy II, the best known Fukuyama congenital muscular dystrophy characterized by seizures, microcephaly, and developmental delay in motor and verbal milestones; congenital muscular dystrophy III and IV with muscle, eye, and brain abnormalities: the milder Finish-type congenital muscular dystrophy (congenital muscular dystrophy III) and the severe Walker-Warburg syndrome (congenital muscular dystrophy IV). The "pure" or classic form of congenital muscular dystrophy does not show any mental retardation or structural changes in brain or eyes. Congenital muscular dystrophy I is divided into two subgroups: A, without white matter hypodensity and with normal merosin, and B, with white matter hypodensity and deficient merosin. Approximately half the children with congenital muscular dystrophy I have recently been shown to have a deficiency of merosin, a component of the extracellular matrix protein laminin-2. Affected children have severe hypotonia, normal intelligence, and central nervous system white matter changes, as noted in our cases. Congenital muscular dystrophy IB (merosin-deficiency congenital muscular dystrophy) is clinically similar to congenital muscular dystrophy IA except for usually more severe clinical expression and course and some dysmorphic features. Leukoencephalopathy on the MRI in our case led us to assay merosin deficiency. In children with merosin-deficiency congenital muscular dystrophy, abnormal somatosensory and visual evoked potentials, as well as abnormal motor nerve conduction, were reported. Partial merosin deficiency in late-onset limb-girdle muscular dystrophy was recently reported in an adult. This case was almost identical with ours. In congenital muscular dystrophy, CPK is usually mildly elevated. Needle EMG shows a myopathic pattern.

MAXIMS

1. Merosin deficiency must be evaluated in any muscular dystrophy patients with leukoencephalopathy on the MRI.
2. Decreased insertional activity is indicative of fibrosis of muscles.

REFERENCES

1. Leyten QH, Gabreëls FJM, Rnier WO, ter Laak HJ. Congenital muscular dystrophy: A review of the literature. Clin Neurol Neurosurg 1996;98:267–280.
2. Vainzof M, Marie SKN, Reed UC, et al. Deficiency of merosin (laminin M or 2) in congenital muscular dystrophy associated with cerebral white matter alterations. Neuropaediatrics 1995;26:293–297.

Index

Page numbers followed by f denote figures; those followed by t denote tables.